THE QUARTERLY JOURNAL OF MEDICINE

mB
IV

NEW SERIES, VOLUME XXIII

(VOLUME XLVII OF THE CONTINUOUS SERIES)

1954

OXFORD

AT THE CLARENDON PRESS

Oxford University Press, Amen House, London E.C.4

GLASGOW NEW YORK TORONTO MELBOURNE WELLINGTON

BOMBAY CALCUTTA MADRAS KARACHI CAPE TOWN IBADAN

Geoffrey Cumberlege, Publisher to the University

PRINTED IN GREAT BRITAIN

AT THE UNIVERSITY PRESS, OXFORD

BY CHARLES BATEY, PRINTER TO THE UNIVERSITY

CONTENTS

NEW SERIES, VOLUME XXIII, NUMBER 89, JANUARY 1954

Neurological Sequelae of Prophylactic Inoculation. By Henry G. Miller and John B. Stanton 1

Sarcoidosis: With Special Reference to Diagnosis and Prognosis. By R. H. Cowdell. With Plates 1 to 3 29

Pulmonary Hypertension in Congestive Heart Failure complicating Chronic Lung Disease. By W. Whitaker 57

The Effects of Peripheral Arterial Embolism. By R. L. Richards 73

Treatment of Polycythaemia Vera with Radiophosphorus. By John D. Abbatt, H. Chaplin, J. M. M. Darte, and W. R. Pitney 91

Clinical Diagnosis of Pulmonary Hypertension in Patients with Mitral Stenosis. By William Whitaker. With Plates 4 to 7 105

NUMBER 90, APRIL 1954

Pulmonary Tuberous Sclerosis, and its Relationship to Other Forms of the Disease. By John Dawson. With Plates 8 to 15 113

Water-losing Nephritis. A Syndrome simulating Diabetes Insipidus. By N. J. Roussak and S. Oleesky. With Plates 16 and 17 147

Osteomalacia in Steatorrhoea. By John Badenoch and Paul Fourman . . 165

Salicylates in Rheumatic Fever: An Attempt to Assess their Value. By R. S. Illingworth, J. Burke, S. A. Doxiadis, J. Lorber, M. G. Philpott, and D. G. H. Stone. With statistical assistance by J. F. Scott 177

Pink Disease: The Autonomic Disorder and its Treatment with Ganglion-blocking Agents. By B. D. Bower. With Plate 18 215

Biological Actions and Therapeutic Applications of Nitrogen Mustard. By J. W. Beattie and Leonard H. Howells 231

NUMBER 91, JULY 1954

Sequential Tests in Prophylactic and Therapeutic Trials. By P. Armitage . 255

Spinal Cord Complications of Tuberculous Meningitis: A Clinical and Pathological Study. By W. D. W. Brooks, A. P. Fletcher, and R. R. Wilson. With Plates 19 to 22 275

Studies of Uropepsinogen Excretion in Gastrointestinal Disorders. By W. Sircus 291

Ascorbic Acid Requirements and Urinary Excretion of *p*-Hydroxyphenylacetic Acid in Steatorrhoea and Macrocytic Anaemia. With a Description of the Paper-Chromatographic Technique for Identification of Hydroxyphenylic Acids. By R. J. Boscott and W. Trevor Cooke 307

Familial Factor V Deficiency: The Pattern of Heredity. By C. S. Kingsley . 323

The Effect of Weight Reduction upon the Blood-Pressure of Obese Hypertensive Women. By A. P. Fletcher 331

A Five-Year Assessment of Patients in a Controlled Trial of Streptomycin in Pulmonary Tuberculosis. Report to the Tuberculosis Chemotherapy Trials Committee of the Medical Research Council. By Wallace Fox, Ian Sutherland, and the late Marc Daniels 347

NUMBER 92, OCTOBER 1954

Electrolyte Depletion in Pyloric Stenosis. By D. A. K. Black and R. P. Jepson 367

Idiopathic Hypoparathyroidism: A Study of Three Cases. By P. K. Robinson, E. Arnold Carmichael, and J. N. Cumings 383

Non-Tuberculous Addison's Disease and its Relationship to 'Giant-Cell Granuloma' and Multiple Glandular Disease. By Anthony G. Rickards and Geoffrey M. Barrett. With Plates 23 and 24 403

'Giant-Cell Granuloma' and the Other Pituitary Granulomata. By Anthony G. Rickards and Peter W. Harvey. With Plates 25 and 26 425

Hypertensive Retinopathy and its Medical Treatment. By Robert Platt. With Plates 27 to 34 441

Proceedings of the Association of Physicians of Great Britain and Ireland, 1954: Forty-eighth Annual General Meeting 451

INDEX OF CONTRIBUTORS

ABBATT, J. D. Treatment of Polycythaemia Vera with Radiophosphorus . 91

ARMITAGE, P. Sequential Tests in Prophylactic and Therapeutic Trials . . 255

BADENOCH, J. Osteomalacia in Steatorrhoea 165

BARRETT, G. M. Non-Tuberculous Addison's Disease and its Relationship to 'Giant-Cell Granuloma' and Multiple Glandular Disease. With Plates 23 and 24 403

BEATTIE, J. W. Biological Actions and Therapeutic Applications of Nitrogen Mustard 231

BLACK, D. A. K. Electrolyte Depletion in Pyloric Stenosis 367

BOSCOTT, R. J. Ascorbic Acid Requirements and Urinary Excretion of *p*-Hydroxyphenylacetic Acid in Steatorrhoea and Macrocytic Anaemia. With a Description of the Paper-Chromatographic Technique for Identification of Hydroxyphenylic Acid 307

BOWER, B. D. Pink Disease: The Autonomic Disorder and its Treatment with Ganglion-blocking Agents. With Plate 18 215

BROOKS, W. D. W. Spinal Cord Complications of Tuberculous Meningitis: A Clinical and Pathological Study. With Plates 19 to 22 275

BURKE, J. Salicylates in Rheumatic Fever: An Attempt to Assess their Value 177

CARMICHAEL, E. A. Idiopathic Hypoparathyroidism: A Study of Three Cases . 383

CHAPLIN, H. Treatment of Polycythaemia Vera with Radiophosphorus . . 91

COOKE, W. T. Ascorbic Acid Requirements and Urinary Excretion of *p*-Hydroxyphenylacetic Acid in Steatorrhoea and Macrocytic Anaemia. With a Description of the Paper-Chromatographic Technique for Identification of Hydroxyphenylic Acid 307

COWDELL, R. H. Sarcoidosis: with Special Reference to Diagnosis and Prognosis. With Plates 1 to 3 29

CUMINGS, J. N. Idiopathic Hypoparathyroidism: A Study of Three Cases . 383

DANIELS, M. A Five-Year Assessment of Patients in a Controlled Trial of Streptomycin in Pulmonary Tuberculosis. Report to the Tuberculosis Chemotherapy Trials Committee of the Medical Research Council . . 347

DARTE, J. M. M. Treatment of Polycythaemia Vera with Radiophosphorus . 91

DAWSON, J. Pulmonary Tuberous Sclerosis, and its Relationship to Other Forms of the Disease. With Plates 8 to 15 113

DOXIADIS, S. A. Salicylates in Rheumatic Fever: An Attempt to Assess their Value 177

FLETCHER, A. P. Spinal Cord Complications of Tuberculous Meningitis: A Clinical and Pathological Study. With Plates 19 to 22 275

—— The Effect of Weight Reduction upon the Blood-Pressure of Obese Hypertensive Women 331

FOURMAN, P. Osteomalacia in Steatorrhoea 165

FOX, W. A Five-Year Assessment of Patients in a Controlled Trial of Streptomycin in Pulmonary Tuberculosis. Report to the Tuberculosis Chemotherapy Trials Committee of the Medical Research Council 347

HARVEY, P. W. 'Giant-Cell Granuloma' and the Other Pituitary Granulomata. With Plates 25 and 26 425

HOWELLS, L. H. Biological Actions and Therapeutic Applications of Nitrogen Mustard 231

ILLINGWORTH, R. S. Salicylates in Rheumatic Fever: An Attempt to Assess their Value 177

JEPSON, R. P. Electrolyte Depletion in Pyloric Stenosis 367

KINGSLEY, C. S. Familial Factor V Deficiency: The Pattern of Heredity . . 323

LORBER, J. Salicylates in Rheumatic Fever: An Attempt to Assess their Value 177

MILLER, H. G. Neurological Sequelae of Prophylactic Inoculation . . . 1

OLEESKY, S. Water-losing Nephritis. A Syndrome simulating Diabetes Insipidus. With Plates 16 and 17 147

PHILPOTT, M. G. Salicylates in Rheumatic Fever: An Attempt to Assess their Value 177

PITNEY, W. R. Treatment of Polycythaemia Vera with Radiophosphorus . 91

PLATT, R. Hypertensive Retinopathy and its Medical Treatment. With Plates 27 to 34 441

RICHARDS, R. L. The Effects of Peripheral Arterial Embolism . . . 73

RICKARDS, A. G. Non-Tuberculous Addison's Disease and its Relationship to 'Giant-Cell Granuloma' and Multiple Glandular Disease. With Plates 23 and 24 403

—— 'Giant-Cell Granuloma' and the Other Pituitary Granulomata. With Plates 25 and 26 425

ROBINSON, P. K. Idiopathic Hypoparathyroidism: A Study of Three Cases . 383

ROUSSAK, N. J. Water-losing Nephritis. A Syndrome simulating Diabetes Insipidus. With Plates 16 and 17 147

SIRCUS, W. Studies of Uropepsinogen Excretion in Gastro-intestinal Disorders 291

STANTON, J. B. Neurological Sequelae of Prophylactic Inoculation . . . 1

STONE, D. G. H. Salicylates in Rheumatic Fever: An Attempt to Assess their Value 177

SUTHERLAND, I. A Five-Year Assessment of Patients in a Controlled Trial of Streptomycin in Pulmonary Tuberculosis. Report to the Tuberculosis Chemotherapy Trials Committee of the Medical Research Council . . 347

WHITAKER, W. Pulmonary Hypertension in Congestive Heart Failure complicating Chronic Lung Disease 57

—— Clinical Diagnosis of Pulmonary Hypertension in Patients with Mitral Stenosis. With Plates 4 to 7 105

WILSON, R. R. Spinal Cord Complications of Tuberculous Meningitis: A Clinical and Pathological Study. With Plates 19 to 22 275

616.8–02:614.47

NEUROLOGICAL SEQUELAE OF PROPHYLACTIC INOCULATION[1]

By HENRY G. MILLER AND JOHN B. STANTON

(From the Royal Victoria Infirmary and the Medical School, King's College, Newcastle upon Tyne)

THIS paper presents a review of the literature of neurological complications of prophylactic inoculation and serum administration, and a report of 12 further recent cases collected chiefly from the medical records of the Ministry of Pensions and from the clinical practice of neurological colleagues. Paralytic poliomyelitis following inoculation and neurological sequelae of Jennerian vaccination are excluded from consideration; the cases reported followed inoculation against tetanus, typhoid-paratyphoid, pertussis, diphtheria, and rabies. Many of these neurological sequelae of inoculation are described in the standard textbooks of neurology. They receive scant attention, and are often entirely ignored, in even the larger works on infectious diseases and preventive medicine. There are several reasons for this omission, with its implication that the parenteral introduction of a miscellaneous variety of biological products is a procedure devoid of risk. Probably the most important is that the patient is rarely treated for the complication by the physician who gave the original injection; the relation between inoculation and subsequent neurological symptoms may pass quite unrecognized. Furthermore, in the days when antiserum was more commonly used in therapy, neurological complications which might more properly be laid at the door of therapeutic inoculation were often attributed to infection (Vogel, 1939). Such cases are admittedly rare, and some experienced workers in the field of immunology and preventive medicine remain quite unaware of their occurrence. They lie in a neglected borderland between the fields of neurology, preventive medicine, and paediatrics, and have been the subject of many isolated case reports but of little systematic study. Finally it must be admitted that, in the heat of the emotional battle provoked by propaganda for and against prophylactic inoculation, there has been a tendency on the part of the medical profession to turn a blind eye to unfortunate individual complications of procedures which have the indisputable sanction of social value. Nevertheless the conditions under discussion are not without practical importance, and they are certainly of great theoretical interest. They are among the few acute diseases of the nervous system in which the main aetiological factor, if not the intimate pathogenesis, is clearly identifiable. Secondly, although neurological illnesses arising after inoculation in apparently identical clinical contexts, and presumably therefore on the basis of similar pathological mechanisms, may affect any

[1] Received May 2, 1953.

or every level of the nervous system, from peripheral nerve to cerebral cortex, the localization of clinical and pathological changes within this wide group is far from capricious. It yields, among more indeterminate cases, several symptom-complexes which are clearly defined both anatomically and in their natural history. Thirdly, all the neurological syndromes which follow inoculation may arise in other patients, either apparently spontaneously, or following specific or banal infections. The nervous system admittedly has a limited repertoire of clinical, as of pathological, response, yet it seems likely that common aetiological and pathogenetic factors are involved in these syndromes, under whatever clinical circumstances they arise. It is at least possible that consideration of the rare cases under discussion may ultimately provide clues to our understanding of the commoner but mysterious disorders of similar type encountered in every-day clinical practice.

Neurological Complications of Serum Administration

Neurological complications of serum treatment form the largest group in the literature, and the description of the first case has been attributed to Engelmann in 1897. In the case he described, however, in which injection of antitetanus serum, with a mild serum reaction, was followed by a slowly developing polyneuritis starting 36 days later, the causal relationship of the injection is somewhat doubtful. Grünberger (1904) and Gangolphe and Gardère (1908) described cases of paralysis in the course of serum treatment, but without definitely relating the two events, and Thaon (1910) appears to have been the first definitely to associate paralysis with serum sickness and serum treatment. It was not until 1919, however, that amyotrophic paralysis and polyneuritis were definitely recognized as complications of serum treatment by Lhermitte, and from this time a number of reports of such cases began to appear in France. In England the first cases were described by Dyke in 1918, in Germany by Katz (1927), and in the United States by Gordon in 1928 and 1932 and Kennedy in 1929, although cases with serum sickness and optic neuritis following serum injection had been previously described in America by Mason (1922) and Brown (1925). There are useful reviews by Young (1932), Doyle (1933), Vogel (1935, 1939), Paillas (1936), and Kraus and Chaney (1937). The early reports incriminated antitetanus serum, but subsequent reports have shown that the antisera of diphtheria, scarlatina, tuberculosis, gas gangrene, pneumococcus, gonococcus, meningococcus, and streptococcus have all produced similar neurological complications, as have plain horse serum, other foreign proteins, for example milk (Zeckel, 1939), and even convalescent poliomyelitic human serum (Schneider, 1946). In many cases the neurological complications ensue after a single injection of serum, but in others they follow second or subsequent injections, often some years after the first. Sometimes neurological symptoms may follow each of several injections. The neurological condition is often, but not invariably, associated with somatic symptoms of serum sickness, such as fever, malaise, headache and vomiting, urticaria, oedema, or pain and swelling of the joints. Local soreness and swelling is often present at the site of the injection, and the Arthus phenomenon has been known to occur (Wilson and Hadden, 1932). The signs of serum sickness usually precede the neurological complications by one or two days, but may coincide with them, or rarely (Dyke, 1918; Etienne, 1928; Hughes, 1944) follow them by one or two days. Of 77 cases reported in the literature up to 1931 and reviewed by Lhermitte and Haguenau (1931), 67 showed signs of serum sickness of more than slight severity. The neurological complications usually appear seven to 10 days after the injection of antiserum, although cases have been described of onset within a few hours (Hahn, 1934) or after as long as 18 days (Sommer, 1936).

Clinical types. The clinical syndromes fall into four main groups, which are not rigidly separated and sometimes overlap: (1) Radiculitis (including radiculoneuritis, mononeuritis, plexitis, shoulder-girdle neuritis). (2) Polyneuritis, polyradiculoneuritis (Guillain–Barré syndrome). (3) Myelitis and Landry's ascending paralysis. (4) Meningeal and cerebral forms. Table I indicates the relative frequency of these syndromes. It will be seen that brachial plexitis is the commonest form, occurring in more than 50 per cent. of cases.

TABLE I

Relative Frequencies of Neurological Syndromes Complicating Serum Administration, Based on 100 Adequately Documented Cases including Cases 1–5 reported below

	Number of cases
1. Radiculitis, including brachial plexitis (59 cases)	74
2. Polyneuritis (7) and Guillain–Barré syndrome (3)	10
3. Landry's paralysis (2) and myelitis (4)	6
4. Cerebral and meningeal types, including optic neuritis (6)	10
Total	100

1. *Signs and symptoms.* The radicular and the *neuritic types* usually begin in a similar fashion, with severe stabbing pains across the shoulders, radiating down the limb or along the course of the affected nerve. The duration of this pain is variable, but is usually two to three days. It may last much longer, even for 30 days. Shortly after the appearance of the pain the patient notices weakness, which becomes rapidly more severe for 24 to 48 hours. On examination flaccid weakness of proximal muscles of the limb, or of muscles supplied by the affected nerve, becomes obvious, and fasciculation and subsequent wasting may occur. The affected muscles may show heightening of the threshold to faradic and galvanic stimuli, or even the reaction of degeneration. The brachial plexus in its upper trunk is most commonly involved, and when the condition is unilateral the right side is affected more often than the left. The muscles innervated from the fifth and sixth cervical segments of the cord, including deltoid, spinati, serratus magnus, biceps brachialis, and triceps, are the most frequently affected, especially the first three of these. Rarely one muscle, such as the deltoid or serratus magnus (Richardson, 1942), is affected alone, or bears the brunt of the disability. If both sides are involved the pattern is not necessarily symmetrical. If the biceps, triceps, and supinator longus are affected,

the corresponding tendon-reflexes may be diminished or abolished. Sensory changes such as hypaesthesia and hypalgesia may occur, often over a limited area on the outer surface of the upper arm. Sometimes vasomotor and trophic changes are seen. The lumbosacral plexus and nerves of the lower limb are less frequently involved. Occasionally the recurrent laryngeal and phrenic nerves may be involved, as in the case reported by French (1938) and in Case 2 described below, although Horner's syndrome is not recorded. Young (1932) and Cutter (1936) both reported cases in which nerve deafness appeared to be the result of serum treatment.

2. *Polyneuritic forms* have been described by Sézary and Dessaint (1923), Babonneix (1924), Kennedy (1929), Etienne (1928), Filotico (1929), and Bourrat (1929). In most cases the development was that of a frank polyneuritis from the outset, with generalized pains, motor weakness, distal paraesthesiae and loss of sensation in the limbs, ataxia, and diminished reflexes. Sometimes polyneuritis may be associated with paralysis of one of the facial nerves, as in Filotico's (1929) case, which closely resembles some examples of the Guillain–Barré syndrome. A classical Guillain–Barré syndrome in serum sickness, with typical findings in the spinal fluid, is reported by Reitman and Rothschild (1950). Sometimes impairment of superficial sensation is absent, and an ataxic picture with clumsiness and loss of tendon-reflexes appears, described by French writers as 'pseudo-tabes'.

3. *Myelitis and Landry's paralysis.* Cases of Landry's type of paralysis complicating serum treatment have been reported by Roger, Poursines, and Recordier (1934) and Kroll (1938), while myelitis occurred in cases described by Bourguignon (1931), Bennett (1939), and Sovena (1947). In the Landry type the usual ascending paralysis rapidly appeared; in the fatal case reported by Roger, Poursines, and Recordier, this led, 10 days after cessation of serum treatment, to flaccid paralysis of all four limbs and abolition of tendon-reflexes, with generalized wasting, pain in the limbs, retention of urine, and facial and ocluomotor palsies, without sensory loss. Bourguignon's (1931) case was that of a boy of eight years who received 10 ml. of antitetanus serum after a wound. Eleven days later he had a severe serum reaction, with meningeal symptoms and strabismus. This was rapidly followed by weakness of both upper limbs, more marked on the left, and three days later weakness of the lower limbs ensued, with exaggerated tendon-reflexes and extensor plantar responses. Musculature of the trunk was also involved, and wasting appeared later in the upper limbs. In this case there was no evidence that the patient was suffering at any time from tetanus. Bennett (1939) mentioned a case of transverse myelitis occurring in a young woman undergoing antiserum treatment for tetanus, and Sovena (1947) has reported a similar case. Cases of myelitis merge with the cerebral forms to give a picture of encephalomyelitis, as in the case of Winkelman and Gotten (1935), mentioned below, and in that of Csermely (1950).

4. *Cerebral forms.* Cases of cerebral type have been described by Mason (1922) and Kennedy (1929), and an encephalomyelitic syndrome by Winkelman and Gotten (1935). These cases usually develop the symptoms and signs of raised

intracranial pressure, with headache, vomiting, papilloedema, and neck stiffness, together with signs of cerebral involvement such as aphasia, alexia, hemianopia, and hemiparesis. In the patient of Winkelman and Gotten papilloedema and jargon aphasia were combined with an ascending sensorimotor paralysis. Mental changes may occur either with the other cerebral manifestations, or alone as in Vogel's (1939) case of a 53-year-old workman who, 10 days after cessation of serum treatment for mild cephalic tetanus, developed typical serum sickness combined with a severe confusional state with restlessness, lasting for several weeks. When seen one year later he showed residual emotional lability, and amnesia for the period of confusion.

Meningeal forms. Meningeal symptoms often accompany the cerebral symptoms, as in Kennedy's Case 3 (1929), or myelitis, as in Bourguignon's patient (*vide supra*), or they may occur alone. Such a case, with severe headache, vomiting, photophobia, nuchal rigidity, and Kernig's sign, was reported by Spaar (1943) in a patient who was having treatment of tetanus with antitoxin. Post-mortem examination revealed widespread meningeal inflammation.

Other forms. A few unusual forms have been described, such as Lhermitte's case (1938) of progressive amyotrophy of the shoulder girdle following serum neuritis, and the case described by Thévenard, Lenormand, Nigoux, and Marquès (1950) of myasthenia developing after injection of antitetanus serum.

Cerebrospinal fluid. In the cases in which records are available the pressure of the cerebrospinal fluid has often been raised, with reduction in the glucose-content and slight increase in the number of cells (5 to 28 per c. mm., mostly lymphocytes, with occasional polymorphonuclears), but little or no increase of protein. Cytoalbuminological dissociation occurs in the Guillain–Barré syndrome. These changes appear to reach their zenith between two and four days after the onset of serum sickness, subsiding towards the end of the first week.

Pathological findings. In the relatively infrequent cases in which death has occurred and post-mortem examination has been carried out (Roger, Poursines, and Recordier, 1934; Winkelman and Gotten, 1935; Spaar, 1943; Sovena, 1947; Csermely, 1950) congestion has been found in the brain, meninges, and cord, with glial and lymphocytic infiltration and areas of necrosis. Vasodilatation, perivascular oedema, and small haemorrhages are common. Neuronophagia is usually absent. In affected nerves and nerve-roots oedema and interstitial neuritis have been described (Roger, Poursines, and Recordier, 1934). There may be evidence of raised intracranial pressure, and in the patient of Roger, Poursines, and Recordier there was gross symmetrical dilatation of the ventricular system. In Sovena's myelitic case (1947), in which paraplegia had developed three weeks after treatment of tetanus with antiserum, and autopsy was performed on the patient's death three and a half years later, plastic leptomeningitis with 'chronic myelitis' was found. Csermely (1950) found *post mortem* in his patient, who had shown a clinical picture of encephalomyelitis following prophylactic antitetanus serum, that there was a perivascular effusion of plasma, with marked demyelination far more extensive than that occasionally seen in cases of clinical tetanus (Baker, 1942). The histological picture in this case was remarkably similar to that seen in cases of para-infectious encephalomyelitis. In the case of Winkelman and Gotten (1935), which was clinically of encephalomyelitic type, there was glial and lymphocytic infiltration of the spinal cord, brain, and meninges, with necrotic areas. In Spaar's case (1943) with predominantly meningeal signs, post-mortem examination revealed widespread inflammatory reaction of the meninges, with perivascular exudation, and erythrocytic and lymphocytic infiltration and swelling of the vessel walls. Small perivascular foci of demyelination were also noted in the corpus callosum and corpora quadrigemina.

Prognosis. Recovery takes place in the majority of the neuritic and radicular types within a few months to two years. About 20 per cent. of patients are left with some residual weakness and wasting (Bennett, 1939). The cerebral and myelitic forms carry a graver prognosis.

Four further cases in which neurological symptoms accompanied serum sickness after the prophylactic administration of antitetanus serum are reported below. They comprise two instances of cervical radiculitis, one of which showed suggestive evidence of slight involvement of the spinal cord, and the other coincident weakness of the diaphragm; a mild polyradicular syndrome; and an instance of transient peripheral neuritis accompanied by bilateral papilloedema. The fifth case in this group is an example of transverse myelitis following the administration of antidiphtheritic serum.

Case 1. Bilateral cervical radiculitis, with probable involvement of the spinal cord, in a man of 30 years, 10 days after prophylactic administration of 3,000 international units of antitetanus serum. Good recovery within four months.

Seven years previously this man had received a similar injection of 3,000 units of A.T.S., without any toxic reaction, after a finger injury. Seven days after suture of a laceration of the chin, sustained on the football field, and injection of 3,000 units of A.T.S. into the right arm, the site of injection became red. On the eighth day generalized urticaria developed, and on the ninth day diarrhoea was accompanied by a syncopal attack. On the 10th day the patient complained of severe pain across the shoulders and down both arms, without neck stiffness. The pain lasted for about 36 hours, leaving profound weakness of the left arm which had appeared within 24 hours of its onset. Examination 48 hours after the onset of symptoms showed weakness of the deltoid, infraspinatus, and wrist and finger extensors on the left side, and of the serratus magnus, finger extensors, and intrinsic hand muscles on the right side. There was an area of sensory loss on the outer side of the left arm, and pain on stretching the right brachial plexus. All deep reflexes in the arms and legs were exceedingly brisk; the left plantar response was flexor, but the right equivocal. The spinal fluid was normal. Electromyography five days later confirmed a neuropathic lesion of the left deltoid. Improvement was slow but progressive. Five weeks later there was some improvement in power in the affected muscles, and the sensory loss was less extensive. Four months later slight weakness in the right infraspinatus and right finger extensors was the only abnormal finding.

Case 2. Cervical radiculitis with weakness of the diaphragm nine days after prophylactic administration of antitetanus serum in a 39-year-old man, subject to hay-fever, with a past history of an acute neurological illness, possibly encephalomyelitic, two years previously. Incomplete recovery seven months later.

This 39-year-old medical practitioner has a long history of hay-fever. Two years previously an 'influenzal' illness was associated with intense headache, nausea, vomiting, nystagmus, and generalized muscular pains, worst in the right arm. The acute illness lasted for a week. There was neither meningism nor disturbance of consciousness, but the illness left marked weakness in the muscles of the right shoulder-girdle, a symptom which remained troublesome for 12 months. Although he received several injections of typhoid-paratyphoid vaccine and tetanus toxoid during military service, A.T.S. had never previously been administered. Seven days after the administration of 3,000 units of A.T.S. after an injury to the thumb, the site of injection became red. In spite of 48 hours of generalized urticaria treated with adrenaline injections, considerable exertion was undertaken during this period (driving in stakes), and subsidence of the urticaria was followed by the appearance of severe pains across the shoulders and down the inner sides of both arms. The pain was so intense as to demand repeated injections of morphia, and weakness of the right arm was progressive over the course of several days, loss of power of abduction at the shoulder being complete. At the same time fasciculation was noted in the right upper arm and the right quadriceps, and paraesthesiae in the two ulnar digits on the right. Marked dyspnoea on lying down and on exertion developed. The pain remained severe for two weeks, but left only extensive tenderness a month later. Examination at this time showed weakness and wasting of the right deltoid, supraspinatus, and infraspinatus, with absence of the triceps-jerk and sensory impairment over the ipsilateral fifth cervical dermatome. Breathing was difficult in the recumbent posture, with inspiratory indrawing of the upper abdominal wall. At this stage the patient returned to work still severely incapacitated. Dyspnoea was very troublesome in bed at night for many months. At present, seven months after the onset, the patient is breathless on stooping or exertion (especially when recumbent), the right shoulder is still weak, and there is still marked wasting of the right deltoid, with sensory loss over the fifth cervical dermatome. Slow improvement continues.

Case 3. Symptoms of a mild polyradiculitis, appearing in a man of 38 years, 11 days after prophylactic injection of 1,500 international units of antitetanus serum, and clearing up in three weeks.

Seven days after the injection of 1,500 units of A.T.S., administered when a puncture of the left forefinger became mildly infected, this medical practitioner developed oedema at the site of injection. The next day a generalized morbilliform rash appeared, and this, together with the local reaction, subsided during the subsequent 36 hours, to give place to painful tingling in arms, hands, legs, and feet, brought on especially by movement. The pain was of an unpleasant stinging character, and left a 'slow' pain after each sharp episode. A characteristic of this stinging pain was that it appeared, for example, in stretching out the hand, or on turning sharply in a chair, but it was not present at rest. The pain was thus brought about frequently, because the likelihood of pain being produced was forgotten, and movement produced an unpleasant surprise. These symptoms became progressively worse, and led to neurological consultation five days later. Findings on examination were rather unsatisfactory. There was hyperaesthesia over the lower part of the left triceps, and over the lower end of the radial surface of the right forearm. There was no alteration of reflexes or of motor power. Fever and systemic upset were absent, and the patient was able to follow his occupation. Unpleasant symptoms continued moderately severe for a further week, and after that time began to subside. A persistent symptom which appeared late was pain down the inner aspect of the left lower arm and forearm. This pain was consistently brought about by a slight sharp extension of the head as the patient adjusted his stethoscope to allow the ear-pieces to fit in the ear. The pain from this movement was quite severe, and left a 'stinging' in its distribution, and slight numbness, which would last for up to five minutes. Similar pain was elicited on flexion of the head to the side. The symptoms in the legs were mild and not localized. For 24 hours there was pain of root distribution in the upper left chest. Symptoms were most troublesome during the second week of the illness, and had disappeared three weeks from the onset.

Case 4. Severe serum sickness with transient peripheral neuritis and bilateral optic neuritis in a man of 29 years, nine days after the injection of 1,500 international units of antitetanus serum.

This patient had never received A.T.S. before, but had developed fever and a painful arm after the injection of tetanus toxoid in 1943; injection of typhoid-paratyphoid vaccine had elicited no reaction. There is a family history of probable food allergy. Nine days after a single injection of 1,500 units of A.T.S., given because of an infected laceration of the forearm, he developed headache, fever, shivering attacks, severe angioneurotic oedema affecting the upper part of the body and the head, and aching pain in the right wrist, feet, and ankles. Several joints were red and swollen. In two days all these symptoms had subsided, but during the next 48 hours he developed intense generalized hyperaesthesia. This was most marked in the feet and hands, which were so painful that he had to have cold compresses applied. It was accompanied by the gradual onset of weakness in the legs, arms, and right side of the face. The peripheral muscles were acutely tender. Examination revealed flaccid weakness of the muscles of all four limbs and of the back. Except for the left biceps-jerk, which was absent, reflexes were everywhere normal. There was muscle tenderness and skin hyperaesthesia below the elbows and knees, with impairment of peripheral discriminatory sensibility, though pin-prick and touch could everywhere be distinguished. There was no complaint of visual impairment, but bilateral papillitis of moderate degree was present, without haemorrhages or exudates. The pressure and composition of the spinal fluid were normal. There was pyrexia of 100·5° F., polymorphonuclear leucocytosis, and a raised erythrocyte sedimentation rate. Improvement began within 12 hours of his admission to hospital, and 24 hours later both pain and weakness were much less pronounced and the temperature had become normal. He was discharged from hospital 10 days after admission, without symptoms, and with receding swelling of the optic disks as the sole abnormal finding, and has subsequently remained well except for a complaint of recurrent frontal headaches.

Case 5. Transverse myelitis following epididymo-orchitis, acute tonsillitis, and administration of diphtheria antitoxin, in a man of 24 years. Fair recovery, with some residual disability six years later.

Six days after the development of an illness characterized by a non-specific left epididymo-orchitis and a follicular tonsillitis, an organism morphologically indistinguishable from the Klebs–Loeffler bacillus was grown from a throat swab. Subsequent daily cultures were all negative, but meanwhile the patient was given two injections of 24,000 units of diphtheria antitoxic serum at an interval of 24 hours. Forty-eight hours after the second injection he developed pain in the back, dysuria, and paraplegia, with disappearance of deep reflexes and lower abdominal responses, extensor plantar reflexes, and patchy impairment of sensation in the legs. The spinal fluid contained 24 lymphocytes per c.mm., but the protein-content was normal. Bladder control returned within a week, and within 14 days the knee- and ankle-jerks reappeared. Sensory impairment, which was partial, disappeared completely during the course of three weeks. During recovery there was some wasting of the legs; the plantar responses could no longer be elicited, and finally became flexor. Six months after the onset recovery was almost complete, except for some exaggeration of the deep reflexes and a tendency to backache and frequency and precipitancy of micturition. Six years later these symptoms and signs were unchanged.

Typhoid-Paratyphoid Vaccine (T.A.B.)

Typhoid-paratyphoid vaccine is used in two distinct ways: either intravenously in artificial fever therapy, or for vaccination. It has been recognized for many years that intravenous T.A.B. may activate latent chronic infections, especially pulmonary tuberculosis, but reports of neurological complications from its use in fever therapy are rare. Cowie (1921) described a case in which hemiplegia occurred the day after intravenous injection of T.A.B. in a patient with polyarthritis and septic endocarditis; more recent examples are Hughes's (1944) Case 4, of a soldier given an intravenous injection of T.A.B. containing 30 million organisms, who had a secondary rise of temperature the next day and developed a complete right musculospiral palsy 10 days later, and Case 1 of Peacher and Robertson (1945), described more fully below. Since inoculation against typhoid was introduced in 1896, the procedure has been carried out millions of times without untoward reactions, and relatively few cases have been reported in which neurological complications have ensued. The earliest report appears to be that of Gubb (1915), and after the war further accounts appeared, particularly in France. Guillain and Barré (1919) described the first fatal case, that of a soldier in whom an acute ascending paralysis of Landry type, following the first injection of T.A.B., led to death after eight days. Further cases were reported by Jumentié (1916), Roussy (1919), Roussy and Cornil (1919), Léri and Boivin (1919), Preti (1919), Souques (1919), Bury (1920), Russell (1924), Benon (1924), Alajouanine, Fribourg-Blanc, and Gauthier (1928), Kennedy (1929), Noïca (1932), Gayle and Bowen (1933), Robinson (1937), Krais (1943), Lemke (1943), Peacher and Robertson (1945), von Keyserlingk (1947), Giffin, Rogers, and Kernohan (1948), Bannwarth (1948), Starý (1948), Tarnay (1948), and Mumme (1950).

The distribution of clinical types is shown in Table II. The neurological manifestations may appear after any of the injections, being most common after the second and rare after the first. Many of the patients whose symptoms appeared after a single injection had been inoculated against typhoid-paratyphoid on earlier occasions and were undergoing revaccination, but not all were in this category, for example Bannwarth's Case 8, whose only previous vaccination had been against smallpox. There is evidence that heroic persistence in giving the remainder of a series of T.A.B. inoculations, after the appearance of symptoms, causes rapid worsening almost at once, as was seen in some of the military patients subsequently examined by Bannwarth. Neurological complications may follow T.A.B. vaccination at intervals varying from a few hours to 14 days, with a maximum incidence at three days. The symptoms vary with the clinical type of neurological involvement. General symptoms include giddiness, fainting, malaise, headache, vomiting, and pyrexia. A local reaction at the site of the injection is common, but generalized urticaria appears to be rare, although it can occur, as in Mumme's (1950) 56-year-old patient who,

TABLE II

Relative Frequencies of Neurological Syndromes Complicating T.A.B. Vaccination, based on 49 Adequately Documented Cases from the Literature and Case 6 of the Present Series

	Number of cases
1. Radiculitis or plexitis (6) and mononeuritis (6)	12
2. Polyneuritis (5) and Guillain–Barré syndrome (3)	8
3. Landry's paralysis (9) and myelitis (1)	10
4. Cerebral (15) and meningeal forms (5)	20
Total	50

after the third T.A.B. injection, developed a generalized rash as a prelude to a polyneuritis. Neurological symptoms include paraesthesiae, hyperaesthesia, weakness and pains in muscles, loss of libido and potency, tenderness to pressure over nerve-trunks, visual disturbances, weakness of one half of the body, cortical sensory loss, speech disturbance, involuntary movements, and mental symptoms. The latter usually consist of the acute organic psychiatric syndrome, with clouding of consciousness, sleepiness, apathy, defects of attention and memory, and lability of mood, occasionally passing into true delirium and coma. In some instances permanent intellectual or personality defects may ensue, as in Souques's (1919) fifth case. The signs vary from those of peripheral neuritis (motor or sensory, or both), of cord involvement, and of meningeal involvement, to those of cerebral disturbances, according to the clinical type of the neurological disorder. The cerebrospinal fluid may be normal, but may show slight increase of cells, or the typical cytoalbuminological dissociation of the Guillain–Barré syndrome (Bannwarth, 1948).

Pathological reports on such cases are few. In the case of Guillain and Barré (1919) with Landry's paralysis, the findings in the nervous system were within normal limits. Gayle and Bowen (1933) demonstrated oedema of the anterior-horn cells of the cord, with degeneration, congestion, and oedema of the peripheral nerves, in their patient who had Landry's paralysis. The first patient of Peacher and Robertson (1945), with a clinical picture of clouded consciousness, headache, papilloedema, and left hemiparesis with twitching of the left hand, showed, at operation for suspected tumour, considerable oedema of the right hemisphere with a large, necrotic, friable subcortical mass involving the frontal and parietal lobes. Sections taken from this region showed areas of focal degeneration with vacuolization, necrosis, perivascular congestion, and oedema. Granular cells and cells laden with lipoid were also present. There was only slight tendency to thrombosis in the smaller blood-vessels. The patient of

Giffin, Rogers, and Kernohan (1948), who had left hemiparesis (including the face), cortical sensory changes in the left arm, left hemianopia, and dysarthria, and died after a period of emotional lability followed by apathy and stupor, was found at post-mortem examination to have intense congestion and oedema of the brain, with subcortical areas of softening in the right frontal and parieto-occipital regions. Microscopical examination of sections from these areas showed perivascular collections of fat-laden phagocytes, with patchy demyelination which was almost complete in the right occipital region. The nerve-cells of the cortex were well preserved, and there was no evidence of thrombi, though there was endothelial proliferation in some of the smaller blood-vessels. Lemke's patient (1943), who had left brachial plexitis, followed later by transverse myelitis at the level of the seventh cervical segment, and died of bulbar and respiratory failure after a period of delirium, proved *post mortem* to have hyperaemia of the meninges of brain and cord, with severe degeneration of the cervical and upper dorsal cord. Microscopic examination showed engorgement of the vessels of the cord, with multiple perivascular haemorrhages, oedema of nerve-fibres, and little glial reaction. There was also oedema of the left brachial plexus. The course and *prognosis* appear to be favourable except in the cases of cord and cerebral involvement, in which the mortality rate may be as high as 50 per cent. according to Robinson (1937). Five of the 50 cases reviewed here proved fatal. Of nine cases of Landry's paralysis, three died.

T.A.B. and tetanus toxoid. Injections of these two preparations are quite often combined, and neurological complications of such injections have been reported, for example by Hughes (1944). In view of the relative rarity of neurological disorders complicating the use of tetanus toxoid alone, this group is included under T.A.B. The complications of the double injection appear to follow the same patterns as those following T.A.B. alone. Of Hughes's three patients, one developed an encephalitic illness with left hemiparesis, nystagmus, and emotional lability, proceeding to moderate recovery; the other two had shoulder-girdle palsies of the type described on page 3.

We report below two further cases in this group—an instance of Landry's paralysis beginning seven days after a second injection of T.A.B., and a rapidly fatal neurological illness two days after a first inoculation with T.A.B. and tetanus toxoid.

Case 6. Landry's syndrome appearing seven days after a second inoculation with T.A.B. vaccine. A very severe illness with respiratory paralysis; recovery almost complete in 12 months.

At an interval of seven days this 21-year-old man was given two injections, each of 0·5 ml. of T.A.B. Seven days after the second injection he complained of numbness and tingling in the right foot. Two days later the left foot was similarly affected. After a further two days both hands became numb and tingling, and within the next 48 hours a flaccid quadriplegia developed, which was most marked in the legs, but was also associated with dysphagia, dysarthria, and increasing dyspnoea. Widespread flaccid weakness was accompanied by disappearance of all deep reflexes and of the plantar responses. The muscles were tender, but the only other sensory change was a slight impairment of superficial sensation to touch and pin-prick over the trunk and limbs. There was no headache, meningism, sphincter disturbance, or change in the spinal fluid. Breathlessness and cyanosis became marked, and the patient was in a respirator for seven days, and dangerously ill for three weeks. After this time improvement was slow but steady. Generalized muscular wasting ensued, most marked in the legs, which were cold and blue; there were similar but lesser changes in the arms. The sensory impairment disappeared completely within three weeks. Six months later he was still completely incapacitated, but improving. Twelve months after the illness bilateral partial foot-drop was the only residual symptom, and two years later some weakness of the ankles, with absent ankle-jerks, was the only evidence of his illness.

Case 7. Fatal cerebral illness of 12 hours' duration, beginning 48 hours after T.A.B. and tetanus-toxoid inoculation.

Two days after his first inoculation with 0·5 ml. of T.A.B. vaccine and 1 ml. of tetanus toxoid, this previously healthy 32-year-old man complained of headache, and became mentally confused. Within a few hours he was deeply comatose, with flaccid quadriplegia, complete disappearance of reflexes including the plantar responses, and incontinence of urine. The spinal fluid was normal. The patient died 12 hours after the onset of headache; autopsy was refused.

Tetanus Toxoid

Tetanus toxoid given alone appears to be one of the least reactive of these biological products. Only a few reactions have been reported in the literature, and such cases as the fatal one of Schittenhelm, quoted by Lemke (1943), occurred at a time when methods of preparation of the toxoid allowed the presence of considerable amounts of foreign protein. Modern methods of producing tetanus toxoid, by the Pillemer or similar processes, leave the preparation virtually free from non-specific fractions. Nevertheless Woolling and Rushton (1950) referred to a case recently seen in the Mayo Clinic, in which a shoulder-girdle syndrome, running a course similar to that seen in serum neuritis, occurred five days after the administration of tetanus toxoid.

Pertussis Inoculation

The possibility of serious neurological complications after inoculation against whooping-cough has been recognized since Madsen (1933) reported from Denmark the deaths of two newborn children after second injections of a pertussis vaccine, given because they had been born into families where pertussis was present. Doull, Shibley, and McClelland (1936) reported three cases of children with transient convulsions after pertussis vaccination. Another case was reported by Taylor (1938), and similar examples by Kendrick and Eldering (1939) and Sako, Treuting, Witt, and Nichamin (1945). In 1947 Brody and Sorley reported the case of a child who had recovered from encephalitis, and was given pertussis vaccine a few months later. After each of the first two injections the encephalitic syndrome returned, and after a third, much diluted, intracutaneous dose the child died. The following year Byers and Moll (1948) reported a series of 15 cases encountered in the Children's Hospital in Boston in a period of eight years. Toomey (1949) added 38 cases discovered by a questionnaire submitted to a large number of practitioners, and Globus and Kohn (1949) reported two further cases. These complications may follow the use of a variety of pertussis vaccines, may occur after first, second, or third injections, and are not dependent on the dosage used. In the series of Byers and Moll five children had reactions after the first, four after the second, and six after the third dose. The age of the infants varied from five to 18 months. Clinically the picture is a striking one, most commonly of convulsions occurring 20 minutes to 72 hours after the injection, followed by coma or hemiplegia, or both. The convulsions may continue throughout the acute stage, which may last from two to 10 days, but they may occasionally be absent. The spinal fluid may show a slight increase of protein and mononuclear cells. In six out of eight patients in whom Byers and Moll performed pneumoencephalography considerable ventricular dilatation was discovered.

Pathology. In one case of Byers and Moll the child died subsequently from pneumonia, and at post-mortem examination the brain showed diffuse atrophy and gliosis. Rather more detail is available in Case 2 of Globus and Kohn (1949). This was a male infant of eight months, who after the second injection of pertussis antigen vaccine (detoxified formolized filtrate) had generalized convulsions and lapsed into stupor. He died after four weeks, during most of which time he had been in a state of decerebrate rigidity with raised intracranial pressure. Post-mortem examination showed a soft and oedematous brain, in which the cortex was devoid of the usual lamellation and none of the cells looked normal. There was a copious accumulation of macrophages with fat-granules in the cortex and subcortex, and to a less extent in the brain-stem, cerebellum, and cord. There were no vascular changes or perivascular lymphocytic infiltration, no haemorrhages, and no necrotic changes in the vessels. Van der Horst (1950), however, considered that perivascular neuroglial cuffs and demyelination are usual features of encephalitis after pertussis vaccination.

Prognosis. Madsen's two patients (1933) and one of the patients of Brody and Sorley (1947) died. Of the 15 patients of Byers and Moll (1948) two died, as did two of Toomey's (1949) 25 patients as to whom full details were available; and one of the two cases of Globus and Kohn (1949) was fatal. One of the most serious features of these complications is the evidence of residual damage to the nervous system. Continued epileptic fits, residual hemiplegia, blindness, mental defect, behaviour disorders, and reversal of sleep rhythm have been reported, and it appears that about two-thirds of the patients who recover from the acute phase are liable to such residua. One of the cases in which Byers and Moll performed pneumoencephalography showed enormous ventricular dilation one month after the incriminated injection.

Combined pertussis and diphtheria immunization. A combined preparation for simultaneous immunization against whooping-cough and diphtheria has been popular in the last few years, and has apparently been successful. Cases of neurological complications from use of these preparations have been reported, and appear to conform to the type found in the cases of pertussis vaccination described above. Thus Werne and Garrow (1946) reported two cases of fatal anaphylactic shock, following the second injection of a combined diphtheria and pertussis vaccine, in identical twins aged 10 months. The first case in this country appears to have been the fatal illness of a male twin aged eight months, who received a combined diphtheria-pertussis prophylactic (first injection) in the morning and died early next day, after a period of irritability and curious movements of one arm (*British Medical Journal*, 1949). Another case was reported by Anderson and Morris (1950), in which severe neurological complications occurred in a boy aged two and a half years. He developed convulsions, followed by coma, 36 hours after the first injection of combined antigen, and investigations eight months later showed gross atrophy of the left cerebral hemisphere. One year later the patient still had a right hemiplegia, his vocabulary was limited, and he was mentally retarded. A further similar case with hemiplegia was reported by Vahrman (1950).

Triple vaccine (pertussis, diphtheria, tetanus toxoid). Grace (1950) described two cases of unilateral convulsions with hemiparesis, occurring in children of seven months and three years respectively, after injection of a triple vaccine for pertussis, diphtheria, and tetanus toxoid. The first child had hemiparesis, petit mal, and disturbances of behaviour, which were still present one year later. A similar triple vaccine appears to have been responsible for comparable neurological complications in the case reported by Escardó and Vazquez (1950).

There appears to be no doubt that these complications of pertussis vaccination are different from those encountered in other prophylactic inoculations in that the illness is always cerebral. No cases have been described in which there were neuritic, myelitic, or Landry types of complication with pertussis vaccine. Two further cases of cerebral illness after inoculation with combined diphtheria-pertussis vaccine are reported below.

Case 8 Right hemiplegia following an apparently acute cerebral illness seven days after a third injection of combined diphtheria-pertussis vaccine, leaving moderate residual disability two years later.

Seven days after her third injection of a combined diphtheria-pertussis vaccine, this previously healthy baby (age not recorded) developed a severe attack of screaming, followed by drowsiness. During the subsequent two days the child remained alternately drowsy and restless, though she was able to take her food. At the end of this period the parents noticed that she was not moving her right arm and leg. Examination revealed a right hemiplegia involving face, arm, and leg, with increased deep reflexes on the right side and bilateral extensor plantar responses. The temperature was 100° F., there was some neck stiffness, and the spinal fluid, otherwise normal, contained 46 lymphocytes per c.mm. Improvement was rapid, and the infant left hospital after two weeks. Two years later right hemiparesis persists. There is difficulty in using the right hand, but the child can walk. General development and intelligence appear to be unimpaired.

Case 9. Neurological illness of 10 days' duration, beginning 24 hours after a second injection of combined diphtheria-pertussis vaccine, and characterized by convulsions and stupor. Complete and rapid recovery.

Twenty-four hours after a second injection of 0·5 ml. of combined diphtheria-pertussis vaccine, this 13-month-old baby developed fever, convulsions, and vomiting. Her identical twin, similarly inoculated for the second time one month after the first injection, had no reaction. Pyrexia settled within 24 hours, but the child remained stuporose, with eyes and head turned to the right, frequent myoclonic twitching, and many frank convulsions. There were no other abnormal physical signs; blood count, biochemical investigations, and examination of the spinal fluid were all negative. Her condition was static for seven days, after which improvement was rapid. Ten days from the onset she appeared normal. Six months later she remained perfectly well and indistinguishable from her twin sister.

Diphtheria Immunization

It is now generally recognized that paralytic poliomyelitis may follow diphtheria immunization, and that the paralysis is more common in the inoculated extremity. Nevertheless, there are rare cases in which the clinical picture, including sensory impairment, cerebral signs, and allergic manifestations, indicates that the cause of the neurological disturbance is not poliomyelitis. There are few published reports of such cases after immunization against diphtheria alone, in spite of the vast number of these inoculations which are performed. Wilkinson (1937) reported the case of an infant of one year who was given 0·5 ml. of alum-precipitated toxoid (A.P.T.). About one week after the injection there developed in the course of a few days a flaccid paralysis of all four limbs, trunk, and neck, with no allergic manifestation, no pain, and no fever. This child had also had an attack of measles two and a half weeks before the injection of A.P.T. Liessens (1949) reported another case of a boy who, after an encephalitic illness of undetermined nature at the age of six months, was vaccinated at the age of three years against smallpox and diphtheria. Five years later he received 0·3 ml. of A.P.T. as a 'booster' dose, and 24 hours later he developed headache, neck stiffness, and strabismus, which lasted for five days. Three days later he had pains in the arms and a fleeting scarlatiniform rash, accompanied by fever. There was rapidly increasing weakness of the right arm and right leg. The next day he complained of severe joint pains, which lasted on and off for a fortnight. These symptoms abated, and when examined two to three months later he had weakness and wasting of the right upper limb, and to a less extent of the right lower limb, with some incoordination in the right leg, and slight weakness of the right palate and right hypoglossal nerve. The case described by Fanconi, Zellweger, and Botsztejn (1944) is a little less certain: a child developed mild diphtheria at the age of five and a half years. He was immunized at the age of seven and a half years in view of a diphtheria epidemic in the neighbourhood. A few hours after the fourth injection of anatoxin (formol toxoid) he complained of severe pain in the right arm and elbow, which lasted for three or four days and was followed by paralysis of the right shoulder. These three are the only cases we have been able to find in the literature in which neurological complications unequivocally followed the use of diphtheria toxoid alone, though there are several reports of such complications following administration of vaccines which combine diphtheria toxoid with pertussis, tetanus, or other vaccines, which are reviewed in another section of this paper. We report below a case of transverse myelitis following administration of diphtheria toxoid.

Case 10. Transverse myelitis following inoculation against diphtheria with alum-precipitated toxoid. Appreciable disability persisted nine years later.

Eleven days after an initial injection of 0·2 ml. of A.P.T. this 22-year-old man complained of weakness and heaviness of the legs and difficulty in passing water. During the subsequent 24 hours he developed a burning pain round the middle of the chest and retention of urine, while the weakness of the legs had become such that he could take only a few steps. Examination revealed a spastic paraplegia, with brisk reflexes, extensor plantar responses, and absent abdominal reflexes. There was complete loss of all forms of sensation below the eighth dorsal dermatome on both sides. During the first few days the level of sensory loss ascended, and at the end of this time there was profound impairment of all forms of sensation below the fourth dorsal segment. The Wasserman reaction was negative, the erythrocyte sedimentation rate was 28 mm. in one hour, and the spinal fluid contained 125 lymphocytes per c.mm., with a normal protein-content. Retention of urine cleared within a week, and sensory improvement began two weeks later and was complete in six weeks. Five months after the onset he was able to walk 200 yards in short strides, but could not sit up unaided, and had occasional bed-wetting and painful cramps in both legs at night. Examination at this time revealed a spastic paraplegia without sensory impairment. Two years later these symptoms persisted, but he was able to walk half a mile. Impotence, nocturnal enuresis, and precipitancy and frequency of micturition persisted. Eight years after the onset there was little change. He still cannot walk more than half a mile, and although he is running a small business his wife does most of the work.

Symptoms and signs. The four cases described above indicate a polymorphic clinical picture—Landry's syndrome, hemiplegia, cervical radiculitis, transverse myelitis. There are no reports of pathological findings in cases of this type. *Prognosis* appears to be good, though there is clearly some risk to life in the Landry and encephalomyelitic forms, and a possibility of permanent muscular wasting or weakness from radicular lesions.

'Neuroparalytic Accidents' of Antirabic Treatment

That neurological complications may ensue in the course of the Pasteur treatment and prophylaxis of rabies has been known since their general adoption, and has been related to the fact that animal nervous tissue is used in the inoculation. The incidence of such complications varies from 1/2,500 (Wilson, 1940) to 1/5,814 (Greenwood, 1945–6), the extreme ages of life being almost immune, although two children five years old were among the cases reported by Stuart and Krikorian (1933). There is evidence (Greenwood, 1945–6) that phenolized antirabic vaccine may reduce the risk (1/8,517). Clinically, the neurological complications tend to appear between the 10th and the 15th days from the time of the first injection (not the bite), with a lower limit of five days (Gros, 1897) and an upper limit of 35 days (Wilson, 1940); this period is shorter than the incubation period of rabies. There are four main clinical forms, which may overlap: (1) mononeuritic; (2) polyneuritic (including the Guillain–Barré syndrome); (3) Landry's paralysis and transverse myelitis; (4) meningoencephalitic and encephalomyelitic forms. The first three forms occur with almost equal frequency, while the last group is less common, comprising about 10 per cent. of all cases.

1. In the mononeuritic type the sciatic, median, ulnar, or various cranial nerves, particularly the facial, may be involved (Rubin and Bowman, 1950).
2. The Guillain–Barré syndrome of polyneuritis, often involving the facial nerve, and showing cytoalbuminological dissociation in the cerebrospinal fluid, has been described as a complication of antirabic treatment by Marinescu and Draganesco (1938), Koenigsfeld (1945), McIntyre and Krouse (1949), and D'Ingianni and Fontenelle (1949).
3. Landry's type of ascending paralysis, resembling the paralytic type of rabies (Hurst and Pawan, 1931) has been encountered complicating antirabic treatment by Avezzù (1928), Remlinger (1928), Babonneix and Sigwald (1929), Stuart and Krikorian (1930), Imrie (1944), Ansell (1948), and Wrightsman (1949). This type usually starts with headache, vomiting, pain in the back, and fever, followed within 48 hours by paralysis of the legs and sphincters, without sensory loss, rapidly extending upwards to involve the trunk, arms, face, and vital centres. The dorso-lumbar myelitic type has been described by Avezzù (1928) and Latimer, Webster, and Gurdjian (1951). In this type the onset is less sudden, with little fever; girdle pains, motor and sensory paralysis in the lower limbs, sphincter disturbance, and loss of reflexes are the main features. The plantar responses may become extensor.
4. Meningoencephalomyelitic forms have been described by Bussell (1946), Redewill and Underwood (1947), Gornicki (1948), Pickar and Kramer (1949), Fisch and Wood (1950), and Latimer, Webster, and Gurdjian (1951). Such cases usually have an acute onset, with fever, raised intracranial pressure, papilloedema, meningism, and signs of diffuse involvement of the central nervous system.

Spinal fluid. The spinal fluid usually shows no change in the neuritic and Landry types, but in the Guillain–Barré forms there is found the typical excess of protein without increase of cells, while in the encephalomyelitic types there may be some increase of cells, the highest reported count being 1,260 cells per c.mm. (Appelbaum, Greenberg, and Nelson, 1953).

Pathology. Pathological reports on neuroparalytic accidents in antirabic treatment have been made by Babès and Mironesco (1908), Fielder (1916), Koritschoner and Schweinburg (1925), Busson (1926), Bassoe and Grinker (1930), Stuart and Krikorian (1933), Latimer, Webster, and Gurdjian (1951), and Smith (1951). The changes found are usually oedema and perivascular congestion, with degeneration of ganglion cells. Perivascular lymphocytic infiltration has been described in the peripheral nerves and neuraxis, with local perivascular demyelination and neuroglial reaction, in at least one case (Bassoe and Grinker, 1930).

Prognosis. The neuritic forms usually lead to good recovery in weeks or months. The dorso-lumbar myelitic type has a mortality of 5 per cent. (Ansell, 1948), but the majority of patients rapidly recover. The Landry type has a mortality of 30 per cent. (Brain, 1951), but the surviving patients improve and become well. The encephalomyelitic form has a similar mortality to the Landry type, and residual damage to hypothalamic function has been described in two such cases (McFadzean, 1952). The overall mortality in neurological syndromes complicating antirabic treatment is in the region of 40 per cent. (Latimer, Webster, and Gurdjian, 1951).

Case 11. High transverse myelitis developing on the eighth day of antirabic therapy in a man of 23 years. Fair recovery, with residual signs five years later.

For seven days after contact with a rabid dog this man was given daily injections of 2 ml. of antirabic vaccine (phenolized rabbit-brain virus). On the eighth day he developed severe generalized headache, and a few hours later fell to the ground when his legs became suddenly weak. Within an hour he developed a profound ascending flaccid quadriplegia, with disappearance of reflex activity and profound sensory impairment below the clavicles. The spinal fluid contained 50 mg. of protein per 100 ml., and 160 cells per c.mm., most of which were polymorphonuclear leucocytes. There was marked dyspnoea, and the patient was in a respirator for 72 hours, at the end of which time he was removed and suprapubic cystostomy was performed in view of persisting retention of urine. Within seven days the temperature fell to normal, and the spinal fluid contained only 25 mg. of protein per 100 ml. and 20 lymphocytes per c.mm. Three weeks later paraesthesiae were present on the inner sides of the legs and thighs, and sensation returned gradually from the toes upwards. There was concurrent improvement of bladder function, and at the end of four weeks from the onset sensation was almost normal, urine was passed voluntarily *per urethram*, and some movement had returned in the right ankle. The plantar responses, previously absent, were now extensor. Slow improvement continued, and within six months the patient was able to walk the length of the ward. Twelve months later, although walking was fair, impotence was complete, and there was some difficulty in emptying the bladder if it was allowed to become over-full. Five years after the onset he was walking well without sticks, and the only remaining disabilities were precipitancy of micturition, constipation, and relative impotence. The plantar responses remained extensor.

Miscellaneous Immunizing Agents

Olmer and Paillas (1935) described a case of Landry's paralysis in a patient who had received an injection of antipneumococcic vaccine. Bannwarth (1948) reported a case of polyneuritis following inoculation against dysentery. The patient received three injections of killed bacterial dysentery vaccine at seven-day intervals. Twenty-four hours after the third injection he developed a classical Guillain–Barré syndrome, with cytoalbuminological dissociation in the cerebrospinal fluid. The same author reported a case of brachial plexitis in a soldier after typhus immunization. Three days after the second injection the patient developed severe pain in the left scapular region, which spread to involve the extensor surface of the left arm and forearm, with marked paraesthesiae in the left hand. Examination revealed tenderness on pressure of the left brachial plexus and nerves of the left arm, with superficial hyperpathia. There was no demonstrable weakness, but the tendon-reflexes of the left upper limb were markedly diminished. Lhermitte and Fribourg-Blanc (1936) reported a case in which a subacute encephalomyelitis followed vaccination against yellow fever. The patient, aged 32 years and in good health, received a single injection of Laigret's vaccine; he developed immediate headache, giddiness, and fever, followed a few days later by paraesthesiae, cramps, and weakness in the lower limbs. These symptoms improved for three weeks, but returned after three months, and spread to involve the medulla and cause death from secondary infection and respiratory failure. Post-mortem examination showed perivascular infiltration, with areas of demyelination. The vaccine used in this case appears to have been prepared from inoculated mouse-brain. Radermecker (1949) reported a case of Landry's ascending paralysis following combined vaccination against typhus, tetanus, and variola.

Neurological Sequelae of Skin-Testing

The child reported by Brody and Sorley (1947) with encephalitis complicating pertussis vaccination had adverse reactions to the first two injections of the vaccine, and therefore received, on the third occasion, a very small dose intracutaneously, which caused a fatal relapse of the encephalitis. A somewhat similar case, fortunately less serious, in which a bulbar encephalopathy followed a Schick test, is described below.

Case 12. Acute bulbar encephalopathy following Schick testing, with some points of similarity to diphtheria.

A 10-year-old boy, who had been Schick-tested regularly every three years, was inoculated against diphtheria in 1940. Ten days later he developed a sore throat, with high fever and joint pains. In 1943 he had a further Schick test, which was negative, and 10 days later developed fever, constipation, posterior cervical adenitis, paralysis of the soft palate for five or six days, blurred vision for four days, and some disturbance of speech. There were no symptoms referable to the limbs. He made a good recovery from the illness, but examination seven months later revealed residual wasting and weakness of the left masseter and temporal muscles, deviation of the jaw to the left on opening the mouth, and difficulty in moving the jaw to the right.

Mérei (1950) described two patients in whom disseminated sclerosis became apparent after a Mantoux test. These two cases appear to fall into a different category from the two discussed above. A third case, however, was of a man aged 23 years, with no previous signs of neurological disease, who developed disseminated leucoencephalomyelitis several days after a positive Mantoux test.

Discussion

The aim of the present paper is to present a clinical account of neurological sequelae of prophylactic inoculation, to compare the syndromes which follow inoculations of different kinds, and to seek evidence as to the pathogenesis of the conditions described. We exclude from this discussion the cases of poliomyelitis following inoculation against pertussis and diphtheria, separately or combined, to which attention has been drawn by McCloskey (1950) and Hill and Knowelden (1950). Not only do such cases differ clinically from the essentially cerebral complications here described as following such inoculations, but the pathological findings of perivascular cuffing and demyelination seen in the fatal neurological illnesses which have followed pertussis vaccination (van der Horst, 1950) are essentially different in nature from the familiar histopathological findings in poliomyelitis or any other virus disease of the nervous system. We have records of several additional cases of poliomyelitis following inoculation. Such cases are recognizably poliomyelitic, and form a clinical group quite distinct from any of the neurological complications discussed in the present paper. If for the moment the sequelae of vaccination against pertussis are excluded, the family resemblance among the other cases described is immediately striking. Radicular, polyneuritic, myelitic, and meningoencephalitic syndromes may all occur after serum administration and T.A.B. and rabies vaccination, and probably, though much more rarely, after inoculation against diphtheria. The interval between the injection and the onset of neurological symptoms tends to be of different average length for each type of inoculation (seven to 10 days in the case of serum injection; two to four days in T.A.B. inoculation; 10 to 15 days in rabies vaccination), and there is evidence that the more severe cerebral illnesses may follow a shorter latent period in each instance.

Only in the groups of complications following serum administration and T.A.B. inoculation is the number of recorded cases adequate to permit comparison of the incidence of the various clinical syndromes. The difference here is immediately striking (Table III). It will be seen that radiculitis is three times as common after serum administration as after T.A.B. vaccination, while a converse

TABLE III

Percentage Distribution of Neurological Syndromes Complicating Serum administration and T.A.B. Vaccination, based on 100 and 50 Recorded Cases Respectively

	Serum administration	*T.A.B. vaccination*
Radiculitis	74	24
Polyneuritis	10	16
Landry's paralysis and myelitis	6	20
Meningo-cerebral syndromes	10	40

relationship holds for myelitic and cerebral syndromes. The most commonly reported cases are those which follow serum administration, and these cases are of special importance also because serum sickness has been extensively studied from the pathological point of view, and because it can be reproduced experimentally (Rich, 1947). On the basis of clinical, pathological, and experimental evidence it is now firmly established that the histopathological basis of serum sickness is an allergic reaction of anaphylactic type, affecting chiefly the vascular tree, and characterized by a disseminated focal infiltrative vasculitis, with focal oedematous-inflammatory reactions in the tissues which are probably secondary to the vascular lesions. The histological findings described above, in the small number of patients who died after neurological complications of serum administration, are entirely in keeping with the occasional occurrence of similar changes in the nervous system. The pathological similarity of these changes to those seen in acute disseminated, for example para-exanthematous, encephalomyelitis is only slightly less striking than the close clinical similarity between the two groups of cases. There is no evidence from any source that the specificity of the antibody involved influences the nature of the pathological reaction to injected serum. The globulin fraction is usually held responsible for the manifestations of serum sickness, but similar reactions may follow massive dosage with serum-albumin (Heyl and Janeway, 1947), and there is evidence that the localization of somatic pathological changes in the recipient may depend on the fraction involved (Hawn and Janeway, 1947).

The extraordinary frequency with which the brachial plexus is involved in serum neuritis, and the special susceptibility to paresis of the muscles innervated by the fifth and sixth cervical roots, has been explained in various ways. Bourguignon (1931) suggested that muscles innervated by nerves with different chronaxies were affected by different antitoxins. He claimed that tetanus antitoxin affects those with low chronaxy (C5 and C6), and diphtheria antitoxin those with medium chronaxy (C8, T1). Analysis of recorded cases shows this hypothesis to be untenable, quite apart from the objection that in the case of serum injection the site of the lesion shows no correlation with the type of antibody involved. An anatomical explanation appears more probable, and is found in the concept of axonal swelling with strangulation of the nerves at their points of exit from the dura, a post-mortem finding in ten cases of the Guillain–Barré syndrome by Scheinker (1947). Sicard and Cantaloube (1923) suggested that similar compression of the nerve in the aponeurotic sheath (neurodocitique) may be an important mechanism in the pathogenesis of mononeuritis. The large size of the fifth and sixth cervical roots relative to their intervertebral foramina may render them more liable to interruption of function by compression; it is possible that the basis of the lesion may, in fact, commonly be a polyradiculitis (as in Case 3 above), the symptoms of which are limited to those arising from a few roots because of some such anatomical factor. The comparison of brachial-plexus lesions which follow serum administration with the 'shoulder-girdle syndrome' described by Spillane (1943), Turner (1944), and Parsonage and Turner (1948), is irresistible, and, as the last two authors state, 'there is complete clinical similarity between the serum cases and the type of case described in this paper (neuralgic amyotrophy), and it is reasonable to assume that they are of similar aetiology'. The fact that T.A.B. vaccination is more rarely complicated by easily recognizable somatic manifestations of hypersensitivity, compared with the injection of foreign serum, may be in part responsible for the small number of cases on record. This circumstance certainly renders diagnosis more difficult. Nevertheless symptomatology, natural history, and histopathological findings all support a very close relationship between these two groups of cases—a relationship qualified by the different proportional incidence of clinical syndromes and of pathological changes within the nervous system.

The 'neuroparalytic accidents' of rabies inoculation are clinically identical with those seen after serum injection and T.A.B. vaccination. The pathological appearances are in general similar, though the actual degeneration of ganglion-cells seen after vaccination against rabies has not been reported after serum or T.A.B. The special point of interest in the rabies cases lies not so much in their symptomatology or histopathology as in the means whereby they are produced. The repeated injection of brain emulsion, used in the prophylaxis of rabies, reproduces to a remarkable degree the conditions of experimental production of 'allergic' encephalomyelitis in the rhesus monkey by injections of heterologous brain-tissue emulsified with Freund adjuvants (Kabat, Wolf, and Bezer, 1947; Morgan, 1947). It has been generally accepted that the experimental encephalomyelitis thus produced is closely analogous with the acute disseminated encephalomyelitis with which we are familiar after Jennerian vaccination and the exanthemata in man. The case of pertussis is in many ways different, though it seems likely that the basic mechanism is the same. As already described, these neurological complications of pertussis vaccination appear to be invariably central, and characterized chiefly by convulsions and hemiplegia. Their incubation period is shorter than that of neurological accidents associated with other inoculations, although it appears that, when similar cerebral syndromes follow other inoculations, they also tend to occur early.

These symptomatological considerations illustrate in a graphic way another relationship which has impressed us in considering these cases. The neurological sequelae of a particular prophylactic inoculation appear to be similar in distribution to the neurological complications of the infective disease concerned. Thus, as Wilson (1940) wrote, 'peripheral neuritis complicating typhoid fever must be regarded as a rarity'. Only 12 examples were found among 3,102 cases of typhoid studied by Rolleston (1929), and two among 385 similar patients in Hloucal's (1949) series. On the other hand hemiplegia, aphasia, and other focal cerebral signs occur with some frequency (Osler, 1900; Williams, 1912; Sen, 1946), and myelitis is uncommon (Renault and Lévy, 1913), but not rare (Sen, 1946; Hloucal 1949). Again, in whooping-cough the most usual neurological complication is convulsion, often accompanied by coma and followed by hemiplegia (over 60 per cent. of cases), dysphasia, choreo-athetosis, and mental defect (Wilson, 1940). A Landry type of paralysis may complicate pertussis (Zamboni, 1915), but is extremely rare. The most frequent neurological complication of diphtheria is a mono- or polyneuritis, often accompanied by paralysis of the soft palate and of accommodation, and less often of the bulbar musculature. Palatal weakness was a feature of Liessens's (1949) case of encephalomyelitis following inoculation with A.P.T., and of Case 12 in the present series, in which encephalomyelitis followed Schick testing.

Consideration of the clinical and pathological findings described above leads us to the conclusion that most neurological illnesses which follow prophylactic inoculation are manifestations of hypersensitivity. In the case of the neurological complications of serum sickness this conclusion seems inescapable. After other inoculations somatic signs of hypersensitivity are somewhat less frequent, yet it appears that only some similar mechanism can adequately account for the observed facts. In favour of this view are the stereotyped 'latent period' associated with the various inoculations, which calls to mind the similar phenomena of acute glomerulonephritis and acute rheumatism; the not infrequent coincidence of frank manifestations of allergy; and the provocation of further neurological symptoms by repeated inoculations (Bannwarth, 1948), which may occasionally be averted by a change in the antigen (Vogel, 1939). Further support is lent by the occurrence of neurological accidents of inoculation in patients who had previously been the subjects of encephalomyelitic illness (Brody and Sorley, 1947; Liessens, 1949; Case 2 above), and by the striking clinical and pathological similarity of the cases described above to the more commonly occurring examples of acute disseminated encephalomyelitis which follow specific or non-specific infections. It is of interest that no case of neurological illness after inoculation is on record in which spontaneous recurrence of symptoms has occurred in the absence of a repetition of the causal inoculation or (very occasionally) a further injection of some other kind. In this feature these illnesses are reminiscent of encephalomyelitis following exanthemata or Jennerian vaccination; encephalomyelitic illnesses which follow banal infections, or appear to arise spontaneously, not infrequently recur, possibly because such infections produce little immunity, and therefore little protection from further exposure to antigen. The view that these various inoculations may activate some latent virus already present in the tissues of the recipient, and give rise to the various syndromes described in a manner analogous to the well-recognized precipitating role of pertussis and diphtheria inoculations in cases of paralytic poliomyelitis, appears to us highly improbable. Such a view could be sustained only by ignoring the clinical differences which we have shown to exist between the sequelae of these various inoculations, or by the postulation of an appreciable number of such latent infective agents. More important still, it encounters the fatal objection that the recorded histopathological findings in cases of the type we describe are quite dissimilar to those seen in virus infections of the nervous system.

If the syndromes under discussion have an allergic basis, the importance of these observations is twofold. Should our view be correct, the prophylaxis and treatment of the conditions under discussion resolves itself into the employment of drugs known to influence hypersensitive reactions. In the case of encephalomyelitis following antirabic vaccination, success has already been claimed in isolated cases for treatment with antihistamine drugs (Pickar and Kramer, 1949) and cortisone (Garrison, 1952). Secondly, and more important, the occurrence in identical clinical circumstances of radicular, polyneuritic, Landry, Guillain–Barré, encephalitic, and myelitic syndromes, separately or in combination, strongly suggests a common denominator in the pathogenesis of these various conditions, whether they occur after prophylactic inoculation or arise, as they more commonly do, in association with preceding infection. There is increasing evidence that this common denominator is anaphylactic hypersensitivity, and the clinical observations put forward in the present paper further suggest that the nature of the antigen involved may be one factor in determining the localization of lesions within the nervous system.

We wish to thank Sir Russell Brain for his kind interest and helpful criticism, as well as for furnishing the records of Case 12; and also the many other colleagues who have helped us in the collection of these cases, especially Dr. R. H. Dobbs (Cases 8 and 9), Professor D. M. Dunlop and Dr. J. K. Slater (Case 4), Dr. G. S. Graveson (Cases 1 and 3), and Dr. Lovell Hoffman (Case 2.).

Summary

This paper reviews the literature concerning neurological complications of serum injection and prophylactic inoculation, and reports 12 further cases following antitetanic and antidiphtheritic sera, typhoid-paratyphoid vaccine, combined diphtheria-pertussis vaccine, alum-precipitated diphtheria toxoid, antirabic vaccination, and Schick testing. Clinically and pathologically these illnesses may involve every level of the nervous system, and they appear to be closely analogous with the acute disseminated encephalomyelitis which follows exanthemata and Jennerian vaccination. The distribution of lesions varies with each inoculation, and shows some correspondence with that seen in the neurological complications of the relevant infection.

It is suggested that the common factor in the pathogenesis of these cases, comprising encephalitic, myelitic, Landry, Guillain–Barré, radicular, polyneuritic, and mononeuritic syndromes, is anaphylactic hypersensitivity, and that a similar mechanism may be involved in many of the identical neurological illnesses which occur independently of preceding inoculation.

REFERENCES

Alajouanine, T., Fribourg-Blanc, A., and Gauthier, (1928) *Bull. mém. Soc. med. hôp. Paris,* **52,** 446.
Anderson, I. M., and Morris, D. (1950) *Lancet,* **1,** 537.
Ansell, I. (1948) *Brit. Med. J.* **2,** 338.
Appelbaum, E., Greenberg, M., and Nelson, J. (1953) *J. Amer. Med. Ass.* **151,** 188.
Avezzù, G. (1928) *Ann. d'igiene* (sper.) **38,** 550.
Babès, V., and Mironesco, T. (1908) *Compt. rend. Soc. biol.* **44,** 965.
Babonneix, L. (1924) Cited by I. M. Allen (1931) *Lancet,* **2,** 1128.
—— and Sigwald, J. (1929) *Ann. méd.* **26,** 114.
Baker, A. B. (1942) *J. Neuropath. Exp. Neurol.* **1,** 394.
Bannwarth, A. (1948) *Arch. Psychiat. Nervenk.* **180,** 531.
Bassoe, P., and Grinker R. R. (1930) *Arch. Neurol. Psychiat.* **23,** 1138.
Bennett, A. E. (1939) *J. Amer. Med. Ass.* **112,** 590.
Benon, R. (1924) *Paris méd.* **51,** 94.
Bourguignon, G. (1931) *Rev. neurol.* **1,** 310.
Bourrat, L. (1929) *Lyon méd.* **143,** 787.
Brain, W. R. (1951) *Diseases of the Nervous System,* London.
British Medical Journal (1949) **2,** 1478. (Medico-Legal Note).
Brody, M., and Sorley, R. G. (1947) *New York St. J. Med.* **47,** 1016.
Brown, A. L. (1925) *Amer. J. Ophthal.* **8,** 614.
Bury, J. S. (1920) *Lancet,* **2,** 844.

Bussell, L. J. (1946) Ibid. **2**, 826.
Busson, B. (1926) *Ztrbl. Bakt.* 1. Abt. **99**, 80.
Byers, R. K., and Moll, F. C. (1948) *Pediatrics,* **1**, 437.
Cowie, D. M. (1921) *New York St. J. Med.* **21**, 395.
Csermely, H. (1950) *Arch. Neurol. Psychiat.* **64**, 676.
Cutter, R. D. (1936) *J. Amer. Med. Ass.* **106**, 1006.
D'Ingianni, V., and Fontenelle, I. L. (1949) *New Orl. Med. Surg. J.* **102**, 45.
Doull, J. A., Shibley, G. S., and McClelland, J. E. (1936) *Amer. J. Pub. Health,* **26**, 1097.
Doyle, J. B. (1933) *Amer. J. Med. Sci.* **185**, 484.
Dyke, S. C. (1918) *Lancet,* **1**, 570.
Engelmann, M. (1897) *Münch. med. Woch.* **44**, 880.
Escardó, F. F., and Vazquez, H. J. (1950) *Arch. pediat. Urug.* **21**, 701.
Etienne, G. (1928) *Rev. méd. de l'est,* **56**, 503.
Fanconi, G., Zellweger, H., and Botsztejn, A. (1944) *Die Poliomyelitis und ihre Grenzgebiete,* Basel.
Fielder, F. S. (1916) *J. Amer. Med. Ass.* **66**, 1769.
Filotico, R. (1929) *Morgagni,* **71**, 718.
Fisch, C.. and Wood D. E. (1950) *J. Indiana Med. Ass.* **43**, 1197.
French S. G. (1938) *J. R. Nav. Med. Serv.* **24**, 349.
Gangolphe and Gardère (1908) *Lyon méd.* **110**, 497.
Garrison, S. C. (1952) *Amer. J. Med.* **12**, 135.
Gayle, R. F., Jnr., and Bowen, R. A. (1933) *J. Nerv. Ment. Dis.* **78**, 221.
Giffin, M. E., Rogers, H. M., and Kernohan, J. W. (1948) *Arch. Neurol. Psychiat.* **59**, 233.
Globus, J. H., and Kohn, J. L. (1949) *J. Amer. Med. Ass.* **141**, 507.
Gordon, A. (1928) *Med. J. and Rec.* **127**, 530.
—— (1932) *J. Amer. Med. Ass.* **98**, 1625.
Gornicki, B. (1948) *Pediat. polska,* **22**, 104.
Grace, H. B. (1950) *Canad. Med. Ass. J.* **63**, 129.
Greenwood, M. (1945–6) *League of Nations Bull. Health Org.* **12**, 301.
Gros, M. C. (1897) *Bull. Acad. méd.* **37**, 797.
Grünberger, V. (1904) *Wien. klin. Woch.* **17**, 736.
Gubb, A. S. (1915) *Med. Pr. and Circ.* **100**, 371.
Guillain, G., and Barré, J. A. (1919) *Rev. neurol.* **35**, 595.
Hahn, E. (1934) *Klin. Woch.* **13**, 1309.
Hawn, C. V., and Janeway, C. A. (1947) *J. Exp. Med.* **85**, 571.
Heyl, J. T., and Janeway, C. A. (1947) *J. Clin. Invest.* **26**, 1185.
Hill, A. B., and Knowelden, J. (1950) *Brit. Med. J.* **2**, 1.
Hloucal, L. (1949) *Neurol. psychiat. čes.* **12**, 32.
Horst, L., van der (1950) *Folia psychiat. neurol. neurochir. neerl.* **53**, 710.
Hughes, R. R. (1944) *Lancet,* **2**, 464.
Hurst, E. W., and Pawan, J. L. (1931) Ibid. **2**, 622.
Imrie, A. (1944) *J. R. Army Med. Corps,* **83**, 196.
Jumentié, J. (1916) *Rev. neurol.* **30**, 582.
Kabat, E. A., Wolf, A., and Bezer, A. E. (1947) *J. Exp. Med.* **85**, 117.
Katz, G. (1927) *Dtsch. med. Woch.* **53**, 1637.
Kendrick, P., and Eldering, G. (1939) *Amer. J. Hyg.* **29**, Sect. B, 133.
Kennedy, F. (1929) *Amer. J. Med. Sci.* **177**, 555.
Keyserlingk, H. von (1947) *Med. Klin.* **42**, 189.
Koenigsfeld, E. G. H. (1945) *J. R. Army Med. Corps,* **85**, 254.
Koritschoner, R., and Schweinburg, F. (1925) *Zts. Immun.-forsch.* **42**, 217.
Krais, W. (1943) *Dtsch. Zts. Nervenheilk.* **155**, 91.
Kraus, W. M., and Chaney, L. B. (1937) *Arch. Neurol. Psychiat.* **37**, 1035.
Kroll, F. W. (1938) *Nervenarzt,* **11**, 252.
Latimer, F. R., Webster, J. E., and Gurdjian, E. S. (1951) *Arch. Neurol. Psychiat.* **65**, 16.
Lemke, R. (1943) *Münch. med. Woch.* **1**, 49.
Léri, A., and Boivin (1919) *Rev. neurol.* **35**, 965.

Lhermitte, J. (1919) *Gaz. hôp. Paris,* **92,** 1053.
—— (1938) *Rev. neurol.* **69,** 375.
—— and Fribourg-Blanc, A. (1936) Ibid. **65,** 391.
—— and Haguenau, J. (1931) Ibid. **55,** 347.
Liessens, P. (1949) *Acta neurol. psychiat. belg.* **49,** 741.
McCloskey, B. P. (1950) *Lancet,* **1,** 659.
McFadzean, A. J. S. (1952) *Arch. Neurol. Psychiat.* **67,** 451.
McIntyre, H. D., and Krouse, H. (1949) Ibid. **62,** 802.
Madsen, T. (1933) *J. Amer. Med. Ass.* **101,** 187.
Marinescu, G., and Draganesco, S. (1938) *Ann. Inst. Pasteur,* **60,** 477.
Mason, V. R. (1922) *J. Amer. Med. Ass.* **78,** 88.
Mérei, F. T. (1950) *Arch. Neurol. Psychiat.* **63,** 249.
Morgan, I. M. (1947) *J. Exp. Med.* **85,** 131.
Mumme, C. (1950) *Dtsch. Zts. Nervenheilk.* **164,** 236.
Noïca, D. (1932) *Bull. mém. Soc. méd. hôp. Paris,* **48,** 1026.
Olmer, J., and Paillas, J. E. (1935) *Paris méd.* **2,** 236.
Osler, W. (1900) *Johns Hopkins Hosp. Rep.* **15,** 397.
Paillas, J. E. (1936) *Marseille méd.* **73,** 7, 49, 97.
Parsonage, M. J., and Turner, J. W. A. (1948) *Lancet,* **1,** 973.
Peacher, W. G., and Robertson, R. C. L. (1945) *J. Nerv. Ment. Dis.* **101,** 515.
Pickar, D. N., and Kramer, H. M. (1949) *South. Med. J.* **42,** 127.
Preti, L. (1919) *Atti Soc. lombarda sci. med. biol.* **8,** 85.
Radermecker (1949) Cited by Liessens (1949).
Redewill, F. H., Jnr., and Underwood, L. J. (1947) *Calif. Med.* **66,** 360.
Reitman, N., and Rothschild, K. (1950) *Ann. Int. Med.* **32,** 923.
Remlinger, P. (1928) *Ann. Inst. Pasteur,* Suppl. p. 71.
Renault, J., and Lévy, P. P. (1913) *Bull. mém. Soc. méd. hôp. Paris,* **36,** 80.
Rich, A. R. (1947) Harvey Lecture, 1946–7, Lancaster, Pa.
Richardson, J. S. (1942) *Lancet,* **1,** 618.
Robinson, L. J. (1937) *New Engl. J. Med.* **216,** 831.
Roger, H., Poursines, Y., and Recordier M. (1934) *Rev. neurol.* **61,** 1078.
Rolleston, J. D. (1929) *Post-Grad. Med. J.* **4,** 153.
Roussy, G. (1919) *Rev. neurol.* **35,** 505.
—— and Cornil, L. (1919) Ibid. **35,** 453.
Rubin, W., and Bowman, N. (1950) *J. Med. Soc. N.J.* **47,** 68.
Russell, J. L. (1924) *Kentucky Med. J.* **22,** 378.
Sako, W., Treuting, W. L., Witt, D. B., and Nichamin, S. J. (1945) *J. Amer. Med. Ass.* **127,** 379.
Scheinker, I. M. (1947) *Trans. Amer. Neurol. Ass.* **72,** 141.
Schneider, G. (1946) Thesis, Bâle.
Sen, S. (1946) *J. Indian Med. Ass.* **15,** 364.
Sézary, A., and Dessaint (1923) *Bull. mém. Soc. méd. hôp. Paris,* **47,** 1375.
Sicard, J. A., and Cantaloube, P. (1923) Ibid. **47,** 1046.
Smith, D. E. (1951) *Amer. J. Med.* (Clinico-Pathological Conference) **11,** 228.
Sommer, R. (1936) *Arch. orthop. Unfall-Chir.* **36,** 443.
Souques, A. (1919) *Rev. neurol.* **35,** 501.
Sovena A. (1947) *Policlinico,* sez. prat. **54,** 218.
Spaar, R. (1943) *Arch. Psychiat. Nervenk.* **116,** 1.
Spillane J. D. (1943) *Lancet,* **2,** 532.
Starý, O. (1948) *Čas. lék. čes.* **87,** 865.
Stuart, G., and Krikorian, K. S. (1930) *Lancet,* **1,** 1123.
—— —— (1933) *Brit. Med. J.* **1,** 501.
Tarnay, B. (1948) *Orv. lapja,* **4,** 1534.
Taylor, H. W. (1938) *Arch. Pediat.* **55,** 572.
Thaon, P. (1910) *Sem. médicale,* **30,** 513.
Thévenard, A., Lenormand, J., Nigoux, R., and Marquès, J. M. (1950) *Rev. neurol.* **81,** 296.

Toomey, J. A. (1949) *J. Amer. Med. Ass.* **139**, 448.
Turner, J. W. A. (1944) *Brit. Med. J.* **2**, 592.
Vahrman, J. (1950) Ibid. **2**, 608.
Vogel, P. (1935) *Nervenarzt*, **8**, 11.
—— (1939) *Dtsch. med. Woch.* **65**, 171.
Werne, J., and Garrow, I. (1946) *J. Amer. Med. Ass.* **131**, 730.
Wilkinson, S. J. (1937) *J. Pediat.* **10**, 180.
Williams, A. W. (1912) *Amer. J. Med. Sci.* **143**, 352.
Wilson, G., and Hadden, S. B. (1932) *J. Amer. Med Ass.* **98**, 123.
Wilson, S. A. K. (1940) *Neurology*, London.
Winkelman, N. W., and Gotten, N. (1935) *Amer. J. Syph.* 19, 414.
Woolling, K. R., and Rushton, J. G. (1950) *Arch. Neurol. Psychiat.* **64**, 568.
Wrightsman, E. C. (1949) *Illinois Med. J.* **95**, 105.
Young, F. (1932) *J. Amer. Med. Ass.* **98**, 1139.
Zamboni, G. (1915) *Riv. Clin. pediat.* **13**, 773.
Zeckel, A. (1939) *Rev. neurol.* **71**, 459.

SARCOIDOSIS: WITH SPECIAL REFERENCE TO DIAGNOSIS AND PROGNOSIS[1]

By R. H. COWDELL

(From the Department of Pathology, the Radcliffe Infirmary, Oxford)

With Plates 1 to 3

SINCE Jonathan Hutchinson in 1875–7 published in his *Illustrations of Clinical Surgery* an account of what has come to be recognized as the first recorded case of lupus pernio, three-quarters of a century have passed. During that time several thousands of articles have been written on various aspects of that enigmatic condition, sarcoidosis, and yet some of the most important facts related to it remain shrouded in mystery. An admirable account of the early history of sarcoidosis is that of Hunter (1936), and the later developments are recorded in the major monographs of Pautrier (1940), Leitner (1949), and Longcope and Freiman (1952). The classical paper on *Multiple Benign Sarkoid of the Skin* by Caesar Boeck (1899) gave rise to the name sarcoidosis, but Boeck, despite the eponymous use of his name, cannot claim priority either of clinical or of histological description, for before he likened the morphological appearance to that of a sarcoma, Tenneson (1892) had examined a biopsy specimen from a patient with lupus pernio, and considered the appearances to be those of tuberculosis. During the first two decades of the present century it was gradually realized that the cutaneous lesions, described under a variety of names by Hutchinson (1875–7, 1898, 1900), Besnier (1889), Tenneson (1892), Boeck (1899), and others, were not the most important manifestations of the disease. For this discovery Schaumann (1914, 1916–17) and Kuznitsky and Bittorf (1915) share much of the credit, but many others contributed to it, and it came to be known that almost any part of the body might be involved.

The capacity of sarcoidosis to manifest itself in many different ways, and also to involve many organs without necessarily producing corresponding symptoms or signs, is well recognized. On the other hand, the first sentence of a definition of the malady issued by a committee of the U.S. National Research Council in 1949 (Ricker and Clark, 1949) remains true today: 'Sarcoidosis is a disease of unknown aetiology.' There are two other fields in which our knowledge is restricted, prognosis and treatment. The course of individual cases has often been described, occasionally over a considerable period of years. The description by Danbolt (1947) of the post-mortem findings in Boeck's first case, 41 years after diagnosis, holds the record in this respect, but there have been few concerted attempts to follow up a large number of patients, and some lack

[1] Received May 2, 1953.

precision owing to uncertainty of the diagnostic criteria used. Similarly, any attempt to obtain a comprehensive picture of the outcome of the disease by a review of the literature is liable to error, owing to variation in the standard of diagnosis and in the width of meaning allowed to the words 'sarcoid' and 'sarcoidosis'. The wide choice of forms of therapy which have been advocated shows that none which has yet had adequate trial has been found ideal, and here also the inconsistencies of results reported by different authors may sometimes be due to different diagnostic standards, although other factors, such as the stage of the disease at the time of treatment, are also important. The purpose of the present paper is to suggest appropriate diagnostic criteria, and subsequently to describe the progress of the disease as seen in a series of 90 patients who conform to these criteria. The subject of aetiology is only approached as far as necessary in discussion of diagnosis, and only a brief commentary on treatment is included. No attempt is made to repeat the wide reviews of the literature already published, such as those of Leitner (1949) and Longcope and Freiman (1952).

Patients Investigated, Age, and Incidence

Of the 90 patients considered, 34 were seen at the Radcliffe Infirmary, Oxford, during the years 1938–50, while the records of 56 were derived from the Oxford Lymph-Node Registry over the same period. The patients in the former group nearly all lived in Oxfordshire or the neighbouring counties. Those of the latter group were widely distributed over the British Isles, but clinical data and histological material were available from all. The age-distribution at the onset of symptoms is shown in Table I. The youngest

TABLE I

Age-distribution in 90 Patients

Age (years)	*Cases*	*Age (years)*	*Cases*
0– 9	3	40–49	16
10–19	12	50–59	10
20–29	23	60–69	4
30–39	22		

patient was first seen at the age of six years, the oldest at 69 years. While sarcoidosis may become apparent at the extremes of life, and patients from three months (Naumann, 1938) to 80 years of age (Leitner, 1949) have been reported, the greatest incidence in this, as in other unselected groups, falls in the third and fourth decades. Forty-four of the patients were male, and 46 female. A slight preponderance of female patients has often been noted, but in the present series there is no significant difference in sex incidence. All the patients were white, and with the exception of one German girl working in England all were of British nationality. The disease occurs in all parts of the world, and estimates of the incidence vary. Robb-Smith (1947) reported a rate of 0·66 per 100,000 among the general population of Oxfordshire. Michael, Cole, Beeson, and Olsen (1950) found 0·88 per 100,000 white people and 17·81 per 100,000 Negroes in the United States Army. In the Swiss Army the presumptive rate in recruits, based on mass radiography, was 13 per 100,000 (Schönholzer, 1947). The higher incidence in military units can be accounted for partly by the high proportion of young men, and partly by routine medical examination, which may discover cases in which medical advice might never be sought in civilian life. The frequency in American Negroes, associated with very scanty reports of the disease in other coloured peoples, remains unexplained, as does the greater incidence in both white and Negro population of rural districts of the United States (Michael, Cole, Beeson, and Olsen, 1950). No relation to occupation has been discovered, although in the present series three patients with pulmonary involvement were workers in dusty occupations, who first presented respiratory symptoms which they attributed to their employment.

Presenting Symptoms and Signs

The presenting symptoms in sarcoidosis are numerous, the most frequent being related to involvement of the lungs, mediastinal lymph-nodes, superficial lymph-nodes, or skin. Severe constitutional symptoms are unusual, but many patients complain of lack of energy or undue fatigue. Fever of more than slight degree was present in only three patients of the present series, two of whom had secondary pulmonary infection, and the third pyelitis. The more important presenting symptoms or signs are shown in Table II. This Table includes only

TABLE II

Presenting Symptoms and Signs in 90 Patients

Referable to chest		44
Chest pain	5	
Cough	18	
Dyspnoea	25	
Lymph-node enlargement		33
Malaise or excessive fatigue		31
Skin manifestations		24
Loss of weight		15
Nasal obstruction		6
Tonsillitis		4
Dysphagia		3
Salivary-gland swelling		6
Abdominal pain or swelling		6
Visual disturbance		8

the factors observed by the patient and causing him to seek medical advice. Some of them, such as lymph-node enlargement, were found much more frequently on examination than is here indicated. Other less frequent presenting features included swelling of a finger (two cases), of a large joint (two), and of the lachrymal glands (one). In four cases erythema nodosum was present. One patient was first seen on account of nodules on tendon sheaths, one with amenorrhoea, one with jaundice, and one with the symptoms of diabetes insipidus. One patient was first seen moribund, with a clinical picture similar to that of Cushing's syndrome, and congestive cardiac failure. Another young woman died suddenly from heart failure, and was found to have cardiac sarcoidosis at autopsy. The disease was discovered during post-mortem examination of an apparently healthy man, who died of pulmonary embolism after synovectomy for post-traumatic synovitis. In some cases sarcoidosis was discovered during investigation of other conditions, including thyrotoxicosis, diabetes mellitus, and iron-deficiency anaemia. In one boy it was recognized when enlarged mediastinal lymph-nodes were seen in a routine radiograph after his sister had developed pulmonary tuberculosis. Another case was revealed in a mass miniature radiography survey.

Organs Involved

Once the concept of sarcoidosis as a generalized disease was firmly established, authors vied with each other to report its presence in diverse situations, so that now it is doubtful whether there is any part of the body which may not occasionally be involved. Table III shows the organs which appeared clinically

TABLE III

Involvement of Organs in 90 Patients

	Clinical	*Radiological*	*Histological*	*Total*
Superficial lymph-nodes	74	..	68	74
Mediastinal lymph-nodes	..	54	5	57
Other deep lymph-nodes	..	..	6	6
Lung	..	37	5	40
Skin	34	..	17	34
Spleen	20	..	9	22
Liver	11	..	5	14
Salivary glands	14	..	1	14
Eye	11	..	..	11
Nasal and pharyngeal mucosa	8	..	4	9
Bone	2	5	..	5
Tonsil	5	..	1	5
Pituitary gland	3	..	1	3
Thyroid	..	..	3	3
Nervous system	2	..	..	2
Tongue	1	..	1	2
Lachrymal gland	1	..	..	1
Epididymis	1	..	..	1
Tendon-sheath	1	..	1	1
Small intestine	1	..	..	1
Kidney	..	..	1	1
Heart	..	..	1	1
Fallopian tubes	..	..	1	1

or radiologically to be affected in the present series, and also those in which histological confirmation was available, or in which the disease was discovered at autopsy although not necessarily clinically suspected. The clinical signs of pulmonary involvement are not sufficiently specific for any figure to be given under this heading. The clinical and radiological appearance of the disease as seen in the more commonly affected organs is well known, and for those more rarely involved reference may be made to the works of Pinner (1938), Pautrier

(1940), Rubin and Pinner (1944), Leitner (1949), and Longcope and Freiman (1952). Colover (1948) has reviewed an interesting collection of cases of involvement of the nervous system.

Diagnosis

To achieve accuracy of diagnosis, a definition of the disease is an essential requirement, and to provide one which will admit every case, and yet not include any example of other conditions, is difficult. The necessity is emphasized by Pautrier (1947), who referred to the danger of sarcoidosis becoming a formless monster without limits. Scadding (1950) correctly criticized those who avoid a formal definition by starting their papers with a historical survey, and answer the question 'What disease are you talking about?' by saying 'The disease that has been described in these classical papers'. As he pointed out, this 'leaves open the question which part of the classical descriptions should be regarded as essential and which incidental, and has made way for much unfortunate wrangling about priority of description and for a confusing variety of eponyms'. The definition proposed by a committee of the U.S. National Research Council (Ricker and Clark, 1949), as Scadding has said, includes many permissive phrases; its only positive statements relate to aetiology and histological characters: 'Sarcoidosis is a disease of unknown aetiology. Pathologically it is characterized by the presence in any organ or tissue of epithelioid-cell tubercles, with inconspicuous or no necrosis, and by the frequent presence of refractile or apparently calcified bodies in the giant cells of the tubercles. The characteristic lesion may be replaced by fibrosis, hyalinization, or both. Clinically, the lesions may be widely disseminated. The tissues most frequently involved are lymph-nodes, lungs, skin, eyes, and bones, particularly of the extremities. The clinical course usually is chronic with minimal or no constitutional symptoms; however, there may be acute phases characterized by a general reaction with malaise and fever. There may be signs and symptoms referable to the tissues or organs involved. The intracutaneous tuberculin test is frequently negative; the plasma-globulins are often increased. The outcome may be clinical recovery with radiographic evidence of residue, or impairment of function of organs involved, or a continued chronic course of the disease.' The weight to be given to the individual sections of this definition merits consideration. Sarcoidosis is a popular disease, and many cases have been reported under its name but with atypical clinical or histological findings. On the other hand, if arbitrary conditions are imposed, it is likely that some genuine cases will be excluded. Most authors have found that the tuberculin test is negative in the majority of their patients, but to make this an absolute requirement, as some have done, excludes cases which are clinically and pathologically typical in every other respect, and it has to be considered whether there is justification for doing so. Equally there is a possibility that routine omission of any case in which necrosis is present in the epithelioid granulomata, in which acid-fast bacilli are found, or which has some of the characteristics of both sarcoidosis and tuberculosis, may perpetuate a lack of knowledge of the aetiology. Even more harm may result from assuming that sarcoidosis is a type of non-caseating tuberculosis when this assumption is unproved, as was done by Pinner (1938). Many other authors have included cases which appear to be sarcoidosis under such terms as chronic miliary tuberculosis (Hoyle and Vaisey, 1937) or tuberculous splenomegaly (Engelbreth-Holm, 1938).

Robb-Smith (1952) considered that 'it is only by studying "proved cases" that increased knowledge of the nature of the disorder can be gained, and consequent upon this a more confident approach to prognosis and treatment'. His requirements were typical clinical and histological features, a Mantoux reaction negative to a dilution of 1:100 old tuberculin, and that a guinea-pig inoculated with material from a biopsy should not have developed tuberculosis in six to eight weeks. These requirements are satisfactory for the purposes specified, but because a patient presents with, for example, some previously unreported clinical feature, it does not follow that he has a different disease. While the introduction of requirements subsequently found to be inessential will not necessarily vitiate observations on the nature of the disease, it may cause errors of diagnosis as far as the individual patient is concerned.

In a few sites the clinical features of the disease are very characteristic, in some they are suggestive but inconclusive, while in others they offer no assistance. A well-developed example of lupus pernio is not easily mistaken, and the other types of cutaneous lesion are usually, but less certainly, distinguishable. The mucosal lesions are said to have recognizable differences from lupus vulgaris, the condition with which they are most liable to be confused (Lomholt, 1934). The superficial lymph-nodes have constant features in that they are discrete, mobile, firm, and not more than slightly tender, but the same condition is found in some of the reticuloses. Clinical signs in the chest are variable, and while certain radiographic appearances here and in the bones are very suggestive, they are not sufficiently specific for positive diagnosis. Combinations of such clinical findings, for example skin lesions accompanied by lymph-node enlargement and radiographic changes in the chest or bones, are of greater value than one alone, and, when the disease is very widespread and well developed, clinical diagnosis may not appear to need ancillary support. It is in just such cases that support is most easily obtainable; lymph-nodes and skin are easily accessible for biopsy, and the inconclusive type of corroborative evidence, such as hyperglobulinaemia, may be present. The patient in whom the disease is only manifested by a single group of enlarged lymph-nodes, especially if they are inaccessible, as in the mediastinum, presents a more difficult problem. While other lesions may appear over a period of years, it is not always convenient to wait for Nature to take her course. It is very doubtful whether absolute reliance should ever be placed on clinical diagnosis, but the clinical picture should certainly be taken into account. Even when the most strict criteria are adopted, the histological appearances of sarcoidosis are occasionally simulated by certain conditions of known aetiology. The great majority of cases in which histology alone might give rise to error are capable of elucidation on clinical grounds.

Histology

The essential histological appearance of sarcoidosis is identical in all parts of the body, and has been well described on many occasions, for example by Pautrier (1940). It may be briefly recapitulated as seen in the lymph-node, the tissue most frequently examined by biopsy. Sharply circumscribed aggregates of epithelioid cells are present, and where involvement is not too far advanced they can be seen to lie in relation to the sinuses. The aggregates may, but do not always, include giant cells. However numerous the epithelioid congeries may be—and they may occupy the node so profusely as almost to exclude lymphoid tissue—they remain discrete, and do not coalesce. They are usually surrounded by a narrow zone of lymphocytes, less extensive and less constant than that seen in tuberculosis. The appearances are illustrated in Plates 1 and 2, Figs. 1 to 3. In the earlier stages there is concentric arrangement of reticulin fibres round the periphery, but no collagen and little or no reticulin extend inwards. Later there is gradual replacement of the cellular elements by fibrous tissue, so that finally there remains a rounded nodule of hyalinized collagen. Some authors (Reisner, 1944) consider that lesions may sometimes resolve completely without fibrosis, and this would be in keeping with the rapid diminution of size seen in many affected lymph-nodes at the time of remission. The healing process has been reviewed by Rosenthal and Feigin (1948). Before the final stage of scarring there may be material which has variously been termed 'fibrinoid' and 'paramyloid' in the central area, but there is no caseation. Some authors, for example Pinner (1938), have not held so strict a view about caseation, but in the present series the criterion of its complete absence has excluded no case which appeared in every other way to be sarcoidosis. Differentiation from tuberculosis may be difficult in biopsy material even if this criterion is adopted, and impossible in some instances if not. It is an entirely different question whether, when tuberculosis develops in a patient with sarcoidosis, pre-existing sarcoid granulomata develop caseation; this problem appears insoluble. Nickerson (1937) considered that the giant cells differed from those of tuberculosis, being usually much larger and with many more nuclei, which are evenly distributed throughout the cell; but many of the giant cells seen in the present series were indistinguishable from Langhans cells. Certain forms of intracytoplasmic inclusion are sometimes seen. Schaumann (1917) described the occurrence of rounded laminated inclusions, which are usually doubly refractile and which are often known as Schaumann bodies. Jadassohn (1914) found sharply defined, clear areas in the cytoplasm of some giant cells, often with a central sphere the staining properties of which were similar to, but not identical with, those of the cytoplasm. Projecting from the sphere in most instances were numerous rays, to produce the appearance of a conventional star up to 25μ in diameter. These structures have been called asteroids. Neither Schaumann bodies nor asteroids are of diagnostic assistance, since neither is regularly present in sarcoidosis, and both may appear in other conditions. Teilum (1948) described homogeneous eosinophile material in and around the granulomata, which he termed 'paramyloid'. This again is of no diagnostic help, since it is inconstant, and there is doubt as to whether it is not merely degenerate collagen. As in the matter of caseation, if the absence of visible acid-fast bacilli is not stipulated in sarcoidosis it is inevitable that cases of tuberculosis will be included. Tuberculosis may develop in a patient with sarcoidosis, but it cannot be considered justifiable to make an initial diagnosis of sarcoidosis if acid-fast bacilli are present in sections, in spite of a few cases like that of Kyrle (1921). In a small number of classical descriptions sarcoid-like lesions have been associated with a finding of objects resembling mycobacteria; interesting though they are in other respects, such descriptions do not affect the position as regards routine diagnosis, and in collecting the present series no patient was found to have any such objects in the available histological material. Further, there was no case which in every other respect showed sarcoidosis, but which was excluded owing to the presence of acid-fast bacilli. Hence the histological standards adopted in the present series are the presence of uniform discrete non-caseating epithelioid granulomata which do not coalesce, which may undergo fibrotic replacement, and which contain no acid-fast bacilli.

The distribution of the granulomata in the spleen is similar to that found in the lymph-nodes. In the lung a peribronchial disposition is frequent, and in the liver the lesions usually lie in the portal tracts (Nickerson, 1937). Histological diagnosis during life is most often based on a biopsy of skin or of a lymph-node. In the present series the tissue or tissues used for initial diagnosis are shown in Table IV. There are patients who have no cutaneous lesions, no enlarged superficial nodes, and no other easily accessible lesion. In such cases liver biopsy by

TABLE IV

Tissues Used for Diagnosis

Lymph-node	64	Thyroid	1
Skin	17	Tendon-sheath	1
Spleen	4	Salivary gland	1
Mucosa	3	Numerous tissues at autopsy	4
Tonsil	1		

needle puncture has been found to give a high proportion of positive results (van Beek and Haex, 1943; van Buchem, 1946; Scadding and Sherlock, 1948). Sternal-marrow biopsy has its advocates (Dressler, 1938; Gormsen, 1948), but on the whole has been found disappointing (Leitner, 1949). We have once made a presumptive diagnosis on bronchoscopic biopsy, later confirmed when lymph-node enlargement appeared, and this method has also been used by Olsen (1946) and Jacobs (1949). The essential point of any biopsy, whatever its site, is that a reasonably large portion of tissue should be available for examination. A lymph-node or an extensive skin lesion provides an adequate specimen, but frequently this is not the case with needle-biopsy material, which may contain only one or a very few granulomata, and may consequently be insufficient to show the general uniformity of pattern which is one of the most important features.

In the absence of tissue accessible to biopsy, an artificial cutaneous lesion may be produced by the Kveim reaction. Skin tests for sarcoidosis based on the intradermal injection of a suspension to tissue from a sarcoid lesion have been described by Williams and Nickerson (1935) and by Kveim (1941). Immediately after injection the site shows slight redness and a little infiltration, which soon disappear. After a latent period of one to two weeks, occasionally longer, a small papule appears, which gradually increases in size and is histologically indistinguishable from natural cutaneous sarcoidosis. Usually the lesion after development remains static for several months, subsequently disappearing in the course of a year or two. Occasionally, however, deep chronic ulceration has developed, which has been very slow to heal (Lomholt, 1943). In the experience of Kveim and of Danbolt (1943, 1946), Putkonen (1943), Lomholt (1943), and Danbolt and Nilssen (1945), the test was positive in nearly all cases of sarcoidosis, whether or not there was cutaneous involvement, and only very exceptionally positive in other conditions. In particular it was nearly always negative in lupus vulgaris and other forms of tuberculosis of the skin. The precise nature of the reaction is obscure, since various non-specific antigens, and even local trauma, may precipitate local lesions in patients with sarcoidosis, but this fact does not affect the value of the method.

Of conditions which may bear a histological resemblance to sarcoidosis, tuberculosis has already been mentioned. While typical sarcoidosis is easily distinguished from caseous or acute miliary tuberculosis, occasional cases appear to lie on the borderline, and these have naturally been used by the proponents of the tuberculous theory of sarcoidosis. Histological differentiation in a very small biopsy specimen may be impossible; but it is much more rare for the general pattern of even-sized discrete granulomata to be simulated by tuberculosis than it is for a single epithelioid-cell collection to be the subject of confusion. Leitner (1949) has discussed in detail the relationship between sarcoidosis, generalized caseous tuberculous lymphadenitis, classical tuberculosis, and 'sepsis tuberculosa acutissima'. Nicolas and Gaté (1934) remarked that the human body has only a limited number of ways in which to react to almost innumerable pathogenic influences, and that in consequence it is not surprising that sarcoid-like lesions may be produced by syphilis, leprosy, leishmaniasis, and various foreign bodies such as oil. While there is much truth in their observation, it is probable that all the conditions they name invariably show adequate points of differentiation from sarcoidosis. Kissmeyer (1934) stated that Boeck confused a case of sarcoidosis with leprosy. No less an authority than Pautrier (1934) described a case of 'leprosy' with the histological appearances of sarcoidosis. The patient, a native of the Belgian Congo, had lesions which were considered to be of the nodular anaesthetic variety of leprosy, but no lepra bacilli were found. The lesions ceased to progress during antileprol therapy. Lomholt (1934) considered that antileprol was successful in treatment of mucosal sarcoidosis. With the tendency to natural remission which is so characteristic of sarcoidosis, almost any therapeutic agent may appear effective, and in Pautrier's patient the diagnosis of leprosy was not proved. Kienböck (1902) attributed sarcoid-like areas of translucency in radiographs of the phalanges to syphilis, and some other authors have done the same. Those who discover patients with sarcoidosis who give positive serological tests for syphilis sometimes attempt to associate these findings (Bernstein, Konzlemann, and Sidlick, 1929), but the Wassermann reaction is rarely positive in sarcoidosis, presumably as an incidental finding (Longcope, 1941), and no lesion has been described which had the appearance of sarcoidosis and could be proved to be due to syphilis. Dupont (1934) described a case of cutaneous leishmaniasis in which the lesions had the general configuration of sarcoidosis, but there was the important difference that the macrophages present were packed with Leishman-Donovan bodies. Longcope (1941) examined many lymph-nodes from patients with sarcoidosis without finding such bodies. Another disease alleged to show occasional histological similarity is brucellosis (Spink, Hoffbauer, Walker, and Green, 1949); but, apart from other differential criteria such as agglutination reactions, the similarity does not appear to be close. Certain mycoses, such as coccidioidomycosis, may also show some resemblance to sarcoidosis (Dickson, 1938). With the exception of some cases of tuberculosis, none of these generalized diseases should give rise to serious difficulty. One must agree with Freiman (1948) that the resemblance of sarcoidosis to leprosy, brucellosis, the mycoses, and leishmaniasis is extremely superficial. The histological differences are not easily illustrated, because no one claims that these other conditions always present a similar picture to sarcoidosis, but only that they may do so. Consequently, if differences are portrayed, it is always possible to argue that dissimilar examples were intentionally chosen. It is possible, however, to indicate the type of distinction by reference to a rare condition, Stengel-Wolbach sclerosis, first described by Wolbach (1911), because it has been asserted (Kay, 1950) that this condition is identical with sarcoidosis, and not merely that it may sometimes be indistinguishable. Robb-Smith (1938) drew attention to features by which the two conditions could be separated, and these were confirmed on subsequent examination of his material. Briefly, although in Stengel-Wolbach sclerosis there are rounded granulomata, they consist of giant cells and histiocytes in much less orderly arrangement than in sarcoidosis. The histiocytes are spindle-shaped cells with a distinct margin, unlike the polyhedral epithelioid cells, with an indistinct cytoplasmic border, of sarcoidosis. Reticulin fibres are never absent from the granulomata of Stengel-Wolbach sclerosis, and tend to run between individual cells, whereas in sarcoidosis the early granulomata may contain no reticulin, and later the reticulin separates groups of cells, before the stage of complete fibrotic replacement is reached. The distinctions are shown in Plate 3, Figs. 5 and 6.

There are other conditions to be considered in which usually a more limited part of the body is involved. These may be divided into two groups: those resulting from the presence of exogenous foreign bodies, and those appearing usually in the neighbourhood of neoplasms or in their regional lymph-nodes, but sometimes in other conditions. The exogenous-foreign-body granulomata can usually be distinguished by their known aetiology or distribution, or because the cause is visible in sections. Perhaps beryllium granuloma deserves special mention, since the skin, the lymph-nodes, the lungs, and rarely the liver may be involved, but I share the view of Dutra (1948) that the histological picture is not identical with that of sarcoidosis, although it may be similar. Once it is recognized that sarcoid-like granulomata may occasionally be found in relation to malignant tumours (Gherardi, 1950; Nadel and Ackermann, 1950; Symmers, 1951), these present no diagnostic problem. There are also a few cases in which isolated lymph-nodes containing this type of granuloma are found incidentally during operations for other conditions. I have seen isolated nodes removed, near the operation site, from a woman undergoing cholecystectomy for chronic cholecystitis, and from another in whom partial gastrectomy was performed for chronic peptic ulcer. In both these cases the histological appearance was in keeping with sarcoidosis, and in the absence of other evidence of the disease the most that could be said was that the diagnosis was unproved.

The usual aetiological theories fall into three main groups: one in favour of an atypical form of tuberculosis, as a result either of abnormally high resistance or of infection by an attenuated organism (Kyrle, 1921, 1927; Pinner, 1938; Schaumann, 1934, 1936, 1941; Warfvinge, 1943); the second, that the disease is due to a single unknown cause, possibly viral, bacterial, or even chemical (Kissmeyer, 1932; Kissmeyer and Nielsen, 1933; Snapper and Pompen, 1938; Pautrier, 1948; Bjørnstad, 1948; Löfgren and Lundbäck, 1950); the third that it is merely a form of tissue reaction which may result from a variety of noxious agents (Nicolas and Gaté, 1934; Teilum, 1948; Freudenthal, 1948; Scadding, 1950). While there is no intention here of entering the lists in favour of either the first or the second school of thought, much of the argument in favour of the third theory is demolished once a sufficiently critical attitude is adopted to the histological appearances. As Pautrier (1948) observed, sarcoidosis 'has all the characteristics of an autonomous disease, a morbid entity, and not a single monomorphic tissue reaction elicited by different causes'.

The Tuberculin Test

The view is generally accepted that in most cases of sarcoidosis the intradermal tuberculin test is negative to 1:100 old tuberculin (Pinner, 1938; Ricker and Clark, 1949), but some go farther and insist on a negative result at this dilution as a necessity (Schaumann, 1936; Robb-Smith, 1952). Whether this is so could best be judged by comparison, from the onset of the disease until death, of two large groups of patients with typical clinical and histological features, one with the Mantoux reaction negative at 1:100 and the other with a positive response at this dilution. Such an investigation has not yet been published, but in the present series it is possible to compare two small groups in which most of the patients are still living. Thirty-two cases are available in which the reaction was negative at 1:100, and 17 in which it was positive (Table V). Three in each group had been in close family contact with tuberculosis. Of the Mantoux-negative patients, two had developed chronic cervical abscesses in childhood, the behaviour of which was very suggestive of tuberculosis. These had healed 25 and 50 years before the onset of the illness diagnosed as sarcoidosis. Three others were found to have frank tuberculosis some years after sarcoidosis, while in two patients probable tuberculous lesions appeared concurrently with Mantoux conversion to strongly positive at 1:10,000. Thus three out of 32 patients developed confirmed tuberculosis, and four others had probable tuberculous lesions, either before or after sarcoidosis. The four deaths in the group include one due to congestive cardiac failure associated with

TABLE V

Relation of Mantoux Reaction in Sarcoidosis to Incidence of Tuberculosis and to Prognosis

	Mantoux reaction at 1:100 dilution	
	Negative (32 *patients*)	*Positive* (17 *patients*)
History of contact with tuberculosis	3	3
Probable previous tuberculosis	2	0
Subsequent tuberculosis	3	0
Probable subsequent tuberculosis	2	0
Present condition:		
Well	10	7
Improved	10	6
Unchanged	6	2
Deteriorating	2	0
Died	4	2
Follow-up period:		
Range (years)	3–21	3–13
Average (years)	8	7

long-standing pulmonary sarcoidosis, one following massive haemoptysis, one due to myocardial infarction, and one attributed to gastroenteritis. Of the 17 Mantoux-positive patients, none had any previous clinically recognizable tuberculous lesion. After the appearance of sarcoidosis, one developed a cavity in the lung, but over 60 examinations, including culture and animal inoculations, failed to reveal tubercle bacilli in the sputum or gastric fluid, and the cavity was almost certainly an emphysematous bulla. In four patients the Mantoux reaction became positive at greater dilution as the sarcoid lesions retrogressed, without clinical or radiological evidence of tuberculosis having appeared. There have been two deaths, one due to right heart failure complicating sarcoidosis, and one to diabetic coma. Clinical progress of the surviving patients has been very similar in the two groups, and the distribution of organ-involvement is almost identical. It is admitted that the number of patients concerned is insufficient to be the basis for any definite views, but it appears that a negative Mantoux reaction is not to be regarded as a diagnostic requirement. No purpose will be served here by entering into the reason why such a finding is frequent. Pickert and Löwenstein (1908) described 'prokutin' and 'antikutin', substances in the serum which when mixed with old tuberculin enhanced or decreased its skin reactivity, and Martenstein (1921) believed that the anergy in sarcoidosis was related to the presence of anticutin. Leitner (1949) further discussed this subject, and a tuberculin neutralization factor was found in many patients with sarcoidosis, and in a few with other conditions, by Wells and Wylie (1949).

Other Diagnostic Tests

It is sufficient to say of the haematological changes that they may be characteristic, but are far too inconstant to be of any diagnostic value. Some patients show slight neutropenia or lymphopenia, moderate eosinophilia, and monocytosis, and the erythrocyte sedimentation rate is often raised. The findings in the present series were similar to those previously described (Kissmeyer, 1932; Longcope, 1941; Reisner, 1944). The frequency of increased serum-globulin was first pointed out by Salvesen (1935), and the increase was shown by Fisher and Davis (1942) to affect the γ-globulin fraction. In the present series the plasma-proteins were estimated in 48 patients, and the globulin fraction exceeded 4 gm. per 100 ml. in 11. Of these patients five had clinical evidence of hepatomegaly, and five had signs of impaired hepatic function, seven showing one or the other feature. Hepatomegaly was seen in only two patients, and impaired hepatic function in one, whose plasma-globulin was less than 4 gm. per 100 ml. It appears possible that the hyperglobulinaemia may bear a relation not to sarcoidosis in general but to hepatic involvement, which is known to occur in many cases without becoming apparent during life (Nickerson, 1937). Other biochemical deviations from normal which occur inconstantly are an increase in the blood-calcium (Harrell and Fisher, 1939) and in serum alkaline phosphatase. The latter substance was increased in 10 of the 22 patients in the present series in whom it was estimated, the highest values occurring in cases of known impairment of hepatic function. Bacteriological investigation assists only by exclusion of tuberculosis, and occasionally of other specific infective processes, so that the only positive diagnostic criteria so far available are clinical and histological. It is submitted that if these are adequately applied they are sufficient.

Course and Prognosis

Fifty-four of the 90 patients studied have been under observation for over five years, and their present state of health is tabulated according to length of follow-up period in Table VI. The majority have received no specific treatment. The question of treatment is considered later. The findings are expressed in a different form in Table VII, to make them easily comparable with those of Longcope and Freiman (1952). The morbidity figures include the occurrence of any symptoms possibly referable to sarcoidosis or subsequent tuberculosis, while those for mortality cover deaths from all causes. Patients described as well are free from symptoms. If they suffered cutaneous lesions, nothing more than faint brown patches remains to indicate the site. In those who had lymphadenopathy no palpable enlargement remains, and in those who had pulmonary or mediastinal involvement radiographs of the chest have reverted to normal. Those who show even slight residual signs or symptoms, other than the scars of healed skin lesions, have been classified as improved, although most patients in this group are in excellent health. The two patients classed as deteriorating both have tuberculosis.

Of 25 patients with skin lesions who have been observed for at least five years, the lesions have gradually diminished to leave only faint scars in 17, while the others have all improved. There is a tendency for one group of lesions to appear as another is regressing, but in general there has been steady improvement with or without treatment, although in a few cases large doses of calciferol

TABLE VI

Progress of 90 Patients

	Follow-up period (years)						
	0–1	*1–2*	*2–5*	*5–10*	*10–15*	*15–25*	*Total*
Well	2	2	7	13	13	2	39
Improved	2	2	3	5	9	1	22
Unchanged	4	2	2	..	2	..	10
Deteriorating	..	..	..	2	..	..	2
Died	2	3	5	7	..	..	17
Total	10	9	17	27	24	3	90

TABLE VII

Progress of 90 Patients Expressed in Form Adopted by Longcope and Freiman (1952)

			Sarcoidosis									
			Active				*Inactive or cleared*					
Follow-up period	*Number of patients*		*Number*		*%*		*Number*		*%*		*Deaths*	
	a	*b*	*a*	*b*	*a*	*b*	*a*	*b*	*a*	*b*	*a*	*b*
Less than 2 years	19	*17*	..	..	..	..	..	..	..	..	5	*1*
2 to 5 years	17	*23*	4	*11*	23	*48*	8	*8*	47	*35*	5	*4*
5 to 10 years	27	*23*	4	*9*	15	*39*	16	*8*	59	*35*	7	*6*
10 to 20 years	24	*19*	8	*8*	33	*42*	16	*10*	67	*53*	0	*1*
Over 20 years	3	*2*	1	*1*	33	*50*	2	*1*	67	*50*	0	*0*
Total	90	*84*										

a = present series.
b = combination of Tables VII and VIII of Longcope and Freiman (1952).

appeared to accelerate the process. While there is much variation, the life-cycle of an individual plaque from first appearance to subsidence, observed in several patients, has nearly always been within the range of six months to three years. Progress of lupus pernio of the ears or fingers was sometimes slower than this; on the other hand regression from a florid lesion may take as little as one or two months, even without treatment. In two patients there was rapid disappearance concurrent with the development of pulmonary or skeletal tuberculosis, a finding similar to that of Schaumann (1936). Lesions of the mucosae tend to regress in much the same way as those of the skin. It has been reported that severe nasal stenosis may occur, but the only residuum in the cases in the present series is slight fibrotic thickening of the submucosa. Of 53 patients with lymphadenopathy who are still alive, in 37 no enlarged nodes are now palpable or visible in radiographs. In 10 the size of the nodes has diminished, and in six the condition is unchanged. Sarcoidosis of the lymph-nodes was not responsible for death in any instance, although the secondary effects of mediastinal or tracheobronchial lymph-node enlargement may be serious. In some cases it was associated with severe dyspnoea, without radiographic evidence of pulmonary involvement, and the dyspnoea disappeared at the same time as the mediastinal mass ceased to be visible in radiographs. One patient developed bronchiectasis after bronchial stenosis which was attributed to enlargement of adjacent lymph-nodes. For three years there were recurrent pyrexial episodes due to secondary infection, although eventually the condition subsided, and he was virtually free from symptoms when seen 10 years after the onset. There is very great variation in the length of time which may elapse before lymph-nodes subside, but spontaneous disappearance may occur in as little as three weeks, a fact which makes it difficult to assess the value of therapy. Some patients gave a history of recurrent attacks of enlargement, which might last a few months and be separated by as much as two or three years. This history is surprising in view of the histological life-cycle of the lesions, but has been met with several times.

Pulmonary sarcoidosis is the form most liable to cause serious effects on general health, although the lesions here, as elsewhere, frequently regress and leave no impairment of function. Of the 40 patients in whom radiological or post-mortem evidence of pulmonary involvement was found, 12 have never had symptoms attributable to it. One such case was discovered as a result of a mass miniature radiography survey, and one by routine radiography when the patient's sister developed pulmonary tuberculosis. This patient conformed to all the diagnostic criteria for sarcoidosis, and his Mantoux reaction was negative at 1:100. In one case sarcoidosis was not suspected before the patient's sudden death from pulmonary embolism after an operation for synovectomy. In five of the others radiographs of the chest were taken on account of some totally unrelated disease; the remaining four patients were seen because of sarcoidosis of other organs. It need hardly be added that a diagnosis of sarcoidosis was never reached by radiography alone, but was confirmed, either at the time or later, by biopsy of lymph-nodes or other organs. Minor degrees of lymphadenopathy had frequently not been noticed by the patient. Among the patients who had pulmonary symptoms there were three in whom these symptoms were related to an acute secondary infective episode, and when this had subsided no chest symptoms remained. The outcome to the present date among the 40 patients is as follows:

No residual pulmonary signs or symptoms .	18 patients
No symptoms; radiograph still abnormal .	6 ,,
Cough or dyspnoea still present . . .	5 ,,
Died	11 ,,

The group with residual symptoms includes one patient who has developed pulmonary tuberculosis. The serious effects of lesions in the lung usually ensue only in the stage of scarring, when pulmonary fibrosis, emphysema, or bronchiectasis may occur (Rubin and Pinner, 1944). These complications may lead to right heart failure, the most common cause of death which can be directly related to sarcoidosis. Of the 11 patients with pulmonary involvement who have died, cardiac failure of this type was responsible in four; one death resulted from haemoptysis, and the other six from causes unrelated to pulmonary sarcoidosis. Extensive fibrosis as judged by radiographs does not necessarily imply a serious outcome. In one case serial radiographs during five years from the onset of symptoms were reported as showing steadily increasing fibrosis, and then for seven years as remaining unchanged, but the patient's general condition has improved throughout the second period, and he has only a very slight residue of his previously severe dyspnoea, which does not now incapacitate him in any way. Although many radiologists feel that the appearance of cavitation precludes the diagnosis of sarcoidosis, the cavities may be of emphysematous and not tuberculous origin, as was seen in one case in the present series, and as reported by Tice and Sweany (1941), Ustvedt (1948), and Scadding (1950). It has not been possible to reveal any correlation between the extent of the original radiographic changes and the severity of symptoms or the subsequent course. In cases showing remission symptoms may abate rapidly, but the radiographic changes have been slower to clear, rarely disappearing in less than two years.

Of other organs, involvement of the eye is the most frequent cause of permanent incapacity in the experience of many authors (Levitt, 1941). The process of healing by replacement fibrosis may increase the degree of visual disturbance. Experience in the present series appears to have been much more favourable than in most of those published, although none but the usual therapeutic methods was employed. The 11 patients with iridocyclitis received local atropine medication, riboflavine by mouth, and in one instance calciferol also. The active phase of the disease lasted in every instance for about two years, and after this had subsided visual acuity began to improve in every case. Of seven patients seen five to twelve years later, one developed secondary glaucoma, which has responded well to iridectomy. None of the remainder has any serious visual defect, although there is a limited reduction in acuity. Severe deformity may follow the bony lesions (Doub and Menagh, 1929; Pautrier, 1940). Experience of skeletal sarcoidosis in the present series is too slight to justify comment. Of five patients with radiographic bone changes, two had phalangeal swellings. In one the swelling has subsided completely in the course of six years; in the other it had almost disappeared at death after eight years. One patient who complained of aching of the shoulder was found to have a group of small areas of translucency in the upper end of the humerus.

Sarcoidosis of the heart is an infrequent cause of morbidity, and a rare cause of sudden death; one such fatality occurred in the present series. Too little is known about the frequency of cardiac involvement in generalized sarcoidosis to permit an assessment of its effect on the prognosis. During life it is not practicable to ascertain whether cardiac irregularity in patients with sarcoidosis is due to direct involvement by this disease. The patient here referred to, a girl aged 21 years, had been working and apparently well until two days before death, although the previous year she had been rejected for military service on account of 'heart disease'. Two days before death she vomited several times, but the next day she felt better. On the day of death she complained of 'dizziness', and went to bed. A few minutes later she became deeply cyanotic and died. Post-mortem examination revealed cardiac enlargement resulting mainly from right ventricular hypertrophy and dilatation. Throughout the myocardium, and particularly in the subpericardial region, were numerous small, discrete, rounded, white foci resembling tubercles. Tortuous bands of similar tissue extended across the ventricular walls, running usually transversely across branches of the coronary arteries, and enclosing areas of hyperaemia. The lumen of the coronary vessels was not narrowed. Microscopically the discrete lesions had the typical appearance of sarcoidosis, and infiltrated the myocardium extensively. The wider bands contained similar granulomata with surrounding fibrosis. There was no evidence of infarction. Pulmonary involvement was widespread, but not so dense as that usually seen in patients who have died with cor pulmonale, and other organs showing the disease were lymph-nodes, liver, spleen, and Fallopian tubes. Comparable cases have been reported by Longcope and Fisher (1942), Scotti and McKeown (1948), and Bates and Walsh (1948).

Splenic sarcoidosis may give rise to abdominal discomfort and dyspnoea, but more often it is symptomless. Of the 22 patients with splenomegaly, only the four in which it was gross suffered discomfort, dyspnoea being also present in two. In three splenectomy resulted in complete relief, the organ weighing 2,600 gm. in one case. In the fourth patient a biopsy specimen was taken, but the spleen was not removed owing to dense surrounding adhesions. Eleven years later the patient still had slight attacks of upper abdominal discomfort, and the size of the spleen has changed little since she was first seen. In the patients in whom splenic enlargement gave rise to no symptoms, it was common for the spleen to cease to be palpable, and the rate of subsidence was sometimes rapid.

Ascites was present at autopsy in one patient shown to have hepatic involvement, but was almost certainly due to congestive cardiac failure. Another patient with generalized sarcoidosis had recurrent attacks of jaundice, but if they were directly caused by sarcoidosis it was probably as a result of biliary obstruction by enlarged lymph-nodes. Slight to moderate hepatomegaly was recognized during life in nine other patients, in two of whom sarcoidosis of the liver was confirmed at autopsy. Four of these patients showed very slight diminution of liver function by tests unrelated to the plasma-protein level, but were without other clinical evidence of liver disease. In another three patients hepatic sarcoidosis, previously unsuspected, was found *post mortem*. Serious effects from involvement of the liver appear to be unusual.

The nervous system and pituitary gland are sites in which sarcoidosis can result in severe disease, and occasionally in death. Colover (1948) was able to find 115 cases of involvement of various sites within this system. In the present series meningeal and peripheral nervous symptoms were thought to be due to sarcoidosis in two patients known to have the disease, but no biopsy was available of the site in question from either patient. There have been two cases of diabetes insipidus; in one patient it produced the presenting symptoms, and the other was already known to have had sarcoidosis for five years. In both cases the condition was controlled satisfactorily with pituitrin. Another patient, a woman of 29 years, was admitted to hospital moribund, with hypertensive cardiac failure and many of the features of Cushing's syndrome. She died two days later, and at autopsy was found to have generalized sarcoidosis, with extensive involvement of the anterior lobe of the pituitary (Plate 2, Fig. 4). There was suprarenal cortical hyperplasia, but whether this was primary or followed the pituitary disease it is not possible to say.

Involvement of the salivary and lachrymal glands may result in secretory failure, dryness of the mouth being usual. The course of the disease in these glands closely resembles that seen in the lymph-nodes. There is often considerable fluctuation in the size of the swellings, even from one day to another, but a sudden change related to food or drink is uncommon. Eventual subsidence occurs in most cases after several months or a few years. No instance of pancreatic involvement has been seen, although it is not unknown in the literature (Leitner, 1949).

Resection has been practised in most of the few reported cases of gastrointestinal sarcoidosis (Watson, Rigler, Wangensteen, and McCartney, 1945; Raven, 1949). It was not done in the one case occurring in the present series. The patient, a girl of 15 years, had recurrent attacks of abdominal colic, which lasted for a day or two and occurred at intervals of several months. A laparotomy revealed structures resembling tubercles, and also larger flat, white plaques, scattered over much of the ileum, with enlarged mesenteric lymph-nodes. Some of the plaques almost surrounded the intestine, and caused narrowing of the lumen. A biopsy showed appearances typical of sarcoidosis. The attacks recurred with considerable severity for a period of eight years, during which time X-ray therapy appeared ineffective, but in the course of a further five years they have almost entirely abated. It seems appropriate to refer briefly to the alleged association between sarcoidosis and regional ileitis. Hadfield (1939) stated that the two conditions had the same histological features, but Watson, Rigler, Wangensteen, and McCartney (1945) could not support this view Examination of sections from 15 cases of regional ileitis in the records of the Radcliffe Infirmary has shown no lesion in the least resembling that of sarcoidosis. The lympho-histiocytic aggregates and giant cells in these cases of Crohn's disease, among which are examples representative of all phases of development, from early changes in the vermiform appendix to the late stage of fibrosis and fistula formation, are quite unlike the discrete sarcoid granulomata. In view of the conflicting opinions, Raven (1949) suggested that the relationship could not be disrupted until a series of cases of Crohn's disease had been observed for 10 years, to see whether signs of generalized sarcoidosis appeared. It has now been possible to follow nine cases for periods varying from eight to 12 years, and in none of them has anything suggestive of sarcoidosis been found.

Lesions of other sites, if superficial, have produced palpable or visible nodules, as in the tongue or tendon-sheaths, but no disturbances of function. Those of other internal organs, including the thyroid, kidney, and Fallopian tube, were only revealed incidentally after surgical removal of the organ or at autopsy.

The above survey is consistent with the general view that sarcoidosis is usually a benign disorder, characterized by spontaneous remissions and often a functional return to normality, with scarring or apparent resolution of the lesions.

TABLE VIII

Causes of Death

Case Number	*Cause of death*	*Years after diagnosis of sarcoidosis*	*Autopsy performed*
6	Pulmonary sarcoidosis, secondary lung infection, right heart failure . . .	3	..
11	Pulmonary sarcoidosis, haemoptysis .	8	..
16	Malignant hypertension, cardiac failure (Pituitary sarcoidosis) . . .	0	Yes
46	Pulmonary sarcoidosis, right heart failure	2	Yes
57	Mediastinal lymphadenopathy, congestive cardiac failure	4	Yes
61	Cardiac sarcoidosis	0	Yes
65	Mediastinal lymphadenopathy, right heart failure	1	..
74	Pulmonary sarcoidosis, right heart failure.	7	..
32	Tuberculous meningitis	3	Yes
10	Hypertensive heart failure	8	..
14	Gastroenteritis	5	..
27	Pulmonary embolism	0	Yes
34	Diabetic coma	7	..
62	Myocardial infarction	7	..
68	Uraemia, pyelonephritis, prostatic hypertrophy	6	..
90	Hodgkin's disease	1	Yes
43	Unknown	2	..

The rate of regression is very variable, and may be rapid, so that only by comparison of large series can therapeutic results be satisfactorily assessed. Of the 17 patients who have died, death appears to have been directly or indirectly attributable to sarcoidosis in eight, and one died of tuberculous meningitis. Seven died of causes not related to the disease, and one other patient is known to have died, but the cause has not been stated. The causes of death are shown in Table VIII. Five of the patients whose death was attributable to sarcoidosis died in cardiac failure, and in four this was characteristically of the right side. Three of them had extensive pulmonary sarcoidosis, known to have been present for from two to seven years, and Case 46 at autopsy showed fibrosis and hyalinization of the pulmonary lesions. In the other two there was massive enlargement of mediastinal lymph-nodes. No autopsy was performed in Case 11, so that the precise cause of haemoptysis remains uncertain, but in a similar case reported by Ricker and Clark (1949) there was fatal haemoptysis without evidence of tuberculosis. Reference has already been made to Cases 16 and 61. The former patient had been a semi-invalid on account of obesity and mental dullness for 17 years, but was in her normal state of health until the onset of dyspnoea five days before death; the latter was well and at work until two days before death. Of the patients grouped together as having died of causes other than sarcoidosis, in all but two this disease had been present for at least five years. One (Case 10) had developed spinal tuberculosis and myxoedema in the latter part of her illness. There is no reason to believe that her eventual hypertension was of sarcoid origin, but permission for autopsy was refused. In Case 34, in which death was due to diabetic coma, the patient had suffered from diabetes mellitus for several years before sarcoidosis was diagnosed on the basis of cutaneous lesions and lymphadenopathy. There was a strong family history of diabetes, so that the likelihood of the cause being pancreatic sarcoidosis is remote. Of the two patients with only a short history of sarcoidosis, one (Case 90) was discovered to have sarcoidosis of the lymph-nodes of one side of the neck when he was seen on account of a much larger mass, due to Hodgkin's disease, on the other side. The second patient (Case 27) was an apparently healthy young man, who died in an orthopaedic hospital from pulmonary embolism three weeks after synovectomy of the knee-joint. There was a history of injury to the knee 10 years previously, and no evidence of sarcoidosis was found in the excised synovia, but the disease was shown to affect many organs at autopsy. In contrast to the patients who died of heart failure, the pulmonary lesions, though widespread, were all in the cellular stage, with only slight fibrosis.

It has already been mentioned that many published reports are insufficiently specific about diagnostic criteria, and this statement applies to records of autopsy findings as well as to those of living patients. The total number of post-mortem reports on patients with sarcoidosis is not large, but there is general agreement on the commoner causes of death. Rubin and Pinner (1944) summarized the findings in 43 cases, and added one of their own. Leitner (1949) tabulated the causes of death in 72 cases, while Ricker and Clark (1949) added a further 22 among American service personnel. Among Leitner's collection, 26 patients died from cardiac failure, 12 from tuberculosis, nine from sarcoidosis of the nervous system, and nine of various secondary infections. Of the remainder, the only deaths which should probably be attributed to the disease were one following haemoptysis and one after rupture of an emphysematous bulla and pneumothorax. In the series of Ricker and Clark the proportion of traumatic deaths was high, but the fatalities related to sarcoidosis showed a similar distribution. In 14 of their 22 cases sarcoidosis was not suspected during life.

The frequency of tuberculosis in the present series is recorded without prejudice to aetiological opinions. Of the 90 patients, eight had a history of close contact with open tuberculosis before the onset of their disease. One of them had calcified hilar lymph-nodes, but the Mantoux reaction was negative at

1:100 old tuberculin, and a guinea-pig inoculated with tissue from a lymph-node showing the morphological features of sarcoidosis remained healthy six months later. Calcified hilar or mesenteric nodes were present in four other patients, while three gave a history of cervical abscesses in childhood which strongly suggested tuberculosis. Five patients are known to have developed tuberculosis after sarcoidosis, involvement being pulmonary in one, skeletal in three, and meningeal in one. A sixth has developed a painless cervical abscess concurrently with reversal of her previously negative Mantoux reaction to positive at 1:10,000 old tuberculin, while four more showed Mantoux conversion as their sarcoid lesions regressed, without developing overt tuberculosis. Published reports have shown that tuberculosis often follows sarcoidosis, whether the two conditions are related or not.

Treatment

Several entirely different forms of therapy have been used in sarcoidosis, but few justify the belief that apparently good results are due to any other factor than coincident spontaneous remission. General supporting treatment is indicated where such symptoms as cough and dyspnoea are prominent, but Hunter's (1936) claim of cure by rest and diet during four and a half years is unconvincing. Many patients with pulmonary sarcoidosis have found their way to sanatoria, and undoubtedly rest is beneficial in reducing the severity of symptoms. It may also reduce the density of radiographic shadows by removing vascular congestion, but there is no good evidence that it produces any fundamental and permanent change. The oral administration of Fowler's solution was in vogue early in the century, and intravenous arsphenamine has had supporters (Kissmeyer, 1932; Snapper and Pompen, 1938). It has even been suggested that arsenic might be of use as a test of diagnosis (Goeckerman, 1928), but its exhibition has not been reported recently, and was of no convincing therapeutic value. Lomholt (1934) was enthusiastic about the effect of antileprol, and a few other authors have used chaulmoogra derivatives, but progress was no better than might have been expected in untreated patients. Tuberculin (Irgang, 1939) and BCG have also been used, with no conspicuous success. One patient in the present series received graduated doses of a suspension of the vole tubercle bacillus. The Mantoux reaction became positive during the course, but there was no clinical benefit. Claims have been made for various forms of light and heat treatment. In addition to local diathermy or other applications to individual cutaneous lesions, which may hasten their course, the Finsen and Kromeyer lamps have been used, chiefly on mucosal lesions by analogy with lupus vulgaris, and Longcope (1941) considered that ultraviolet light might be of value.

Opinions on the value of X-ray therapy are varied. Bernstein and Oppenheimer (1942) thought the results encouraging, and felt that they were better in the earlier stages of the disease. Katz, Cake, and Reed (1943) observed reduction in the size of hilar lymph-nodes in one case. Pohle, Paul, and Clark (1945) noted rapid clinical improvement after the treatment of mediastinal nodes; this was followed after two to four months by decrease in the radiographic shadows. Donlan (1948) treated 11 patients who had lesions in sites including the lungs, lymph-nodes, eyes, and skin. Some cutaneous plaques disappeared rapidly, but the results were poor as far as the general course of the disease was concerned. It is interesting to observe to what extent the views of different authors on the aetiology of sarcoidosis appear to influence their choice of treatment and appraisal of its results. Mediastinal sarcoidosis is not infrequently confused clinically with Hodgkin's disease, and some patients have received radiotherapy on the basis of this diagnosis before histological confirmation was obtained. In the present series 20 patients have received X-ray therapy. The results cannot be compared exactly with the untreated group, owing to variation in the extent of involvement and in the behaviour of the disease among untreated patients, but there is evidence to suggest that, while sometimes regression is hastened, this treatment may have a seriously detrimental effect in some cases. The organs irradiated, the immediate effect, and the final course are shown in Table IX. No response was seen in two patients with cutaneous lesions, although these lesions subsided spontaneously a few years later. Of 16 patients with enlarged superficial or mediastinal lymph-nodes, regression was evident in 10 within two to 12 weeks after commencement of treatment. This rate of regression appears to be more rapid than would be expected to occur spontaneously, but there was recurrence in two cases, and the distribution of results in the final outcome is comparable with that found in untreated patients. The Mantoux reaction changed from negative at a dilution of 1:100 old tuberculin to strongly positive in three patients, one of whom developed a cervical abscess which was probably tuberculous. Another patient died of tuberculous meningitis, but this was not until three years after treatment. While the possibility is still entertained that sarcoidosis may be a manifestation of tuberculosis, and in the certain knowledge that patients with sarcoidosis frequently develop tuberculosis, any method of treatment suspected of ability to precipitate such a happening is open to criticism. It is also noteworthy that of the 10 patients with mediastinal or pulmonary involvement four have died of cardiac failure, compared with one of the 38 with untreated lesions of these sites.

Surgery finds a limited place in the treatment of sarcoidosis. While it does not affect the general disease process, it may effectively relieve the only serious symptoms in some cases, particularly when the spleen or the gastrointestinal tract is involved. Splenectomy is well tolerated (Friedman, 1944; Kay 1950), and was performed with success in three cases of the present series. Gastrectomy (Gore and McCarthy, 1944) and resection of segments of the small intestine and colon (Raven, 1949) have produced a satisfactory result in the few cases reported.

While some authors regard calciferol therapy as valuable, there is unanimity with regard to its frequent toxicity, which appears much more often than when it is used in the treatment of lupus vulgaris. Dowling and Thomas (1946) found no favourable response to the drug, and Meyer, Grupper, and Gaulier (1949) spoke of its abuse. Curtis, Taylor, and Grekin (1947) treated five patients with calciferol and dihydrotachysterol. The results were said to be generally satisfactory, but toxic reactions were severe. Nelson (1949) attempted a controlled experiment, eight patients with active sarcoidosis receiving calciferol and eight

TABLE IX

Effects of Radiotherapy

Case Number	*Organs irradiated*	*Early effect*	*Outcome*
42	Superficial and mediastinal LN	Smaller in 3 weeks	Well
45	Superficial LN	Little change	?Tuberculous adenitis. Mantoux 1:10,000 positive. Now well
53	Superficial LN	Not palpable in 3 months	Well
55	Palate and pharynx	Steady regression within 2 weeks	Well
60	Mediastinal LN and lungs	Regression within 2 weeks	Mantoux 1:100,000 positive at end of course. Now well
66	Skin	No change	Well
72	Mediastinal LN	Gradual regression for 9 months	Mantoux 1:1,000 positive when regression complete. Now well
73	Mediastinal LN	Not visible after 3 months	Well
79	Superficial LN	Not palpable in 1 month	Well
80	Mediastinal LN and lungs	Gradual regression for 5 years	Well
8	Ileum and mesenteric LN	No change	Improved
18	Skin	No change	Improved
70	Superficial LN	Smaller within 2 weeks of end of each of 4 courses; recurred each time	Improved
13	Deep LN. Lungs. (Trunk bath)	Little change	Unchanged
6	Mediastinal LN	Smaller within 6 weeks	Died: right heart failure
32	Superficial and mediastinal LN	Smaller within 3 months	Died: tuberculous meningitis
46	Mediastinal LN and lungs	No change	Died: right heart failure
57	Superficial and mediastinal LN	Smaller within 3 months after each of two courses	Died: cardiac failure
62	Superficial LN	Not palpable after 3 months	Died: myocardial infarction
74	Superficial and mediastinal LN. Lungs	Little change	Died: right heart failure

LN = lymph-nodes.

being untreated. The results in the two groups showed very little difference, and he concluded that calciferol is of no value. Foster (1952) was impressed by its effect on the ocular manifestations, and Scadding (1950) considered that it deserved further trial. In the present series six patients received calciferol. It was soon abandoned in two cases owing to intolerance. Two patients tolerated it well in doses of 100,000 to 150,000 units daily, but derived no benefit. In one patient the dose was gradually reduced from 100,000 to 10,000 units daily in view of thirst, nausea, and malaise, but there was concurrent improvement in cutaneous and pulmonary sarcoidosis, which had been present and virtually static for 10 years. The sixth patient had only cutaneous lesions, and these subsided during three months' treatment with 150,000 units daily. The only conclusion that can be drawn is that the value of calciferol remains very doubtful. The use by Snider (1948) of nitrogen mustard only emphasizes the absence of a therapeutic agent of known efficiency. Reports on the effect of streptomycin are not numerous, although Hedvall (1950) was enthusiastic about its value. Gernez-Rieux, Breton, Bonte, and Delwaulle (1948) reported successful treatment of one patient, but the history is confused by the presence of tuberculosis. Pulaski and White (1948) treated seven patients who had pulmonary sarcoidosis with streptomycin, without success. Sarcoidosis, at least in its earlier stages, appears to show a dramatic immediate response to treatment with cortisone. Siltzbach, Posner, and Medine (1951), Lovelock and Stone (1951), and Small (1951) reported a very rapid effect, and only a small residuum of scarring, which would be a great asset in the treatment of ocular and pulmonary lesions. Several more recent papers, including that of Siltzbach (1952), have described subjective and objective improvement during treatment, but a high rate of relapse shortly after its completion. Klemperer (1951) stated that 'within two to five weeks the epithelioid tubercles are transformed into hyaline nodules which in the untreated cases are seen only after months or years'. In the absence of detailed information about his methods it is impossible to give any views on this statement, since varying degrees of fibrosis and hyalinization may be seen early in the clinical course of the disease in some cases, and the general tendency of cortisone is to inhibit fibrosis. It is certainly clear that further trial should be given to cortisone in cases in which the severity of the disease is such as to justify the use of so potentially dangerous a substance. Small, however, (1951) gave a timely reminder of a possible danger, in that one of his patients developed vertebral tuberculosis shortly after completion of treatment. Whatever form of therapy is adopted, allowance should be made for the tendency to spontaneous remission in assessing results. The state of the lesions must be considered, because a remedy efficient in the granulomatous stage may not affect the final scar-tissue. Finally, the danger of replacing a usually relatively innocuous malady by active tuberculosis must not be forgotten.

It is a pleasure to express my indebtedness to Dr. A. H. T. Robb-Smith for his encouragement, and for making available to me the records of the Oxford Lymph-Node Registry; also to the physicians and surgeons of the Radcliffe Infirmary, in particular Professor L. J. Witts, who have kindly allowed me to study cases under their care. Finally, I wish to thank the many patients and their medical advisers who have replied to my inquiries. This paper is based on part of a dissertation submitted for the degree of D.M., Oxford, in Trinity Term, 1952.

Summary

1. A review is given of the clinical findings in 90 patients with sarcoidosis.

2. The requisite diagnostic criteria are discussed, with special reference to the need for accurate histological interpretation. A negative Mantoux reaction, while frequent, is not regarded as essential.

3. The progress of the patients is recorded. It is shown that sarcoidosis is usually a relatively innocuous condition, although involvement of certain organs or systems, notably the lungs, heart, eyes, and central nervous system, may have serious or fatal results. The tendency to spontaneous remission, which may affect the assessment of therapeutic results, is emphasized.

4. A brief review is given of methods of treatment. Certain apparent dangers of radiotherapy are mentioned. Further trial of cortisone in suitable cases is required.

REFERENCES

Bates, G. S., and Walsh, J. M. (1948) *Ann. Int. Med.* **29**, 306.
Beek, C. van, and Haex, A. J. C. (1943) *Acta med. scand.* **113**, 125.
Bernstein, M., Konzlemann, F. W., and Sidlick, D. M. (1929) *Arch. Int. Med.* **44**, 721.
Bernstein, S. S., and Oppenheimer, B. S. (1942) *J. Mt. Sinai Hosp.* **9**, 329.
Besnier, E. (1889) *Ann. dermat. syph.* **10**, (Ser. 2), 333.
Bjørnstad, R. T. (1948) *Acta tuberc. scand.* **22**, 142.
Boeck, C. (1899) *J. Cut. Genito-Ur. Dis.* **17**, 543.
Buchem, F. S. P. van (1946) *Acta med. scand.* **124**, 168.
Colover, J. (1948) *Brain,* **71**, 451.
Curtis, A. C., Taylor, H., and Grekin, R. H. (1947) *J. Invest. Dermat.* **9**, 131.
Danbolt, N. (1943) *Acta med. scand.* **114**, 143.
—— (1946) *Nord. med.* **29**, 118.
—— (1947) *Schweiz. med. Woch.* **77**, 1149.
—— and Nilssen, R. W. (1945) *Acta derm.-venereol.* **25**, 489.
Dickson, E. C. (1938) *Amer. Rev. Tuberc.* **38**, 722.
Donlan, C. P. (1948) *Radiology,* **51**, 237.
Doub, H. P., and Menagh, F. R. (1929) *Amer. J. Roentgenol.* **21**, 149.
Dowling, G. B., and Thomas, E. W. P. (1946) *Brit. J. Dermat.* **58**, 45.
Dressler, M. (1938) *Klin. Woch.* **17**, 1467.
Dupont, A. (1934) *Bull. Soc. fr. dermat.-syph.* **41**, 1291.
Dutra, F. R. (1948) *Amer. J. Path.* **24**, 1137.
Engelbreth-Holm, J. (1938) *Amer. J. Med. Sci.* **195**, 32.
Fisher, A. M., and Davis, B. D. (1942) *Bull. Johns Hopkins Hosp.* **71**, 364.
Foster, J. (1952) *Brit. Med. J.* **1**, 318.
Freiman, D. G. (1948) *New Engl. J. Med.* **239**, 664, 709, 743.
Freudenthal, W. (1948) *Brit. J. Tuberc.* **42**, 11.
Friedman, M. (1944) *Amer. J. Path.* **20**, 621.
Gernez-Rieux, C., Breton, A., Bonte, G., and Delwaulle (1948) *J. fr. méd. chir. thorac.* **2**, 376.
Gherardi, G. J. (1950) *Arch. Path.* **49**, 163.
Goeckerman, W. H. (1928) *Proc. Staff M. Mayo Clin.* **3**, 125.
Gore, I., and McCarthy, A. M. (1944) *Surgery,* **16**, 865.
Gormsen, H. (1948) *Acta med. scand.* Suppl. **213**, 154.
Hadfield, G. (1939) *Lancet,* **2**, 773.

Harrell, G. T., and Fisher, S. (1939) *J. Clin. Invest.* **18**, 687.
Hedvall, E. (1950) *Arch. tisiol.* **5**, 5.
Hoyle, C., and Vaisey, M. (1937) *Chronic Miliary Tuberculosis*, Oxford.
Hunter, F. T. (1936) *New Engl. J. Med.* **214**, 346.
Hutchinson, J. (1875–7) *Illustrations of Clinical Surgery*, London, **1**, 42.
—— (1898) *Arch. Surg.* **9**, 307.
—— (1900) Ibid. **11**, 205.
Irgang, S. (1939) *Arch. Dermat. Syph.*, **40**, 35.
Jacobs, E. (1949) *Acta clin. belg.* **4**, 301.
Jadassohn, J. (1914) *Arch. Dermat. Syph.*, Berlin, **119**, 10.
Katz, S., Cake, C. P., and Reed, H. R. (1943) *New Engl. J. Med.* **229**, 498.
Kay, S. (1950) *Amer. J. Path.* **26**, 427.
Kienböck, R. (1902) *Zts. Heilk.* **23**, 130.
Kissmeyer, A. (1932) *La Maladie de Boeck*, Copenhagen.
—— (1934) *Bull. Soc. fr. dermat.-syph.* **41**, 1327.
—— and Nielsen, J. (1933) *Acta derm.-venereol.* **14**, 283.
Klemperer, P. (1951) *Amer. J. Path.* **27**, 710.
Kuznitsky, E., and Bittorf, A. (1915) *Münch. med. Woch.* **62**, 1349.
Kveim, A. (1941) *Nord. med.* **9**, 169.
Kyrle, J. (1921) *Arch. Derm. Syph.*, Berlin, **131**, 33.
—— (1927) *Vorlesungen über Histo-Biologie der menschlichen Haut und ihrer Erkrankungen*, Berlin, **2**, 207.
Leitner, S. J. (1949) *Der Morbus Besnier–Boeck–Schaumann*, Basel.
Levitt, J. M. (1941) *Arch. Ophthal.* **26**, 358.
Löfgren, S., and Lundbäck, H. (1950) *Acta med. scand.* **138**, 71.
Lomholt, S. (1934) *Bull. Soc. fr. dermat. syph.* **41**, 1142.
—— (1943) *Acta derm.-venereol.* **24**, 447.
Longcope, W. T. (1941) *J. Amer. Med. Ass.* **117**, 1321.
—— and Fisher, A. M. (1942) *J. Mt. Sinai Hosp.* **8**, 784.
—— and Freiman, D. G. (1952) *Medicine*, **31**, 1.
Lovelock, F. J., and Stone, D. J. (1951) *J. Amer. Med. Ass.* **147**, 930.
Martenstein, H. (1921) *Arch. Derm. Syph.*, Berlin, **136**, 317.
Meyer, J., Grupper, C., and Gaulier, J. (1949) *Bull. Soc. fr. dermat. syph.* **56**, 195.
Michael, M., Cole, R. M., Beeson, P. B., and Olsen, B. J. (1950) *Amer. Rev. Tuberc.* **62**, 403.
Nadel, E. M., and Ackermann, L. V. (1950) *Amer J. Clin. Path.* **20**, 952.
Naumann, O. (1938) *Zts. Kinderheilk.* **60**, 1.
Nelson, C. T. (1949) *J. Invest. Dermat.* **13**, 81.
Nicolas, J., and Gaté, J. (1934) *Bull. Soc. fr. dermat. syph.* **41**, 1011.
Nickerson, D. A. (1937) *Arch. Path.* **24**, 19.
Olsen, A. M. (1946) *Ann. Otol. Rhin. Laryng.* **55**, 629.
Pautrier, L. M. (1934) *Bull. Soc. fr. dermat. syph.* **41**, 1284.
—— (1940) *La Maladie de Besnier–Boeck–Schaumann*, Paris.
—— (1947) *Presse méd.* **55**, 293.
—— (1948) *Brit. J. Tuberc.* **42**, 1.
Pickert, M., and Löwenstein, E. (1908) *Dtsch. med. Woch.* **34**, 2262.
Pinner, M. (1938) *Amer. Rev. Tuberc.* **37**, 690.
Pohle, E. A., Paul, L. W., and Clark, E. A. (1945) *Amer. J. Med. Sci.* **209**, 503.
Pulaski, E. J., and White, T. T. (1948) *Arch. Int. Med.* **82**, 217.
Putkonen, T. (1943) *Acta derm.-venereol.* Suppl. **10**, 1.
Raven, R. W. (1949) *Ann. Roy. Coll. Surg.* **5**, 3.
Reisner, D. (1944) *Amer. Rev. Tuberc.* **49**, 289, 437.
Ricker, W., and Clark, M. (1949) *Amer. J. Clin. Path.* **19**, 725.
Robb-Smith, A. H. T. (1938) *J. Path. Bact.* **47**, 457.
—— (1947) In *Recent Advances in Clinical Pathology*, ed. S. C. Dyke, London, p. 350.

Robb-Smith, A. H. T. (1952) *Modern Practice in Tuberculosis*, Vol. 2, London, p. 262.
Rosenthal, J., and Feigin, I. (1948) *Arch. Path.* **45,** 681.
Rubin, E. H., and Pinner, M. (1944) *Amer. Rev. Tuberc.* **49,** 146.
Salvesen, H. A. (1935) *Acta med. scand.* **86,** 127.
Scadding, J. G. (1950) *Brit. Med. J.* **1,** 745.
—— and Sherlock, S. (1948) *Thorax,* **3,** 79.
Schaumann, J. (1914) *Mém. presenté à la Société franç. derm. pour le prix Zambaco,* Stockholm.
—— (1916–17) *Ann. dermat. syph.* **6** (Ser. 5), 357.
—— (1917) *Nord. med. Ark.* **49,** Part 2, 17.
—— (1934) *Bull. Soc. fr. dermat. syph.* **41,** 1296.
—— (1936) *Brit. J. Dermat.* **48,** 399.
—— (1941) *Acta med. scand.* **106,** 239.
Schönholzer, G. (1947) *Schweiz. med. Woch.* **77,** 585.
Scotti, T. M., and McKeown, C. E. (1948) *Arch. Path.* **46,** 289.
Siltzbach, L. E. (1952) *Amer. J. Med.* **12,** 139.
—— Posner, A., and Medine, M. M. (1951) *J. Amer. Med. Ass.* **147,** 927.
Small, M. J. (1951) Ibid. **147,** 932.
Snapper, I., and Pompen, A. W. M. (1938) *Pseudo-tuberculosis in Man,* Haarlem.
Snider, G. E. (1948) *South. Med. J.* **41,** 11.
Spink, W. W., Hoffbauer, F. W., Walker, W. W., and Green, R. A. (1949) *J. Lab. Clin. Med.* **34,** 40.
Symmers, W. St. C. (1951) *Amer. J. Path.* **27,** 493.
Teilum, G. (1948) Ibid. **24,** 389.
Tenneson, M. (1892) *Bull. Soc. fr. dermat. syph.* **3,** 417.
Tice, F. and Sweany, H. C. (1941) *Ann. Int. Med.* **15,** 597.
Ustvedt, H. J. (1948) *Tubercle,* **29,** 107.
Warfvinge, L. E. (1943) *Acta med. scand.* **114,** 259.
Watson, C. J., Rigler, L. G., Wangensteen, O. H., and McCartney, J. S. (1945) *Gastroenterology,* **4,** 30.
Wells, A. Q., and Wylie, J. A. H. (1949) *Lancet,* **1,** 439.
Williams, R. H., and Nickerson, D. A. (1935) *Proc. Soc. Exp. Biol. Med.* **33,** 403.
Wolbach, S. B. (1911) *J. Med. Research,* **24,** 243.

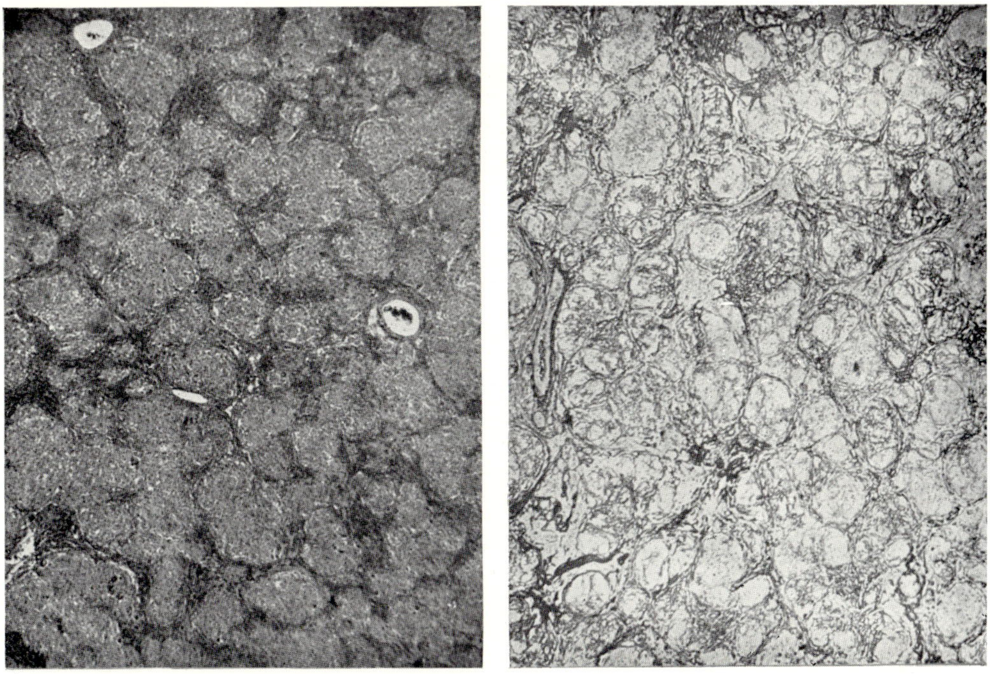

a *b*

FIG. 1. Low-power view of lymphadenoid sarcoidosis to illustrate the general pattern (*a*, haematoxylin and eosin, ×35; *b*, Robb-Smith's modification of Foot's reticulin method, ×35)

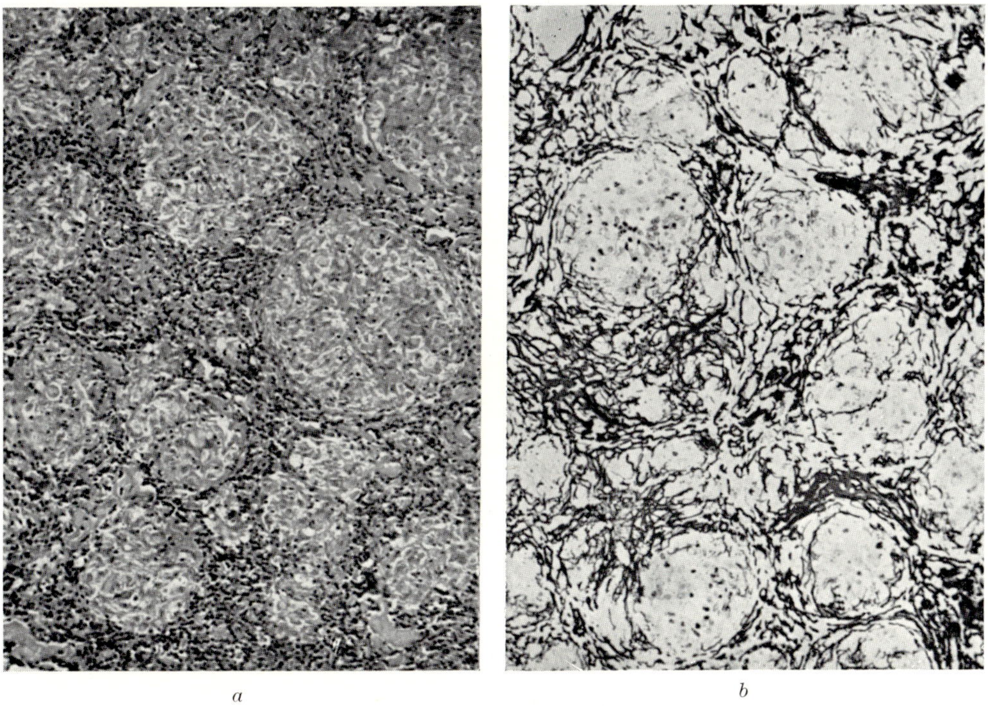

a *b*

FIG. 2. Lymphadenoid sarcoidosis in the cellular phase. Some of the granulomata contain no reticulin, others very little (*a*, haematoxylin and eosin, ×150; *b*, reticulin, ×150)

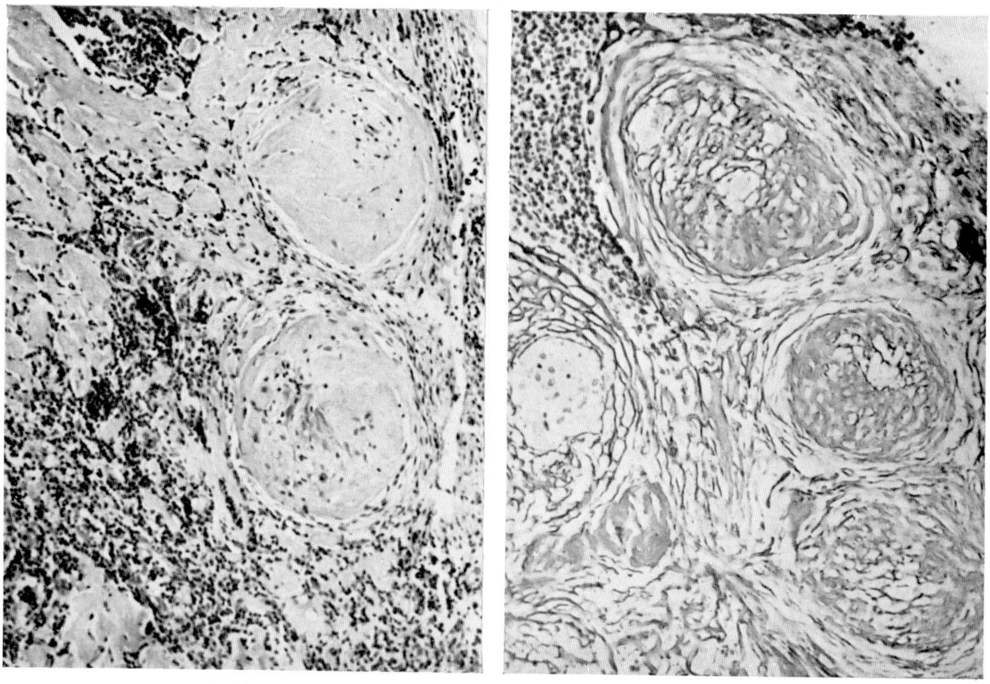

a *b*

FIG. 3. Fibroid replacement of epithelioid granulomata in a lymph-node (*a*, haematoxylin and eosin, ×100; *b*, reticulin, ×180)

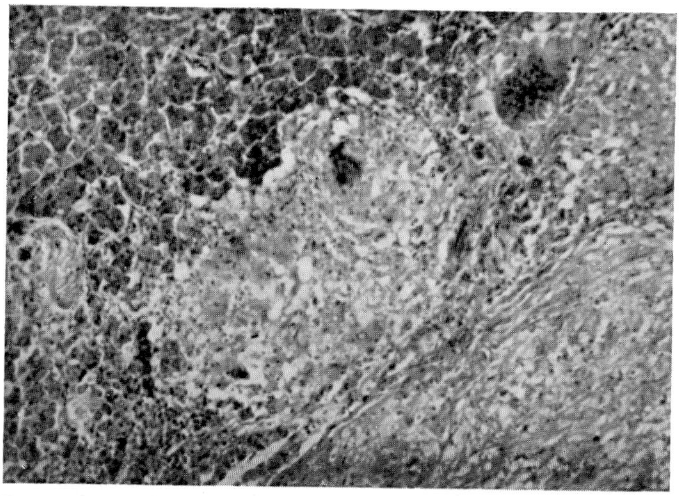

FIG. 4. Infiltration of the pituitary by epithelioid granulomata (haematoxylin and eosin, ×180)

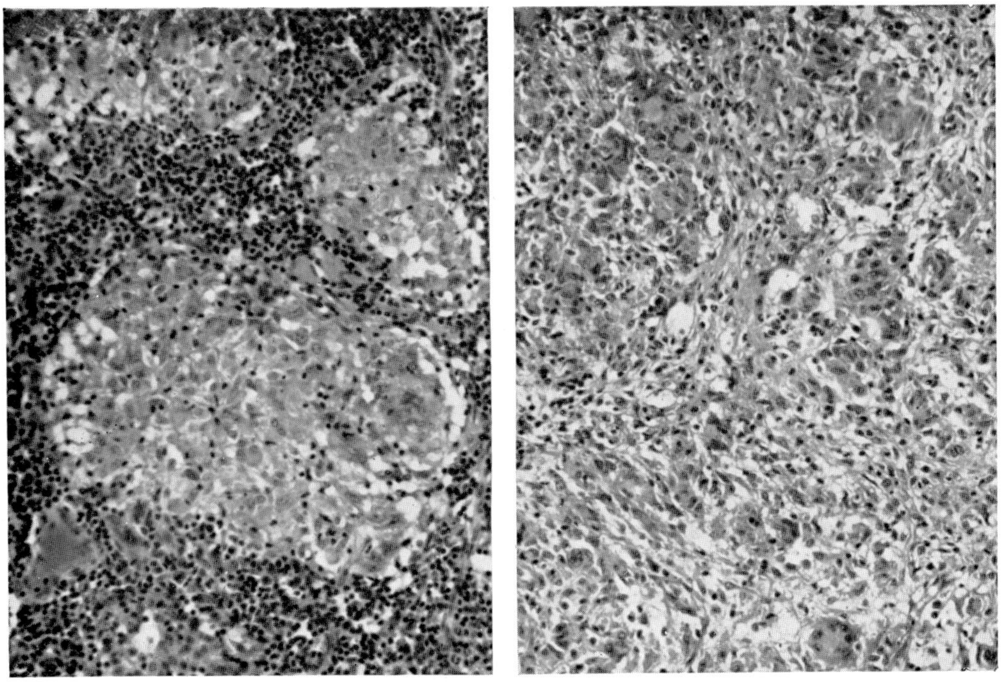

a b

FIG. 5. (a) Spleen in sarcoidosis. (b) Spleen in Stengel-Wolbach sclerosis. In sarcoidosis the characteristic cells are epithelioid cells with a poorly defined cytoplasmic margin. In Stengel-Wolbach sclerosis they are sharply defined elongated histiocytes (haematoxylin and eosin, ×200)

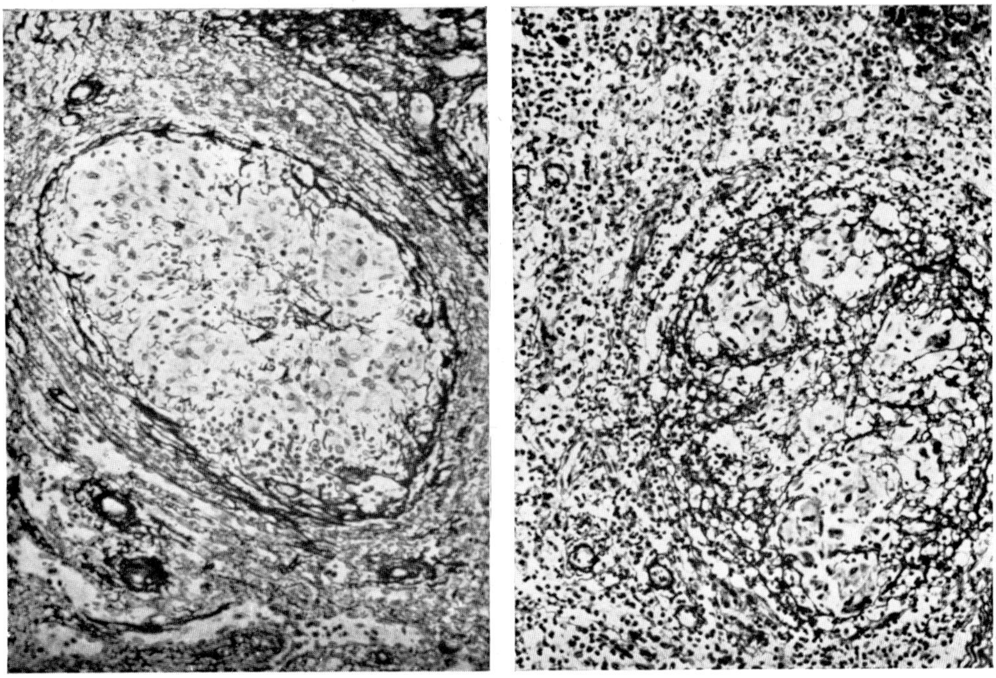

a b

FIG. 6. (a) Spleen in sarcoidosis. (b) Spleen in Stengel-Wolbach sclerosis. In sarcoidosis there may be little or no reticulin in the granulomata. Where there is more, it tends to form central clumps with fibres separating groups of cells, while in Stengel-Wolbach sclerosis the histiocytic aggregates are divided by reticulin fibres running between individual cells or very small groups (reticulin, ×200)

616.131–008.21:616.24

PULMONARY HYPERTENSION IN CONGESTIVE HEART FAILURE COMPLICATING CHRONIC LUNG DISEASE[1]

By W. WHITAKER

(From the University Department of Medicine, The Royal Hospital, Sheffield)

In chronic lung disease pulmonary hypertension has long been considered to be the important factor in the production of congestive heart failure. This view, which was recently restated by Bedford (1951), received support from the work of Cournand (1950), who showed that pulmonary hypertension was present in patients who had congestive heart failure complicating chronic lung disease. Recently, however, Ferrer, Harvey, Cathcart, Webster, Richards, and Cournand (1950) and Mounsey, Ritzmann, Selverstone, Briscoe, and McLemore (1952) found that pulmonary hypertension usually disappears when such patients recover from congestive heart failure, a fact which suggests that the primary cause of heart failure is not pulmonary hypertension. The increase in pulmonary artery blood-pressure which occurs with congestive heart failure may produce some of the features associated with heart failure, but must itself be the product of some more fundamental disturbance. The present investigations were made to determine the relation between pulmonary artery blood-pressure and the right auricular blood-pressure, the blood gases, the cardiac output, and the haematocrit value in patients with chronic lung disease with and without congestive heart failure.

Method of Investigation

The patients investigated were selected from a larger group of patients with chronic lung disease by excluding those with associated ischaemic heart disease, chronic rheumatic heart disease, or hypertensive heart disease. Each patient was studied at least two hours after a light meal, while resting in a semi-recumbent position. Cardiac catheterization was performed under fluoroscopic control, and the catheter tip was passed into the pulmonary artery. Blood-pressures were recorded in the pulmonary artery and subsequently, when the catheter was withdrawn, in the right ventricle and right auricle. In the early investigations mean pressures were recorded on a saline manometer, but later a condenser manometer was used, which gave in addition to mean pressures a graphic record of systolic and diastolic pressures. A level 5 cm. behind the frontal plane passing through the sternal angle was chosen as the zero position from which all blood-pressures were measured. A respiratory variation in intra-thoracic blood-pressures, noted previously by Borden, Wilson, Ebert, and Wells (1950) in patients with pulmonary emphysema, was observed in many patients

[1] Received March 4, 1953.

in this series, and the pressures reported are the average pressures recorded in a respiratory cycle. Oxygen consumption was measured by analysis of expired air collected in a Douglas bag for at least four minutes at the time of cardiac catheterization. During the collection of expired air, samples of mixed venous blood from the pulmonary artery and of arterial blood from an indwelling brachial arterial needle were withdrawn into 20 ml. syringes wetted with heparin. The haematocrit reading, haemoglobin-content, and oxygen-saturation of each blood sample were determined. The haemoglobin-content was measured by a photoelectric colorimeter, and from this the oxygen capacity was calculated; the percentage oxygen-saturation was measured by a direct spectrophotometric method, and from these results the oxygen-content of the sample was calculated. In many samples the oxygen and carbon dioxide contents were also determined by a Van Slyke manometric apparatus, and there was close agreement between the values of the oxygen-content determined by the two methods. From the oxygen consumption and the oxygen-contents of the arterial and mixed venous blood the cardiac output was calculated by the Fick principle. The effects produced on the pulmonary artery blood-pressure by acute changes in arterial blood oxygen-saturation were studied by giving patients 100 per cent. oxygen, or 10 per cent. oxygen and 90 per cent. nitrogen, through a B.L.B. oronasal mask for 10 minutes, and then recording the pulmonary artery blood-pressure and the blood oxygen-saturation. Pure oxygen was given to patients with heart failure to produce an acute increase in blood oxygen-saturation; the gas with low oxygen-content was given to patients without heart failure to produce acute anoxia. No patient was distressed by the administration of either gas at the time of catheterization, but in several the effect of anoxia was not investigated, as a trial administration of the gas with low oxygen-content caused distress. In the majority of patients a simple estimation of ventilatory function was made by recording the vital capacity and the maximum breathing capacity. These tests were performed after recovery from heart failure in patients who suffered from this complication.

Results

The clinical diagnoses, radiological findings, and results of the simple ventilatory function tests in 26 patients investigated are shown in two groups in Table I. Patients with chronic pulmonary disease of similar aetiological and anatomical type are present in each group, but the 13 patients in Group A had complicating congestive heart failure, while the 13 patients in Group B had not. The criteria for the existence of congestive heart failure were elevation of the jugular venous pressure above the sternal angle in all phases of respiration and the presence of peripheral oedema. In Group A the vital capacity averaged 1·86 litre and had a range of 0·9 to 3·2 litres, and the maximum breathing capacity averaged 32·5 litres per minute and had a range of 22 to 52 litres per minute, while in Group B the vital capacity averaged 2·08 litres and had a range of 1·4 to 2·8 litres, and the maximum breathing capacity averaged 35·6 litres per minute and had a range of 24 to 64 litres per minute.

TABLE I

Ventilatory Function and Clinical and Radiological Diagnoses in Patients Investigated

Case number	*Age (years)*	*Sex*	*Body-surface area (sq. m.)*	*Vital capacity (l.)*	*Maximum breathing capacity (l./min.)*	*Radiological diagnosis of lung disease*	*Clinical diagnosis of chronic lung disease*
Group A. Patients with a history of congestive heart failure:							
1	24	M	..	..	..	Extensive bilateral bronchiectasis	Bronchiectasis
2	52	M	1·59	1·8	29	Basal emphysema	Chronic bronchitis and emphysema
3	48	M	1·66	1·5	25	Basal emphysema	Chronic bronchitis and emphysema
5	36	F	1·67	1·7	23	Extensive bilateral bronchiectasis	Bronchiectasis
10	49	M	..	..	..	Fibrosis of upper lobes with basal emphysema	Chronic bronchitis and emphysema
11	59	M	1·57	1·7	22	Emphysema	Chronic bronchitis and emphysema
13	54	M	1·41	1·6	26	Emphysema	Chronic bronchitis and emphysema
14	54	M	1·69	..	..	Emphysema	Chronic bronchitis and emphysema
15	53	M	1·74	1·7	36	Emphysema	Chronic bronchitis and emphysema
16	61	F	1·69	0·9	40	Emphysema	Emphysema and mild chronic bronchitis
20	42	M	1·87	3·2	52	Emphysema	Chronic bronchitis and emphysema
21	45	M	1·55	2·1	33	Emphysema. Slight generalized fibrosis	Chronic bronchitis and emphysema
26	45	M	1·59	2·4	39	Emphysema	Chronic bronchitis and emphysema
Group B. Patients with chronic pulmonary disease not complicated by congestive heart failure:							
4	26	F	1·33	1·4	52	Pulmonary fibrosis	Chronic giant-cell pneumonia (lung-biopsy diagnosis)
6	28	M	1·42	2·0	29	Bronchiectasis of right upper lobe	Asthma. Bronchiectasis
7	53	M	1·55	..	..	Nodular silicosis	Silicosis with emphysema
8	48	M	1·76	2·3	30	Mild cylindrical bronchiectasis	Chronic bronchitis and emphysema
9	45	M	1·72	2·3	24	Bilateral basal bronchiectasis	Bronchiectasis
12	68	M	1·74	2·3	64	Normal lung fields	Chronic bronchitis and emphysema
17	64	M	1·38	1·9	33	Emphysema	Chronic bronchitis and emphysema
18	62	M	1·64	2·1	36	Emphysema	Chronic bronchitis and emphysema
19	32	M	1·73	1·8	..	Bronchiectasis of left lower lobe	Asthma. Bronchiectasis
22	49	M	1·68	2·3	32	Emphysema	Chronic bronchitis and emphysema
23	57	M	1·66	2·8	45	Emphysema	Chronic bronchitis and emphysema
24	43	F	1·5	2·0	58	Pulmonary fibrosis	Non-industrial pulmonary fibrosis (lung-biopsy diagnosis)
25	63	M	1·52	1·8	24	First stage of pneumoconiosis	Miner's pneumoconiosis

Observations on the circulation in patients at rest (Tables II and III). Ten patients with congestive heart failure were studied, and six of these were re-investigated after receiving treatment for at least a month, when they were free from oedema and venous congestion. Three other patients recovering from congestive heart failure, who were not investigated with failure, and 13 patients without congestive heart failure, were studied on only one occasion.

Table II

Results of Observations on the Circulation in Patients with Chronic Lung Disease at Rest

Case number	*Arterial blood-pressure (mm. Hg)*	*Mean pressure in pulmonary artery (mm. Hg)*	*Mean pressure in right auricle (mm. Hg)*	*Arterial oxygen-saturation (%)*	*Mixed venous oxygen-saturation (%)*	*Mixed venous CO_2 content (vols. %)*	*Arteriovenous oxygen difference (ml./100 ml.)*	*Oxygen consumption (ml./min.)*	*Cardiac output (l./min.)*	*Cardiac index (l./min./sq. m.)*	*Haemoglobin (gm./100 ml.)*	*Haematocrit reading*
I. Patients in congestive failure:												
1	110/80	59	5	..	..	67	..	..	..	..	..	..
20	140/85	57	15	66	51	64	2·9	237	8·1	4·3	16·0	55
16	110/75	56	6	56	37	61	3·9	285	7·4	4·4	17·1	54
14*	110/70	55	8	71	24	..	8·8	170	1·9	1·1	13·8	47
11*	120/65	52	10	72	44	..	5·1	184	3·6	2·1	13·6	44
15*	140/85	51	16	62	46	..	3·6	153	4·3	2·5	17·6	58
2*	110/80	49	16	57	38	72	4·4	255	5·8	3·5	18·0	58
3	150/95	47	8	70	46	63	5·7	..	..	..	16·4	53
26*	105/55	42	11	70	54	64	3·3	235	7·1	3·9	14·8	52
13*	125/95	37	4	67	38	..	5·9	260	5·3	3·8	14·9	45
II. Patients in recovery phase of congestive failure:												
14*	..	47	4	83	54	..	4·9	263	5·4	3·2	12·9	42
21	110/65	39	2	83	69	59	3·5	206	5·9	3·8	18·6	59
2*	130/95	31	3	77	62	67	3·8	..	..	..	18·6	60
10	140/95	30	3	93	62	..	5·6	220	3·9	..	13·3	46
15*	130/80	27	2	82	69	58	3·6	196	5·4	3·1	18·3	58
11*	120/85	26	−2	88	60	..	5·0	210	4·2	2·7	13·9	46
5	110/70	26	2	89	70	..	4·7	..	..	..	14·2	46
13*	115/80	24	−2	87	60	..	7·1	267	3·8	2·7	15·5	47
26*	120/80	24	−4	84	64	58	4·3	214	5·0	3·1	15·4	49
III. Patients with no history of congestive failure:												
7	135/80	33	5	95	73	56	4·3	200	4·6	3·0	15·9	48
9	125/85	27	3	95	72	53	4·8	255	5·6	3·3	14·8	44
17	145/95	26	−2	83	60	60	4·9	114	2·3	1·7	16·0	47
6	120/70	26	4	88	66	49	4·7	..	..	..	14·9	42
4	115/70	25	4	83	63	51	3·4	..	..	..	12·8	..
19	120/70	22	1	93	76	52	4·4	205	4·7	2·7	18·8	61
22	115/75	21	1	93	67	54	5·7	203	3·6	2·2	14·9	43
23	130/80	21	0	90	62	..	5·2	194	3·8	2·3	13·3	43
8	120/75	20	2	94	65	53	5·3	225	4·2	2·4	13·8	42
12	160/100	17	3	94	75	..	3·4	285	8·4	4·8	13·8	41
25	115/70	14	0	94	64	44	5·8	222	3·8	2·5	14·0	44
24	105/75	12	−1	91	66	42	4·5	155	3·4	2·3	13·9	40
18	180/110	8	−2	93	72	50	4·1	158	3·9	2·4	14·7	40

* Patients investigated twice.

Effects of breathing abnormal gas mixtures (Table IV). The change in pulmonary artery mean blood-pressure and in arterial blood oxygen-saturation was observed in four patients with congestive heart failure who were given pure oxygen, and in four patients without heart failure who were given a gas mixture of 10 per cent. oxygen and 90 per cent. nitrogen.

TABLE III

Statistical Analysis of Results of Circulatory Studies at Rest

	Mean pressure in pulmonary artery (mm. Hg)	*Mean pressure in right auricle (mm. Hg)*	*Arterial oxygen-saturation (%)*	*Mixed venous oxygen-saturation (%)*	*Mixed venous CO_2 content (vols. %)*	*Arteriovenous oxygen difference (ml./100 ml.)*	*Oxygen consumption (ml./min.)*	*Cardiac output (l./min.)*	*Cardiac index (l./min./sq. m.)*	*Haemoglobin (gm./100 ml.)*	*Haematocrit reading*
I. Ten patients in congestive failure:											
Mean of values	50·8	9·7	65·7	42·0	65·2	4·34	222·4	5·43	3·20	15·09	51·8
Range . . .	37–59	4–16	56–72	24–54	61–72	2·9–8·8	153–285	1·9–8·1	1·1–4·4	13·6–18·0	44–58
Standard deviation	±7·1	±4·4	±6·0	±9·9	±3·16	±2·2	±46·5	±2·04	±1·15	±1·36	±4·7
Standard error of mean . .	±2·25	±1·4	±2·0	±3·3	±1·25	±0·7	±13·3	±0·73	±0·40	±0·45	±1·6
II. Nine patients in recovery phase of congestive failure:											
Mean of values .	30·4	0·9	85·1	62·9	60·5	4·72	225·1	4·80	3·10	15·63	50·3
Range . . .	24–47	−4 to 4	77–93	54–70	58–67	3·5–7·1	196–267	3·8–5·9	2·7–3·8	12·9–18·6	42–60
Standard deviation	±7·76	±2·90	±4·7	±5·23	±4·4	±1·3	±38·2	±0·83	±0·45	±2·27	±6·8
Standard error of mean . .	±2·59	±0·97	±1·57	±1·71	±2·2	±0·43	±14·4	±0·32	±0·21	±0·76	±2·3
III. Thirteen patients with no history of congestive failure:											
Mean of values .	20·9	1·5	91·3	68·5	51·3	4·65	201·6	4·40	2·60	14·74	44·6
Range . . .	8–33	−2 to 5	83–95	60–76	42–60	3·4–5·8	114–285	2·3–8·4	1·7–4·8	12·8–18·8	40–61
Standard deviation	±6·8	±2·24	±4·2	±3·9	±4·78	±0·75	±47·5	±1·53	±0·75	±1·73	±5·8
Standard error of mean . .	±1·9	±0·63	±1·2	±1·1	±1·4	±0·21	±14·4	±0·5	±0·23	±0·43	±1·7

Discussion

Harvey, Ferrer, Richards, and Cournand (1951) found that 15 mm. Hg was the upper limit of the pulmonary artery mean blood-pressure in normal subjects. In the present series the pulmonary artery mean blood-pressure of patients

TABLE IV

Results of Breathing 100 per cent. Oxygen or 10 per cent. Oxygen and 90 per cent. Nitrogen

Case number	*Content of inspired air*	*Arterial oxygen-saturation* (%)	*Mean blood-pressure in pulmonary artery* (*mm. Hg*)
A. Patients with heart failure:			
11	Air	72	52
	100 % oxygen	90	48
13	Air	67	37
	100 % oxygen	89	39
15	Air	69	51
	100 % oxygen	95	45
16	Air	56	57
	100 % oxygen	94	49
B. Patients without heart failure:			
18	Air	93	8
	10 % oxygen	78	13
19	Air	93	22
	10 % oxygen	60	36
23	Air	90	21
	10 % oxygen	74	27
25	Air	94	14
	10 % oxygen	92	14

without heart failure ranged from 8 to 33 mm. Hg, while that of patients with heart failure was consistently higher, ranging from 37 to 59 mm. Hg. During recovery from heart failure a fall of pulmonary artery blood-pressure occurred; in five of the six patients investigated twice, the mean pressure fell to the levels recorded in patients with uncomplicated chronic lung disease, and in two of the three patients investigated only during recovery the pressure was also of this order (Table II; Fig. 1). A statistical analysis of the pulmonary artery mean blood-pressures showed that patients with the complication of congestive heart failure had higher pressures than patients without this complication when they were in failure, but not when they were recovering from failure (Table III). Similar results have been obtained by other workers; Hickam and Cargill (1948), Riley, Himmelstein, Motley, Weiner, and Cournand (1948), Borden, Wilson, Ebert, and Wells (1950), and Harvey, Ferrer, Richards, and Cournand (1951) found pulmonary hypertension in some patients with chronic lung disease without heart failure, while Ferrer, Harvey, Cathcart, Webster, Richards, and

Cournand (1950) and Mounsey, Ritzmann, Selverstone, Briscoe, and McLemore (1952) noted in addition higher pulmonary artery pressure in patients with the complication of congestive heart failure, and found that this pressure fell to levels seen without heart failure as the patients recovered. All these observers considered destruction of the pulmonary vascular bed by emphysema to be the

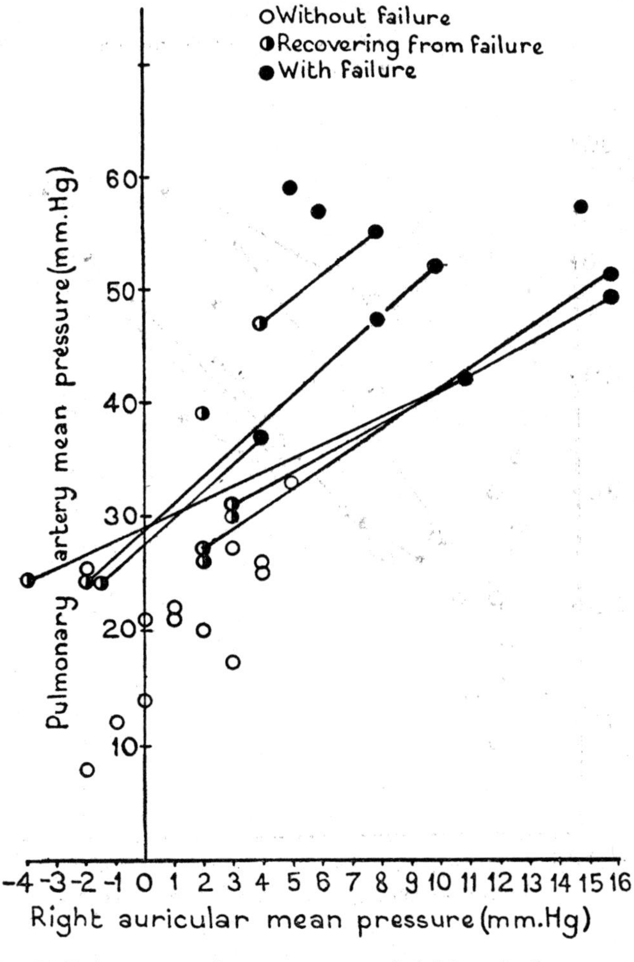

FIG. 1. Pulmonary artery pressure and right auricular pressure in chronic lung disease with, without, and during recovery from congestive heart failure. Where two values are joined by a line, they refer to the same patient.

cause of the mild degree of pulmonary hypertension seen in patients without heart failure, and no new evidence on this point is provided by the present observations. Various possible causes were suggested by Ferrer, Harvey, Cathcart, Webster, Richards, and Cournand (1950) and by Mounsey, Ritzmann, Selverstone, Briscoe, and McLemore (1952) for the increase of pulmonary artery blood-pressure occurring with congestive heart failure; these included anoxia, carbon dioxide retention, increased cardiac output, and increased blood viscosity, which will now be considered in relation to the present investigations.

Anoxia. In the present series the highest pulmonary artery pressures occurred with the most severe degrees of anoxia in patients with congestive heart failure, the lowest pressures occurred with the least degrees of anoxia in patients with

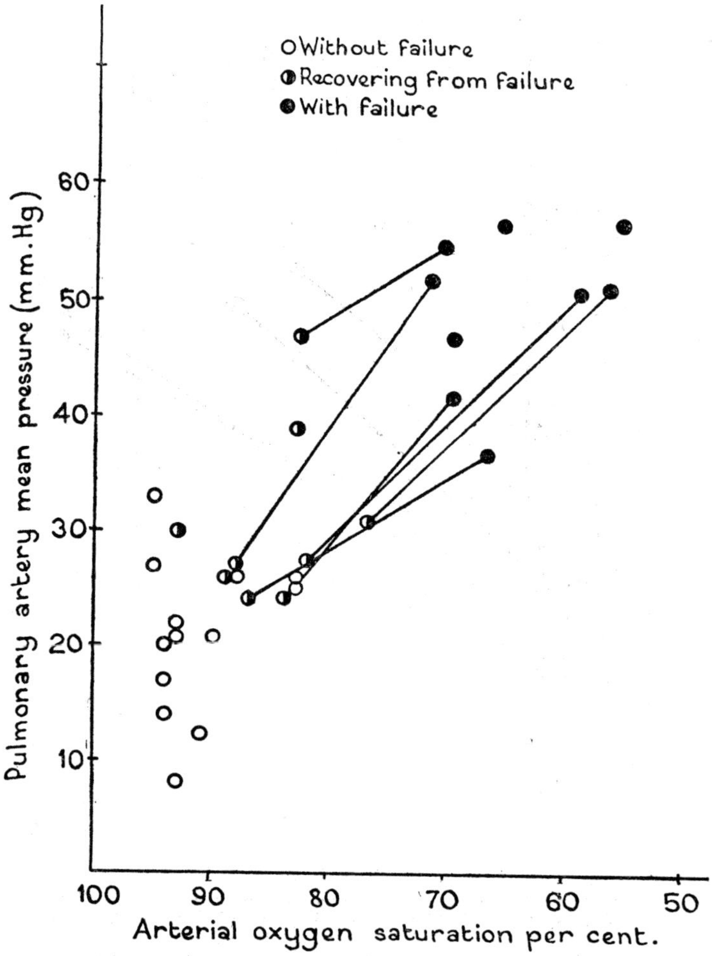

FIG. 2. Pulmonary artery pressure and arterial oxygen saturation in chronic lung disease with, without, and during recovery from congestive heart failure. Where two values are joined by a line, they refer to the same patient.

no heart failure, and the fall of pressure with recovery from failure was invariably accompanied by an increase of blood oxygen-saturation (Tables II and III; Figs. 2 and 3). A statistical analysis of 31 observations of the pulmonary artery mean blood-pressure and blood oxygen-saturation gave correlation coefficients of —0·83 between pressure and arterial oxygen-saturation and of —0·75 between pressure and mixed venous oxygen-saturation, suggesting more than a coincidental relation between these features. More direct evidence that

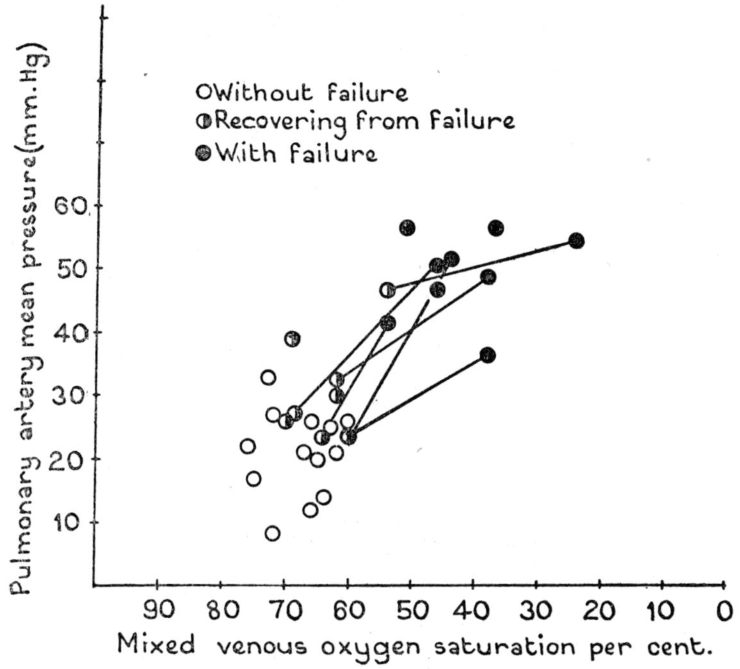

FIG. 3. Pulmonary artery pressure and mixed venous oxygen saturation in chronic lung disease with, without, and during recovery from congestive heart failure. Where two values are joined by a line, they refer to the same patient.

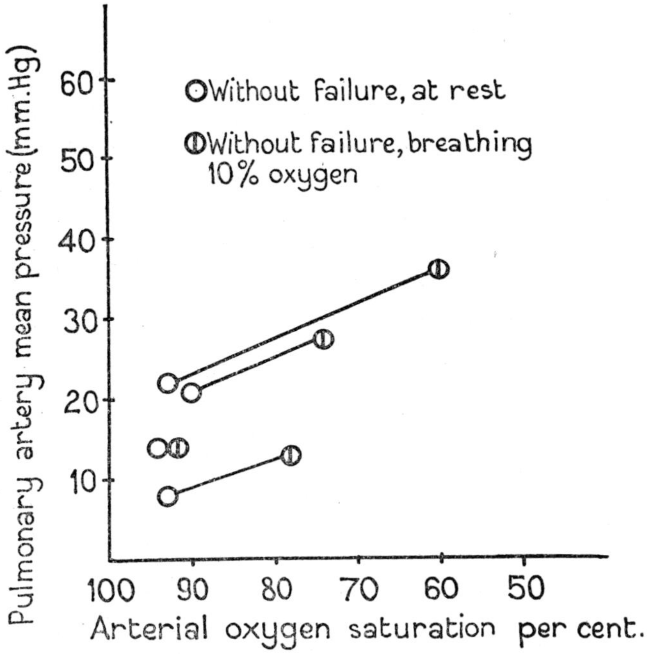

FIG. 4. Pulmonary artery pressure and arterial oxygen saturation in patients with chronic lung disease, without congestive failure, breathing (1) normal air and (2) 10 per cent. oxygen.

anoxia is a cause of pulmonary hypertension was provided by the observations of the effect of acutely induced anoxia. There was a rise of pulmonary artery mean blood-pressure in three patients breathing 10 per cent. oxygen who became anoxic, but no change of pressure in a fourth, in whom there was no significant alteration of blood oxygen-saturation (Table IV; Fig. 4). Similar

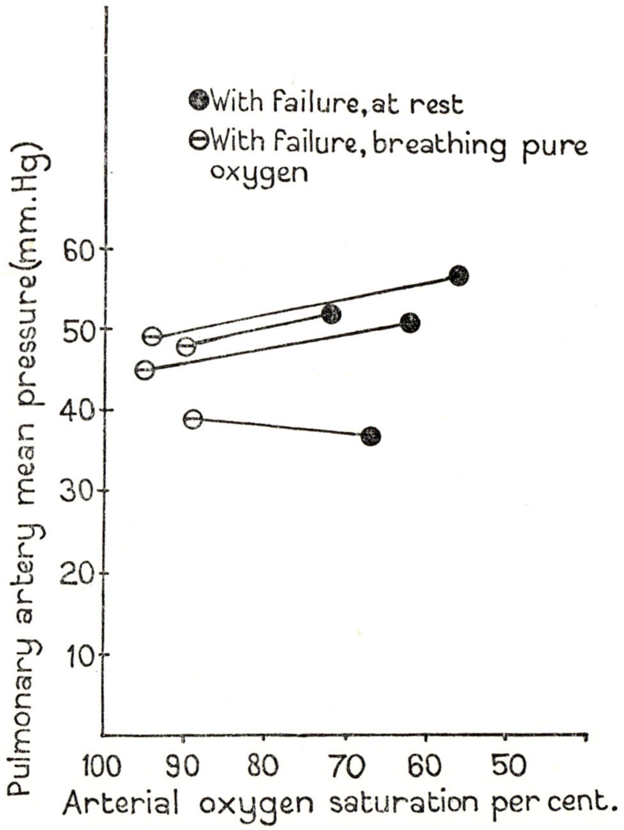

Fig. 5. Pulmonary artery pressure and arterial oxygen saturation in patients with chronic lung disease and congestive heart failure breathing (1) normal air and (2) pure oxygen.

observations of the induction of pulmonary hypertension by acute anoxia have been recorded in animals by von Euler and Liljestrand (1946), and in man by Motley, Cournand, Werkö, Himmelstein, and Dresdale (1947) and Doyle, Wilson, and Warren (1952). The latter observers suggested that anoxia causes an increase in pulmonary artery pressure by a direct vasoconstrictor effect of the low oxygen tension in the mixed venous blood on the pulmonary arterioles. No opinion can be expressed on the relative importance of arterial or mixed venous anoxia in producing pulmonary hypertension, as similar abnormalities of oxygen-saturation were invariably present in arterial and mixed venous blood in the present observations. While it is probable that anoxia is an important cause of pulmonary hypertension in congestive heart failure complicating chronic lung disease, as was suggested by Cournand (1950) and Harvey, Ferrer, Richards, and Cournand (1951), it is unlikely that pulmonary hypertension is due solely to vasoconstriction caused directly by anoxia, since restoration of normal blood oxygen-saturation by the administration of oxygen to patients with heart failure does not produce a fall in pulmonary artery blood-pressure

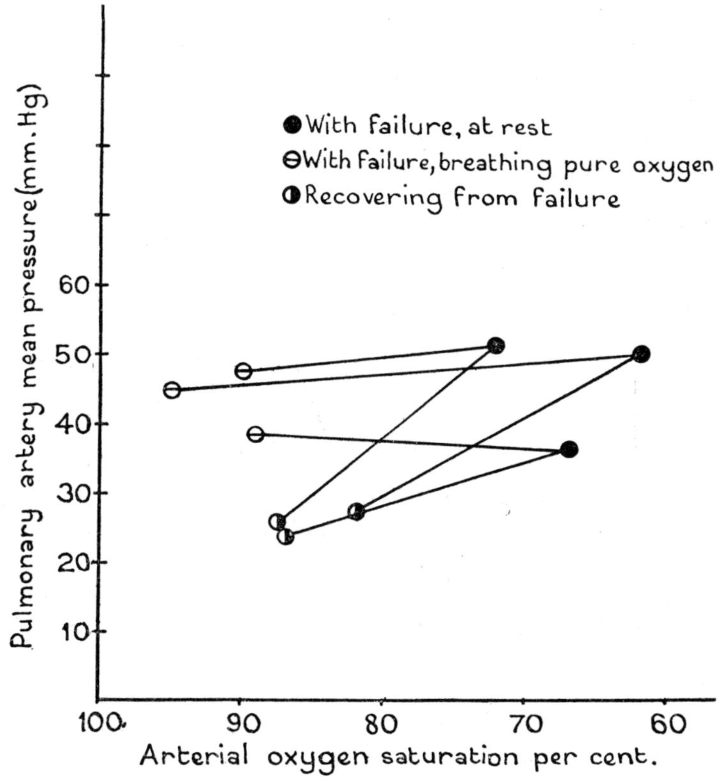

FIG. 6. Pulmonary artery pressure and arterial oxygen saturation in patients with chronic lung disease and congestive heart failure, breathing normal air and breathing pure oxygen, compared with the values obtained during recovery from failure.

comparable to that which occurs with recovery. When pure oxygen was administered to four patients (Cases 11, 13, 15, and 16) with congestive heart failure, the pulmonary artery mean blood-pressure fell in three and rose in one (Table IV; Fig. 5), but when pulmonary blood-pressures were subsequently recorded in three of these patients (Cases 11, 13, and 15) during recovery from failure (Table II), much lower values were found than had been observed during oxygen breathing, although there was not so great a rise in the oxygen-saturation of the arterial blood (Fig. 6).

Carbon dioxide retention. The possibility of carbon dioxide retention being a cause of pulmonary hypertension in chronic pulmonary heart disease was suggested by Cournand (1950). Evidence for this possibility is that carbon dioxide retention occurs in patients with congestive heart failure complicating chronic lung disease (Platts, 1953), and that carbon dioxide retention causes pulmonary hypertension in animals (von Euler and Liljestrand, 1946). The present results also support this view. The carbon dioxide content of mixed venous blood was higher in patients with pulmonary hypertension and heart failure than it was in those with lower pressures and no history of this complication, and furthermore,

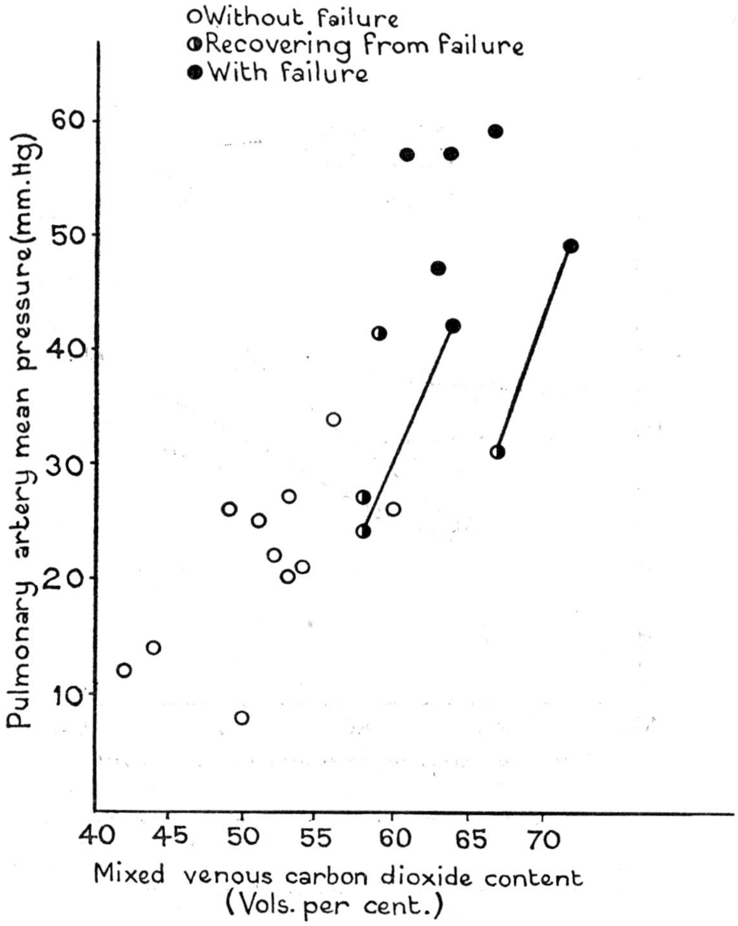

FIG. 7. Pulmonary artery pressure and carbon dioxide content of mixed venous blood in patients with chronic lung disease, with, without, and recovering from congestive heart failure. Where two values are joined by a line, they refer to the same patient.

in two patients who were studied twice, the fall of pulmonary artery pressure with recovery was associated with a fall of the carbon dioxide content of mixed venous blood (Table III; Fig. 7). For 21 observations the correlation coefficient between pulmonary artery mean blood-pressure and the carbon dioxide content of the mixed venous blood was 0·94. A pulmonary vasoconstriction produced by carbon dioxide may be partly responsible for the anomalous pressure changes which occur in patients with chronic pulmonary heart disease breathing pure oxygen, since Taquini, Fasciolo, Suarez, and Chiodi (1948) found that the carbon

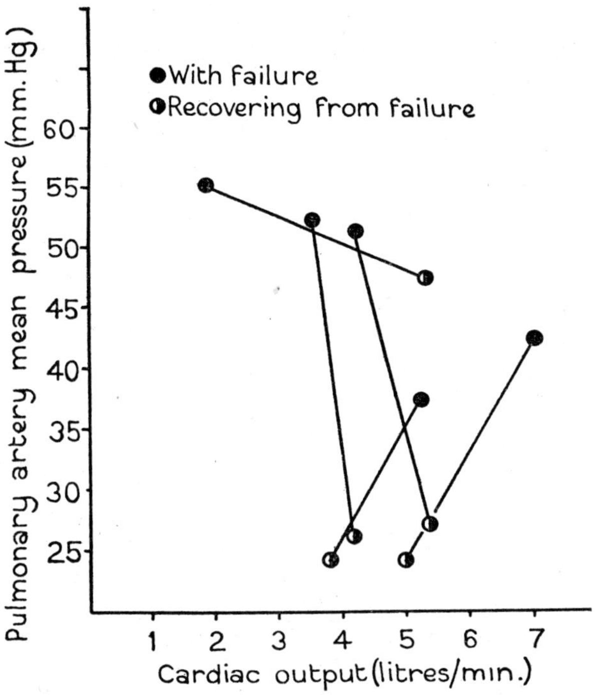

FIG. 8. Pulmonary artery pressure and cardiac output in patients with chronic lung disease, during congestive failure and during recovery.

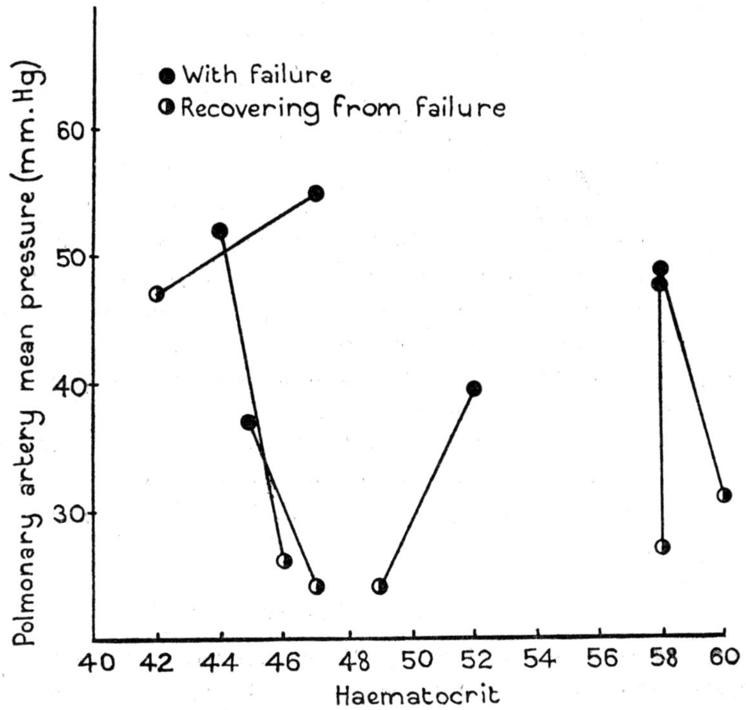

FIG. 9. Pulmonary artery pressure and haematocrit reading (per cent.) in patients with chronic lung disease, during congestive failure and during recovery.

dioxide of the arterial blood increased when emphysematous subjects breathed gas mixtures with a high oxygen-content. When there is no fall, or a rise, of pulmonary artery blood-pressure in patients with chronic pulmonary heart disease breathing pure oxygen, it is possible that a pulmonary vasoconstrictor effect due to retention of carbon dioxide has been equal to or greater than any dilator effect from the relief of anoxia.

Cardiac output. Since Hickam and Cargill (1948) and Riley, Himmelstein, Motley, Weiner, and Cournand (1948) had shown that increasing the pulmonary blood-flow by exercise caused a sharp rise in pulmonary artery blood-pressure in patients with chronic lung disease, and since McMichael and Sharpey-Schafer (1944) and Richards (1945) had found a high cardiac output in patients with congestive heart failure complicating chronic lung disease, it was reasonable for Cournand (1950) to suggest that this high cardiac output was a cause of pulmonary hypertension. In more recent observations, however, on the circulation in chronic pulmonary heart disease by Dexter (1949), Mounsey, Ritzmann, Selverstone, Briscoe, and McLemore (1952), and Fowler, Westcott, Scott, and Hess (1952), and in the present series, the cardiac output has usually been normal, and in the present series the cardiac output occasionally rose as the pulmonary artery blood-pressure fell during recovery (Tables II and III; Fig. 8). A high cardiac output cannot therefore be considered a consistent cause of pulmonary hypertension which develops with congestive heart failure. Mounsey and his colleagues (1952) criticized the use of the term 'high-output failure' to describe congestive heart failure complicating chronic lung disease, and in view of the reports of a normal cardiac output cited above, the view that the cardiac output is always or usually raised in this condition is now untenable. The present results, and those of Fowler, Westcott, Scott, and Hess (1952) indicate that the cardiac output in congestive heart failure complicating chronic lung disease may be high, low, or normal, but that it is usually normal (Tables II and III).

Blood viscosity. An increase in blood viscosity does not appear to be an important cause of pulmonary hypertension in congestive heart failure complicating chronic lung disease, since in the present series the disappearance of pulmonary hypertension during recovery from failure was not always accompanied by a fall in haematocrit value (Table II; Fig. 9).

Ventilatory function. The results of the simple ventilatory function tests were similar in patients with and without congestive heart failure. This observation supports the opinion of Harvey, Ferrer, Richards, and Cournand (1951) that there is no direct correlation between impairment of ventilatory function and the development of congestive heart failure in chronic lung disease.

Acknowledgements

I wish to thank Professor C. H. Stuart-Harris and Dr. C. Darke for permission to investigate patients under their care, Drs. M. W. A. Gatman and M. M. Platts for technical assistance, and Dr. C. E. Davies for much helpful advice in the preparation of the results for publication.

Summary and Conclusions

1. The pulmonary artery blood-pressure was recorded by cardiac catheterization in patients with chronic pulmonary disease with, recovering from, and without congestive heart failure, and simultaneous observations were made on the right auricular blood-pressure, the blood oxygen and carbon dioxide content, the haematocrit value, and the oxygen consumption.

2. Studies were made of 10 patients with heart failure, of six of these patients and three others recovering from failure, and of 13 without failure.

3. The relation between acute changes of blood oxygen-saturation and pulmonary blood-pressure was observed by giving pure oxygen to four patients with heart failure and a gas mixture containing 10 per cent. oxygen to four patients without failure.

4. Patients without heart failure had pulmonary artery mean blood-pressures which ranged from normal to twice normal, 8 to 33 mm. Hg, and patients with heart failure had pressures consistently higher than this, in the range 37 to 59 mm. Hg.

5. Recovery from heart failure was accompanied by a fall of pulmonary artery blood-pressure, and the majority of pressures in patients studied during recovery were within the range recorded in patients without failure. This observation indicated that heart failure was not caused by irreversible pulmonary hypertension.

6. Arterial and mixed venous anoxia was present in all patients with congestive heart failure, and recovery from failure was accompanied by an increase of blood oxygen-saturation. For these reasons, and since acutely induced anoxia raised the pulmonary artery blood-pressure, anoxia appeared to be a probable cause of pulmonary hypertension in patients with congestive heart failure.

7. Oxygen breathing in patients with congestive heart failure did not reduce the pulmonary artery blood-pressure to the levels recorded during recovery, although higher degrees of oxygen-saturation were achieved. Hence the pulmonary hypertension of congestive heart failure did not appear to be due solely to a pulmonary vasoconstriction produced directly by anoxia.

8. Carbon dioxide retention appeared to be a possible cause of the pulmonary hypertension of congestive heart failure, since it occurred in patients with heart failure, and since experimental work in animals had shown that such retention caused pulmonary hypertension.

9. A high cardiac output was not a consistent feature of patients with congestive heart failure complicating chronic lung disease, and the pulmonary hypertension of heart failure was not dependent upon an increase in cardiac output.

10. An increase in blood viscosity did not appear to be a cause of the pulmonary hypertension of congestive heart failure.

11. There was no significant difference in ventilatory function between the groups of patients with and without the complication of congestive heart failure.

REFERENCES

Bedford, D. E. (1951) *Proc. R. Soc. Med.* **44,** 597.
Borden, C. W., Wilson, R. H., Ebert, R. V., and Wells, H. S. (1950) *Amer. J. Med.* **8,** 701.
Cournand, A. (1950) *Circulation,* **2,** 641.
Dexter, L. (1949) *Bull. New Engl. Med. Center,* **11,** 240.
Doyle, J. T., Wilson, J. S., and Warren, J. V. (1952) *Circulation,* **5,** 263.
Euler, U. S. von, and Liljestrand, G. (1946) *Acta physiol. scand.* **12,** 301.
Ferrer, M. I., Harvey, R. M., Cathcart, R. T., Webster, C. A., Richards, D. W. Jnr., and Cournand, A. (1950) *Circulation,* **1,** 161.
Fowler, N. O., Westcott, R. N., Scott, R. C., and Hess, E. (1952) Ibid. **6,** 888.
Harvey, R. M., Ferrer, M. I., Richards, D. W. Jnr., and Cournand, A. (1951) *Amer. J. Med.* **10,** 719.
Hickam, J. B., and Cargill, W. H. (1948) *J. Clin. Invest.* **27,** 10.
McMichael, J., and Sharpey-Schafer, E. P. (1944) *Quart. J. Med.* N.S. **13,** 123.
Motley, H. L., Cournand, A., Werkö, L., Himmelstein, A., and Dresdale, D. (1947) *Amer. J. Physiol.* **150,** 315.
Mounsey, J. P. D., Ritzmann, L. W., Selverstone, N. J., Briscoe, W. A., and McLemore, G. A. (1952) *Brit. Heart J.* **14,** 153.
Platts, M. M. (1953) *Clin. Sci.* **12,** 63.
Richards, D. W. Jnr. (1945) *Federation Proc.* **4,** 215.
Riley, R. L., Himmelstein, A., Motley, H. L., Weiner, H. M., and Cournand, A. (1948) *Amer. J. Physiol.* **152,** 372.
Taquini, A. C., Fasciolo, J. C., Suarez, J. R. E., and Chiodi, H. (1948) *Arch. Int. Med.* **82,** 534.

616.13–005.7

THE EFFECTS OF PERIPHERAL ARTERIAL EMBOLISM[1]

By R. L. RICHARDS

(From the Gardiner Institute of Medicine, University of Glasgow)

Introduction

THE conception of embolism as we know it today is approximately a hundred years old. According to Welch (1910): 'Between the years 1846 and 1856 Virchow constructed the whole doctrine of embolism upon the basis of anatomical, experimental and clinical investigations which for completeness, accuracy and just discernment of the truth must always remain a model of scientific research in medicine.' During the past century much has been written on the subject but, at least so far as embolism of the peripheral arteries is concerned, the literature deals principally with the sources of emboli, with their sites of lodgement, and with the treatment of the condition. The clinical picture produced by the lodgement of an embolus in a peripheral artery has received relatively little attention. Most clinicians think of embolism as a condition with a dramatic onset, often accompanied by severe pain, and followed by numbness, loss of power, and pallor or lividity of the affected extremity. The effects of embolism are worthy of closer study, for the condition affords a unique opportunity for observing the effects of uncomplicated acute ischaemia in man. The purpose of the present paper is to review the effects of embolism of the peripheral arteries. The paper is based on a survey of the literature and on personal observations made in 52 cases of peripheral arterial embolism. Details of the cases are given in Table I.

TABLE I

Details of 52 Patients with Peripheral Arterial Embolism

		Treatment		*Results*			
Artery	*Number of emboli*	*Conservative*	*Embolectomy*	*Died*	*Loss of limb*	*Recovery with ischaemia*	*Complete recovery*
Aorta	12	8	4	9	0	2	1
Common iliac	1	0	1	1	0	0	0
External iliac	2	1	1	0	1	1	0
Femoral	25	15	10	8	2	10	5
Popliteal	5	4	1	1	1	2	1
Axillary	2	1	1	1	0	0	1
Brachial	9	8	1	0	0	2	7
Total	56*	37	19	20	4	17	15

* Four patients were seen in two separate embolic episodes.

[1] Received July 9, 1953.

Morbid Physiology

Before clinical features are considered, it is important to have a clear conception of the events which follow the lodgement of an embolus. The majority of emboli which obstruct systemic arteries are portions of blood-clot detached from a parent thrombus in the heart. The discussion which follows is concerned only with this type of embolism, but there is no reason to believe that similar emboli from other sources, such as clot in an aneurysm, or paradoxical emboli, behave differently. Lewis (1936) was the first to point out that an embolus of this nature is soft, and has approximately the same specific gravity as blood, and that therefore it cannot have a pronounced physical effect on the arterial wall. Immediately the embolus is arrested, however, with each cardiac systole it is subjected to a hammering effect by the onward thrust of the blood proximal to it. The force of this hammering depends on the efficiency of the patient's circulation at the time the embolus is thrown off; in a young patient with a well compensated mitral stenosis the force may be considerable; in a patient with congestive cardiac failure and a low blood-pressure from a transmural myocardial infarction it may be feeble. The effect of this hammering is either to dislodge the embolus and carry it forward to a more distal bifurcation, or to impact it firmly into its present site. In the latter instance the physical effects upon the arterial wall cannot be dismissed so readily. When the site of impaction of an embolus is exposed at operation, the onward thrust at each pulse is often striking, and, if embolism has occurred some hours previously, it is not unusual to find that the artery is slightly distended and its wall a little oedematous. Histological confirmation of these findings has been obtained by Fiolle (1937) and Haimovici (1937) in experimental embolism in dogs. They found swelling and oedema of the arterial wall in the early stages, followed later by cellular infiltration most marked in the adventitia and sometimes affecting the adjacent vein.

The lodgement of an embolus is followed by certain other events which have considerable influence upon the clinical picture. An embolus occludes only a short length of an artery. If a short length of a main artery is temporarily occluded by pressure, the blood-flow in the limb distal to the block falls temporarily to zero, but within a few minutes has returned to a normal level (Shepherd, 1950). The restoration of the circulation is effected through collateral channels. When arterial embolism occurs, the development of a collateral circulation may be hindered by any or all of three mechanisms:

1. *By occlusion of collaterals by the embolus.* Since an embolus usually lodges at an arterial bifurcation, it often occludes not only the main artery, but also the orifice of at least one major branch; the main artery cannot then be refilled by a collateral circulation utilizing that branch.

2. *By arterial spasm.* The idea that arterial spasm always follows the lodgement of an embolus, and that it may affect the main artery either proximal or distal to the embolus, and also involve collaterals, is one that is widely held.

3. *By consecutive thrombosis.*[2] Once an embolus is firmly impacted, thrombosis may occur either proximal to it or distal to it or in both sites. If anti-coagulants are not given, some degree of thrombosis distal to an embolus is almost invariable, but its extent is unpredictable. If embolectomy is delayed for some hours, a long 'tail' thrombus is frequently extracted from the artery distal to the embolus. Such a thrombus may be present within two hours of the onset of symptoms (Reynolds and Jirka, 1944); but even without anticoagulants thrombosis may be absent after five days (Nystrom, 1936). Distal thrombosis is favoured by the slowing of the blood-stream which inevitably follows the obstruction produced by the embolus, and will be further favoured if there is any disease, such as atheroma, of the artery. It is uncertain whether distal thrombosis begins immediately beyond the embolus or peripherally. The removal of a 'tail' thrombus at embolectomy indicates that thrombosis begins at the distal end of the embolus and is propagated centrifugally; but in cases coming to autopsy it is often found that the state of affairs in the affected artery is (1) embolus with its 'tail' thrombus, (2) an open segment, and (3) further occlusion by fresh thrombus, which suggests that thrombosis may also begin peripherally and spread backwards. Thrombosis proximal to an embolus is seldom extensive unless the circulation is failing, and is rarely of sufficient length to occlude a major branch (Linton, 1941). The importance of consecutive thrombosis is twofold: first it makes the block in the main artery irreversible; secondly, either by occluding their orifices or by extending into their lumina, it may occlude important collaterals through which the circulation to the limb might have been restored.

The occurrence and the importance of the first and third of these mechanisms are not disputed, but, although the majority of writers on the subject postulate that arterial spasm occurs, there are those who believe that the importance of spasm is overestimated, and that the clinical features which are attributed to spasm may all be explained by the occlusion produced by the embolus and consecutive thrombosis. Pickering (1951) in particular has called attention to the fact that 'the idea of severe and localized contraction of an artery, vascular spasm, occurring in the absence of a recognizable stimulus is entertained too freely and uncritically in current thought and writing'. It is therefore important to consider the evidence upon which the idea of arterial spasm associated with embolism is based. There are three observations which seem to indicate that arterial spasm does occur in these cases: (1) the finding of constricted arteries at operation; (2) the delay in the return of pulses after successful embolectomy, and (3) the condition known as 'pseudo-embolism'.

1. 'The extreme narrowing of both the external and the internal iliac arteries distal to the embolus should be noted. At operation this constriction extended as far as the vessels could be traced distally, that is to the inguinal ligament and into the pelvis, a distance of several centimeters' (Linton, 1941). 'The artery immediately peripheral to the occlusion is always in spasm by the time direct observation of the vessel is possible' (Reynolds and Jirka, 1944). 'In most of the common femoral embolectomies performed by the author spasm

[2] I prefer this term to secondary thrombosis, since the latter is also used to designate the thrombosis that may occur after embolectomy (McClure and Harkins, 1943).

of the superficial femoral artery just distal to the site of the occlusion was observed as soon as surgical exposure was effected' (Holden, 1952). These statements, selected at random from the recent literature, are typical of many observations. I have personally seen such distal arterial constriction on several occasions (for example, Case 4). It is doubtful, however, whether the arterial narrowing is due to spasm, if by spasm is meant a sudden and violent contraction of the arterial wall which is outside the normal range of vasoconstriction. When an embolus occludes an artery, the blood-pressure distal to it falls rapidly. A reduction in the calibre of the artery may merely reflect this fall in blood-pressure. Kinmonth (1952), who has recently studied the physiology of arterial spasm, has stressed the point that alterations in arterial diameter due to changes in arterial pressure should not be mistaken for spasm. Moreover Burton (1952) has pointed out that blood-vessels are distensible tubes, and as such have a 'critical closing pressure'; if the intraluminal pressure falls below this level, marked reduction in calibre is bound to follow. In the arm this critical closing pressure may be as high as 70 mm. of mercury. It is not difficult to imagine that the mean arterial pressure distal to an embolus, both in the main artery and in collaterals, may fall below this level. If this is the mechanism of arterial constriction distal to an embolus, it is certainly incorrect to refer to it as spasm. Some authors have stated that arterial spasm may also affect the artery proximal to an embolus, but I have not personally seen such an occurrence, and have been able to find only one record in which it has been clearly described: 'The common iliac artery above the embolus was also narrowed, but of utmost importance was the fact that contrary to the constriction distalward, it was very sharply localized so as to involve less than a centimeter of the artery' (Linton, 1941). More often the artery is seen to be pulsating vigorously down to the point at which the embolus is impacted.

2. If the records of cases in which embolectomy has been successfully performed are carefully scrutinized, it is remarkable that it is very seldom stated that pulsation reappeared immediately in the distal arteries. Although the circulation may return rapidly, as judged by improvement in the colour and temperature of the limb, it is often hours, days, or even weeks before the pulses can be felt. Nystrom (1936) discussed this delay in the return of the peripheral pulse, and attributed it to arterial spasm. If his hypothesis is accepted, it must be postulated that in some cases arterial spasm may persist for several days. Smooth muscle in the walls of other hollow viscera does not behave in this way, and Kinmonth (1952) in his experiments found that traumatic arterial spasm passed off after two to three hours. Once the embolus, and 'tail' thrombus, if present, have been removed, the artery will be open to systemic blood-pressure. This should not take long to open the distal arteries, unless opposition is offered either by active contraction of the circular muscle-fibres in the arterial walls or by occlusion of the lumina by thrombus. It is difficult to believe that the former could delay the return of the pulses for more than a few hours. When the brachial or axillary artery is ligated the radial pulse is often palpable within 24 hours, and when the femoral artery is tied the posterior tibial pulse may be felt

within seven to ten days. In these instances the return must be through collateral channels. These observations suggest that, in the majority of instances in which the peripheral pulses do not return within 24 hours of embolectomy, the cause of the delay is not arterial spasm but organic occlusion in the main artery distal to the embolus. A further observation relating to the return of circulation, which seems to indicate that an embolus may provoke arterial spasm, is the following. When an embolus occludes the aortic bifurcation, the lower half of the abdominal wall, which is supplied by the inferior epigastric artery, is rendered ischaemic. A knowledge of anatomy suggests that there should be a readily available collateral supply to this area through the superior epigastric branch of the internal mammary artery and the subcostal arteries (Quiring, 1949). Yet my experience has been that after aortic embolism the lower abdominal wall may remain ischaemic, as judged by the persistence of pallor and the absence of bleeding when the tissues are incised, for as long as nine hours. I have seen an analogous persistence of unilateral ischaemia in a case of embolism of the common iliac artery, and Holden (1952) has observed a similar phenomenon in a case in which a small embolus was eventually found at the bifurcation of the popliteal artery. Active arterial constriction provoked by the lodgement of the embolus seems to be the only adequate explanation for these findings, but the evidence suggests that it is not a myogenic arterial spasm, but a neurogenic reflex constriction which can be relieved by spinal anaesthesia or paravertebral block.

3. The condition known as 'pseudo-embolism' is one in which all the features of embolism except the embolus are present. There are a number of well authenticated cases of this condition on record, such as those of Atlas (1942) and Learmonth (1948). So far as I am aware, the condition has not been reported in a patient who has not either a history of other definite embolic episodes, or else a possible source of an embolus. It has therefore been assumed that the condition is due to spasm of a main artery provoked by the lodgement of a small embolus in one of its branches. Some instances of pseudo-embolism are undoubtedly due to emboli which first occlude a main artery, and then slip into a branch where their presence cannot be detected clinically, for example the profunda femoris, as in a case reported by Pickering (1951, Case 2). I do not think this can be the explanation in all cases. I have seen a case in which the initial features were those of occlusion of the bifurcation of the aorta and in which, without operation, complete recovery occurred, with return of all the peripheral pulses. It is difficult to believe that an embolus large enough to occlude the aortic bifurcation could disappear so completely. Burt, Learmonth, and Richards (1952) have recorded two other cases in which the initial symptoms of aortic occlusion were followed by rapid and complete recovery in one lower limb and slow recovery in the other. This occurrence might suggest that the embolus had been dislodged into the limb which recovered more slowly; but in one such limb the femoral and popliteal arteries were explored without finding an embolus. Active arterial constriction seems to be the most satisfactory explanation of the symptoms in these cases also.

In conclusion, there is good evidence that arterial constriction occurs in most cases of embolism, but it is debatable whether this constriction comes within the category of arterial spasm. The physiology of arterial spasm is poorly understood, but it is a direct response of the smooth muscle in the arterial wall, and has to be differentiated from any reduction in arterial calibre due to a fall in intraluminal pressure, and from vasoconstriction due to reflex nervous activity. The stimuli which are known to cause arterial spasm are sudden arterial distension (Haimovici, 1937) and mechanical stimuli such as pinching or traction (Kinmonth, 1952). In embolism only the first of these stimuli could be present, and in some cases it may provoke true myogenic arterial spasm, but in most cases the so-called arterial spasm has a simpler explanation.

Clinical Features

1. *Onset.* The idea that embolism is a condition with a dramatic onset invariably associated with pain is one which dies hard. Haimovici (1950), in a recent review of 330 cases of embolism of the arteries of the limbs, found that 82 per cent. had a sudden onset, 12 per cent. had a slowly progressive onset, and 7 per cent. were 'silent'. My own experience has been somewhat similar. Of 48 cases of embolism in which data regarding the onset are adequate, the onset was sudden in 37. The initial symptom is most often pain, but numbness or coldness of the extremity, either sudden or progressive, precedes pain in about one-third of the cases.

2. *Pain* is generally considered the most prominent symptom in cases of peripheral embolism, but there has been much controversy about the incidence, the character, and the cause of the pain in such cases (Table II). Even in those instances in which pain is not the initial complaint, it usually develops within a matter of minutes, and rapidly becomes the dominant symptom. Painless embolism of a peripheral artery is not unknown; I have seen three cases of proved embolism (one of aortic embolism and two of embolism of the brachial artery) in which I am certain that the condition was painless. The character of the pain in cases of embolism is disputed. Most continental writers refer to it as a sudden sharp pain: like a 'stab with a dagger' (Nystrom, 1936); 'un véritable coup de fouet' (Haimovici, 1937). British and American authors, while admitting the severity of the pain, are inclined to describe it as a burning, throbbing, or aching type of pain. The problem of the character of the pain is inevitably linked with that of its causation. Until 1936 it had always been assumed that the sudden onset of pain signalled the impaction of the embolus in the artery, and that the pain was due to a stimulus set up in the arterial wall (Table II). This view was strongly challenged by Lewis in his Gibson Lecture to the Royal College of Physicians of Edinburgh (Lewis, 1936). He suggested that the pain of embolism was the result of ischaemia of muscle, and that its appearance did not indicate the moment of lodgement of the embolus. In support of this hypothesis he put forward cogent arguments which may be summarized as follows:

(1) Pain is not invariably the initial symptom of peripheral embolism.

(2) When pain is the initial symptom, it is followed too rapidly by numbness and paralysis for these to be due to a period of ischaemia starting at the moment of pain.
(3) Pain occurs only when an embolus occludes an artery supplying a muscular organ; compare embolism of the limbs or heart with cerebral or pulmonary embolism.
(4) Pain is felt not at the site of impaction of the embolus, but distally, usually in a muscular portion of the limb.
(5) When embolectomy is successful, pain is not relieved by the removal of the embolus, but only when the circulation is restored.

It might be expected that the opinion of such an authority, supported by these observations, would be generally accepted. A survey of the literature relating to embolism since 1936 shows that this is not so (Table II). Only Reynolds and Jirka (1944), and to a lesser extent Rykert and Graham (1938), have accepted Lewis's hypothesis. Until recently I was convinced that Lewis's view that ischaemia was the cause of the pain in cases of embolism was correct, and that the idea of a sudden embolic ictus with pain was erroneous. A short time ago, however, I had the good fortune to see a case in which I was certain that the onset of a sudden, sharp pain in the groins marked the moment of lodgement of bilateral femoral emboli (Case 1). In this case pain in the legs did not appear until after the anterior tibial and calf muscles were exercised. This experience has convinced me that, as Rykert and Graham (1938) have suggested, in some cases of embolism there are two distinct pains: an initial pain which is sharp, worst at the onset, and felt at the site of occlusion, and a later pain which comes

TABLE II

Pain in Peripheral Arterial Embolism

Author	*Type of pain*	*Site of pain*	*Cause*
Welch (1910)	Like a painful blow	Site of lodgement	Distension of artery. Irritation of nerve-endings in arterial wall
Seifert (1931)	Like a whip lash	Site of lodgement	Arterial spasm
Danzis (1933)	Sharp and persistent	Site of lodgement	Spasm of artery and branches
Lewis (1936)	Continuous ache	Distal in muscular portion of limb	Muscle ischaemia
McKechnie and Allen (1936)	Sudden and severe	Difficult to localize	Arterial spasm
Funck-Brentano (1937)	At first local, sharp. Later diffuse	Initially at site of lodgement, then spreading diffusely distalward	Distension of artery and irritation of peri-arterial sympathetic plexus
Rykert and Graham (1938)	Initial pain: sharp, worst at onset	Site of lodgement	Arterial spasm
	Later pain: prolonged distress	Distal	Muscle ischaemia
Lesser (1943)	..	Anywhere distal to site of occlusion	Spasm of main artery and collaterals
Reynolds and Jirka (1944)	Constant and agonizing	Distal, referred to muscular area	Muscle ischaemia
Haimovici (1950)	..	Region of lodgement	Arterial spasm
Holden (1952)	Burning 'Pins and needles'	Zone between ischaemic and normal tissues	Arterial spasm. Acute ischaemia

on gradually, but rapidly becomes severe, situated distal to the site of occlusion and aggravated by movement of the limb. The initial pain is probably often not recorded because, unless the patient is seen within a few minutes, the later severe and progressive pain will be present and will claim the patient's full attention. In cases in which numbness or coldness is the first symptom the initial pain must be absent or slight. Its occurrence may depend upon the innervation of the segment of artery which is occluded; Wilde (1951) has shown that the femoral artery has a very rich sensory nerve-supply. An alternative suggestion is that the initial pain occurs only when the occlusion is immediately complete; in those instances in which it is absent the embolus may not occupy the entire lumen of the artery, and the block is slowly completed by consecutive thrombosis. Several authors (Haimovici, 1937; de Takats, 1942) have commented on the fact that painless embolism is most often seen in patients who are gravely ill as a result of their cardiac disease.

With regard to the cause of the pain, the impaction of a soft blood-clot in the artery cannot, as already stated, have much physical effect on the vessel wall. A large embolus may distend an artery. According to Brun (1952) it is well established that distension of an artery causes pain, but it has to be admitted that Moore and Moore (1933), in their careful experiments on arterial sensation, found that distension did not cause pain. The idea that arterial spasm is the cause not only of the initial pain, but also of the later pain, is one that is widely held (Table II). Fiolle (1937) suggested that the lodgement of an embolus is followed by a wave of spasm spreading distally along the artery and its branches, an arterial colic. The pain of embolism, however, does not resemble that of either renal or intestinal colic. The idea that arterial spasm is of itself a painful condition is one for which there is no good evidence. Unequivocal arterial spasm is most often seen as a sequel to trauma. I have seen a number of patients with traumatic arterial spasm, and my impression is that they do not experience much pain until the effects of ischaemia are well established. Even if arterial spasm occurs in cases of arterial embolism, I think it is unlikely that it is a cause of pain. For reasons already given I agree with Lewis (1936) that ischaemia is the principal cause of pain in cases of embolism, but I doubt whether muscle is always the tissue from which the pain arises. Pain is sometimes most severe on the dorsum of the foot or in the palm of the hand, relatively non-muscular areas (for example in Case 2). This later pain is indistinguishable from that experienced in other types of acute ischaemia of a limb, as in acute arterial thrombosis or gunshot wounds involving the main arteries. Thus the initial pain of embolism, when it occurs, may be due to sudden arterial distension, but the later pain is certainly due to ischaemia.

3. *Vascular disturbances.* Next to pain, the most striking features of arterial embolism are the vascular disturbances. Of these the most important is the absence of pulsation in arteries distal to the level of occlusion. Unfortunately the state of the peripheral pulses in the limbs of patients who have cardiac lesions which predispose to embolism is seldom recorded before a frank embolic episode is suspected. In such cases the peripheral arteries should be examined

as a routine, and it will often be found that one or more of the important pulses, especially in the lower limbs, is absent, probably as the result of a 'silent' embolism. When a patient with heart disease complains of pain, numbness, or coldness in a limb, and it is found that one or more of the pulses in that limb cannot be felt, a presumptive diagnosis of embolism can be made. It is then important to determine the most proximal level at which pulsation is absent, so as to localize the site of impaction of the embolus. For this purpose an oscillometer or a sphygmomanometer cuff may be helpful. A possible source of error, which is not well recognized, is that the downward thrust of each pulse on the impacted embolus may be transmitted along the artery for some distance (Nordentoft's sign) and be mistaken for a pulse; I have seen the popliteal artery explored in error because it was thought that pulsation was present in the lower thigh, when in reality the embolus was lodged at the origin of the profunda femoris. Changes in the colour and objective coldness of the affected extremity are well recognized signs. In the early stages pallor is more often seen than lividity, but after a few hours cyanotic patches develop, and give the limb a mottled appearance. To palpation there is often quite a sharp change between the zone of normal temperature and the area of coldness, but this line of demarcation is seldom a useful guide to the level of occlusion. The condition of the superficial veins of the limb is of interest. Soon after the occlusion they are found to be empty, or if emptied by light pressure they do not refill even when the limb is a little below the level of the heart. Nystrom (1936) has picturesquely described this as 'the sign of the dried up river-bed'. Later, however, even when the occlusion remains complete, the superficial veins are found to be full of blood, and if emptied will refill slowly. My observations lead me to believe that this change takes place about eight to twelve hours after the onset. I am not sure why the change occurs, but Haimovici (1950) has commented on the frequency with which deep venous thrombosis occurs in cases of embolism, and it may be that when this happens there is a damming back of any small trickle of blood which still enters the limb.

The fate of the limb is usually decided within the first 72 hours. If medical or surgical treatment is not instituted, either a collateral circulation develops which is adequate for the basic needs of the limb, or gangrene ensues. In the latter event the limb becomes swollen, blood is extravasated into the skin, and subcutaneous tissues and blisters may form. This is followed by drying and shrinking of the tissues, and finally by necrosis. Occasionally, when all appears to be going well, gangrene develops insidiously several days later (Case 2).

4. *Motor disturbances.* In the majority of descriptions of the effects of peripheral embolism, loss of power is the only disturbance of muscular activity that is recorded. Although paralysis certainly occurs, there are other changes in the muscles which are of equal or greater importance in assessing the prognosis. The degree of paralysis in cases of embolism varies considerably. It may appear rapidly; Reynolds and Jirka (1944) mentioned that peripheral paralysis may be complete within half an hour of the onset. I have seen complete paralysis of both lower limbs within one and a half hours of aortic occlusion (Burt,

Learmonth, and Richards, 1952). The paralysis is often patchy; for example, in a case of femoral embolism the long flexors of the toes continued to be active for several hours after all other muscles in the leg were paralysed, and in a case of axillary embolism only the extensors of the fingers and of the thumb were paralysed. This peculiarity suggests that ischaemia of muscle rather than of nerve is the cause of the paralysis. If the tone and consistence of the affected muscles are examined after embolism, it will be noticed that they show a relatively constant series of changes (Table III). As paralysis develops the muscle-

TABLE III

Peripheral Arterial Embolism: Effects of Ischaemia

Time (hours)	*Muscles and joints*	*Prognosis (if circulation restored)*
0 to 6	Onset of paralysis. Consistence of muscles normal. Tenderness +++. Joints slightly flexed; slight elastic resistance to extension	Complete or almost complete recovery
6 to 48	Paralysis fully developed. Muscles firm, and tenderness ++. Marked flexion-contracture of digits and ankle (or wrist). Tendons stand out as tight cords. Marked resistance to passive movement, which causes pain	Limb may be saved, but complete functional recovery unlikely
48 et seq.	Persisting paralysis. Muscles become soft and only slightly tender on deep pressure. Joints lax, and passive movement easily performed. Swelling of limb	Muscles dead. Motor recovery impossible. Amputation probable

bellies become tender to palpation. At first their consistence is normal, but after about six hours they become firm and contractures develop, which are more pronounced in the flexor muscles, so that a flexion deformity of the digits and wrist or ankle appears, and the tendons stand out as firm cords. Attempts to overcome these contractures by passive movement meet with resistance, and cause pain in the stretched muscles. This stage passes more slowly into one in which the muscles soften and are no longer tender except on deep pressure, and the joints now become lax. The times at which one stage passes into the next are not fixed, and vary from patient to patient; factors such as the level of occlusion, the completeness of the occlusion, and the state of the collateral vessels influence the rapidity of their development, but in untreated patients the three stages are invariably present. By recognizing the stage which has been reached it is possible to assess the need for urgent treatment, and to give some estimate of the likely outcome. There is little information in the literature about the reflexes in peripheral arterial embolism. It is recognized that when paralysis is complete the tendon reflexes are absent (Welch, 1910), but my experience has been that the reflexes are lost early, even before paralysis is extensive (for example in Case 1). I have never observed the reflexes to be other than absent or diminished, although Rothstein (1935) stated that they may be increased.

5. *Sensory disturbances*. Pain, coldness, and numbness are the commonest

subjective complaints of patients who have an embolic occlusion of a peripheral artery. Paraesthesiae of the 'pins and needles' type are seldom experienced. This is not altogether surprising, for it has been found that when the circulation to a limb is interrupted ischaemic paraesthesiae last for a few minutes only, no matter how long the period of ischaemia (Merrington and Nathan, 1949). The occasional persistence of paraesthesiae for more than a few minutes is in my experience a favourable sign; such paraesthesiae are of the post-ischaemic variety, and indicate a developing collateral circulation. Objective sensory loss characteristically begins in the digits and spreads centripetally. All modes of sensation are affected. On two occasions I have been able to observe loss of appreciation of passive movement of the toes when pain and touch sensation were still intact (for example in Case 5). The distribution of the cutaneous sensory loss is almost always of the glove, stocking, or slipper pattern. A 'slow pain' response may be elicited long after all other modes of sensation are absent, and pain on stretching or compressing ischaemic muscles can frequently be elicited from a segment of limb which has lost all cutaneous sensation.

6. *Factors influencing the clinical picture.* It is well recognized that there is no clear-cut clinical picture which can be looked upon as diagnostic of the lodgement of an embolus at a given site. Numerous factors, for example the pre-existing cardiac or other lesion, the state of the peripheral arteries, and the rapidity with which consecutive thrombosis develops, modify the situation. A factor which is often present in cases of embolism, and which influences the picture in a rather unexpected way, is the presence of an old and often unsuspected embolism in the limb. In a case of aortic embolism reported previously (Burt, Learmonth, and Richards, 1952, Case 15) the patient was not seen until 24 hours after the onset of symptoms. At this time it was noticed that, although the clinical picture was clearly that of aortic embolism, the right lower limb was considerably less affected than the left. At autopsy it was found that there were old emboli in the right external iliac and femoral arteries (Fig. 1). In another patient (Case 1) the history and initial clinical findings indicated the lodgement of bilateral femoral emboli. Within three hours the left lower limb had returned to normal, although the pulses were still absent; on the right the foot remained ischaemic, and eventually became gangrenous. *Post mortem*, in addition to the two recent emboli, an old organized clot was found occluding the left popliteal bifurcation (Fig. 2). It therefore appears that the presence of a previous arterial occlusion helps to protect a limb from the effects of an acute ischaemia produced by a more proximal obstruction. At first sight this appears paradoxical, but the explanation must be that the old occlusion has already stimulated the formation of collateral channels in the limb, which is thereby more favourably placed to withstand the second embolic episode. A second factor may operate in the same direction: as a sequel to the first occlusion the tissues of the limb may have become adapted to a reduced blood-supply.

7. *The late effects of embolism.* Cases of peripheral arterial embolism in which embolectomy is not successfully performed may follow one of four courses: (1) The patient dies soon after the embolic episode, from the combined effects

of the embolism and the primary disease. (2) The patient survives, but the affected limb becomes gangrenous and has to be amputated. (3) The limb is preserved, but there is some persistent loss of function. (4) Complete recovery occurs. The first two groups account for about half of all the cases of embolism that are recognized clinically: 40 per cent. in Haimovici's (1950) series, and 24 of the 52 cases in the present series. The last two groups comprise the cases

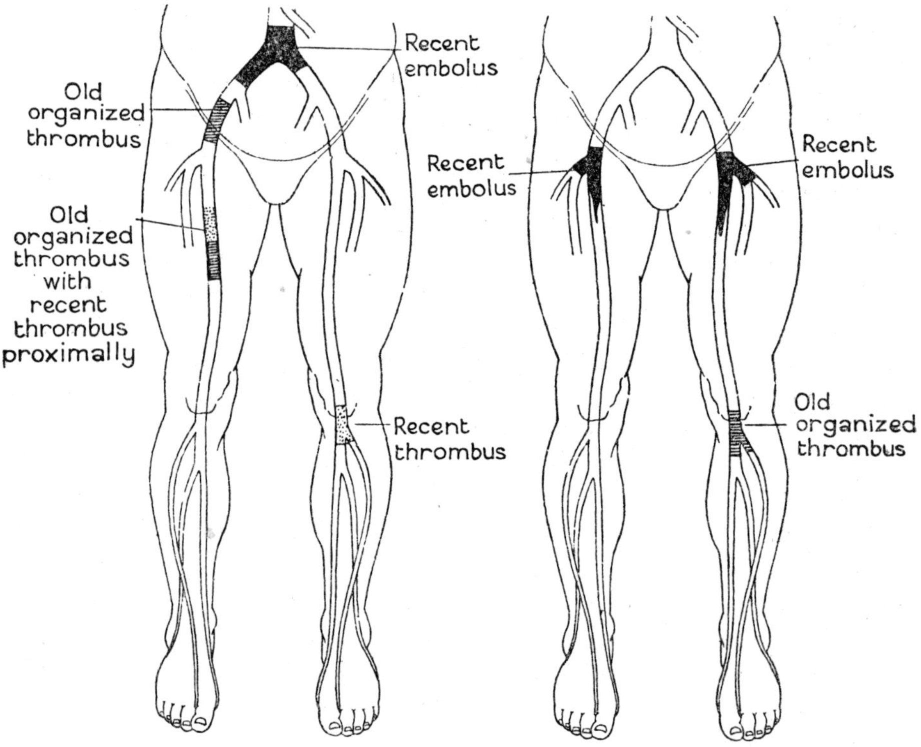

FIG. 1. Case of aortic embolism with old occlusions in the right external iliac and femoral arteries.

FIG. 2. Case of bilateral femoral embolism with an old occlusion in the left popliteal artery.

which are referred to as 'embolismes manqués' by Fiolle (1937). Few cases fall into the fourth group, probably because the majority of such cases are not recognized. I have seen only four cases in which, without embolectomy, recovery of function in the limb was complete within 72 hours of the first symptom, and these were all cases in which the upper limb was affected. The third group comprises the cases which show the clinical picture of chronic post-embolic ischaemia. The manifestations of this condition are varied. Often the patient complains that his limb is persistently cold and is painful. The pain may be that of intermittent claudication or that of ischaemic neuropathy (Richards, 1951). Contractures similar to Volkmann's ischaemic contracture of the forearm flexors are sometimes seen, as Griffiths (1940) pointed out. Paralysis often persists; this may be due to muscle ischaemia, in which case it often has a patchy distribution; but it may also be the result of an ischaemic nerve lesion.

I have seen several instances of femoral or popliteal embolism in which the residual disability was a lateral popliteal nerve palsy (for example Case 3), and elsewhere two cases of aortic embolism have been described in which the late effects appeared to be those of a root lesion (Burt, Learmonth, and Richards, 1952). These late effects are often very troublesome; they may recover slowly in a period of months, but sometimes remain as a permanent disability.

Treatment

The choice lies between conservative treatment and embolectomy. The aim of the former is to provide the best conditions for the development of a collateral circulation. The position of the ischaemic limb is important, and the advice given by Hippocrates, 'neither raised very high up, nor inclined much downward, but rather upward' (Adams, 1939) is still sound. Pain must be relieved; for this morphine is the best drug, and also has some vasodilator action (Himmelsbach, 1944). In my experience other vasodilator drugs are seldom helpful. Papaverine was given either intravenously or intra-arterially in some of the cases in the present series, but Kinmonth (1952) has clearly shown that, to be effective in relieving arterial spasm, this drug has to be applied locally to the arterial wall. In two recent cases tolazoline hydrochloride ('priscol') was given by intra-arterial injection, but I was not convinced that it influenced the outcome. The prevention of consecutive thrombosis is the most important objective. Immediately the diagnosis of embolism is made, 10,000 units of heparin should be given intravenously, and thereafter its administration should be continued at intervals of four to six hours until either embolectomy is to be performed or the fate of the ischaemic limb is decided. In the former event, before operation, the effect of the heparin can be neutralized by an injection of protamine sulphate. The difficulty is that the heparin penetrates only slowly to the place where it is most needed, the arteries distal to the site of occlusion.

Embolectomy is theoretically the ideal treatment; early removal of the embolus should allow rapid restoration of a normal circulation. It has already been pointed out that in practice this result rarely happens. Nevertheless embolectomy is the treatment of choice in aortic embolism, from which spontaneous recovery is rare (Milwidsky, Ehrenfeld, and de Vries, 1952), and probably also in embolism of the common iliac artery. In smaller arteries embolectomy is technically more difficult, especially for a surgeon who is not expert in arterial surgery. In the upper limb the results of conservative treatment are so good that I doubt whether embolectomy is ever indicated. The decision for or against embolectomy is most difficult in cases of femoral embolism. Many successes have been reported from embolectomy, but I believe that equally good results may be achieved if the patient is seen early and treated medically by modern methods. In the present series (Table I), of the five patients who recovered completely after femoral embolism, three had embolectomy and two were treated conservatively; both the patients who lost their limbs had previously been operated upon for removal of the embolus, and of the eight deaths, two followed embolectomy and four occurred in patients who were considered too ill for operation. Three of the 10 patients who had post-embolic ischaemia of the affected limb had been operated upon; the remainder were treated conservatively. These figures, although small, do not provide convincing evidence in favour of embolectomy. If the operation is to be performed, it should be done early; after 10 hours the number of successful results falls rapidly (Nystrom, 1936; McClure and Harkins, 1943). At this stage one cannot be certain whether spontaneous recovery will occur and, if one waits, the chance of obtaining the best result by embolectomy may be lost. The best policy seems to be a compromise. When a patient is seen within eight hours of the onset, medical treatment should be instituted. If after two to three hours it is apparent that the condition of the limb is not improving—and it is at this time that the state of the muscles and joints provides the best guide—then, if the patient's general condition does not preclude operation, embolectomy should be advised.

APPENDIX

Case Reports

Case 1. Bilateral femoral embolism; immediate pain; old left popliteal embolism.

A male patient aged 27 years, suffering from rheumatic heart disease and auricular fibrillation, was convalescent from an attack of congestive cardiac failure, and had been up and about for a week. He was sitting on the edge of his bed, and had just had his temperature and pulse taken by a nurse, who noted nothing abnormal. He got up to walk up the ward, and 'felt something give in his heart'. Immediately thereafter he experienced a sharp pain in both groins, which caused him to cry out and fall back on his bed. When he was seen within a few minutes there was no local abnormality in the groins, but neither femoral pulse was felt. By the time his shoes and socks were removed his feet were already pale. He could move his feet and toes normally, and sensation was not impaired. The knee- and ankle-jerks were present. While he was being examined he stated that the pain had moved down to his calves, and approximately 10 minutes after his first symptom he complained of numbness of the toes. The pain in the legs rapidly became severe, and soon overshadowed all other symptoms. Thirty minutes after the onset the right knee- and ankle-jerks were absent, appreciation of passive movement of the toes was lost, and there was a level of sensory loss to pin-prick just above the malleoli. He could still plantar-flex and dorsiflex the right foot, and there was slight voluntary flexion of the toes. On the left side there was only slight weakness of dorsiflexion of the toes, with hypalgesia of the distal two-thirds of the foot and diminished tendon-reflexes. At one hour, on the right side there was complete paralysis and sensory loss, except for deep sensation, distal to the knee. At three hours the left lower limb was normal apart from the absence of pulses. Some recovery had also taken place on the right side: plantar flexion of the foot and slight dorsiflexion of the toes could be performed, and the level of sensory loss had receded again to the ankle. Because of this favourable progress embolectomy was not attempted. The improvement was not maintained; a commencing contracture of the calf muscles was noticed at seven hours, and by 12 hours was fully developed. Shortly after this his general condition suddenly deteriorated and, 48 hours after the embolic episode, he died. At autopsy recent emboli were found in both femoral arteries at the level of the origin of the profunda femoris; 'tail' thrombi extended distally from both emboli for a distance of 3 cm. on the left and 2 cm. on the right. Distal to this point the arteries were patent on the right, but on the left the popliteal artery was found to be occluded for a distance of 4 cm. by an old, firmly adherent, fibrous thrombus. The presence of mitral stenosis was confirmed, and 60 gm. of clot were removed from the left atrium. A recent occlusion, probably embolic, of a penetrating branch of the left coronary artery was found; this was thought to be the cause of the sudden deterioration in his general condition.

Case 2. Embolism of left external iliac artery; little pain; delayed onset of gangrene.

A 33-year-old housewife, who was known to have rheumatic heart disease, was admitted to hospital five days after an episode in which her left leg had suddenly become heavy and stiff, 'as though I had been lying on it for too long'. She was in bed at the time, and did not experience any pain. Her husband massaged the foot, and about three hours later the leg felt 'more normal' and she got up. She was able to walk, but when she did so experienced a burning feeling on the dorsum of the foot. This pain was severe enough to make her go back to bed. Thereafter she had recurrent attacks of this burning pain in the foot, always most intense on the dorsum, and frequently awakening her at night. Persistent coldness of the foot was her only other complaint. Examination on admission showed that she had mitral stenosis and auricular fibrillation. In the left lower limb all the pulses were absent, whereas on the right they were easily felt. There were no contractures, and a full range of active and passive movement, with normal power, was present. The left ankle-jerk was diminished, but other reflexes were normal. There was hypalgesia of the anterior half of the left foot, and vibration was not appreciated on the tip or at the metatarsophalangeal joint of the great toe, but sensation of passive movement was normal. The left foot felt ice-cold and was slightly cyanotic, with abnormal pallor of the toes. The veins were full, and refilled slowly after emptying. For 18 days the objective condition of the foot did not change appreciably, although she continued to complain of pain on the dorsum of the foot, especially on the inner side. Twenty-three days after the onset of her symptoms the great toe developed a persistent cyanosis, and slowly became gangrenous. The area of necrosis spread to involve the dorsum of the foot and the tip of the second toe, but remained localized. Eventually amputation of all the toes was performed, but the patient has a useful foot, and is able to get about as well as her cardiac disability will allow.

Case 3. Popliteal embolism; ischaemic palsy of lateral popliteal nerve.

A 41-year-old woman, with long-standing mitral stenosis and auricular fibrillation, had a right hemiplegia, presumably due to cerebral embolism. She was admitted with a complaint of sudden, severe pain in the left leg of several hours' duration. The left foot was pale, the veins were collapsed, and the popliteal, posterior tibial, and dorsalis pedis pulses were absent, but the femoral pulse could be felt down to the adductor hiatus. All muscles of the leg were paralysed and, although there was no contracture, the calf and anterior tibial muscles were tender on pressure. The ankle-jerk could not be elicited. Position sense in the toes was lost, and there was a 'sock' area of analgesia. Spontaneous recovery occurred; by next morning there was a noticeable degree of dropped foot, with slight contracture of the calf muscles; active plantar flexion of the foot and toes was present, but the peronaei and all the anterior tibial group were still paralysed. Sensory loss was now confined to the dorsum of the foot and toes. Within the next 48 hours the posterior tibial muscles recovered full power and the ankle-jerk returned, but 10 days passed before any voluntary power was found in the anterior tibial group of muscles. Progress thereafter was slow; three months after the embolic episode she was still experiencing pain in the foot suggestive of ischaemic neuropathy, and the dorsiflexors of the foot and toes, especially extensor hallucis longus, were weak.

Case 4. Right femoral embolism; embolectomy; recovery.

A housewife, aged 48 years, with established mitral stenosis and auricular fibrillation, was admitted to hospital because of increasing dyspnoea. She responded well to rest in bed and an increased dosage of digitalis. After tea on the day before she was to go home she was restless, and about an hour later noted numbness of her right foot. When she felt the foot it was cold, and within a few minutes she experienced a gnawing pain in the front of the leg, which rapidly became severe. Two hours later pain was still present, but had been eased by an injection of morphine sulphate gr. $\frac{1}{4}$. The right foot was blanched, and the veins empty. A strong femoral pulse was felt, but the popliteal, posterior tibial, and dorsalis pedis pulses were absent on that side. Tenderness was elicited at the apex of the femoral triangle in the line of the femoral artery. Below the knee the only voluntary movement was weak plantar flexion of the foot. There were no contractures, but even gentle palpation of the calf and of the anterior tibial muscles was painful. The ankle-jerk was absent, the knee-jerk present. The level of analgesia was at approximately mid-leg. Appreciation of passive movement was absent in the toes. A diagnosis of embolism of the right femoral artery was made. Because her general condition was good, and because only two hours had elapsed since the onset, embolectomy was advised. At operation (four hours after the first symptom) the right femoral artery was exposed under local anaesthesia. The common femoral artery was pulsating strongly to the point where it divided. At this level it appeared a little distended, and it was obvious that there was a solid mass within the lumen. Distally the superficial femoral artery was constricted; its diameter was estimated to be about a quarter of that of the artery proximal to the block. The profunda artery was also constricted; the vessel appeared so small that at first it was mistaken for an anomalous lateral femoral circumflex artery arising directly from the common femoral trunk. The constriction affected both arteries as far distally as they were exposed. The embolus was easily removed from the bifurcation, and a gush of blood from the proximal artery followed. Only a sluggish flow of dark blood issued from the distal arteries, but no further thrombus could be extracted. The artery was sutured, and before the wound was closed it was noticed that the profunda was pulsating slightly. After operation there was a rapid improvement in the limb. A pink flush was noticed to spread slowly downwards from the knee. Because of the amount of sedation the patient had received it was difficult to ascertain when her pain disappeared, but four hours after operation it was certainly gone. She then said that her foot felt warm and tingled, and she could move her toes. Next day the limb was apparently normal, but the ankle-jerk was still absent, and the pulses in the foot had not yet returned. Complete recovery followed, but six weeks later she had a fatal cerebral embolus.

Case 5. Left popliteal embolism.

A young man with auricular fibrillation was seen as an out-patient, complaining of numbness and tingling in the left foot, of sudden onset. On examination the only abnormalities were absent pulses in the foot, loss of position sense in the great toe, and an absent ankle-jerk. A diagnosis of popliteal embolism was made, and he was advised to come into hospital, but refused. Two days later he was admitted to another hospital with acute abdominal pain, and a diagnosis of mesenteric embolism was made. He died, and at autopsy multiple visceral infarcts were found. Unfortunately the vessels of the limbs were not examined.

Summary

The events which follow the lodgement of an embolus in a peripheral artery are reviewed in detail. Impaction of an embolus is followed by constriction of the main artery and its branches distal to the level of the embolism. This constriction, which is often referred to as spasm, may be due entirely to the fall in blood-pressure caused by the sudden interruption of the flow along the main artery. Arterial constriction proximal to an embolus is sometimes present, and is probably due to a nervous reflex. It is doubtful whether true myogenic arterial spasm occurs in cases of embolism. Consecutive thrombosis in the arterial tree distal to the embolus, rather than arterial constriction, is the factor which interferes most with the development of a collateral circulation.

The clinical features of peripheral arterial embolism have been studied, and certain points are emphasized. The onset is not always sudden, and pain need not be the initial symptom. In some cases a brief, sudden, sharp pain is felt at the site of lodgement of the embolus. The cause of this pain is uncertain, but it must arise from stimulation of nerve-endings in the arterial wall; distension rather than spasm is favoured as the stimulus. The principal pain of embolism develops gradually, and is felt distal to the site of occlusion; it is due to ischaemia of muscle and other tissues. The muscles and joints of the ischaemic limb pass through a regular sequence of changes. These are described in detail, and from a knowledge of the stage which has been reached a reasonably accurate prognosis may be given. It has been found that the presence of a previous, often unsuspected, embolus in a limb helps to minimize the effects of a second, more proximal, embolism. In a number of cases chronic post-embolic ischaemia of the limb may follow; the manifestations of this condition are variable, and often very troublesome to the patient. The principles of treatment are outlined.

REFERENCES

Adams, F. (1939) *The Genuine Works of Hippocrates*, Baltimore and London.
Atlas, L. N. (1942) *Surg. Gynec. Obstet.* **74**, 236.
Brun, G. C. (1952) In *Visceral Circulation*, ed. G. E. W. Wolstenholme, London.
Burt, C. C., Learmonth, J., and Richards, R. L. (1952) *Edin. Med. J.* **59**, 65.
Burton, A. C. (1952) In *Visceral Circulation*, ed. G. E. W. Wolstenholme, London.
Danzis, M. (1933) *Ann. Surg.* **98**, 249.
Fiolle, J. (1937) *J. chir.*, Paris, **50**, 460.
Funck-Brentano, P. (1937) Ibid. **50**, 433.
Griffiths, D. L. (1940) *Brit. J. Surg.* **28**, 239.
Haimovici, H. (1937) *Les Embolies artérielles des membres*, Paris.
—— (1950) *Angiology*, **1**, 20.
Himmelsbach, C. K. (1944) *J. Pharmacol.* **80**, 343.
Holden, W. D. (1952) *Acute Peripheral Arterial Occlusion*, Springfield, Ill.

Kinmonth, J. B. (1952) *Brit. Med. J.* **1,** 59.
Learmonth, J. R. (1948) *Edin. Med. J.* **55,** 449.
Lesser, A. (1943) *J. Amer. Med. Ass.* **122,** 285.
Lewis, T. (1936) *Clin. Sci.* **2,** 237.
Linton, R. R. (1941) *New Engl. J. Med.* **224,** 189.
McClure, R. D., and Harkins, H. N. (1943) *Surgery,* **14,** 747.
McKechnie, R. E., and Allen, E. V. (1936) *Surg. Gynec. Obstet.* **63,** 231.
Merrington, W. R., and Nathan, P. W. (1949) *J. Neurol. Neurosurg. Psychiat.* **12,** 1.
Milwidsky, H., Ehrenfeld, E. N., and de Vries, A. (1952) *Angiology,* **3,** 275.
Moore, R. M., and Moore, R. E. (1933) *Amer. J. Physiol.* **104,** 259.
Nystrom, G. (1936) *Lectures on Embolism and Other Surgical Subjects,* Baltimore.
Pickering, G. W. (1951) *Lancet,* **2,** 845.
Quiring, D. P. (1949) *Collateral Circulation,* London.
Reynolds, J. T., and Jirka, F. J. (1944) *Surgery,* **16,** 485.
Richards, R. L. (1951) *J. Neurol. Neurosurg. Psychiat.* **14,** 76.
Rothstein, J. L. (1935) *Amer. J. Dis. Child.* **49,** 1578.
Rykert, H. E., and Graham, D. (1938) *Amer. Heart J.* **15,** 395.
Seifert, E. (1931) *Dtsch. Zts. Chir.* **232,** 187.
Shepherd, J. T. (1950) *Clin. Sci.* **9,** 355.
Takats, G. de (1942) *Surg. Clin. N. America,* **22,** 199.
Welch, W. H. (1910) In Allbutt and Rolleston, *A System of Medicine,* London, vol. vi, p. 809.
Wilde, F. R. (1951) *Brit. J. Surg.* **39,** 97.

616.155.191–085: 539.165

TREATMENT OF POLYCYTHAEMIA VERA WITH RADIOPHOSPHORUS[1]

Haemological Studies and Preliminary Clinical Assessment

By JOHN D. ABBATT, H. CHAPLIN, J. M. M. DARTE, and W. R. PITNEY

(From the Medical Research Council's Radiotherapeutic Research Unit and Blood Tranfusion Research Unit, and the Department of Pathology, Post-graduate Medical School of London)

The treatment of polycythaemia vera with radioactive phosphorus is now established as the most effective method which has been employed up to the present time (Tinney, Hall, and Giffen, 1943; Erf and Jones, 1943; Reinhard, Moore, Bierbaum, and Moore, 1946; Lawrence, 1949; Wiseman, Rohn, Bouroncle, and Myers, 1951). As indicated by Lawrence (1949), this method of treatment must not be regarded as curative. It is rather a form of maintenance therapy which, by inducing remissions, eliminates the causes of polycythaemic death and is thus able to extend the patient's expectation of life to one approaching normal for his age. The present paper reports the method of radioactive phosphorus therapy which has been employed at Hammersmith Hospital since 1950, and the preliminary results obtained. The general pattern of response confirms that previously reported by a number of American workers (Lawrence, 1949), and will not be reported in detail. We were particularly concerned to ascertain whether the platelet response was comparable to that which follows external X-irradiation, and whether there was any correlation with the clinical response. Therefore during the observation of our patients the early haematological response was studied in considerable detail. Accurate observations of red-cell mass and plasma-volume have been relatively infrequently reported (Prentice, Berlin, and Lawrence, 1952; Wilson and Boyle, 1952). Careful measurements of plasma-volume and red-cell mass were made in order to ascertain whether any constant pattern was present in patients suffering from polycythaemia vera, and to define the type of response which followed treatment with radiophosphorus.

Patients Investigated

The 27 patients investigated have been sufferers from polycythaemia vera, unselected except by their reference to Hammersmith Hospital. All are alive at the present time; their ages range from 37 to 82 years, and the sex ratio is three female to two male patients. Four patients are of Eastern European

[1] Received June 15, 1953.

Jewish origin. The duration of the condition when the patients were first seen varied from 16 years to six months. Eleven had received previous treatment by methods other than venesection, that is, by external irradiation or by haemolytic drugs. No patient has so far developed leukaemia or myelosclerosis; but one has had a 'leukaemoid' blood picture, which has remained unchanged throughout the period of observation and treatment (four years). All patients fulfilled the usual clinical and haematological criteria for the diagnosis of polycythaemia vera. One presented a diagnostic problem when first admitted to the Hospital, and illustrates the type of case liable to be misdiagnosed unless the possibility of polycythaemia vera is borne in mind. Because of the unusual features her case history is briefly presented.

Case 15. A woman aged 65 years was seen on account of peripheral vascular disease and gangrene of a toe. The spleen was palpable. Examination of the blood revealed an iron-deficiency anaemia; the red blood-cell count was 4,000,000 per c.mm., the haemoglobin 9·3 gm. per 100 ml. (63 per cent.), the haematocrit level 32 per cent., reticulocytes 3·6 per cent., white-cell count 15,000 per c.mm., and platelets 1,600,000 per c.mm. In view of the characteristics of this anaemia, search was made for a site of bleeding, and the stools were found to contain altered blood. The very high platelet count made the diagnosis of polycythaemia vera probable. Many megakaryocytes were present in the sternal marrow. Blood-volume studies revealed a 24 per cent. increase above normal. After a period of observation the red-cell count rose to 6,900,000 per c.mm., and the haematocrit level to 51 per cent. After treatment with ^{32}P her platelet count has become stabilized at about 300,000 per c.mm., and the haematocrit level has remained at 44 per cent. for six months. The patient is now in good health.

Methods

1. *Technique of treatment.* Before 1950 the method of treatment at Hammersmith Hospital generally involved a small preliminary venesection followed by a course of two injections (of 2 to 4 millicuries each) of ^{32}P, with a 10-day interval between injections. In 1950 the method was changed, and, since all the original patients have relapsed and have been treated again on one or more occasions since 1950, they are now included in the interim results of response to the standard technique which is described below. During the course of diagnosis a careful clinical assessment was made, and base-line observations were obtained which included complete blood counts, marrow examination, a chest X-ray, and, where possible, blood-volume estimations. The patient then received a single intravenous injection of 5 to 8 millicuries of ^{32}P as inorganic phosphate, without preliminary venesection. It was considered that venesection would be indicated only if there were signs of an impending vascular accident. The patient was discharged from hospital on the third or fourth day after injection, when the urinary excretion of ^{32}P had reached a safe level (100 microcuries or less in 24 hours).

2. *Follow-up procedure.* Where possible the patient was seen, and blood counts made, at least weekly for the first three months or longer, until the full response to treatment was assessable. At this time the patient's condition was

evaluated to decide whether a satisfactory remission had been induced. If relief of the symptoms and signs of the disease was inadequate, a further injection of ^{32}P was given. Once a satisfactory remission had been obtained, the patients were seen at intervals of one to two months.

3. *Haematological methods.* Blood counts were performed from venous samples. Haemoglobin estimations, haematocrit readings, red- and white-cell counts, and reticulocyte counts were carried out by methods described by Dacie (1950). Double the usual quantity of diluting fluid was used when enumerating red cells. Platelet counts were performed by a modification of Kristenson's method (Lempert, 1935). All platelet counts were made by one observer. The diluting fluid was freshly mixed and filtered daily; in this way satisfactory preparations and consistent values could always be obtained. The normal platelet range in health by this method is 150,000 to 300,000 per c.mm. Bone-marrow aspiration was carried out on all patients when they were first seen. In a few patients this examination was repeated one week after administration of ^{32}P. All marrow aspirations were taken from the sternum. The material aspirated was usually very viscid, containing many fragments. It was found advantageous to mix the fragments with a drop of the patient's serum on a slide before films were made. Marrow films were stained with a combination of May–Grünwald and Giemsa stains at pH 6·8.

4. *Blood-volume measurements.* (1) *Red-cell volume* (RCV^{32P}) was measured by the radioactive-phosphorus method of Reeve and Veall (1949) as modified by Chaplin (1953).

(2) *Plasma-volume* (PV) was measured by the injection of Evans blue (T1824) after at least 12 hours of starvation. The light-absorption by the dye in heparinized plasma, from samples taken at 15, 30, and 45 minutes after injection, was measured in a photoelectric colorimeter, using a deep red filter (combination of Ilford 803 and 205). The concentration of the dye at 'zero time' was obtained as described by Chaplin, Mollison, and Vetter (1953). The dye-disappearance curves obtained from all but two of the present group of patients were not demonstrably different from those obtained in this laboratory with the same batch of Evans blue in a large series of normal and anaemic subjects. It can be concluded that the blood-sampling schedule described above generally gives adequate time for mixing to occur, in spite of the increased viscosity of polycythaemic blood. In two patients, whose haematocrit readings were 78 per cent. and 82 per cent., a steady decrease in the plasma dye-concentration did not become established until 20 to 30 minutes after injection, and consequently the value of the 15-minute sample was ignored in these two instances. By taking care not to allow drying of the blood on the walls of the test-tubes, pipettes, and syringes, haemolysis was successfully avoided in all cases, and thus did not contribute any error to the colorimetric estimations.

5. *Estimation of red-cell volume from plasma-volume.* Heparinized blood was used in all cases. Haematocrit levels were determined in Wintrobe tubes spun at 3,000 r.p.m. for 30 minutes in a centrifuge of radius 15 cm. The 'true venous haematocrit value' was obtained by correcting observed values for plasma

trapping, using a calibration curve, as described by Chaplin and Mollison (1952). In calculating red-cell volume from plasma volume (RCV^{PV}) the 'body haematocrit value' was determined by multiplying the 'true haematocrit value' by the constant 0·91, as described by Chaplin, Mollison, and Vetter (1953). Thus:

$$PV\ (T\ 1824) \times \frac{100}{100 - \text{body hct. value}} = \text{total blood volume } (BV^{PV});$$

$$RCV^{PV} = BV^{PV} - PV^{PV}.$$

Haematological Results

1. *Standard procedures*

Values before treatment (Table I). Red-cell counts ranged from 6,000,000 to 12,000,000 per c.mm., with a mean of 7,900,000 per c.mm. Haematocrit values

TABLE I

Blood Findings Before Treatment

Test	*Number of patients*	*Mean*	*Range*
Red-cell count (millions/c.mm.)	27	7·9	6·0–12·0
Haematocrit value (%)	26	64	48–82
Reticulocytes (per 100 red cells)	20	2·5	0·9–4·4
Platelet count (per c.mm.)	24	490,000	210,000–1,200,000
White-cell count (per c.mm.)	27	16,500	7,900–34,000

ranged from 48 to 82 per cent., with a mean of 64 per cent. The lower haematocrit values were generally found in patients who had a history of either gastro-intestinal haemorrhage or therapeutic venesections; in these cases the red cells were hypochromic and microcytic. Throughout the series mean corpuscular volumes were on the low side of normal, even in patients with no history or evidence of loss of blood. The average reticulocyte count was 2·5 per 100 red cells; in view of the high average total red-cell count this is striking evidence of increased red-cell production. Total white-cell counts before treatment ranged from 7,900 to 34,000 per c.mm. The leucocytosis, when present, was predominantly polymorphonuclear, neutrophils making up 90 per cent. of the white cells. The neutrophils showed a shift to the left; a few metamyelocytes, and occasionally myelocytes, were observed in films of peripheral blood. It should be noted that in nine cases (33 per cent.) the leucocyte count was 11,000 per c.mm. or less. Seven patients (26 per cent.) had platelet counts within the normal range when first seen, that is, not greater than 300,000 per c.mm. by Lempert's method. In the remainder of the series the platelet counts were elevated, in two patients to 1,000,000 or more per c.mm. The marrow was hypercellular in all cases; the fragments were solidly packed with cells, and the fat-spaces were much reduced. Erythropoeisis was normoblastic in all cases. Megaloblasts were not seen. The myeloid:erythroid ratio was usually within the normal range, indicating that the marrow had undergone a general hyperplasia. Megakaryocytes were usually prominent in the films. Although megakaryocyte counts were not attempted, it was our impression that these cells were especially numerous in cases showing very high platelet counts.

Response to treatment. The platelets were the first cellular element of the peripheral blood to be depressed, though this depression was generally not obvious until about 20 days after administration of ^{32}P. The lowest levels were not reached until 30 to 50 days, and in one case not until 62 days, after the

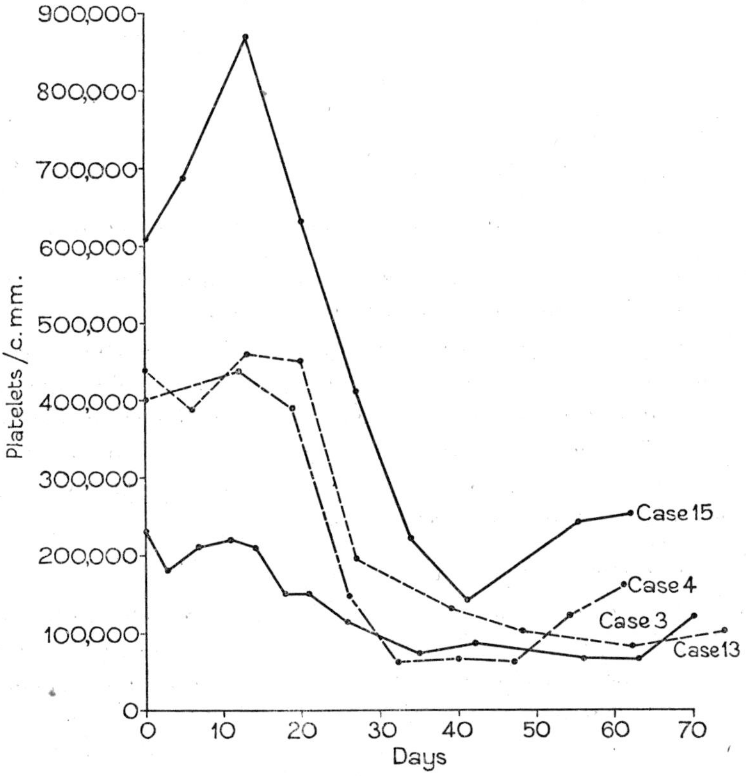

Fig. 1. Typical platelet responses to radiophosphorus.

radiophosphorus injection. The platelet counts illustrated in Fig. 1 are representative of the type of response which preceded a satisfactory remission. In patients who did not respond to ^{32}P the pattern of platelet response was similar, but the degree of depression was not as great as in the successful cases. This relation between the degree of depression of the platelets and the response to therapy is further illustrated by Table II, in which it is shown that the mean platelet level reached by patients having a successful remission was 75,000 per c.mm., as opposed to a mean of 136,000 per c.mm. in patients having only a partial remission. It was noticed that if the platelet count fell below 100,000 per c.mm. a remission usually ensued, and that if the count failed to fall below this level a satisfactory remission was usually not attained. This relationship, however, was not without exception. In the cases in which a remission was attained the platelet count settled at a figure considerably lower than before the injection. The average platelet count in patients who attained a remission, when examined six months after injection, was 210,000 per c.mm., compared with an average count of 640,000 per c.mm. before injection. No similar correlation was discernible between the degree of total or differential leucocyte depression and the subsequent remissions. The white-cell count was much

TABLE II

Extent of Platelet Depression after a Single Injection of ^{32}P

Group	*Number of patients**	*Platelets per c.mm.* *Mean*	*Range*
Full remission	7	75,000	20,000–140,000
Partial remission	4	136,000	95,000–190,000

* Only patients whose progress has been followed weekly are included.

more variable in its behaviour than the platelet count. The total white-cell count fell at a variable time, usually shortly after the platelet depression, and rose more slowly. About the sixth to eighth week the haematocrit level began to drop; it usually became stabilized three to four months after treatment (see Fig. 2*b*). Fig. 2 (*a* and *b*) shows the haematological response of one patient to 6·0 millicuries of ^{32}P, plotted in one instance weekly and in the other monthly. It illustrates the necessity of weekly haematological observations if the full extent of the early platelet response is to be assessed.

2. *Blood-volume measurements*

Levels before treatment. The blood-volumes of 17 patients were measured before they were treated. None of the patients was in congestive failure. In 10 patients simultaneous measurements of red-cell volume and plasma-volume were made. In the remaining seven patients total blood-volume was calculated from the measurement of plasma-volume alone. The results are shown in Table III. By means of the 'body haematocrit value' ('true venous haematocrit value'×0·91) the total blood-volume (BV^{PV}) and red-cell volume (RCV^{PV}) were calculated from plasma-volume in all cases. Where red-cell volume measurements were made simultaneously with plasma-volume measurements, these values are also given (RCV^{32P}). It can be calculated that the mean variation of the measured RCV^{32P} from the calculated RCV^{PV} is 6 per cent. in the 18 instances in which simultaneous measurements of red-cell volume were made. All 17 patients had elevations of the red-cell volume and total blood-volume above the expected values for normal adults of equivalent weight and surface area. It is remarkable, however, that the magnitude of the increase in blood-volume is poorly correlated with the elevation of the haematocrit value in the range 45 to 75 per cent. In Table IV the cases are arranged in the order of increasing haematocrit values. The total blood-volume (BV^{PV}) of each patient is expressed as a percentage increase above the expected normal value as defined by Gibson and Evans (1937). It will be seen that for the five patients with observed haematocrit values in the range 45·0 to 60·0 per cent. the mean increase in total blood-volume was 43 per cent. For the nine patients with haematocrit values from 60·0 to 75·0 per cent. the mean increase in blood-volume was 54 per cent. But within these two groups there were many cases

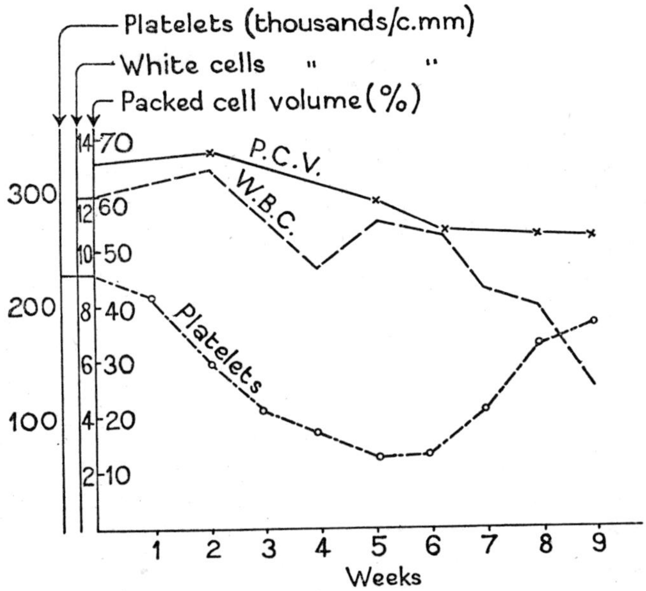

FIG. 2*a*. Haematological response to radiophosphorus, measured weekly.

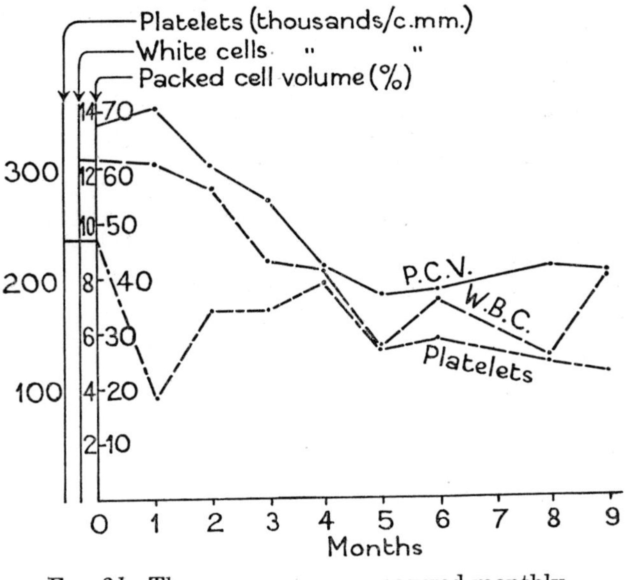

FIG. 2*b*. The same response measured monthly.

which did not follow this general trend. The most striking examples of these discrepancies are Case 17, with a haematocrit value of only 57 per cent. but with an 85 per cent. increase in blood-volume, and Case 1, with a haematocrit value of 71·5 per cent. and an increase in blood-volume of only 4 per cent. (see also

TABLE III

Blood-Volume Data Before Treatment in 17 Patients with Polycythaemia Vera*

Case number	*Body-weight (kg.)*	*Body-surface area (sq.m.)*	*'True venous haematocrit value'* (%)	*Plasma-volume PV(T1824) (ml.)*	*Red-cell volume* *RCV32P (ml.)*	*RCVPV (ml.)*	*Blood-volume BVPV (ml.)*
1	78·2	1·95	67·7	2,202	..	3,536	5,738
2	59·5	1·70	65·0	2,810	..	4,075	6,885
3	57·3	1·67	66·2	2,658	..	4,022	6,680
4	51·0	1·63	73·1	2,037	4,325	4,163	6,200
5	52·8	1·55	46·3	2,392	1,740	1,740	4,132
6	43·7	1·40	67·8	1,903	3,197	3,077	4,980
7	50·0	1·48	67·7	2,341	..	3,759	6,100
8	56·8	1·56	68·5	1,950	..	3,227	5,187
	56·8	1·56	35·3	2,499	..	1,181	3,680
9	66·5	1·75	54·8	2,767	..	2,753	5,520
	65·5	1·73	39·3	2,945	..	1,643	4,588
10	61·8	1·70	75·3	2,458	..	5,372	7,830
	64·1	1·72	28·1	3,949	1,519	1,361	5,310
11	64·0	1·64	47·7	3,660	3,085	2,805	6,465
	72·3	1·72	50·4	2,618	2,827	2,222	4,840
12	66·2	1·78	67·8	2,550	4,242	4,130	6,680
	64·9	1·77	54·7	2,915	2,818	2,893	5,808
13	59·5	1·86	61·1	2,950	3,724	3,695	6,645
	62·3	1·90	45·6	3,205	2,289	2,275	5,480
14	46·7	1·53	77·6	2,355	5,890	5,662	8,017
	47·8	1·55	51·6	3,238	2,813	2,867	6,105
15	47·8	1·41	43·3	2,403	1,691	1,564	3,967
	51·8	1·46	39·8	2,397	1,366	1,365	3,762
16	75·0	1·88	59·0	3,635	3,758	4,220	7,855
	70·0	1·82	61·5	3,508	3,972	4,467	7,975
17	67·9	1·87	54·4	4,920	4,432	4,820	9,740
	71·8	1·92	53·5	4,300	4,283	4,085	8,385

* Wherever two values are given, the second value refers to studies during the stable phase after treatment (see text).

TABLE IV

Elevation in Total Blood-Volume Before Treatment in Relation to Packed-Cell Volume

Case number	*Observed haematocrit value* (%)	*Variation of total blood-volume from normal** (%)	
15	45·3	+24	
5	48·6	+12	
11	51·0	+49	Mean:
17	57·0	+85	+43
9	57·7	+40	
16	62·4	+96	
13	64·6	+28	
2	69·0	+76	
7	69·9	+77	Mean:
3	69·9	+71	+54
1	71·5	+ 4	
12	71·6	+36	
6	71·8	+55	
8	72·4	+40	
4	77·3	+43	Mean:
10	79·9	+101	+84
14	82·3	+108	

* These values refer to the figures for the total blood-volume in normal adults in relation to surface area, after Gibson and Evans (1937).

Fig. 3). Examination of the values for plasma-volume shed some light on this interesting problem. The response of the plasma-volume to the increase in red-cell volume is variable in these patients. In six out of 16 cases a partial compensatory decrease in plasma-volume below normal was observed. In five cases the plasma-volume was normal, while in the remaining five cases it was moderately to markedly increased in spite of the increase of red-cell volume. Case 17

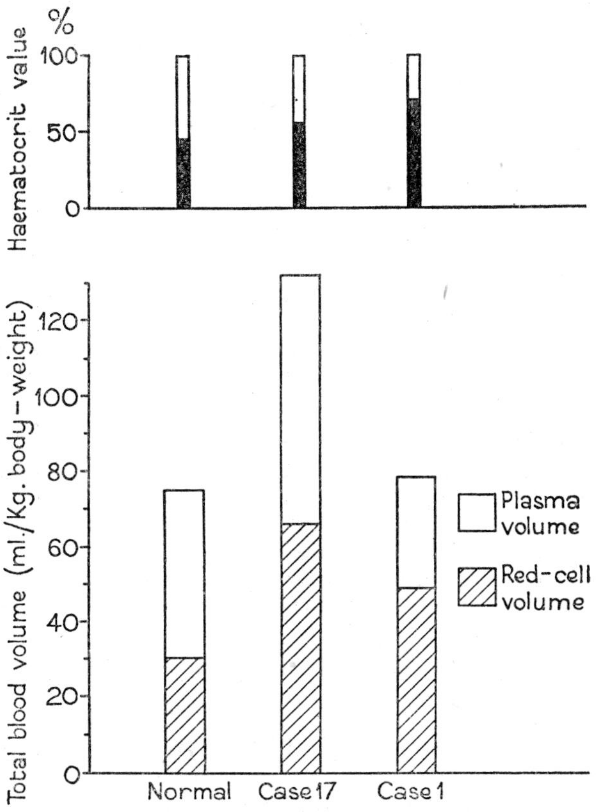

FIG. 3. Poor correlation between haematocrit value and blood-volume.

was an instance of a concomitant marked elevation in plasma-volume occurring in spite of a massive increase of red-cell volume. The result was a very large total blood-volume but a relatively small increase in the haematocrit level. Case 1, on the other hand, showed a marked compensatory shrinkage in plasma-volume, so that in spite of a moderate increase in red-cell volume the rise in total blood-volume was small, but was accompanied by a strikingly elevated haematocrit level.

Changes in blood-volume after treatment. There was no apparent correlation between the time and degree of the patient's response to therapy and the nature or magnitude of the blood-volume abnormality before treatment. The blood-volume measurements of 10 patients were repeated within three to 10 months of treatment with ^{32}P. Whenever possible the second determination was carried out when the patient's haematocrit level had become stable at the new value attained after treatment. The results are shown in Table V. The various types of response serve to emphasize again the difficulty of assessing the true state of

TABLE V

Changes in Total Blood-Volume Following a Single Course of ^{32}P Therapy

Case number	*Time of measurement*	*Observed haematocrit value* (%)	*Variation of total blood-volume from normal** (%)
8	Before treatment	72·4	+ 40
	After 4 months	36·7	0
13	Before treatment	64·6	+ 28
	After 3 months	47·6	+ 2
15	Before treatment	45·3	+ 24
	After 6½ months	40·7	+ 10
11	Before treatment	51·0	+ 49
	After 7 months	52·8	+ 4
9	Before treatment	57·7	+ 40
	After 10 months	40·6	+ 16
14	Before treatment	82·3	+108
	After 3 months	54·1	+ 54
10	Before treatment	79·9	+101
	After 4 months	29·0	+ 36
12	Before treatment	71·6	+ 36
	After 8 months	56·2	+ 20
17	Before treatment	57·0	+ 85
	After 4½ months	55·0	+ 55
16	Before treatment	62·4	+ 96
	After 6½ months	63·4	+102

* These values refer to the figures for the total blood-volume in normal adults in relation to surface area, after Gibson and Evans (1937).

the blood-volume by means of the haematocrit alone. For example, the following patterns of response were observed:

(1) Fall of the haematocrit value and blood-volume to normal (Cases 8, 13, and 15);
(2) Fall of the haematocrit value to normal, but an incomplete fall in blood-volume towards normal (Case 9);
(3) Fall of the haematocrit value to subnormal, with only a moderate fall in the massively enlarged blood-volume (Case 10);
(4) No apparent change in the haematocrit value, but a fall in blood-volume to normal (Case 11), or a partial fall in blood-volume towards normal (Case 17);
(5) Partial fall of the haematocrit value towards normal, with a partial, but not always proportionate, fall in total blood-volume towards normal (Cases 12 and 14).

The explanation of these discrepancies can be found in the behaviour of the plasma-volume after treatment. The plasma-volumes in all the patients who had subnormal values before treatment rose to normal, or above normal, after treatment. In patients who had normal plasma-volumes before treatment there was generally no significant change after treatment, though in one case (Case 14) the plasma-volume rose to a strikingly elevated level in the stable phase after treatment, in spite of the persistence of a marked elevation in red-cell volume. In patients whose plasma-volume before treatment had been increased, it tended to decrease towards normal after treatment, but this response was often partial, and varied from patient to patient.

Clinical Results

Response to treatment. The full pattern of a satisfactory response to a single injection of ^{32}P was not manifest for three or four months after treatment; but marked symptomatic relief frequently occurred within a few days of the injection, and before any objective evidence of response was obtained. From the sixth to the 16th week enlargement of the spleen, if it had been present, regressed, and haemorrhagic and thrombotic tendencies disappeared, together with other symptoms such as pruritus. A remission of variable duration then

TABLE VI

Treatment of Polycythaemia Vera with ^{32}P (Patients Treated for Six Months or Longer)

		Number of patients	%
No response		1	3·7
Symptomatic response (without full remission of signs)		4	14·8
Full remission (duration six months or longer):			
one injection	18	22	81·5
two injections	4		
Total		27	100

ensued. The criteria of full remission which have been adopted are that for a period of six months, or longer, the patient must have complete freedom from all symptoms and signs of polycythaemia vera, including reversion to normal of the peripheral blood picture. Chronic peripheral vascular disease, hypertension, and the residua of previous vascular accidents have not been considered to be reversible. As shown in Table VI, 22 of the 27 patients fulfil the above requirements for full remission, 18 after a single injection of radioactive phosphorus. It is much too early to assess the ultimate results, since the majority of these patients remain in remission at the present time. On a few occasions, when a moderately satisfactory partial remission had been obtained, it was considered undesirable or impracticable to endeavour to obtain a full remission by a second injection of ^{32}P. It should thus be noted that some of the detailed haematological studies which are reported have been made on patients who did not obtain a full remission after the dose of ^{32}P, the response to which was studied. Four patients obtained a partial remission, with full symptomatic relief, but without a complete reversion of the blood picture to normal, or with persistent objective signs such as a palpable spleen. One patient attained only partial symptomatic benefit, associated with a slight platelet depression after the injection of ^{32}P. (This patient, after further treatment with radioactive phosphorus, is now beginning to respond.)

Discussion

1. *Correlation of platelet response with remission.* It has been shown (Brown, 1949) that the platelets are the most sensitive element of the peripheral blood to external X-irradiation, and are probably the best guide to marrow radiation tolerance. We are not aware of any detailed report of the platelet response and its correlation with clinical and other findings after internal irradiation with ^{32}P. Wiseman, Rohn, Bouroncle, and Myers (1951) have given the most complete data so far published, but these workers made few platelet studies during the first month after treatment. In the series now reported the platelets have been shown to be the cellular element of the peripheral blood most sensitive to the administration of ^{32}P. A correlation between the degree of platelet depression and the incidence and completeness of ensuing remissions has been observed. This correlation has been sufficiently close to suggest the possibility of an ensuing remission long before any change in haematocrit values could be expected. As further data regarding early platelet response accumulate, they may become a useful guide in the prompt assessment of patients who will require additional treatment. In the work reported in the present paper, valid evidence of platelet 'peaks' immediately after the administration of ^{32}P was not obtained, probably because it was not possible to perform daily blood counts, as was done during external radiation by Brown (1949). Work at present in progress suggests that in fact platelet 'peaks', and possibly leucocyte and erythrocyte 'peaks', similar to those observed after external wide-field X-irradiation, do occur after internal irradiation with ^{32}P, though on a different time scale. It was suggested by Erf and Jones (1943) that the long delay in response as shown by the haematocrit may be attributed in part to the long life of the normal red cell, which averages 120 days (Mollison, 1951). This factor is unlikely to be the only cause of the latent period, and in our own patients we have observed latent periods much longer than 120 days; moreover, the depression in the platelet and white-cell counts occurred after periods considerably exceeding the known life-spans of these cells in the peripheral blood (Stefanini and Chatterjea, 1951; Stefanini, Chatterjea, Dameshek, Zannos, and Santiago, 1952; Osgood, 1937; Erf, 1940). Inorganic phosphorus is known to be most rapidly concentrated at first in tissues which are the site of active mitosis, and hence where there is active nucleic-acid metabolism. A reasonable hypothesis might be that ^{32}P, when administered as inorganic phosphate to a polycythaemic patient, exerts its prime effect on a primitive stem-cell precursor of the cellular elements of the blood in the marrow, and not on any immediate peripheral-cell precursor.

2. *Blood volume studies.* The poor correlation of elevation in haematocrit values with elevation in total blood volume was of special interest. It was seen to be dependent on the wide variation from patient to patient in the response of the plasma-volume to the elevation in red-cell volume. These findings are in agreement with those of Prentice, Berlin, and Lawrence (1952) and Wilson and Boyle (1952), and emphasize the unreliability of the haematocrit as a measure

of the total blood-volume abnormality in this disease. The physiological interpretation of the changes in blood-volume observed after treatment with ^{32}P is difficult, and the factors determining them are as yet unknown. The variable responses of the plasma-volume during treatment suggest that in some patients the expanded vascular bed is easily able to resume a normal capacity, thus allowing the plasma-volume to change as required to restore a more normal total blood-volume, while in others the expanded vascular bed can make only a partial and slow return towards normal capacity, and the plasma-volume remains elevated or increases to fill the space formerly occupied by red cells. Plasma replacement, with either plasma or a plasma substitute, is probably not necessary after routine therapeutic venesection in polycythaemia vera. There is, however, one circumstance in which plasma replacement may prove useful. As was suggested by Barbour (1950), polycythaemic patients who require surgery benefit by having their haematocrit levels reduced to near normal before operation. If rapid massive venesection is resorted to in these circumstances and there is insufficient time for spontaneous physiological readjustment to take place, plasma replacement is probably desirable to minimize the possibility of surgical shock.

It had been noticed that some patients with polycythaemia vera reported a marked symptomatic improvement within two to four weeks of radiation therapy, before any change in haematocrit values had occurred. It was thought possible that this improvement might be due to a true decrease in the total blood-volume, brought about by proportional diminution in both red-cell volume and plasma-volume, and hence unaccompanied by any change in the haematocrit level. Two patients with very high haematocrit readings (Cases 4 and 14) reported considerable symptomatic relief soon after ^{32}P-therapy, but their haematocrit readings were unchanged. Their plasma-volumes were estimated again at this time, three weeks after treatment; no change in the total blood-volume was demonstrable in either case.

3. *Therapy and response.* A number of different techniques of treating polycythaemia vera with radioactive phosphorus have been described, some of which combine venesection, or limitation of dietary iron intake, or both, with one or more injections of radioactive phosphorus. We were not satisfied that the merit of any one of these methods was well enough established to warrant its adoption; consequently we have employed the single-injection method described above. Since the red cells of most of our polycythaemic patients were initially hypochromic and microcytic, there did not appear to be any valid reason for restricting iron in the diet, at least on the present British dietary intake. A normal or low venous haematocrit level is not a very uncommon finding in polycythaemia vera. This is not surprising when it is remembered that haemorrhage is one of the commonest initial signs of the condition. It is particularly important that patients who are liable to haemorrhage be diagnosed and treated as early as possible, since if untreated they are liable to further haemorrhage and its attendant dangers, whatever the haematocrit level may be. Moreover, it is probably the patient with haemorrhagic and thrombotic tendencies who derives

the most benefit from treatment, if benefit be measured in terms of prolongation of life. While the preliminary results obtained are encouraging, we do not claim that ours is necessarily the best possible method. It has the merit of simplicity, and it allows evaluation of the effects of a single injection of ^{32}P. It is too early for final assessment of the clinical results obtainable by the present method of treatment, since a prolonged period of observation is necessary before a final opinion can be expressed. We have been encouraged to continue to use this simple method, since a full remission has followed a single injection of radiophosphorus in 18, or two-thirds, of the 27 patients. The preliminary clinical results now reported are at least equal to the best reported by other workers, and confirm our belief that at the present time the use of radioactive phosphorus, as inorganic phosphate, in the treatment of polycythaemia vera is the method of choice.

Summary

1. The preliminary results of treatment with ^{32}P in 27 patients suffering from polycythaemia vera are reported. Of these patients 22, or 81 per cent., underwent a full remission lasting six months or longer, 18 of them after a single injection of ^{32}P.

2. The remaining five patients underwent partial remissions.

3. The method of treatment is described, and consists essentially of a single intravenous injection of ^{32}P as inorganic phosphate without previous venesection.

4. A correlation was observed between the degree of platelet depression and the ultimate clinical response.

5. Blood-volume measurements before treatment are reported for 17 of the patients. The blood-volume was measured again after response to treatment in 10 patients. Some implications of the blood-volume abnormalities are discussed.

REFERENCES

Barbour, C. M. (1950) *Anesthesiology*, **11**, 155.
Brown, W. M. C. (1949) *Acta radiol.* **32**, 407.
Chaplin, H. (1953). To be published.
—— and Mollison, P. L. (1952) *Blood*, **7**, 1227.
—— —— and Vetter, H. (1953). To be published.
Dacie, J. V. (1950) *Practical Haematology*, London.
Erf, L. A. (1940) *Amer. J. Med. Sci.* **200**, 1.
—— and Jones, H. W. (1943) *Ann. Int. Med.* **19**, 587.
Gibson, J. G., Jnr., and Evans, W. A., Jnr. (1937) *J. Clin. Invest.* **16**, 317.
Lawrence, J. H. (1949) *J. Amer. Med. Ass.* **141**, 13.
Lempert, H. (1935) *Lancet*, **1**, 151.
Mollison, P. L. (1951) *Blood Transfusion in Clinical Medicine*, Oxford.
Osgood, E. E. (1937) *J. Amer. Med. Ass.* **109**, 933.
Prentice, T. C., Berlin, N. I., and Lawrence, J. H. (1952) *Arch. Int. Med.* **89**, 584.
Reeve, E. B., and Veall, N. (1949) *J. Physiol.* **108**, 12.
Reinhard, E. H., Moore, C. V., Bierbaum, O. S., and Moore, S. (1946) *J. Lab. Clin. Med.* **31**, 107.
Stefanini, M., and Chatterjea, J. B. (1951) *J. Clin. Invest.* **30**, 676.
—— —— Dameshek, W., Zannos, L., and Santiago, E. P. (1952) *Blood*, **7**, 53.
Tinney, W. S., Hall, B. E., and Giffin, H. Z. (1943) *Proc. Staff M. Mayo Clin.* **18**, 227.
Wilson, S. J., and Boyle, P. (1952) *Arch. Int. Med.* **90**, 602.
Wiseman, B. K., Rohn, R. J., Bouroncle, B. A., and Myers, W. G. (1951) *Ann. Int. Med.* **34**, 311.

616.131–008.21 : 616.126.421

CLINICAL DIAGNOSIS OF PULMONARY HYPERTENSION IN PATIENTS WITH MITRAL STENOSIS[1]

By WILLIAM WHITAKER

(From The University Department of Medicine, The Royal Hospital, Sheffield, and The Regional Cardiovascular Department, The City General Hospital, Sheffield)

With Plates 4 to 7

Pulmonary hypertension is a factor which requires consideration in the assessment of patients with mitral stenosis for surgical treatment, and for this reason direct measurements of pulmonary-artery blood-pressures by cardiac catheterization have been made in this and many other centres. Griffith, Miller, Cosby, Levinson, Dimitroff, Zinn, Oblath, Herman, Johns, Meyer, and Jones (1953), discussing the selection of patients for mitral valvotomy, stated that direct measurement of the pulmonary artery blood-pressure is desirable, because of difficulty in evaluating clinically the degree of pulmonary hypertension, but Baker, Brock, Campbell, and Wood (1952) considered it possible to recognize pulmonary hypertension clinically in patients who have mitral stenosis. The purpose of the present study was to determine whether there is sufficient correlation between pulmonary-artery mean blood-pressure and clinical, electrocardiographic, and radiological signs, in patients with mitral stenosis, to make possible a clinical evaluation of pulmonary hypertension.

Methods

Twenty-five patients with mitral stenosis as their sole or dominant lesion have been studied clinically, electrocardiographically, radiologically, and by cardiac catheterization. In the clinical examination particular attention was paid to a history of haemoptysis and nocturnal dyspnoea, to inspection of the jugular venous pulse, to palpation over the right ventricular outflow tract, and to auscultation at the base of the heart. The symptoms of haemoptysis and nocturnal dyspnoea were studied because there appeared to be a possible relation between these symptoms of pulmonary congestion and pulmonary hypertension, since Dexter, Dow, Haynes, Whittenberger, Ferris, Goodale, and Hellems (1950) have shown that pulmonary hypertension in patients with mitral stenosis is associated with a raised left auricular pressure. Although it is often possible, from a history of blood-streaked or frothy pink sputum accompanied by cough and orthopnoea, to recognize haemoptysis occurring

[1] Received April 23, 1953.

from pulmonary congestion, and to distinguish it from haemoptysis due to pulmonary infarction and from the massive haemorrhages which occur unexpectedly in patients who are otherwise well, no attempt was made to separate these various forms of haemoptysis. As Wood (1950) has recently described prominent auricular waves in the jugular venous pulse of patients with pulmonary hypertension, the pulsation of the internal jugular veins was examined, and the pulse-waves were timed by palpation of the carotid artery. These venous pulsations were most carefully scrutinized in patients with sinus rhythm for the presence of prominent auricular waves, which occur as flicking presystolic expansions dwarfing the other waves. The venous pulse was assessed by naked eye, but on several occasions a permanent record was made of the pulsation (Plates 4 and 5, Figs. 1 and 2). In a review of the signs of pulmonary hypertension, Bedford (1951) stated that the first clinical signs were due to enlargement of the outflow tract of the right ventricle, which produced a systolic lift in the second or third left intercostal spaces and a palpable second heart-sound in the same area. In the present investigation the systolic lift of the right ventricular outflow tract was detected by the tips of the fingers in the second and third left interspaces, and, although thrusts of widely varying intensity were encountered, this sign was assessed as either present or absent. The palpable second heart-sound occurred in the same area, and its short vibrations were best felt with the medial side of the palm of the hand. To detect a systolic lift and a palpable second heart-sound, the most satisfactory method was simultaneous palpation, with the tips of the fingers of the right hand in the third left intercostal space and with the medial side of the left palm in the second left intercostal space. The systolic lift of the fingers of the right hand was then followed by a sharp tap felt by the left hand. On auscultation, an assessment was made of the character of the second heart-sound in the pulmonary area, and of the occurrence of a Graham-Steell murmur. Four grades of pulmonary second heart-sounds were recognized: normal sounds; loud sounds, which were louder than the aortic second sound; loud split sounds, which were louder than the aortic sound and more than normally split; and split sounds with the second element louder than the first (Plate 5, Fig. 2). High-pitched short diastolic murmurs immediately following loud pulmonary second sounds, and heard best in the third and fourth left interspaces, were considered to be Graham-Steell murmurs in the absence of other signs of aortic incompetence. Electrocardiographic examination consisted of a recording of the standard leads, the augmented unipolar limb leads, and the precordial leads V_1 to V_6, but the present investigation was restricted to the ventricular complex in the right chest lead, V_1. Each patient had a five-foot postero-anterior chest radiograph taken, from which it was estimated whether the prominence of the main branches of the pulmonary arteries was normal, increased, or extreme. As pointed out by Campbell (1951), the right pulmonary artery is the best measure for this purpose, because the left pulmonary artery is too often hidden by the heart shadow. The pulmonary-artery blood-pressures were measured directly by cardiac catheterization, with the patient resting in a semi-recumbent position. The mean blood-pressures were recorded on either a saline or a condenser manometer, and the results were expressed in mm. Hg above a plane 5 cm. behind the sternal angle.

Results

Table I shows the results, with the pulmonary-artery mean blood-pressures arranged on a descending scale. In Plate 6, Fig. 3 the pulmonary-artery mean blood-pressures are again shown, on a descending scale, below the corresponding ventricular patterns in lead V_1 of the electrocardiogram.

TABLE I

Resting Pulmonary-artery Mean Blood-pressures, and Clinical, Electrocardiographic, and Radiological Features of 25 Patients with Mitral Stenosis

		Palpation over right ventricular outflow tract		*Auscultatory signs*					
Resting pulmonary-artery mean blood-pressure (mm. Hg)	*Jugular venous pulse*	*Systolic lift*	*Palpable second sound*	*Pulmonary second heart-sound*	*Graham-Steell murmur*	*Ventricular complex in lead V_1 of electro-cardiogram*	*Prominence of pulmonary arteries on radiological examination*	*Haemoptysis*	*Nocturnal dyspnoea*
108	*a*	+	+	IV	+	R, T↓	++	+	+
104	*a*	+	+	IV	+	R, T↓	++	—	—
88	*a*	—	+	III	+	Rs, T↓	++	—	+
81	*a*	+	+	IV	—	Rs, T↓	+	+	+
80	N	+	+	II	+	Rs, T↓	++	+	—
78	*a*	+	+	III	+	Rs, T↓	++	+	—
75	*a*	+	+	III	+	Rs, T↓	++	+	+
70	A.F.	+	+	IV	+	rSr, T↓	+	+	—
69	N	+	+	III	—	R, T↓	+	+	+
65	T.I.	+	+	III	—	Rs, T↓	+	—	—
55	N	+	+	IV	+	Rs, T↓	+	+	+
52	*a*	+	+	III	+	R, T↓	+	+	—
50	N	+	+	IV	—	Rs, T↓	+	+	+
47	A.F.	+	—	III	—	rsR, T↓	+	+	—
46	A.F.	—	—	III	—	rS, T↓	+	—	—
40	A.F., T.I.	+	—	III	—	rSR, T↓	+	+	—
40	N	—	+	III	+	rS, T↓	+	+	—
40	A.F.	+	+	IV	A.I.	rS, T↑	N	+	+
34	N	+	+	III	+	rS, T↑	+	—	—
33	N	+	—	III	—	rS, T↑	+	—	+
32	N	—	—	III	A.I.	RS, T↑	N	+	—
32	A.F.	+	—	III	—	rS, T↓	N	—	+
22	A.F.	—	—	I	—	rS, T↑	N	—	—
18	N	—	—	III	—	rS, T↑	N	—	—
16	A.F.	+	—	I	—	rS, T↑	N	+	—

Jugular venous pulse: *a* = prominent auricular wave; A.F. = auricular fibrillation; T.I. = tricuspid incompetence; N = normal pulse wave.

Prominence of pulmonary arteries on radiographic examination: ++ = extreme, + = increased, and N = normal prominence of the main branches. In other columns + is used to signify presence and — absence.

Pulmonary second sound: I = normal; II = loud; III = loud and abnormally split; IV = split with a loud second element.

A.I. = aortic incompetence.

Discussion

The resting pulmonary-artery mean blood-pressures, which were between 16 mm. Hg and 108 mm. Hg, varied from the upper limit of the normal range to levels higher than the pressures in the systemic arteries, and were similar to pressures reported by Baker, Brock, Campbell, and Wood (1952) and by Griffith, Miller, Cosby, Levinson, Dimitroff, Zinn, Oblath, Herman, Johns, Meyer, and Jones (1953) in patients with mitral stenosis. Pulmonary hypertension was arbitrarily considered mild in seven patients with pulmonary-artery mean blood-pressures less than 40 mm. Hg, moderate in 10 with pressures between 40 and 69 mm. Hg, and severe in eight with pressures of 70 mm. Hg or over.

Haemoptysis and nocturnal dyspnoea. A history of haemoptysis was obtained from 16 patients: from six of the eight with severe, eight of the 10 with moderate, and two of the seven with mild pulmonary hypertension. Nocturnal dyspnoea occurred in 10 patients: in four of eight with severe, four of 10 with moderate, and two of seven with mild pulmonary hypertension. These results show that haemoptysis and nocturnal dyspnoea were more common in patients with moderate or severe pulmonary hypertension than in patients with mild pulmonary hypertension; but they also indicate that little value can be placed on these symptoms alone in assessing the degree of pulmonary hypertension. It must not be denied that some patients with tight mitral stenosis and moderate to severe pulmonary hypertension give a characteristic history of recurrent attacks of acute pulmonary oedema, with the expectoration of frothy blood-stained sputum and orthopnoea, as described by Bayliss, Etheridge, and Hyman (1950), Baker, Brock, Campbell, and Wood (1952), and Wade, Werkö, Eliasch, Gidlund, and Lagerlöf (1952).

Jugular venous pulsation. Seven out of eight patients with severe pulmonary hypertension had sinus rhythm, and six of these seven had prominent auricular waves in the jugular venous pulse (Plate 4, Fig. 1). These waves occurred in only one of the 11 other patients with sinus rhythm, and this patient had moderate pulmonary hypertension, a result which indicates that prominent auricular venous waves are a valuable sign of severe pulmonary hypertension in patients with mitral stenosis and sinus rhythm. This sign is especially useful, since patients with mitral stenosis and severe pulmonary hypertension frequently have sinus rhythm (Wade, Werkö, Eliasch, Gidlund, and Lagerlöf, 1952).

Palpation of the right ventricular outflow tract. A systolic lift was present over the right ventricular outflow tract in seven of eight patients with severe, in eight of 10 patients with moderate, and in four of seven patients with mild pulmonary hypertension. The occurrence of this sign with mild pulmonary hypertension indicates that it is of little value as a positive index of the degree of pulmonary hypertension. A systolic lift over the right ventricular outflow tract was, however, almost invariably found in patients who had moderate or severe pulmonary hypertension, so that the absence of this sign makes these complications improbable. A palpable second heart-sound was present in all eight patients with severe, in seven of 10 patients with moderate, and in only one patient with mild pulmonary hypertension; this patient was the one who had the highest pressure, 34 mm. Hg, of the seven. This sign therefore appears to be an important indication of moderate and severe pulmonary hypertension in patients with mitral stenosis. If on palpation over the right ventricular outflow tract of a patient with mitral stenosis there is a systolic lift, there is possibly pulmonary hypertension; but if there is also a palpable second heart-sound, the patient probably has severe or moderate pulmonary hypertension.

Auscultatory signs. The pulmonary second heart-sound was abnormal in all patients except two, in whom the pulmonary-artery mean blood-pressure was 22 mm. Hg and 16 mm. Hg respectively. This finding supports Bedford's (1951) statement that with pulmonary hypertension there is a loud, and often duplicated, second sound. The occurrence of a loud second sound with all degrees of pulmonary hypertension supports the view expressed by Wade, Werkö, Eliasch, Gidlund, and Lagerlöf (1952) that the intensity of the pulmonary second sound is an unreliable guide to the degree of pulmonary hypertension. A loud second element of a split second sound was described by Wood (1950) as a sign of pulmonary hypertension; this was observed in four of eight patients with severe, in three of 10 patients with moderate, and in none of the patients with mild pulmonary hypertension. This fact suggests that in patients with mitral stenosis this type of second sound is a definite, though inconstant, sign of moderate or severe pulmonary hypertension (Plate 5, Fig. 2). A Graham-Steell murmur was present in seven of eight patients with severe, in three of 10 with moderate, and in one of seven with mild pulmonary hypertension. Two patients had aortic incompetence. The high incidence of a Graham-Steell murmur with severe pulmonary hypertension is impressive; but because of difficulty in excluding aortic incompetence in patients with mitral stenosis, it is not desirable that an early diastolic murmur to the left of the sternum should be regarded as evidence of pulmonary hypertension unless accompanied by other signs of this complication, in which case such a murmur may be regarded as an indication of severe pulmonary hypertension.

Electrocardiographic patterns in lead V_1. The electrocardiographic patterns in lead V_1 (Plate 6, Fig. 3) showed evidence of right ventricular hypertrophy in seven of eight patients with severe, in five of 10 patients with moderate, and in none of the patients with mild pulmonary hypertension. This indicates that in patients suffering from mitral stenosis electrocardiographic evidence of right ventricular hypertrophy in lead V_1 is usually present when there is severe pulmonary hypertension, frequently present when there is moderate pulmonary hypertension, and rarely present when there is mild pulmonary hypertension. A ventricular pattern of a large R wave, with or without a small S wave, followed by an inverted T wave, in lead V_1 appears to be an important sign of moderate or severe pulmonary hypertension, since this pattern did not occur with a pressure below 52 mm. Hg, and was present in nine of 12 patients with pressures over 50 mm. Hg.

Prominence of pulmonary arteries on radiological examination. The prominence of the main branches of the pulmonary arteries on radiological examination was extreme in six patients with severe pulmonary hypertension, increased in two with severe, in nine with moderate, and in two with mild pulmonary hypertension, and normal in one with moderate and five with mild pulmonary hypertension. These findings show a rough correlation between prominence of the

TABLE II

Clinical, Electrocardiographic, and Radiological Signs Characteristic of Severe, Moderate, and Mild Pulmonary Hypertension Complicating Mitral Stenosis

Degree of pulmonary hypertension	*Jugular venous pulse*	*Palpation over right ventricular outflow tract*		*Auscultatory signs*		*Lead V_1 of electrocardiogram*	*Prominence of pulmonary arteries on radiological examination*
		Systolic lift	*Palpable second heart-sound*	*Pulmonary second sound*	*Graham-Steell murmur*		
Severe (mean pressure 70 mm. Hg or over)	Prominent auricular waves in patients with sinus rhythm	Present	Present	Split with loud second element, or loud and split	Present	Right ventricular hypertrophy; R, T↓, or Rs, T↓ ventricular patterns	Extreme or increased
Moderate (mean pressure 40–69 mm. Hg)	Normal, or auricular fibrillation	Present	Usually present	Loud and split, or split with loud second element	Occasionally present	Right ventricular hypertrophy, or normal	Increased
Mild (mean pressure < 40 mm. Hg)	Normal, or auricular fibrillation	Present or absent	Absent	Loud and split, loud, or normal	Absent	Normal	Normal

main pulmonary arteries and degree of pulmonary hypertension, and are in agreement with the observations of Campbell (1951) and the angiocardiographic studies of Goodwin, Steiner, and Lowe (1952). Extreme prominence of the main branches of the pulmonary arteries is an indication of severe, increased prominence of moderate or severe, and normal prominence of mild pulmonary hypertension (Plate 7, Fig. 4). A difficulty in interpreting extreme prominence of the main branches of the pulmonary arteries as a sign of severe pulmonary hypertension complicating mitral stenosis is that an atrial septal defect, a ventricular septal defect, or a patent ductus arteriosus can produce a similar radiological picture, with clinical signs of pulmonary hypertension and an apical diastolic murmur; and exclusion of these lesions may be impossible without cardiac catheterization.

Conclusion. The incidence of the three degrees of pulmonary hypertension in relation to clinical, electrocardiographic, and radiological signs has been discussed. Certain of these signs are so often associated with mild, moderate, or severe pulmonary hypertension as to be considered characteristic of that degree of pulmonary hypertension complicating mitral stenosis (Table II). From clinical, electrocardiographic, and radiological findings in patients with mitral stenosis, it is possible to assess complicating pulmonary hypertension as severe, moderate, or mild, and direct measurement of pulmonary-artery blood-pressure is unnecessary as a routine investigation before operation.

Acknowledgements

I wish to thank Professor C. H. Stuart-Harris, Dr. J. W. Brown, and Mr. J. T. Chesterman for permission to investigate patients under their care, and Dr. C. E. Davies for much helpful advice in the preparation of the results for publication.

Summary

1. Resting pulmonary-artery mean blood-pressures were recorded by cardiac catheterization in 25 patients who had mitral stenosis. Pulmonary hypertension was arbitrarily considered mild in seven patients with pulmonary-artery mean blood-pressures less than 40 mm. Hg, moderate in 10 patients with pressure between 40 and 69 mm. Hg, and severe in eight with pressures of 70 mm. Hg or over.

2. In the three groups with mild, moderate, and severe pulmonary hypertension the incidence of the following features was determined: a history of haemoptysis and nocturnal dyspnoea; abnormalities of the jugular venous pulse; a systolic lift and a palpable second heart-sound over the right ventricular outflow tract; an abnormal second heart-sound and a Graham-Steell murmur on auscultation; evidence of right ventricular hypertrophy in lead V_1 of the electrocardiogram; and increased or extreme prominence of the main branches of the pulmonary arteries on radiological examination.

3. Haemoptysis and nocturnal dyspnoea occurred in patients in all three groups, and, although these symptoms were more common with moderate or severe than with mild pulmonary hypertension, they appear to be of little value in assessing its degree.

4. Prominent auricular venous waves, which were present in six of seven patients with sinus rhythm and severe pulmonary hypertension, and in only one other patient who had moderate pulmonary hypertension, are a valuable indication of severe pulmonary hypertension.

5. A systolic lift over the right ventricular outflow tract was usual in patients in whom pulmonary hypertension was moderate or severe, and common in patients in whom it was mild. This sign is of little value as a positive index of the degree of pulmonary hypertension, but its absence makes severe and moderate pulmonary hypertension improbable.

6. A palpable second heart-sound was usually present in patients in whom pulmonary hypertension was moderate or severe, but occurred in only one patient in whom it was mild, and therefore appears to be a sign of moderate or severe pulmonary hypertension.

7. Loud, and loud and split, second sounds occurred with all degrees of pulmonary hypertension, and are unreliable indices of its degree; but split sounds with loud second elements, which occurred only in patients who had moderate or severe pulmonary hypertension, and normal sounds, which occurred only in patients in whom it was mild, are of diagnostic importance.

8. A Graham-Steell murmur, which was usual with severe, and uncommon with moderate and mild pulmonary hypertension, is not regarded as an important sign of pulmonary hypertension, because of difficulty in excluding

aortic incompetence; but when this murmur accompanies other signs of pulmonary hypertension it indicates that the degree is severe.

9. Electrocardiographic evidence of right ventricular hypertrophy in lead V_1 of the electrocardiogram was present in seven of eight patients with severe, in five of 10 patients with moderate, and in no patient with mild pulmonary hypertension; this pattern therefore is evidence of moderate or severe, and a normal pattern of mild or moderate, pulmonary hypertension.

10. All patients who showed extreme prominence of the pulmonary arteries on radiological examination had severe pulmonary hypertension; the majority of patients who showed increased prominence had moderate or severe pulmonary hypertension; and all patients who showed normal pulmonary arteries, except one, had mild pulmonary hypertension. Prominence of the pulmonary arteries is therefore an index of degree of pulmonary hypertension.

11. The relation between clinical, electrocardiographic, and radiological features and pulmonary hypertension is such as to make possible an assessment of the degree of pulmonary hypertension from these features.

REFERENCES

Baker, C., Brock, R. C., Campbell, M., and Wood, P. (1952) *Brit. Med. J.* **1**, **1043.**

Bayliss, R. I. S., Etheridge, M. J., and Hyman, A. L. (1950) *Lancet,* **2**, 889.

Bedford, D. E. (1951) *Proc. R. Soc. Med.* **44**, 597.

Campbell, M. (1951) *Brit. Heart J.* **13**, 438.

Dexter, L., Dow, J. W., Haynes, F. W., Whittenberger, J. L., Ferris, B. G., Goodale, W. T., and Hellems, H. K. (1950) *J. Clin. Invest.* **29**, 602.

Goodwin, J. F., Steiner, R. E., and Lowe, K. G. (1952) *J. Fac. Radiol.* **4**, 21.

Griffith, G. C., Miller, H., Cosby, R. S., Levinson, D. C., Dimitroff, S. P., Zinn, W. J., Oblath, R. W., Herman, L. M., Johns, V. J., Jnr., Meyer, B. W., and Jones, J. C. (1953) *Circulation,* **7**, 30.

Wade, G., Werkö, L., Eliasch, H., Gidlund, A., and Lagerlöf, H. (1952) *Quart. J. Med.* N.S. **21**, 361.

Wood, P. (1950) *Diseases of the Heart and Circulation,* London.

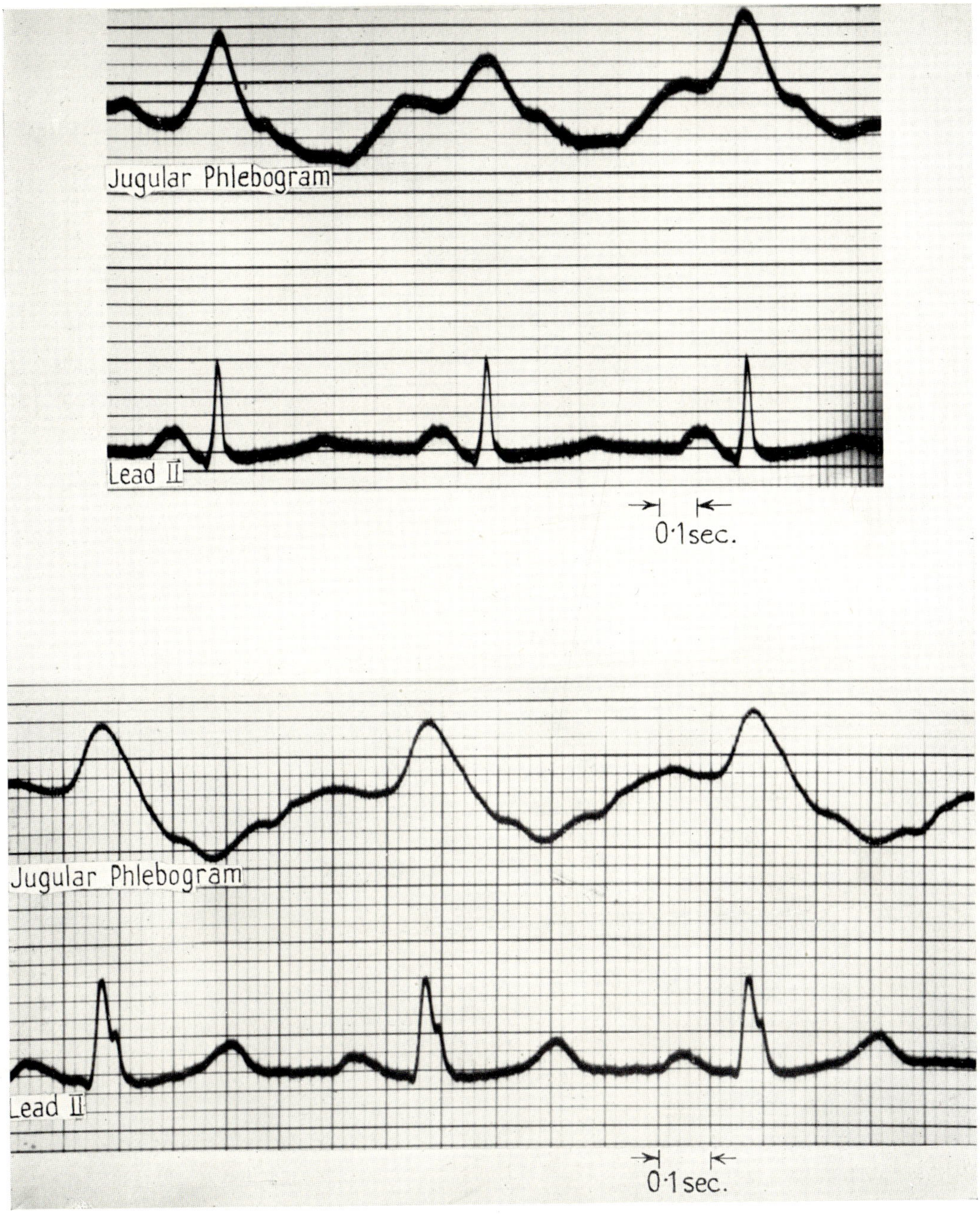

FIG. 1. Synchronous recordings of lead II of the electrocardiogram and of the jugular venous pulse, showing prominent auricular waves, in two patients with mitral stenosis and severe pulmonary hypertension

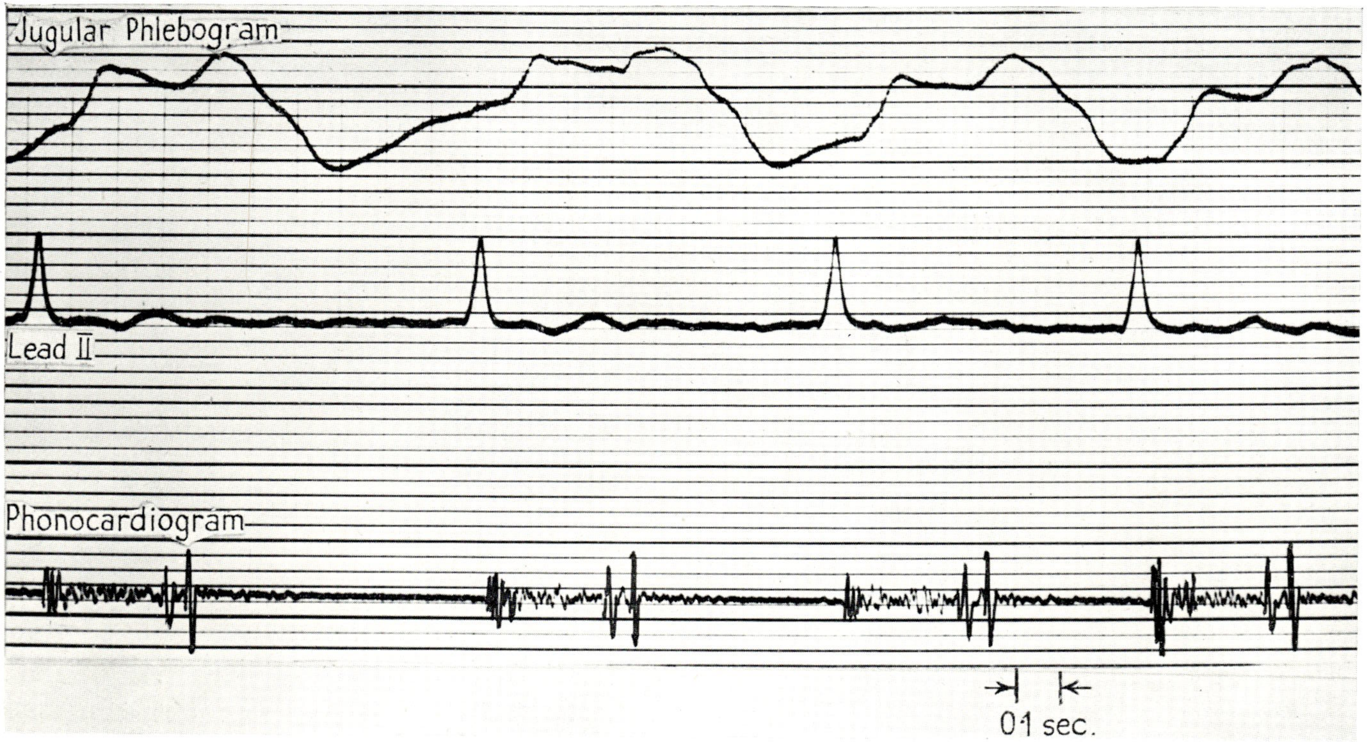

FIG. 2. Synchronous recordings of the jugular venous pulse, lead II of the electrocardiogram, and a low-frequency phonocardiogram from the pulmonary area of a patient with mitral stenosis, auricular fibrillation, and moderate pulmonary hypertension. There is no auricular component of the jugular venous pulse. The phonocardiogram shows a split second sound in which the second element is louder than the first

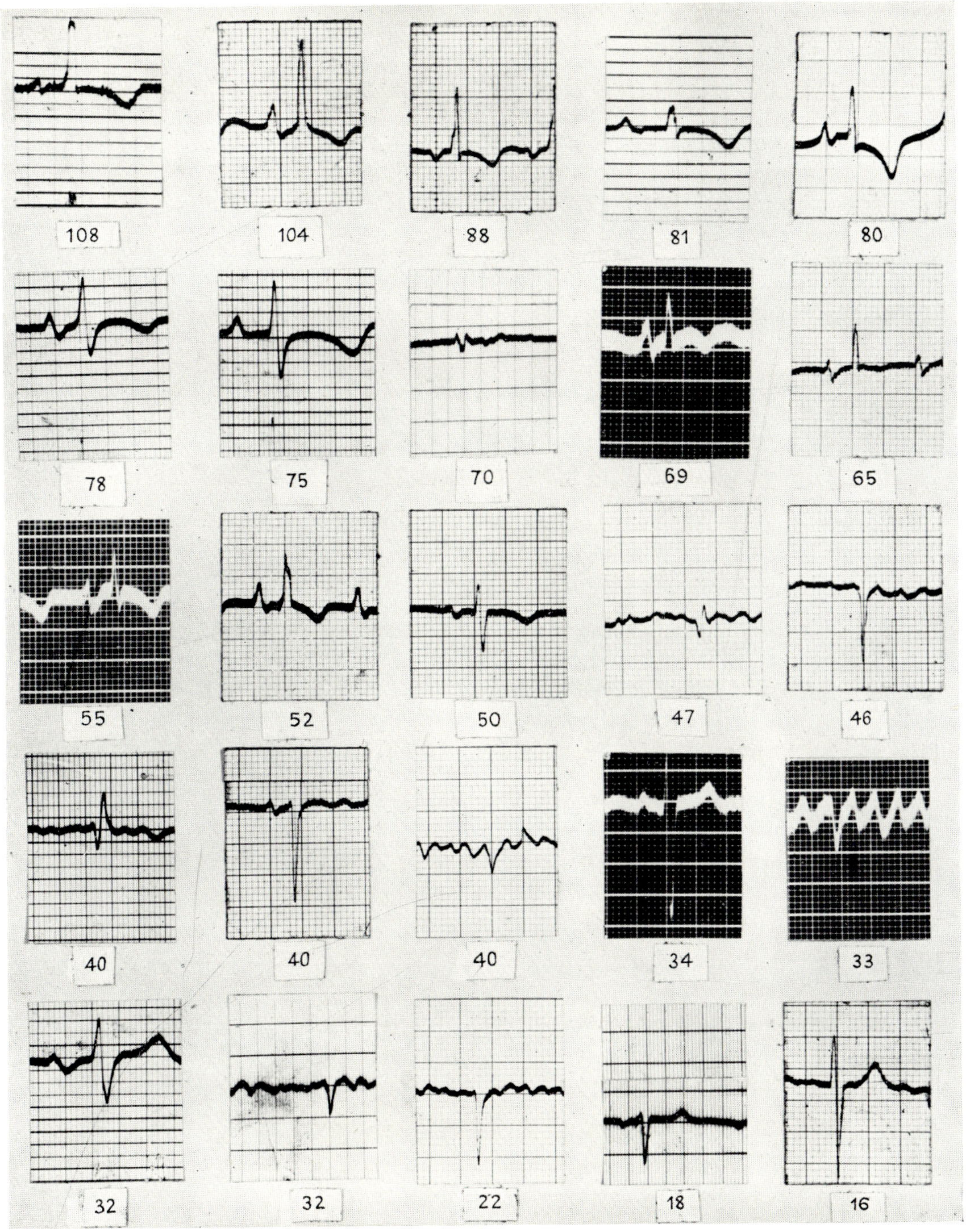

FIG. 3. Records of lead V_1 of the electrocardiogram and the resting pulmonary-artery mean blood-pressure in 25 patients with mitral stenosis. The pressures in mm. Hg are arranged on a descending scale

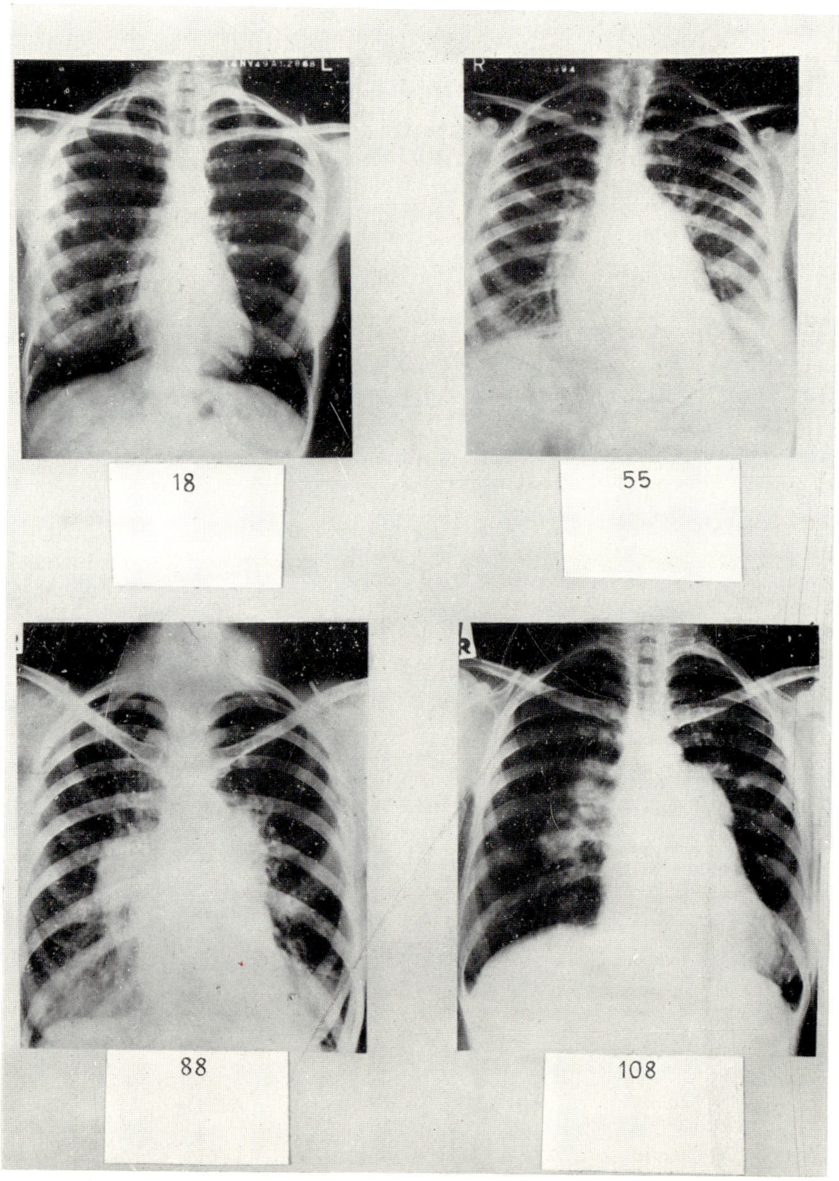

FIG. 4. Chest radiographs and resting pulmonary-artery mean blood-pressures in four patients with mitral stenosis. The prominence of the main branches of the pulmonary arteries is normal in a patient with mild, increased in a patient with moderate, and extreme in two patients with severe pulmonary hypertension

616.831–004.4: 616.24

PULMONARY TUBEROUS SCLEROSIS[1]

And its Relationship to Other Forms of the Disease

By JOHN DAWSON

(From King's College Hospital and Brompton Hospital, London)

With Plates 8 to 15

TUBEROUS sclerosis, a hereditary disorder of the growth of tissues, affects many parts of the body. The first account of it affecting the lungs was given by Berg (1938), since when eight other examples have been recorded. Four more are described in the present paper, which is concerned especially with this feature of the disease and with its relation to the other forms.

Historical Review of Tuberous Sclerosis

Von Recklinghausen (1862) gave the first description of cerebral tuberous sclerosis in a still-born child with numerous rhabdomyomata of the heart, noting briefly many sclerotic areas in the brain. Two years later Virchow (1864–5) found similar widespread changes in a child whose sister had died of a cerebral tumour. These 'scleromas', as he called them, were then regarded as gliomas. Credit for the first account of the clinical and pathological features of tuberous sclerosis goes to Bourneville (1880–1), who described an epileptic imbecile who had died of the disease in a Paris mental hospital. He coined the name 'sclérose tubéreuse', and by 1900 had recorded nine other examples, some of them with the facial and renal stigmata, though he did not appreciate the diagnostic significance of these changes. He noticed also that epilepsy and 'facial eczema' sometimes afflicted their relatives. The characteristic facial eruption was portrayed in colour by Rayer as long ago as 1835, with the title of 'végétations vasculaires'. In 1851 Addison and Gull recorded as 'a case of lichen' in a woman of 24 'a peculiar eruption, extending across the nose and slightly affecting both cheeks. It consisted of shining tubercles, varying in size . . . to that of ordinary acne. They were of lightish colour with . . . superficial capillary veins meandering over them giving them a faint rose tinge.' The moulage is still in the museum at Guy's Hospital with Addison's original label (Plate 8, Fig. 1), but it represents undoubtedly the facial changes seen in tuberous sclerosis. Balzer and Ménétrier (1885), who are usually credited with the first account (Kothe, 1904; Butterworth and Wilson, 1941; Borberg, 1951), gave the name of adenoma sebaceum to this eruption, and their names are still attached to this type of adenoma sebaceum with very few angiomata on and among the papules. By contrast Pringle (1890) in this country described

[1] Received June 18, 1953.

a case with obvious and widespread telangiectasia. Hallopeau and Leredde (1895) first noted another characteristic skin change, 'an avascular plaque in the lumbar region confined within the skin and free from the deep structures', a lesion now known as peau chagriné, or shagreen patch (Plate 8, Fig. 2). They pointed out that Balzer and Pringle had described the same morbid state, and that the differences arose from varying amounts of vascular and 'adenomatous' tissue. The relation between these skin lesions and cerebral tuberous sclerosis was not recognized clearly until Vogt published his paper in 1908; until then no certain diagnosis had been made in life. Sherlock (1911) coined the word 'anoia', which he later changed to 'epiloia' to comprehend the syndrome of epilepsy, mental defect, and adenoma sebaceum, but the term is now becoming obsolete. In the same year Fowler and Dickson (1910–11) collected 28 cases of tuberous sclerosis from the literature, among them examples of tumours in the heart, duodenum (Sailer, 1898), and thyroid gland (Volland, 1909). Van der Hoeve first described the characteristic retinal tumours in 1921. In 1938 Berg published an example of cystic disease of the lungs which, as he showed later (Berg and Vejlens, 1939), was associated with other manifestations of tuberous sclerosis.

Present Investigation

The present investigation consists of two parts. In the first part 72 cases of tuberous sclerosis, and seven others of normal intellect with adenoma sebaceum, have been surveyed. The mentally deficient patients were in the care of mental hospitals in the London area within a period of 21 years. The general and sex incidences of the disease have been calculated from these cases. Clinical and radiological examination established the frequency of the pulmonary form and of the main features of classical tuberous sclerosis. The second part is concerned with a detailed study of four patients with lung changes. Two were taken from the general survey, and two came under medical care with pulmonary symptoms.

Survey of Cases with Mental Deficiency and Adenoma Sebaceum

General incidence. Of the 72 patients with mental deficiency, 69 entered, or were already in, special hospitals in or near London between June 1, 1930, and June 1, 1951. In this time 21,579 patients were admitted, or were already in hospital in 1930, so that tuberous sclerosis accounted for one in 300 admissions. This ratio is similar to that reported by Penrose (1938), who found one case in 250 admissions to a hospital for the mentally defective. Brushfield and Wyatt (1926) found a ratio of one in 150 at a more specialized hospital for defective children. In the areas covered by all these investigations one per 1,000 of the population is admitted to an institution for mental defect (Board of Control, Annual Reports, 1935, 1945); therefore the incidence of tuberous sclerosis with mental defect is of the order of one in 300,000 in the general population. The seven patients with adenoma sebaceum and normal intellect were all that could be found from the out-patient departments of four London hospitals during a period of five years. Two were large general hospitals, the third a special hospital for diseases of the skin, and the last for diseases of children. These hospitals together serve about 140,000 new patients each year, so that this form of the disease is obviously very rare. There are no accurate data for calculating the frequency of less severe forms of the disease, but a rough estimate made from the number of afflicted relatives in this group would indicate that

TABLE I

Incidence of Lung Involvement

Type of case		*Records satisfactory*	*Radiological examination of lungs* — *No evidence of tuberous sclerosis*	*Radiological examination of lungs* — *Evidence of tuberous sclerosis*	*Necropsy findings* — *No pulmonary tuberous sclerosis*
Mental defect with tuberous sclerosis	Alive	39	38	1	..
	Dead	25	..	..	25 (6 with histological examination)
Total 72 patients*					
Adenoma sebaceum		7	6	1	..
Total		71	44	2	25

* Eight cases with inadequate records, discarded.

A total of 71 cases of tuberous sclerosis, including seven without mental symptoms, were examined, and two only were found to have associated pulmonary changes.

these *formes frustes* occur about as often as the major disease (Table III). Gunther and Penrose (1935) also considered that mild and severe forms occurred equally often. If so, the incidence of all forms of the disease would be of the order of 1:150,000.

Sex distribution. Twenty-eight of the mentally defective patients were male and 36 female (Table II). This rough equality agrees with the findings of previous authors (Gunther and Penrose, 1935; Cockayne, 1933; Vaas, 1940). In those over 20 years of age the female patients were more numerous (16 male and 28 female patients), but their predominance was much greater among the patients who showed pulmonary changes (two male and 11 female patients).

Incidence of pulmonary form. Seventy-two mentally defective patients were investigated, 39 living and 33 dead. The documents relating to eight of the dead contained incomplete information about the lungs, and were therefore discarded, leaving 25 whose records were adequate and included post-mortem examination (Table I). The 39 living subjects were investigated clinically and radiologically, and only one (Case 2) was found to have any relevant pulmonary abnormality. Three had healed pulmonary tuberculosis, and two had active disease, one with cavitation and one with enlarged glands which resolved in 18 months. Among the 25 patients who had been examined fully after death, no record was found suggesting changes in the lungs due to pulmonary tuberous sclerosis. Histological sections of the lungs were available in six cases only: none showed evidence of tuberous sclerosis. Thus, of the total of 64 mentally defective patients whose records were adequate, only one was found to have the lungs affected. Seven patients with adenoma sebaceum were also examined; one of them (Case 4) was found to have lung involvement (Table I). So far the only figures relating to the incidence of pulmonary changes have been given by Borberg in his recent clinical and genetic study of tuberous sclerosis (1951). His survey covered the whole of Denmark, where he collected 37 cases of all types found in a period of 20 years. Twenty-six showed the classical features including severe mental disturbance, and 11 others showed only cutaneous or,

TABLE II

Sex and Age Distribution

Type of patient	*Total*	*Sex* *M*	*F*	*Age (years) at death or on June 1, 1951* *0–9*	*10–19*	*20–29*	*30–39*	*40–49*	*50–59*
A. Mental defect and adenoma sebaceum:									
Mentally defective (alive and dead)	64	28	36	8	14	17	14*	7	4
With adenoma sebaceum (alive)	7	2	5	2	1	1	2	..	1*
Total	71	30	41	10	15	18	16	7	5
B. Pulmonary tuberous sclerosis:									
Present series	4	1	3	..	..	1	2*	..	1*
Previously recorded	9	1	8	..	..	2	5	..	2

* Cases 2 and 4 are included in Sections A and B.

occasionally, other visceral abnormalities. None of the mentally defective patients had involvement of the lungs, but four of the other 11 patients were found to have cystic changes, confirmed at necropsy. Three of these four cases had already been recorded by Licht (1942), Samuelsen (1942), and Rosendal (1942). The diagnosis in Rosendal's case is not absolutely certain, as there was no evidence of tuberous sclerosis outside the lungs; it is included in Appendix B. Borberg's findings and my own show that the pulmonary changes are hardly ever met with in patients who have severe mental disturbance, and that they usually come to light because of pulmonary symptoms in patients who are then found to have other stigmata of tuberous sclerosis. In view of the late onset of pulmonary symptoms, and presumably of detectable lung changes—24 years being the youngest recorded age at onset of symptoms—the patients in the present inquiry have been grouped in decades (Table II). The ages of the patients with pulmonary involvement in the present series and in those previously recorded are shown for comparison. One-third of them were over 30 years of age, and more than half over 20 years of age. The figures reveal that an adequate number of the mentally defective group reached the age at which lung changes are found. Early death does not explain why the mental and lung forms of the disease are so seldom seen in the same patient.

Clinical and necropsy findings. The clinical features of the surviving patients are summarized in Table III, and the clinical and necropsy findings in those who had died, with the causes of death, in Tables IV and V. The number of patients with a family history of the disease is certainly too small, because relatives were not examined for minor signs of the disease, and because of the tendency of patients and their relatives to overlook lunatic members of the family and those dying during infancy. The incidence of renal and retinal tumours in the mentally abnormal group is probably higher than the findings suggest, because of poor co-operation during examination. All the patients

TABLE III

Clinical Findings in 39 Cases of Tuberous Sclerosis with Mental Defect and Seven Cases of Adenoma Sebaceum

Type of case	*Total numbers*	*Family history of tuberous sclerosis*	*Mental defect*	*Adenoma sebaceum*	*Epilepsy*	*Palpable renal tumours*	*Subungual fibromas*	*Peau chagriné*	*Retinal tumours*	*Radiological abnormalities: Lungs*	*Radiological abnormalities: Bones*
Cerebral tuberous sclerosis	39*	7 patients (34) 31 relatives	39	39	29 (34)	3 (25)	20 (34)	27 (34)	6 (21)	1	0 (5)
Adenoma sebaceum	7	4 patients 15 relatives	2†	7	1	2	2	1	0	1	2

* Five patients were not available for clinical examination.
† High-grade defectives living normal lives.

The figures in parentheses indicate the number of patients examined for the feature in question, when it differed from the total.

TABLE IV

Clinical and Necropsy Findings in 25 Cases of Tuberous Sclerosis

	Clinical			*Necropsy*			
	Mental defect	*Adenoma sebaceum*	*Epilepsy*	*Renal tumours*	*Cerebral tuberous sclerosis*	*Cardiac tumours*	*Tumours elsewhere*
Number of cases .	25	24	22	5 (13)	25	3	Spleen, eye, liver, thyroid: 1 each

The figures in parenthesis indicate the number of patients examined for the feature in question, when it differed from the total.

TABLE V

Causes of Death in 25 Cases of Tuberous Sclerosis

Tuberculosis: Pulmonary	5
Other	1
Bronchopneumonia or pulmonary suppuration .	10
Status epilepticus	5
Cerebral abscess	1
Cerebral tumour	1
Carcinoma of uterus	1
,, ,, ovary	1

with mental defect due to tuberous sclerosis had adenoma sebaceum, except one, in whom the diagnosis was made at necropsy; the brain alone was affected.

Cases of Pulmonary Tuberous Sclerosis in the Present Series

Only two examples of the pulmonary form were found among the 71 cases of known tuberous sclerosis. Two others were discovered in patients who came for advice about pulmonary symptoms.

Case 1. I. D., a single woman 30 years of age, came under medical care after a visit to a miniature radiography unit in February 1950. Since 1947 she had had four attacks of pain in the chest, followed by breathlessness for a few days; the pain was twice on the right side, and twice on the left. In December 1949 a nasal catarrh was followed a few days later by severe cough, producing a small amount of mucoid sputum, twice streaked with blood. Shortly after starting to cough she felt a sharp pain in the back of the left side of the chest, radiating round to the front and accompanied by considerable breathlessness. She retired to bed for four days, but was still breathless on resuming work a week later. Because of these recurrent attacks she went to a miniature radiography unit in February 1950, where the film revealed a partial pneumothorax. At this time her sputum was again streaked with blood. Soon afterwards a sixth episode occurred, with pain localized to the epigastrium, and breathlessness lasting about two weeks. She was referred to hospital, and in June was admitted for investigation. This patient was the fourth of a family of seven, six of whom were alive and well. Her father had died of carcinoma of the bowel in 1940. There had been no miscarriages, but one girl had died, aged four years, from diphtheria. None of her five siblings had suffered from fits, nor was any known to have any facial eruption or mental disorder. Three of the siblings and the mother were available for examination; all were normal on physical examination, and the chest radiograph showed no evidence of disease. In the previous generation I. D.'s father and his sister had no stigmata of tuberous sclerosis. Her mother was an only child. Six of the patient's nieces and nephews, aged 22, 19, 18, nine, eight, and five years, were alive and well, without significant medical histories. The patient's early life had been uneventful. She was said to have been a healthy infant, delivered naturally without undue delay or instrumental help; breathing and feeding had been readily established. At the age of five years a facial eruption had developed, and had become more conspicuous during the next five years. From eight to 10 years of age she had suffered from recurrent Jacksonian convulsions, usually affecting the left arm and face only, but sometimes the left leg as well; she had never lost consciousness. From the age of 10 years until the present illness she had been well and free from further fits. Her mother believed her to be as intelligent as the rest of her family, though of a more retiring nature. She was of dark complexion and slight build, weighing 50 kg., her height being 160 cm. She was a quiet, restrained girl, who readily co-operated in the investigation and treatment. The skin of the nose and adjacent cheek and, to a lesser extent, of the chin and forehead, was disfigured by a symmetric eruption (Plate 8, Fig. 3). It consisted of numerous skin-coloured papules of lentil size, mostly half embedded but occasionally pedunculated. They were crowded together centrally, but scattered at the periphery. Over and between these nodules were numerous fine blood-vessels, which could make the eruption flush to a dull red colour when the patient was hot or excited, but there was very little obvious telangiectasia. In the left lumbar region was a small patch of peau chagriné about 5 cm. in diameter (Plate 8, Fig. 2). The nails of three fingers and eight toes were deformed by warty swellings arising from the lateral edges of the nail-base (Plate 8, Fig. 4). Some of the nails were ridged longwise and unduly brittle. No clinical abnormality was found in the cardiovascular, respiratory, or central nervous systems. The ocular fundi contained three pale, very slightly raised swellings of about one-third the diameter of the optic disk. They were all in the periphery, two in the right eye and one in the left. The kidneys were moderately enlarged, and deformed by several rounded lumps. Examination of the urine showed no abnormality.

Special investigations. Radiographs of the chest showed a fine mesh-work, uniformly distributed, when both lungs were fully expanded. The films of April 1950 revealed a small left pneumothorax with a little pleural effusion (Plate 9, Figs. 5 and 6). A right bronchogram was not grossly abnormal, though the more distal bronchi were narrower than usual. Tomograms showed clearly the abnormal mesh-work shadowing, but no cysts were seen. All the bones were examined radiologically: the left fibula had subperiosteal thickening and an oval translucency at its lower end, the size of a small bean (Plate 9, Fig. 7). Several of the phalanges also showed subperiosteal nodes. The skull bones were normal; there was no intracranial calcification. Excretion urography confirmed the renal enlargement, and showed deformity of the lower calyces on the right side; concentration of the dye was not impaired. An electrocardiogram showed low-voltage deflections with inverted TV_3 and TV_4, but was otherwise normal. An electroencephalogram was normal. Intelligence tests indicated average ability. The Wechsler index and Rorschach record revealed no evidence of intellectual deterioration or organic damage. The haemoglobin was 76 per cent. (11·3 gm. per 100 ml.), red blood-cells 4,600,000 per c.mm., and white cells 10,200 per c.mm., with a normal differential count. Plasma-cholesterol, serum-proteins, and blood-urea were normal. Three gastric washings contained no acid-fast organisms, and one culture failed to grow any. The Mantoux test was positive at 1/10,000 dilution. A small piece of one of the finger tumours was taken for examination.

Course and treatment. After three weeks the patient returned home, nothing fresh having arisen while she was in hospital. She remained well and at work until December 28, 1950, when she had a further spontaneous pneumothorax on the left side, confirmed radiologically. The lung re-expanded after two weeks' rest, and she returned to work. She remained well for the next nine months except for one small haemoptysis. On October 3, 1951, she had an eighth attack of pain and breathlessness; the pain this time was on the right side. The symptoms were much more severe than they had been on previous occasions, causing her considerable distress, and were accompanied by vomiting. She was admitted to hospital as an urgent case and when seen was restless, cyanotic, and suffering considerable pain. The pulse was rapid, and the blood-pressure normal. She had obvious signs of a right pneumothorax, and a radiograph showed complete collapse of that lung. Five hundred ml. of air were removed from a positive-pressure pneumothorax, with some relief to the patient, but within 12 hours the breathlessness and vomiting returned. More air was removed, but this procedure failed to maintain the negative pressure, so proving the existence of bronchopleural fistula. During the next three weeks, in spite of the continual use of an underwater drain and repeated aspiration of the air, the lung would not expand fully. A thoracotomy was therefore performed. The lung was deeply coloured a dark blue shade, and its surface showed lentil-sized miliary nodules paler than the rest of the lung, and probably caused by small subpleural blebs. On the lateral aspect of the upper lobe there was one surface bulla, 1·5 cm. in diameter, but not obviously leaking. The lung substance felt firmer than normal and rather gritty. A small piece was taken from the upper lobe. Both layers of the pleura were painted with 5 per cent. silver nitrate solution. After operation the lung rapidly expanded, and one month later the patient left hospital to continue convalescence. In December 1951 she was free from symptoms, and able to walk two miles without breathlessness. One month later pneumothorax recurred on the left side, and she again entered hospital for treatment. The chest was opened on the left; the appearance of the lung was the same as on the other side. There were numerous short string- and band-adhesions scattered widely over both lobes, but they were long enough to allow considerable collapse of the lung. Another small biopsy specimen was taken from the interlobar fringe of the upper lobe; the specimen was removed and fixed between clamps to avoid distortion from loss of air. Both pleural layers were painted with 5 per cent. silver nitrate solution. The lung was fully expanded five days after operation. The patient left hospital a week later, and when last seen in November 1953 was well, except for some breathlessness on hurrying, which was noted for the first time apart from her attacks of pneumothorax.

Histological reports. The right lung biopsy specimen (Prof. H. A. Magnus) (Plate 10, Fig. 8) showed condensed lung tissue with several cyst-like spaces, at least two of which were incompletely lined by cuboidal epithelium. No muscle or cartilage was seen. All the alveoli and cyst-like spaces contained large numbers of macrophages filled with iron pigment. There was no obvious angiomatous formation. The finger biopsy specimen showed a squamous-celled papilloma. The left lung biopsy specimen (Prof. H. A. Magnus) consisted of a triangular portion of lung tissue, 2·5 cm. by 2·5 cm. by 2 cm. The pleural surface appeared normal. The cut surface presented a spongy appearance due to the presence of small spherical cysts, the largest measuring 0·2 cm. in diameter. Section of the piece of lung tissue showed a number of small cystic spaces, situated mainly at the periphery. They were lined by a low columnar or cuboidal epithelium. The walls of the cysts contained very many dilated blood-vessels of the size and structure of small venules or arterioles. The central part of the specimen presented a more solid appearance. There was a number of unexpanded alveolus-like structures, lined by large cuboidal cells with a well-developed reticulin framework. In addition there were completely solid areas, composed of similar large cuboidal cells together with small bands of smooth muscle-fibres and of fibroblasts (Plate 10, Fig. 9); there was relatively little collagen. No striated muscle or vasoformative tissue was demonstrable. Throughout the section there were vast numbers of iron-pigment-containing macrophages, lying both free in the cysts or alveoli and within the lung parenchyma (Plate 10, Fig. 10). There was no evidence of an inflammatory basis for the changes observed, and the histological picture was highly suggestive of a developmental anomaly. The iron pigment seen in the sections from both lungs was probably due to haemorrhages from the vascular walls of the lung cysts.

Case 2. G. A. M., a man aged 38 years and a patient in Botley's Park Hospital, suffered from mental defect and epilepsy, which were considered to be due to tuberous sclerosis because he also had adenoma sebaceum. He had been admitted in 1932, at the age of 20 years, under the Mental Deficiency Act, 1913, Sect. III, and the following history had been given by his stepmother. Nothing was known about the circumstances of his birth, but at the age of one year he had fallen in a fit and been 'unconscious' for several days. He then suffered from repeated epileptic fits, and did not walk or talk until the age of five years. It had been impossible to educate him, but he had been kept at home until he had become too difficult to control. None of his family was known to be afflicted by tuberous sclerosis. His father was normal, his mother unknown, and nothing could be discovered about his siblings. Since admission he had been very dull, childish, and unable to attend to his own needs, except for feeding himself. He was ignorant of common fact; his mental age was estimated at four and a half years. He suffered from an average of four epileptic seizures each month. No respiratory symptoms had been noticed, and he was not unduly susceptible to respiratory catarrh. During examination he was stolid and cheerful. His face was covered with adenoma sebaceum of gross degree and showing considerable telangiectasia. In the right lumbar region was a well-marked patch of peau chagriné, a sheet of nodular thickened skin about 10 cm. square, of normal colour. Elsewhere on the back were several intracutaneous fibromas about the size of half a cherry. On four of the toes of the right foot were typical subungual fibromas and ridged nails. He had considerable gingivitis and dental caries, but the mouth was otherwise normal. The chest and cardio-vascular systems were normal. The left kidney could be felt, and was slightly enlarged, its surface being grossly irregular. Apart from mental defect, the central nervous system showed no abnormality. The ocular fundi were normal. Investigations were limited by the patient's inability to co-operate.

Special investigations. Radiographs of his chest showed an ill-defined mottling throughout both lung fields, more prominent in the lower half of the right lung (Plate 11, Fig. 11). No definite cysts were seen in the straight films, but tomograms confirmed the presence of mottling, and in the lower part of the right lung cystic change was apparent. The skull and long bones were radio-logically normal. Excretion urography was unsuccessful.

Case 3. G. B., a married woman aged 41 years, first developed sustained respiratory symptoms when 38 years old. In childhood she had been anaemic, and had suffered from occasional attacks of petit mal, in which she had sometimes bitten her tongue. In recent years these fits had been infrequent. She had four sisters, who had no significant illnesses, and her father and mother had died of carcinoma of the lung and heart failure respectively. One brother, aged 48 years, had suffered from fits in childhood, and recently laryngofissure had been done to remove two soft oedematous sessile polyp-like swellings, one on each vocal cord. The tumours showed overgrowth of loose myxomatous tissue, apparently granulation tissue, and not neoplastic. The chest radiograph was normal. Her only child was born when she was 27 years old, and now, at the age of 15 years, was perfectly healthy. At the age of 32 years she had suffered from 'pleurisy'; the pain started suddenly when she was stooping to open a drawer, and was immediately accompanied by considerable breathlessness, but she had no fever. During the following week she noticed a beating noise and sensation in the neighbourhood of her heart, which even her husband could hear. Her symptoms gradually improved, and when she was examined by fluoroscope two weeks after the onset nothing abnormal could be seen. She remained well for five years, and then, in 1948, began to feel breathless after moderate exertion, and her voice became husky. A chest radiograph showed a shadow at the left apex, which was thought to represent an old tuberculous lesion; her sputum contained no *M. tuberculosis*. During the next two years her breathlessness steadily increased, and an irritable cough developed. In October 1950, when 39 years old, she coughed up a fleck of bright red blood for the first time. Another radiograph showed an increase of the shadowing at the left apex, but her sputum still contained no *M. tuberculosis*. Her symptoms of cough and breathlessness increased and, because of their disproportion to the radiological extent of her supposed tuberculosis, the diagnosis was reviewed. She entered hospital in February 1951 for investigation. At this time she had troublesome cough, but no sputum. The least movement made her breathless and caused discomfort over the lower part of the sternum, and she tired easily. Her voice was husky. She had no other symptoms, and had not lost weight. She was a well-built woman, weighing 55 kg., with a sparse symmetrical papular eruption in the nasal grooves and on the adjoining cheeks, with little telangiectasia (Balzer type). She also had subungual fibromas on three toe-nails.

She was slightly breathless even at rest, and a few scattered crepitations could be heard in the lungs. Nothing abnormal was found in the cardiovascular or central nervous systems. The liver, spleen, and kidneys could not be felt. The urine was normal.

Special investigations. Chest radiographs of August 1948 showed ill-defined patchy mottling in the left upper lobe (Plate 11, Fig. 12). In retrospect some diffuse infiltration was just apparent in the periphery of the right lower zone. By October 1950 the shadow in the left upper lobe had become much heavier, and new confluent infiltration could be seen throughout both lungs. On the right side a circumscribed shadow was seen at the base of the periphery of the upper lobe. Many rounded translucent areas, varying from 1 to 3 mm. in diameter, had appeared. They were most conspicuous in the upper lobes, and were presumably due to 'cysts' or areas of emphysema. In February 1951 all the changes previously seen were intensified, and the contrast between translucent emphysema and the denser infiltration was heightened (Plate 12, Fig. 13). The largest cysts, about six in number, were now 5 mm. in diameter, and their walls were well defined. The changes in the lower lobes appeared as heavy reticulation, the contained spaces being very small. The outlines of the lung-roots, and the heart and the bones, were normal. The erythrocyte sedimentation rate on January 8, 1951, was 59 mm. in one hour. No *M. tuberculosis* were seen in the sputum or in two gastric washings. None were grown in two cultures. Examination of the larynx (Prof. F. C. Ormerod) showed small nodules on each vocal cord. Bronchoscopy (Mr. R. C. Brock) was normal. Lung biopsy (Mr. R. C. Brock): a small piece of middle lobe, containing a firm nodule surrounded by small bullae, was removed.

Course and treatment. Ten days after she left hospital a right pneumothorax developed, and the symptoms were so severe that she was taken to hospital for treatment. Mr. P. R. Allison examined her by thoracoscope, and found numerous bullae of different sizes. The scar of the biopsy performed in February was seen to be well healed. Silver nitrate solution was painted over the bullae. The lung rapidly expanded and became adherent to the chest wall, but a loculated pneumothorax persisted, with air at the apex and base. When she again left hospital at the end of May she was still very breathless at rest. In July she had acute bronchitis, and became even more short-winded; the right partial pneumothorax was still present. She recovered from this attack, and improved steadily, so that she was able to move slowly about her house and garden. On October 10, while sitting in a chair, she developed another pneumothorax, and died of asphyxia within an hour. Permission for necropsy was refused.

Histology of lung biopsy specimen (Dr. J. W. Clegg) (Plate 12, Fig. 14). The specimen measured 2 cm. by 1 cm. Section showed well aerated lung. Many alveolar walls were ruptured, so that numerous emphysematous vesicles were formed. Scattered throughout the section were occasional pedunculated nodules attached to the alveolar walls. They were covered by a single layer of cuboidal cells, and consisted almost entirely of elongated cells with cylindrical nuclei; no collagen was demonstrated. The blood-vessels were normal in form and number, and no free iron was present. The bronchi were also normal. There was no evidence of inflammatory change.

Case 4. J. T., a married woman of 50 years, was interviewed and examined together with two of her children because they were all suffering from tuberous sclerosis. She was one of a family of 12 children; all the others had died in early infancy, and details of their illnesses were unknown. Nothing could be discovered about the health of her father and mother, both of whom were dead. She herself had 12 children, and only three were apparently unaffected by the disease. Seven had died at the ages of 23, 15, 11, seven, and three years, six months, and at birth, respectively; during life they had all suffered from fits, and the first three had been mentally defective. Of these seven children necropsy reports were available as to the three oldest and the three-year-old; the lungs had shown no gross evidence of cystic change or tumour. Five children

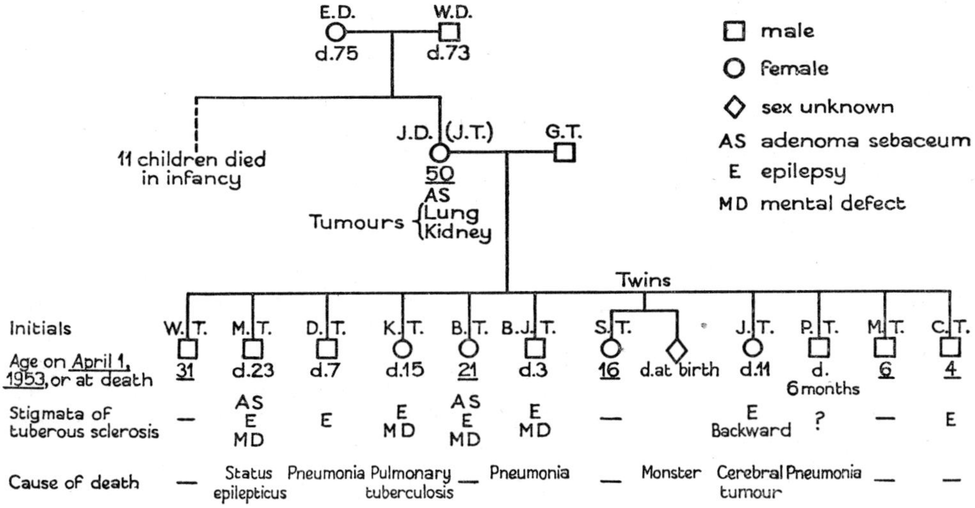

Family of J. T. (Case 4).

survived, and of these one was mentally defective and suffered from fits, one suffered from fits only, and three were apparently normal. Two of these five, aged 21 and four years, were available for examination. The elder, under care in a mental defective hospital, showed many characteristic changes. The younger had suffered from continuous fits from the age of two months, having at the present time as many as 20 seizures in a day, uncontrolled by anticonvulsant drugs; the only other stigma he showed was a lumbar patch of peau chagriné. The chest radiographs of both these sibs were normal. J. T., the mother of these children, had led a healthy life, and her 11 confinements, one a twin birth, had been uneventful. She said she herself had never had fits. She had no respiratory symptoms except occasional winter cough. She was of average height and build. Her level of intelligence was below average, but she was a good and attentive mother within the limits imposed by the size of her family and a small income. Her face was disfigured by a diffuse symmetrical eruption, composed of many small blue capillary naevi and a lesser number of millet-sized papules between and beneath these vessels. These blemishes were concentrated on the parts of the cheeks adjacent to the nose, and gradually diminished in number on the fringes of the eruption. Scattered over the neck and back were several reddish filiform papillomas and flesh-coloured cutaneous fibromas. There was no peau chagriné. Two finger-nails on each hand were deformed by subungual fibromas and longitudinal ridges; both big toes showed similar tumours. Just above the right knee on the lateral side of the thigh was a soft lobulated swelling 7 cm. in diameter, probably a lipoma. In the left eye were five white nodules, and several smaller ones, in the periphery of the inferior part of the fundus (Plate 15, Fig. 20); the larger ones were each about one-sixth of the size of the optic disk. The rest of the central nervous system was normal. The right kidney was enlarged to about twice normal size, and its surface was coarsely nodular. The urine was normal. No clinical abnormality was found in the respiratory or cardiovascular systems.

Special investigations. Radiographs of the chest showed a lobulated circumscribed shadow, 3 cm. in diameter, lying in the anterior segment of the right middle lobe (Plate 13, Fig. 15). No evidence of reticulation or cystic change was seen elsewhere. The hilar shadows were not enlarged. Tomograms confirmed the presence of the mass in the middle lobe. Its outline was clear, and the density even. Stereoscopic views of the skull showed one rounded calcified mass in the region of the basal ganglia (Plate 13, Fig. 16). Radiographs of the long bones were normal, but the hands showed a small cystic space, 3 mm. across, in the base of the second phalanx of the left middle finger. The index finger had similar, less conspicuous, changes in the same site (Plate 14, Fig. 17). Excretion urography revealed that the right kidney was generally enlarged. The blood-cells and the blood-urea were normal.

Course and treatment. The shadow in the right middle lobe did not alter during a period of one year. Nevertheless, because of the possibility that it might be due to a carcinoma, the middle lobe was then removed. The patient left hospital in three weeks, and was well when seen 10 months after operation.

Pathological report (Dr. J. W. Clegg). 'There is a dumb-bell shaped peripheral tumour, about 3 cm. long, situated in the peripheral portion of this middle lobe.' (Plate 14, Fig. 18.) 'The tumour is sharply demarcated from the surrounding lung tissue, and presents a homogeneous yellowish white surface. Section shows an adenoma composed of columnar cells with a tendency to acinar arrangement.' (Plate 14, Fig. 19.) 'Stains with periodic acid show the presence of mucin granules in many of the tumour cells, and there are focal collections of mucin in the somewhat irregular acini. The tumour would appear to be a benign mucin secreting adenoma.'

Discussion

The forms of tuberous sclerosis

The term tuberous sclerosis strictly applies only to particular changes in the brain; by usage, however, it has become accepted as the generic name for diverse clinical forms of the same underlying disease. Several systems are usually affected, and when lung changes have been present characteristic deformities have been found elsewhere. These can be grouped as involving the brain and the eye, the skin, the viscera, and the bones; they will be discussed before considering the lungs themselves. Most sufferers from tuberous sclerosis come under medical care either for mental disorder or for skin eruptions. Of the 78 cases collected from the literature by Bielschowsky and Gallus (1913), 33 patients were mentally defective, many being epileptic, and 59 had adenoma sebaceum, 13 of these being also mentally defective. Now and then the disease has first attracted attention for other reasons, such as the appearance of a renal tumour (Kirpicznik, 1910; Hyman, 1922; Feriz, 1930), a cerebral tumour (Globus, Strauss, and Selinsky, 1932; Parr, 1948), or a retinal tumour (Loewenstein and Steel, 1941); and sometimes it has caused neonatal death (von Recklinghausen, 1862; Hartdegen, 1881; Pratt-Thomas, 1947).

The cerebral changes declare themselves by epilepsy beginning usually, but not invariably, from infancy, and by mental defect of imbecile or idiot grade. Each may occur alone and may be the sole manifestation of the disease (Stewart, 1935), as once in the present series; the diagnosis can then be made only from the family history, or after death. Critchley and Earl (1932) investigated in detail both the neurological and the psychotic features of 29 cases of tuberous sclerosis, describing a characteristic schizophrenic behaviour often out of proportion to the degree of mental defect. Focal disorders are surprisingly uncommon unless malignancy complicates the picture (Globus, Strauss, and Selinsky, 1932) and cerebral tuberous sclerosis does not produce characteristic changes in the electroencephalogram. Sometimes the 'sclerotic' areas in the brain calcify (Marcus, 1924; Dalsgaard-Nielsen, 1935) and can be seen radiologically as 'cotton-balls' asymmetrically distributed and of various size. The masses in the brain lie in the gyri, raising the surface and confined between two sulci. They vary in size and in number from half a dozen to several score. They are whiter, more opaque, and firmer than the surrounding brain tissue, and are scattered mainly throughout the cortex; diffuse enlargement of the convolutions also occurs. The nodules consist mainly of glial fibres with few cell-bodies, but scattered here and there are large bipolar or multipolar giant cells of astroglial origin. The retinal tumours, first described by van der Hoeve (1921), are rarer than cerebral or skin changes. There are two varieties: one a glistening whitish or grey nodular mass protruding into the vitreous, about the size of the disk, and usually lying near the nerve-head, the other a flat white or grey-white plaque about half the size of the first kind, and often multiple (Plate 15, Fig. 20). Van der Hoeve named these tumours phakomata because of their flat lentil-like appearance. These retinal masses usually penetrate no deeper than the nerve-fibre layer, and consist of nerve-fibres and large cells of uncertain origin and of varying shape with large nuclei. The facial eruption, already described in the words of Addison, along with the subungual fibromas (Kothe, 1904) and the peau chagriné (Hallopeau and Leredde, 1895), are alone peculiar to tuberous sclerosis. Subungual fibromas are firm flesh-coloured or dull-red growths, emerging from the groove of the nail-bed to lie on the nail-plate (Plate 8, Fig. 4); they vary in shape, can be as large as a pea, and usually appear during adolescence. The nail-plate often shows unduly prominent ridging. Peau chagriné is a sheet of thickened nodular skin, of normal colour, often about the size of a man's palm (Plate 8, Fig. 2), situated in the lumbar or lower thoracic region. These skin changes usually accompany adenoma sebaceum, but may precede it, as in one of our patients, a two-year-old epileptic. Adenoma sebaceum usually appears between the ages of five and 13 years, but sometimes as late as 20 years. The facial eruption may be the only clinical sign of tuberous sclerosis, but it is not known whether the brain tissue is then inevitably, though silently, involved. Many other types of blemish are also seen: naevoid plaques, brown or red tags, fibromas which may be miliary, papular, or subcutaneous, and large 'café-au-lait' spots, or more diffuse pigmentation or vitiligo. In the mouth fibrous nodules are sometimes found on the gums, palate, or tongue. Adenoma sebaceum consists of overgrown sebaceous glands embedded in

Table VI

Clinical Features of Pulmonary Tuberous Sclerosis

Case number	*Authors*	*Age when first seen (years)*	*Age at death (years)*	*Sex*	*Respiratory symptoms*	*Cause of death*	*Family history*	*Fits or mental defect*	*Adenoma sebaceum (A.S.); subungual fibromas (U.F.)*	*Other organs affected clinically*
I	Berg (1938); Berg and Vejlens (1939)	30	32	F	Cough; loss of weight; dyspnoea 2 years; S.P. (2), recurrent	Right heart failure	+	..	A.S.	..
II	Samuelsen (1942)	36	49	F	Haemoptysis; expectoration; cough; breathlessness. 11 years	Cerebral haemorrhage	?	Mental defect	..	Bones of hands (X-ray)
III	Licht (1942)	63	67	F	Dyspnoea 1 year; sputum; cough	Right heart failure	+	..	..	..
IV	Warren and Warvi (1943)	24	26	F	Dyspnoea	S.P.	..	Mental defect	A.S.	Kidneys (albuminuria and uraemia)
V	Berg and Nordenskjöld (1946)	29	33	F	Dyspnoea 1 year; loss of weight; S.P.	Progressive dyspnoea; debility and right heart failure	+	..	A.S., U.F.	Vagina (myoma); retina (phakoma); skull (bone sclerosis)
VI	Paliard, Plauchu, Galy, and Papillon (1946)	39	Surviving	F	Haemoptysis	..	..	..	A.S., U.F.	Brain; intracranial calcification
VII	Oswald and Parkinson (1949)	31	Surviving	F	Dyspnoea (moderate) 5 years	..	..	..	A.S., U.F.	Kidneys; heart (doubtful); bones (X-ray)
VIII	Inglis (1950)	33	41	F	'Asthma' 8 years; severe dyspnoea 3 years	S.P.; asphyxia	..	..	A.S.	Kidneys (albuminuria)
IX	Borberg (1951)	64	66	M	Dyspnoea 2 years; cough; sputum 2 months; cyanosis	Heart failure; asphyxia; pneumonia	+	..	..	..
Present series:										
1		30	Surviving (32)	F	Dyspnoea; S.P. (2); haemoptysis	..	..	Fits	A.S., U.F.	Kidneys; bones
2		38	Surviving (39)	M	None	..	..	Fits Mental defect	A.S., U.F.	Kidneys
3		38	41	F	Dyspnoea; cough; S.P. (2); haemoptysis	S.P.; asphyxia	+	Fits	A.S., U.F.	..
4		50	Surviving	F	None	..	+	..	A.S., U.F.	Kidneys; bones

S.P. = spontaneous pneumothorax: (2) = bilateral.

hypertrophied connective tissue, with a varying number of blood-vessels; these ingredients form the substance of the other skin abnormalities. The nail-bed tumours are usually described as fibromas covered by normal dermis (Butterworth and Wilson, 1941). Occasionally, as in Case 1, they are papillomas. Renal tumours are the commonest of the visceral manifestations of the disease. In one series (Bielschowsky and Gallus, 1913) 41 of 78 sufferers from tuberous sclerosis had abnormal growths in the kidney at necropsy. The tumours are mostly bilateral, multiple, and of yellow colour. They consist of varying mixtures of renal epithelium and fatty, fibrous, and vascular tissue, and, like the cerebral lesions, they occasionally become malignant (Kirpicznik, 1910; Hyman, 1922; Feriz, 1930). Tumours have been found in many other organs, the commonest being rhabdomyomas in the heart (Farber, 1931). The limb bones also may show radiological changes consisting of nodular periosteal thickening and single cyst-like spaces (Gottlieb and Lavine, 1935). The skull bones may be thickened or mottled by ill-defined areas of increased density (Dalsgaard-Nielsen, 1935). The pathology of these bony changes is still uncertain.

The pulmonary form

Nine examples of tuberous sclerosis affecting the lungs have previously been recorded. Five of them were found in Denmark or Sweden, but none had been recognized in this country until Oswald and Parkinson described a case in 1949. They all showed a fairly uniform clinical and radiological picture in the lungs, and in seven cases characteristic changes were found after death. Summaries of these records (Cases I–IX) are collected in Appendix A. Table VI gives the main features of these cases and those in the present series. The diagnosis of tuberous sclerosis depended on finding typical lesions elsewhere, except in two instances (Cases III and IX) in which the discovery of afflicted relatives made exact diagnosis possible. These two cases raise the important question of whether tuberous sclerosis can affect the lungs without involving the brain, for hitherto cerebral changes have been considered an essential feature of post-mortem studies in this disease. In the past, six other patients have been described whose histories of respiratory disease have been in every way comparable with cases of acknowledged pulmonary tuberous sclerosis. At necropsy the gross and minute changes in the lungs were similar to those found in authentic examples. In addition three of these patients had renal tumours of a type known to occur almost exclusively in tuberous sclerosis. Because characteristic cerebral sclerosis was not found, usually because it was not sought, the relation of this group to the well-founded cases is doubtful; they are therefore recorded and briefly discussed in Appendix B. To return to the proved examples of pulmonary tuberous sclerosis with evidence of the disease outside the lungs: six patients had adenoma sebaceum, and three of these also had subungual fibromas; no other skin lesions were recorded. Mental changes were by no means the rule, and were only once (Case IV) definitely due to the disease, the only other instance (Case II) being due in part to vascular as well as sclerotic lesions; no patient had suffered from epilepsy, and retinal tumours were only noted once (Case V), though it is not certain that every patient was examined from this point of view. Renal tumours were discovered clinically once only (Case VII) but they were found in five others (Cases I, II, IV, V, and VIII) at necropsy. Radiological examination of the bones was probably undertaken in four patients only, all of whom, however, showed typical abnormalities. Periosteal thickening and small cysts were present in the hands or long bones of Cases II and VII. The skull was examined in three cases only: one (Case VI) showed intracranial calcification, and another (Case V) parietal bone sclerosis. Other members of the family were affected by the general form of the disease in two instances, while Berg's two patients were sisters, both of whom suffered from pulmonary tuberous sclerosis.

All four patients in the present series had widespread abnormalities apart from the lungs. In two cases other members of the family were affected. Three patients had had fits, and the fourth showed intracranial calcification as evidence that the brain was involved; in two patients intelligence was impaired. Retinal tumours were seen twice (Cases 1 and 4). All four patients had characteristic changes in the face and nails, and two also had lumbar peau chagriné. Three had palpable renal tumours, which were demonstrated radiologically in two. The abnormal T waves in the electrocardiogram in Case 1 may have been caused by rhabdomyomas in the myocardium, but there was no supporting evidence. Only one of the two patients whose bones were examined showed the typical combination of cystic and sclerotic changes.

The lungs. Of the total 13 patients, 10 came under medical care for respiratory symptoms. The other three were examined incidentally because members of their families suffered from tuberous sclerosis; one of these three later developed respiratory symptoms, from which she died. The most striking and indicative features in the nine cases from the literature were spontaneous pneumothorax (four cases) and eventual breakdown of lung function (four cases). Next to these was congestive heart failure, seen in three of the nine. Breathlessness was the paramount symptom, as well as the earliest one. It steadily increased to the point of severe disability in most cases, preceded or punctuated in four by brief episodes of more intense dyspnoea from sudden deflation of the lung. In the later stages cyanosis usually appeared. Pain was mentioned only as a symptom of the onset of pneumothorax. Cough developed late, and was prominent in only two cases, in which it was also productive from complicating bronchitis. None of the other patients had sputum. Two (Cases II and VI) had haemoptysis of small amount, a symptom which might have been expected more often, considering the vascularity of the abnormal tissue in the lung and the quantity of iron pigment in it.

On physical examination the chest usually appeared normal, except in the presence of a pneumothorax, or of bronchitis in the later stages. In spite of cyanosis and extensive lung disease, clubbing of the fingers was never noted. This may have been because infection in the lung was nearly always absent, or at least no more than terminal. Two of the four patients who had had spontaneous pneumothorax suffered bilateral attacks, which contributed to their death. Heart failure was the end in four of the seven who died, and necropsy showed a large right ventricle or dilated pulmonary artery, evidence of pulmonary hypertension (Cases I, III, V, and VIII) which is not surprising in view of the extensive disorganization of the vascular bed in the lung. The radiological appearance of the lungs in every case was similar, although the density of the abnormal shadows varied. The abnormality consisted of a mesh-work of lines, variously described as reticulation when the pattern was close-knit or as honeycombing when it was more open, or even as cyst-like when it was coarser still. When the intersections of the lines or shadows were sufficiently prominent, as in two of the present series, their appearance merited the term 'miliary'. The radiological changes were widespread and fairly symmetrical, with the single exception of Case VI, in which they were confined to the left upper and right middle zones. In Cases III and VI tomograms revealed cystic changes not otherwise readily discerned, the cysts being only about 3 mm. in diameter. Successive radiographs were described in Cases I, II, V, and VII over periods of two years, eight years, two years, and four years. In Case I the appearance changed from barely perceptible reticulation, only in retrospect thought to be abnormal, to obvious honeycomb shadowing. In Cases II, V, and VII the appearance of the lung fields did not change, though in Case V 'veiling' appeared in the last three years of life, and was thought to be due to pleural thickening. A bronchogram, done in one case, was normal. The hilar glands were never large enough to be seen radiologically.

Two patients in the present series showed most of the characteristic features of the few previous records, especially the recurring atacks of breathlessness due to spontaneous pneumothorax. One of these patients had the lungs so heavily involved as to cause crippling lack of breath, and finally death from asphyxia after another attack. These two patients had small haemoptyses; in one this occurred on several occasions. As in the cases recorded in the literature, infection was absent or late, an important point for diagnosis. The other two patients had no respiratory symptoms; one (Case 2) had characteristic radiological changes in the lungs, and the other a circumscribed shadow in the middle lobe. The reasons for believing that this tumour was an expression of tuberous sclerosis will be discussed when the pathology is considered. The radiological changes in the chest conformed to previous descriptions in two cases. In places the generalized miliary shadowing enclosed minute 'cysts', often only 1 mm. and seldom more than 3 mm. in diameter. They were difficult to discern without close scrutiny of every part of the lung field. It has been said that sometimes the cysts are more conspicuous in the presence of a pneumothorax, presumably because the normal lobules deflate but the air-filled cysts do not. Slight clarification of the radiological pattern was observed in Case 1 under these conditions. Case 3 showed changes which were at first localized to one part of the lung field, forming a picture not hitherto recorded, though Paliard, Plauchu, Galy, and Papillon (1946) described cystic shadows confined to one lobe in each lung. These focal shadows were of moderate density and quite uniform; they did not suggest the presence of small cysts in the lung. The subsequent changes led to a typical fine cystic and miliary appearance, the nature of which was proved by biopsy. The shadow in Case 4 was a circumscribed mass lying in lung that was otherwise radiologically normal.

Pathology. Seven of the patients with pulmonary tuberous sclerosis described in the literature had died, and were examined at necropsy. Small pieces of lung tissue from three of our own patients were also examined. The essential changes are set out in Table VII.

The lungs. In all these cases the naked-eye and microscopic appearances showed a similar and distinctive pattern affecting the whole of both lungs. The outer surface was covered in each instance with numerous small rounded elevations produced by subpleural cysts. Usually the pleural surfaces were loosely adherent to each other, and a pneumothorax was present in three cases. The cut surface was riddled with cavities varying in size from that of a pin's head to that of a pea. Most contained air, but some were filled with fluid. These cysts were set in a matrix of tissue, more or less completely replacing the normal crepitant lung. The cyst walls varied from brown-red to dark grey in colour and were rather firm, giving the whole lung an indurated consistency. The main bronchi were never grossly dilated, and in one case only showed a terminal infection. The bronchial lymph-nodes were mentioned once only (Case VIII), where they were infiltrated with elongated cells resembling those seen in the lung itself. The microscopic appearances have been fully described, except in Cases IV and IX; little normal tissue could be seen, the alveolar pattern having been replaced almost completely by thick-walled 'cysts' surrounded by new tissue of varying structure. Only a few areas of normal alveoli remained, and these areas were mostly atelectatic. The 'cysts' embedded in this tissue were often without an epithelial lining; others were invested with flattened or cuboidal cells or, less commonly, with ciliated epithelium. Vejlens (1941) studied the 'cysts' carefully in his case, but did not find any special relationship to the bronchial tree, although some of them communicated with the finer bronchi. The new tissue consisted of a varying mixture of old and new fibrous tissue, smooth muscle fibres, and blood-vessels. Fibrous tissue was the chief ingredient in Cases II and III, but smooth muscle cells were most prominent in the others. These muscle-fibres were larger than normal, and their cell outlines were irregular. In some places they were intimately fused with, and apparently arising from, the walls of blood-vessels; in others they were more compactly arranged, forming definite nodes or 'myomas'. In no case has any unusual growth of cartilage been described. Abnormal blood-vessels were conspicuous, except in Case II: they were described as 'angiomatous' because of their many haphazard branches and the variable thickness of their walls. Except in Cases III and VIII a conspicuous amount of iron-containing pigment was seen. It lay both in the cyst walls and in the spaces, either as free granules or in macrophages. There was no record of endarteritis or vascular thrombosis in any of these cases.

Lung tissue from three of our patients was available for examination, two

Table VII

Morbid Anatomy and Histology

Case numbers	*Lungs* — *Naked eye appearance*	*Lungs* — *Microscopic appearance*	*Hilar nodes*	*Kidneys* — *Naked eye appearance*	*Kidneys* — *Microscopic appearance*	*Other organs involved*
I (Berg and Vejlens, (1939)	Pneumothorax; sponge-like tissue, pea-sized cysts, air- or fluid-filled	Cysts usually without epithelium; walled by bundles and tumours of smooth muscle. Haemorrhages and iron pigment	No record	Multiple leiomyomata	Smooth muscle cells	Brain. Splenículus. One cervical lymph gland
II (Samuelsen, 1942)	Pleural adhesions; millet- to pea-sized cysts with brown walls, air-filled	Partly atelectatic; alveolar septa thickened by connective tissue and muscle cells or bundles. Much iron pigment	No record	Multiple small tumours	Mixed tumours containing smooth muscle, connective tissue, and angiomata	Brain
III (Licht, 1942)	Roughly pea-sized cysts. Brown indurated lung	Smooth-walled cavities lined by vascular connective tissue. Dilated bronchi in left lower lobe; unusually prominent bronchial musculature	No record	No record	..	Brain, no record
IV (Warren and Warvi, 1943)	Left pneumothorax. Congenital cystic lung disease	No record	No record	Multiple small tumours	No record	Brain. Ovaries and retroperitoneal tissue
V (Berg and Nordenskjöld, 1946)	Pleural adhesions. Pea- to pinhead-sized cavities, some containing fluid	Fibrous induration rich in vessels; extensive angiomyomatous new formations throughout alveolar walls; many cysts. Haemorrhages and haemosiderin; and tuberculosis, some recent	No record	Bilateral tumours	No record	Brain
VIII (Inglis, 1950)	Right pneumothorax. Bullous emphysema of both lungs. Miliary white nodules, 1–2 mm. diameter	Groups of spindle-shaped cells in nodules. Haemosiderin in tissues and air spaces. Some connective tissue	Infiltrated with elongated cells	Multiple small tumours and cysts	Fat, angiomatous tissues, and many elongated cells	Brain, no record
IX (Borberg, 1951)	Diffuse cystic change except right upper lobe	No record	No record	No record	No record	Brain, no record
Present series:						
1 (Biopsy)	Atelectasis and fine cystic change	Cysts set in solid collapsed lung; great increase in connective tissue, with many blood-vessels and some smooth muscle. Haemosiderin present. Emphysematous vesicles	..	..	..	..
3 (Biopsy)	No obvious cysts in specimen	Alveolar walls thickened by nodes of muscle cells and fibroblasts. No increased vascularity	..	..	..	..
4 (Operation specimen)	Tumour in R. middle lobe	Mucus-secreting adenoma	..	..	..	..

blocks from Case 1 (Plate 10, Figs. 8, 9, 10) and one each from Cases 3 and 4 (Plates 12 and 14, Figs. 14, 18, 19). The pathological findings in Case 4 are unique in this disease, for no single circumscribed tumour of the lung has so far been described. The appearances were of a mucus-secreting adenoma (Plate 14, Fig. 19) unconnected with a bronchus and lying in peripheral lung tissue. This adenoma was one of many new growths afflicting this patient; others had been found in the brain, eyes, kidneys, and skin. It is reasonable to infer that this tumour, of unusual situation and cellular composition, was an expression of the same fundamental abnormality of growth. The usual changes were found in the sections from Case 1, in which the right lung showed collapse and 'cyst' formation but little new tissue; but in the specimen from the left side the normal alveolar architecture was solidly replaced by vascular fibrous tissue containing muscle-fibres, and there was much free iron pigment lying within the macrophages and outside them. The section from Case 3 seemed to represent a yet earlier stage of the disease process. A few alveolar walls were broken down, forming emphysematous vesicles, but there was little collapse, and the only new tissue present was localized in nodes within the alveolar walls. It is evident that the architectural changes and the components of the new tissue vary in different parts of the same lung, a point to bear in mind when only a small piece of tissue can be examined. Another notable feature was the extreme vascularity of the new tissue, without formation of haemangiomas. The large amount of iron pigment found in the lungs (Case 1) is presumably the residue from recurrent haemorrhage. There was no general tendency to bleeding, and no clinical evidence of a general rise of blood-pressure in the pulmonary vessels. Moreover, though the kidneys contain vascular tumours, neither Feriz (1930) nor the authors who have described the pulmonary cases have mentioned haemorrhage or deposits of pigment as conspicuous features of the renal changes. It is therefore difficult to account for the evidence of bleeding, unless an increased blood-flow through the new tissue, brought by the bronchial arterial system (Wright, 1938), raises the pressure in the pulmonary capillaries, leading to their rupture. These abnormal tissues, muscular, connective, and vascular, are the components of normal lung, which in response to some stimulus have grown out of the ordinary proportions. Such indiscriminate hypertrophy of the lung connective tissues, including the smooth muscle, was described by Buhl (1872), who called this condition muscular cirrhosis. Both his and subsequent cases (Buchmann, 1911; von Stossel, 1937) have also shown chronic inflammatory changes, and presumably the smooth muscle proliferated in response to this stimulus. Occasionally overgrowth of muscle in the alveolar-duct walls occurs in rheumatic heart disease, when it is associated with congestion of the pulmonary circulation (Engel and Newns, 1939). Apart from these few exceptions, the discovery of an excess of muscle with varying amount of fibrous and vascular tissue is strongly in favour of tuberous sclerosis, and should lead to a search for signs of that disease in the brain and elsewhere. It is probable that the lungs alone may be affected, as in Case III, in which the gross and microscopic changes were those of pulmonary tuberous sclerosis. In six other cases in the literature the appearances were similar. Three of these cases also showed multiple renal tumours like those described in this disease. The evidence for considering them to be examples of tuberous sclerosis is discussed in Appendix B. Certainly, when such cases come under review, all the organs should be carefully examined for the characteristic abnormalities before concluding that this disorder is not present.

Other organs. The brain was examined in four of the seven cases, and was found to show the gross and microscopic changes characteristic of tuberous sclerosis in each instance. Occasionally the disease produces no gross change, and the increased glial tissue can then only be detected microscopically. *The kidneys*, examined in five of the seven cases, were all found to contain numerous small tumours composed of mixtures of fat, smooth muscle, and connective tissue. In Cases I and IV the tumours were seen to be penetrating the renal capsule. No haemorrhages or iron deposits have been described. *Lymph-glands.* There is no record of examination of the lymph-glands draining the kidneys. In Case I a lymph-gland in the parathyroid region was found to be infiltrated with smooth muscle cells, but the capsule was intact.

Diagnosis. The evidence already given has shown that the lungs may be affected by tuberous sclerosis, and that when they are affected the patients most often come under observation owing to respiratory symptoms, usually breathlessness, and sometimes with spontaneous pneumothorax. They are then found to have radiographic changes in the lungs, either reticulation or honeycombing, the nature of which may be deduced either from evidence of tuberous sclerosis elsewhere or from the histological appearance of the lung. The commonest and most obvious stigma is adenoma sebaceum, readily diagnosed at sight and confirmable by biopsy; this alone is proof of tuberous sclerosis. Subungual fibromas and peau chagriné do not occur in any other condition, but their diagnostic value is no higher than that of adenoma sebaceum, because usually they are found only when this condition is already present. The kidneys have been involved in every instance except three (Cases III, VI, and IX), and excretion urography is therefore valuable in every suspected case, though a normal renal outline does not exclude their presence (Case V). Although polycystic disease of the kidneys gives a similar appearance and may be associated with cysts in the liver and pancreas, simultaneous changes in the lungs are not recognized (Oppenheimer, 1934) though one case of localized cystic lung disease and polycystic kidneys has been described (Madonick, Savitsky, and Hochfeld, 1946). Conversely Schenck (1937), reviewing 381 cases of congenital cystic disease of the lungs, did not mention the coexistence of these abnormalities. Thus a combination of renal deformities and typical changes in the lungs would at present be strong evidence in favour of tuberous sclerosis. The presence of radiological changes in the bones, and of retinal tumours, would also add weight to the diagnosis. Surprisingly, the neurological portents are less specific, and in this particular series gave little help. Two patients only had had fits, two were mentally defective, and two had intracranial calcification. When stigmata of tuberous sclerosis are readily found, diagnosis usually gives no difficulty;

but when none is present, as occasionally happens (Cases III and IX), it may be made, as in these examples, by finding relatives with adenoma sebaceum and mental defect or with other features of the disease.

When respiratory symptoms and reticular or miliary shadowing are the sole abnormalities, other diseases are much more likely causes. Among the commoner conditions which give such appearances, the dust-inhalation diseases are distinguished chiefly by their accompanying history of exposure. Miliary tuberculosis and sarcoidosis of the lungs rarely cause pneumothorax, and often affect other organs distinctively. Moreover, their histological appearance is characteristic, and should be sought from a biopsy of the liver, if other sources are not readily at hand. Lymphangitis carcinomatosa can produce radiological shadows similar to those of tuberous sclerosis, but there is usually a rapid downward course and intense breathlessness, and often pleural effusion or other signs of metastasis in an older subject. In cases with an appearance of widespread small cysts, and often a history of pneumothorax, the diagnostic problem centres mainly on the diseases producing honeycomb lung (Oswald and Parkinson, 1949), though all of these, at least in their early stages, may show only miliary shadows without discernible cysts. Tuberous sclerosis is one of the causes of this uncommon alteration in lung structure. Features in favour of this disease would be an onset of symptoms between the ages of 25 and 40 years, a history not longer than five years, progressive dyspnoea punctuated by acute episodes of spontaneous pneumothorax, and absence of both cough and sputum, of finger clubbing, and of abnormal signs in the chest, with possibly recurrent small haemoptyses. Foremost among the other causes of honeycomb lung is a group of disorders of the reticulo-endothelial system known as the 'generalized eosinophilic granulomas' (Thannhauser, 1950). This comprehensive title, based on anatomical and histological grounds, includes the three diseases described by Letterer (1924) and Siwe (1933), Hand (1921) (Hand-Schüller-Christian disease), and Otani and Ehrlich (1940). The finding of foam cells in the last two syndromes led them to be classed at first with other lipoidoses. These accumulations of lipoid in the cells are now thought to be a degeneration following reticulo-endothelial hyperplasia, the serum-lipoids always being normal. All these disorders may cause cystic lung changes. The other hyperlipaemic 'essential xanthomatoses', and the lipoid-storage disorders excepting the Niemann-Pick type, do not do so. The three types of primary reticulo-endothelial disorder, in contrast to pulmonary tuberous sclerosis, usually afflict children, often run a rapid course, and affect the lymph-glands and spleen as well as the lungs. Bone radiographs may show large erosions, especially in the skull, appearances which help to distinguish the few cases occurring in adults (Currens and Popp, 1943; Ackermann, 1944). Other examples of honeycomb lung in adults, which may be related to this group, were associated with diabetes insipidus or other endocrine disorder (Oechsli and Miles, 1934; Oswald and Parkinson, 1949; Spillane, 1952). Various disturbances of pituitary function have been recorded in tuberous sclerosis, but not diabetes insipidus (Krabbe, 1922; Borberg, 1951). Scleroderma of the lungs has occasionally produced widespread small cystic shadows (Dostrovsky, 1947; Church and Ellis, 1950), though in this case the main radiological changes are in the bases, and pulmonary involvement is usually but not invariably (Hayman and Hunt, 1952) preceded by vasospastic or sclerodermal signs in the skin. Some patients with diffuse pulmonary fibrosis, the causes of which are unknown, may show the same radiological appearances. They show no distinguishing features except that they often have clubbing of the fingers. They can be differentiated only by examination of actual lung sections, which reveal granulomatous tissue in the alveolar walls, containing in the earlier stages a variety of inflammatory cells, which are replaced by fibrous tissue as the disease progresses. No abnormal blood-vessels, muscle tissue, or iron are present (Cunningham and Parkinson, 1950). Productive cough is the prime symptom of respiratory infection such as chronic bronchiolitis and diffuse cystic bronchiectasis, which may on other grounds, chiefly radiological, be confused with tuberous sclerosis of the lungs. Breathlessness often develops much later in these conditions, and their symmetrical reticulate or cystic shadows are usually coarser than those of the honeycomb type of lung. Moreover, generalized dilatation of the bronchial tree has not so far been recorded in tuberous sclerosis, an important distinction from these primary bronchial disorders which a bronchogram readily reveals. When the disease reaches the stage of congestive heart failure, other causes of chronic cor pulmonale can be excluded only on account of general features, especially as any distinctive pattern of the lung fields is then obscured by congestion and oedema. Sometimes the diagnosis remains no more than a probability subject to correction or confirmation by necropsy.

Course and treatment. The outlook in tuberous sclerosis depends on which tissues are affected most. The skin nodules may go on enlarging slowly for many years, but they interfere with no vital function, and are never dangerous. The renal tumours may enlarge at any time (Hyman, 1922), occasionally because of malignancy, and death may follow from this condition or from uraemia (Kirpicznik, 1910). Apart from mental deficiency and epilepsy, the changes in the brain may cause symptoms of tumour (Globus, Strauss, and Selinsky, 1932) or, rarely, lead to sudden and unexpected death (Stewart, 1935; Warrack, 1950). In contrast with the skin and cerebral features, the pulmonary effects appear late. The youngest age at which respiratory symptoms have started is 24 years, by which time as a rule the evil potentialities of the brain lesions are spent. At least one may say for the pulmonary cases that, if mental symptoms are absent, they are not likely to arise in future, nor, similarly, are new skin lesions likely to appear. Also patients with pulmonary symptoms are likely to die from them before other lesions can cause harm. With three older exceptions, all the patients who had the pulmonary disease so far have come under observation between 24 and 39 years of age, and they have lived about three years longer, having had persistent dyspnoea for an average of five years. The expectation of life is unrelated to the age at onset, but its limits may be gauged from the duration of symptoms in the recorded cases. Dyspnoea has been present from one to 11 years in the eight fatal cases, including one of the present series; of the five surviving patients two have not been breathless, and the longest known record of symptoms among them is five years. Spontaneous pneumothorax caused severe symptoms in Case I, and a double pneumothorax contributed to death in Case 3. Four patients died in their first attack of congestive heart failure, though the records suggest that it was difficult to decide whether failure of the heart or of the lungs was the chief cause. At the present time no treatment designed to prevent the progressive increase of fibrous and muscle tissue in the lungs has been tried. It is possible that cortisone or adrenocorticotrophic hormone might halt the process temporarily, but in a disease of genetic origin their effects would probably not be permanent. Secondary infection is not usually present in these cases, and chemotherapy is not necessary. When spontaneous pneumothorax recurs frequently, it requires treatment by pleurodesis; the presence of many superficial bullae in our patient did not interfere with the effectiveness of this operation.

Nature of Tuberous Sclerosis

When this disorder was first described, Bourneville and others thought that it was due to diffuse encephalitis occurring during foetal development. Hartdegen (1881) recorded his case as an example of a new type of cerebral tumour which he named glioma gangliocellulare, a mixed ganglion-cell and glial neoplasm. As the frequency of tumours elsewhere became apparent, the idea of a widespread developmental disorder suggested itself to many. Pellizi (1901) considered it to be an example of generalized teratomatous changes. Bielschowsky and Gallus (1913) and Bielschowsky (1923–4), concentrating their attention on the central nervous system, thought that the disease was due to a mixture of malformation and new formation related genetically to neurofibromatosis, the one with mainly central, the other with chiefly peripheral changes. Their views were based on studies of histiogenesis in both diseases, and on a unique case recorded by Orzechowski and Nowicki (1912), which seemed to show central neurofibromatosis and tuberous sclerosis together. In criticism of his theory Bielschowsky wrote that 'what one believes depends on whether one is certain that the anatomical (histological) data are proof of the existence of pathogenic relationship'. At the present time the sciences of genetics and embryology have modified and broadened the conception of developmental abnormalities in general. It is no longer possible to think of tuberous sclerosis as a disorder confined to one germinal layer, for the ectoderm produces the abnormalities of skin and brain, while mesoderm contributes the malformed tissues of the kidneys, lung, and heart. The earlier, rather rigid architectural interpretations of embryonic growth, which stressed the destination of particular germ layers and their contribution to the different organs, is now made more flexible by the knowledge acquired from biochemical and transplantation experiments in the embryo. These studies (Spemann, 1938) have shown that the growth and differentiation of regions of embryonic tissue, which include all primitive layers, are controlled by organizer groups of cells; their mode of action is gradually being translated into terms of protein and enzyme activity

(Needham, 1942). This approach will probably reconcile the rival views which have looked upon tuberous sclerosis as an example of new growth, on the one hand, and of congenital deformity on the other. No matter how the disease produces its widespread changes, the cause is certainly inherited, as was first observed by Kirpicznik (1910). Many examples have since been recorded with up to five generations affected (Fuhs, 1925). The pattern of inheritance has been investigated precisely by Gunther and Penrose (1935) and Penrose (1938). They described families in which the disease was transmitted by a dominant gene, explaining any exceptions by presuming the existence of modifying genes in the same zygote. This mechanism was thought to account for abortive forms, or even for complete masking of the disease-bearing gene. Penrose also found that half of his patients had no relatives affected by the disease, and calculated that these examples, which were usually severe, had arisen by mutation. Were this not so the disease would have died out rapidly, for most of the patients recorded are mentally defective and sterile. He found no evidence to suggest that the disorder occurred with increasing severity in succeeding generations, a view with which my experience agrees. On the contrary, the tendency in some families is for the pattern of the disease to remain constant, for instance when renal tumours have occurred in two generations (Kirpicznik, 1910); and I have seen two sisters with renal symptoms due to tuberous sclerosis, in one of whom, who died with uraemia, characteristic changes were found. Other such examples are the two sisters with cystic lungs described by Berg and Nordenskjöld (1946), and a brother and sister with laryngeal polyps (Case 3). The two types, renal and pulmonary, as well as the mental cases, have their separate symptomatology. Adenoma sebaceum may occur alone or with any of the three types; together they form the chief ways in which adults are affected. When pulmonary changes are present they usually dominate the clinical picture, and it remains to be seen whether they often occur without the characteristic lesions in the brain or skin. The relative incidence of these varieties of the disease cannot be truly estimated from past records, but we may expect to recognize more examples of the pulmonary type as its features become better known.

Acknowledgements

I wish to thank the Medical Superintendents of Cell Barnes, Darenth, The Fountain, Harperbury, Leavesden, and St. Lawrence's, Caterham, Mental Hospitals for permission to examine their patients, and Dr. Crawford, the Medical Superintendent of Botley's Park Mental Hospital, for permission to record Case 2 and for much useful advice. My thanks are also due to Professor H. A. Magnus and his staff, and to Dr. J. W. Clegg, for the reports on the biopsy sections, to Dr. Denis Hill and his department for the psychiatric investigations, and to Mr. W. P. Cleland who gave surgical treatment to Cases 1 and 4. I am greatly indebted to Dr. N. C. Oswald for permission to record Case 3, and for his counsel and criticism. I am grateful to Professor L. S. Penrose, and to Dr. W. S. Maclay, of the Board of Control, for advice about the vital statistics. I wish especially to thank Dr. Clifford Hoyle for permission to record Case 1, and for his invaluable advice and criticism and constant encouragement.

APPENDIX A

Case I (Berg and Vejlens, 1939). A woman aged 32 years. There was no record of fits, but adenoma sebaceum from the age of 17 years. Two siblings had tuberous sclerosis. Spontaneous pneumothorax was confirmed radiologically two years before, and there was subsequent recurrent pneumothorax on either side, with progressive dyspnoea. She died at 32 years from asphyxia and congestive heart failure. Radiographic changes progressed from fine symmetric reticulation to obvious honeycomb shadowing.

Necropsy (Vejlens, 1941). *Brain.* Tuberous sclerosis. *Lungs.* Pneumothorax; both lungs transformed into spongy tissue with thick-walled cysts, all about the size of a pea, containing air or fluid. *Heart.* Hypertrophied and dilated, especially the right side. *Kidneys.* Bilateral leiomyomata. *Spleen.* One small tumour. *Histology.* Lungs: little normal tissue. A few cysts were lined with ciliary or cubical epithelium, but most were unlined. Cysts were surrounded by bundles and tumours of smooth muscle, with a little very vascular connective tissue. Haemorrhages and iron pigment were present. One cervical gland was replaced by a leiomyoma.

Case II (Samuelsen, 1942). A woman aged 49 years. There was no record of fits: she had adenoma sebaceum. No family history was given. Haemoptysis occurred at 36 years; mitral stenosis was diagnosed. At 40 years she had cough, expectoration, fatigue, and dyspnoea. At 41 years widespread close-set miliary opacities were seen in a radiograph, the Mantoux reaction was negative, and the heart normal. Chronic miliary tuberculosis was diagnosed. At 46 years the lung fields were unchanged: oval rarefactions, with some opacities and periosteal thickenings, were seen in the phalanges; the eyes were normal. Imbecility, not previously recorded, was noted. Six months before death veiling of the left basal lung field suggested pleural affection. She died, aged 49 years (in 1941), of cerebral haemorrhage.

Necropsy. Brain. Several recent infarcts; tuberous sclerosis. *Lungs.* Left pleural adhesions and effusion; both lungs showed subpleural air-filled bullae, the size of a millet seed to that of a pea. The cut surface showed air-cysts with dark-brown walls. Hilar glands normal. *Heart.* Slight mitral stenosis. *Kidneys.* Mamillated surface due to millet- to olive-sized elastic nodes. *Histology.* Lungs: partly normal, partly atelectatic. Alveolar septa thickened by much connective tissue, containing muscle-cells lying singly or in small bundles. Much iron pigment present, both in cells and lying free. Kidneys: foci of bundles of smooth muscle, with fine strands of connective tissue and conspicuous blood-vessels of haemangiomatous appearance.

Case III (Licht, 1942). A woman aged 63 years. Previously healthy, she had had increasing breathlessness for one year, cough and sputum for nine months, and pain in the left chest and down the left arm, related to effort, for a few months. A daughter was epileptic, and had adenoma sebaceum. There was slight cyanosis and orthopnoea, some cardiac enlargement, and moist sounds in both lungs. Symptoms progressed to complete incapacity, and death in 10 months from cardiac failure. A radiograph showed a well-marked open network in both lungs. Tomograms showed cystic change. Clinical diagnosis: bronchiolitis with interstitial change.

Necropsy. Brain not examined. *Lungs.* Surface brown, covered with nodules the size of half a pea, but larger over left upper lobe; firm consistency; airless. The cut surface showed dilated bronchi containing little secretion, and numerous small close-set cavities, with smooth walls of greyish tissue. *Heart.* Right-sided hypertrophy. *Kidneys.* No record. *Liver.* 'Nutmeg' change. *Histology.* Lungs: much connective tissue between the alveoli; bands of vascular fibrous tissue beside thin-walled arteries. Bronchiolar musculature thickened in some places, and occasionally invaded by inflammatory tissue. Mucosa thin, covered with flattened cells; only a few cuboidal cells seen. Some bronchioles contained pus. Left lung: conspicuous increase in bronchial muscle, especially near the hilum; mucosal glands and cartilage rings intact; bronchioles showed similar changes.

Case IV (Warren and Warvi, 1943). A woman aged 26 years. Mental deficiency and adenoma sebaceum dated from infancy. Her physical condition was good until two years before death, when she became breathless. Just before death albuminuria and uraemia developed. She died from a spontaneous pneumothorax.

Necropsy. Brain. Tuberous sclerosis. *Lungs.* Congenital cystic disease, with left pneumothorax. *Heart.* No record. Tumours also found in the kidneys, ovaries, and retroperitoneal tissues. The skin showed adenoma sebaceum and multiple fibromata. *Histology.* No record.

Case V (Berg and Nordenskjöld, 1946). A woman aged 29 years, seen because she was sister to Case I. There was no mental defect or history of fits, but adenoma sebaceum, subungual fibromata, a retinal phakoma, and a vaginal tumour. Radiographs showed a honeycomb appearance in both lungs, and tomograms distinct 'cysts'; an intravenous pyelogram was normal; the skull showed parietal sclerosis; the long bones were normal. A bronchogram was normal. When aged 31 years she became dyspnoeic and cyanotic, with slight loss of weight; a vaginal embryoma was removed. Radiographs showed a small pneumothorax, and a very slight increase of infiltration. At the age of 32 years she died from progressive dyspnoea and debility.

Necropsy. Brain. Tuberous sclerosis. *Lungs.* Loose pleural adhesions; brownish-red colour; even distribution in both lungs of pinhead- to pea-sized cavities filled with air or fluid. *Heart.* Hypertrophy of right ventricle. *Kidneys.* Bilateral tumours. *Histology.* Lungs: little normal tissue, very vascular fibrous induration; large vascular areas with dilated thin-walled vessels spread diffusely through alveolar walls and peribronchial regions. Leiomyomatous tissue issuing from walls of some blood-vessels, but in other parts more compact. Cysts not connected with bronchi. Haemorrhages in alveolar remnants and interstitium. Many haemosiderin-laden pigment cells. Few old and fresh tubercles. Bronchi normal. Kidneys: a mass of leiomyomatous tissue which penetrated the renal capsule in many places; some striated muscle cells were seen.

Case VI (Paliard, Plauchu, Galy, and Papillon, 1946). A woman aged 39 years had haemoptysis and purulent sputum after pharyngitis. The family history is not recorded. She had no history of fits or mental defect, but when aged 18 years had adenoma sebaceum and subungual fibromata. No eye or renal lesions were found. There were moist sounds at the left apex. Radiographs showed a cystic and honeycomb appearance of the left upper lobe; the size of the cysts was variable and the walls thin. Tomograms showed oval, thin-walled cysts in the right mid-zone. The skull showed intracranial calcification.

Case VII (Oswald and Parkinson, 1949). A woman aged 31 years had had dyspnoea on exertion for five years. There was no familial nervous disorder, and she had had no fits. Adenoma sebaceum dated from the age of three years, and subungual fibromata were present. The eyes were normal; the heart had an apical diastolic murmur; both kidneys were palpable. Radiographs showed diffuse reticulation of both lungs, and in the long bones periosteal reaction in the tibiae and a small cortical erosion in one phalanx. Intravenous pyelography showed a left renal tumour.

Case VIII (Inglis, 1950). A married woman aged 41 years, with four children. She had had adenoma sebaceum of the nose and cheeks since infancy. At 32 years she had recurrent attacks of 'asthma', which became more severe when she was 38 years old. Intelligence was normal. She had dyspnoea, cyanosis, and albuminuria; red blood-cells 6,800,000 per c.mm.; haemoglobin 141 per cent. The cause of death was presumably asphyxia. Radiographs showed a right pneumothorax, generalized mottling of the left lung, and a large pulmonary artery.

Necropsy. Brain not examined. *Lungs.* Right pneumothorax due to ruptured bulla. Left lung and apex of right lung showed striking bullous emphysema. Both lungs contained many white nodules 1 to 2 mm. in diameter. 'Lower part of right lung was solid with blood.' *Heart.* Pulmonary artery dilated, larger than aorta. Right ventricle: no record. *Liver* congested. Some small white nodules in right lobe. *Kidneys* both studded with small yellow and white tumours; a few cysts in left kidney. *Uterus.* Many small white nodules 1 mm. in diameter. *Histology. Lungs*: large areas of collapsed air sacs, containing much haemosiderin in walls and air spaces. Nodules composed mostly of elongated cells, described as neurilemmoblastic tissue; others showed hyaline bands. Tracheal lymph-nodes enlarged by collections of elongated and round cells like those in lung. 'Liver nodules' were composed entirely of fat-laden cells. 'Uterine nodules' were collections of elongated cells. The renal tumours were made up of fat, vascular tissue, and 'elongated cells'.

Comment. The paper in which this case is recorded seeks to prove that tuberous sclerosis is a form of 'neurilemmoblastosis'. All the elongated cells, which in photomicrographs seem to be smooth muscle, are interpreted as being neurilemmal cells in active division. The same criticism applies to Case XV, Appendix B.

Case IX (Borberg, 1951). A man aged 64 years, with no record of fits. His son aged 39 years was feebleminded; a daughter aged 34 years was epileptic, with pedunculated fibromas on the nape of the neck and in the axilla, and diffuse café-au-lait spots. He had severe dyspnoea and cough for two years, then fever, cough, and sputum; he died in two weeks from cardiac insufficiency and hypostatic pneumonia.

Necropsy. Lungs. Slight induration; generalized cystic change, except in right upper lobe. Cysts the size of a pea, empty or filled with fluid. *Brain* not examined. *Histology.* No record.

APPENDIX B

There are in the literature six other cases, with clinical histories characteristic of diffuse cystic lung disease, and with gross and microscopic changes in the lungs similar to those of pulmonary tuberous sclerosis. Three of these patients had multiple renal tumours, which were thought to be malignant, though in two (Cases X and XII) the evidence of malignancy is unsatisfactory, depending as it does solely upon invasion of the renal capsule and of a local lymph-gland, without distant metastases. Invasion of the capsule and the development of pararenal foci are common characteristics of renal embryomas (Cases I and V, and Feriz, 1930). Even the discovery of distant 'metastases' may be due rather to the development of multifocal embryomas (Case I, and Mittasch, 1922). Lutembacher (Case X) held that the pulmonary changes were due to metastatic tumour-cells, in spite of the diffuse pattern confined to the interstitium of the lung, 'not anywhere invading the alveoli or bronchi'. The actual cells are not described in detail, but he likened them to 'granulation tissue'. The pattern expected in miliary pulmonary metastases is recorded by Kirpicznik (1910) in a case of tuberous sclerosis with a malignant renal embryoma; at necropsy the lungs were full of miliary metastases of spindle-cell sarcoma. Similar deposits were found in the hilar lymph-glands. Case XI was recorded with two diagnoses, congenital bronchiectasis and leiomyosarcoma of an uterine fibroid involving the kidney, although the primary growth was never discovered. The honeycomb lungs were diffusely infiltrated with smooth muscle. Case XII had bilateral renal embryomas, and honeycomb lungs infiltrated with granulation tissue and many iron-containing macrophages. Berg, who saw the microscopic sections, thought they were identical with those taken from his own cases. The brains in these three cases (X, XI, and XIII) were not examined, but the coexistence of multiple renal embryomas and honeycomb lungs strongly suggests that they were examples of pulmonary and renal tuberal sclerosis.

The other three similar cases of cystic lung showed no evidence of generalized disease outside the lungs; in two there was no record of examination of the brain or kidneys, and in the third these organs were normal. The lungs in each case contained unusual quantities of smooth muscle or fibrous tissue and, in Case XIV, of blood-vessels. These lung changes were identical with those found in pulmonary tuberous sclerosis, both in their diffuse honeycomb pattern and characteristic histology, and also in the absence or slight extent of chronic inflammation. The presence of muscle and abnormal blood-vessels in the hilar glands (Case XIV) suggests a process of multifocal overgrowth of these tissues, such as is found in tuberous sclerosis. Case XV concerned a woman, with epilepsy in the family, whose lungs and hilar lymph-nodes were infiltrated with elongated 'neurilemmal cells', which appear in the accompanying photographs to have the same shape and size as smooth muscle-fibres. The hilar glands also contained 'elongated cells'. It is impossible in retrospect to be certain whether these three cases represent the pulmonary manifestations of tuberous sclerosis; but, in spite of the lack of characteristic changes elsewhere, the appearances of the lungs were very similar to those found in authenticated cases. Other examples of over-developed muscle tissue have been associated with chronic infection (Buhl, 1872; Buchmann, 1911; von Stossel, 1937), but the changes were localized, except in the last instance, in which the bronchi were dilated and surrounded by inflammatory and fibrous tissue; the lungs themselves contained many cysts surrounded by granulation tissue and muscle-fibres. The presence of inflammatory tissue in this case probably explains the increase in the amount of muscle.

Case X (Lutembacher, 1918). A woman aged 36 years, who at 34 years had had a spontaneous pneumothorax. She had a history of afebrile pleurisy for two months, a cough, and slight loss of weight. She was admitted with severe dyspnoea and cyanosis, and died in two days from bilateral pneumothorax.

Necropsy. Brain. No record. *Lungs.* Bilateral pneumothorax; sponge-like cut surface; many cysts from size of a bead to that of a nut; widespread pulmonary artery thrombosis. *Heart* small. *Kidneys.* Yellowish-white tumours, 15 on one side, three on the other. *Spleen* of normal size; no tumours. *Histology.* Lungs: no tumours, but diffuse infiltration of both lungs by cells 'like granulation tissue' enveloping alveoli and bronchi, but not anywhere invading them; widespread arteriolar thrombosis. 'Some pigmentary debris.' Hilar glands: no record. Kidneys: fibro-lipo-vascular tumours; larger tumours differentiated into nephrons with cortical and medullary zones, the inner layer composed of connective tissue only. Spleen: diffuse infiltration with 'tumour cells'. Author's diagnosis: renal sarcoma with lung metastases.

Case XI (Burrell and Ross, 1937). A woman aged 36 years. Family history not recorded. She had no record of fits, but progressive attacks of 'dyspnoea' for two years, and was admitted with extreme dyspnoea and cyanosis. There was a left pleural effusion and congestive heart failure. Radiography not recorded.

Necropsy. Brain. No record. *Lungs.* Honeycomb appearance. *Heart.* Enlarged on the right side; pulmonary artery atheromatous and dilated. *Abdomen.* Many large soft glands; large neoplastic mass involving the left kidney, the thoracic duct, and extending down to the pelvic brim. *Histology.* Lungs: diffuse infiltration with smooth muscle-fibres, and diffuse dilatation of all bronchioles. Abdominal glands infiltrated with smooth muscle. Author's diagnosis: malignant change in uterine fibroid which looked innocent, and congenital bronchiectasis with right heart failure.

Case XII (von Stossel, 1937). A woman aged 43 years. Family history not recorded. There was no history of fits. She had secondary syphilis at 34 years, at 37 years a left pleurisy, and at 39 years sanatorium treatment for tuberculosis, but no fever or sputum. When aged 42 years she had increasing fatigue, breathlessness, cough, and sputum, and lost 15 lb. of weight. She had no fever; there were basal crepitations and generalized rhonchi, and no tubercle bacilli in the sputum. Radiographs showed a left pneumothorax with adhesions, and numerous grain-sized shadows all over the right lung and left upper lobe. She died seven months later from heart failure, with a loud pulmonary second sound and enlarged supraclavicular lymph-glands.

Necropsy. Brain not examined. *Lungs.* Honeycomb pattern; hilar gland enlargement. *Heart.* Large right ventricle; pulmonary artery atheromatous. *Abdomen.* Chronic congestion in all organs. *Kidneys* normal. *Histology.* Lung: coarse-pored appearance: narrow bands of connective tissue, surrounding cylindrical spaces lined by cubical epithelium; conspicuous amount of smooth muscle tissue. Bronchi normal. Lymph-glands: increase in collagen, hyaline and reticular fibres, and reticular and giant cells. Author's diagnosis: muscular cirrhosis.

Case XIII (dos Santos and Wohlwill, 1942). A woman aged 40 years. She had had bronchitis since childhood, and renal symptoms at 31 years. Tumours of the left kidney were diagnosed. Arteriography showed two highly vascular tumours, one in each kidney. At 33 years she had left nephrectomy for recurrent pain and enlarging tumour. She was well until the age of 40, when pulmonary symptoms rapidly developed; a radiograph showed a cystic appearance of the lung fields.

Necropsy. Brain not examined. *Lungs.* Many small empty cysts. *Right kidney.* One tumour. Left nephrectomy site: no local recurrence of tumour. *Histology.* Lungs: cystic spaces separated by septa containing fibrocytes, fibroblasts, and lymphocytes; few capillaries seen, and many iron-containing macrophages; some giant cells described. One area showed cells like those of the renal tumour. Right kidney: liposarcomatous tumour with angiomatous interspersions. Left kidney region: no local recurrence. Left kidney (operation specimen): liposarcoma, perirenal tissue involved. Lymph-glands (right renal region): some metastases. Author's diagnosis: congenital malformation of lung and kidney; ? tuberous sclerosis. (Berg examined the lung sections, and found that they corresponded with Case I.)

Case XIV (Rosendal, 1942). A woman aged 51 years had had progressive dyspnoea for seven years, with periodic exacerbations, probably due to recurrent spontaneous pneumothorax. A radiograph at 45 years showed veiling of the lung bases, with a suggestion of early honeycomb change. She was admitted with severe breathlessness and slight haemoptysis. She died, aged 51, after one month's terminal pulmonary infection. A radiograph showed a diffuse, small, spotted, net-like tracing surrounding pea-sized 'cysts' in both lungs.

Necropsy. Brain normal, but no histological record. *Lungs* oedematous, with dense pleural adhesions, considerable interstitial thickening, generalized honeycomb design, and scattered pneumonic foci. Bronchi not dilated. Hilar glands enlarged. *Heart, liver, spleen,* and *kidneys* normal. *Histology.* Lungs: dilated alveoli and bronchioli up to the size of a pea, separated by solid septa of bundles of smooth muscle cells lying in a little connective tissue. These septa contained much iron and anthracotic pigment. Lymph-glands replaced by smooth muscle cells; unusual number of small blood-vessels seen. Author's diagnosis: ? tuberous sclerosis.

Case XV (Inglis, 1950). A woman aged 32 years. Her father's brother was epileptic. There was no previous mental disorder. She had been breathless for four years on the least exertion, and had had haemoptysis at 29 and 30 years. She became more breathless and cyanotic, and died.

Necropsy. Brain not examined. *Lungs.* Right pneumothorax. The whole of each lung consisted of communicating cavities 2 mm. to 1 cm. in diameter. Right lung engorged with blood. Hilar glands not enlarged. *Heart.* Right-sided hypertrophy. *Liver* small and fatty; gross ascites. *Kidneys* congested. *Histology.* Lung: thick-walled cysts composed of spindle-shaped and elongated cells, which sometimes formed nodules. Hilar lymph-nodes: strands of cells like those in lung.

Comment. See note on Case VIII.

Summary

The history and diverse features of tuberous sclerosis are reviewed. The incidence is estimated at one per 150,000 of the population. Seventy-two asylum patients with the disease are surveyed, only one of whom was found to have the lungs affected, an indication of its rarity, especially among sufferers from mental disorder, in whom this finding was not accounted for by early death. Seven cases of adenoma sebaceum were also investigated, one of which showed pulmonary changes.

Four new cases of pulmonary tuberous sclerosis are described and compared with the nine already reported in the literature. The chief features are the predominance of women among those affected; the onset of symptoms in adult life, contrasting with the cutaneous and cerebral features of the disease; chronic progressing breathlessness, recurrent pneumothorax, occasional haemoptysis, diffuse miliary or small cystic shadows, and an absence, or at most a late development, of concomitant infection. Death follows about five years after the onset of symptoms, and is due to asphyxia from lung destruction, to spontaneous pneumothorax, or to right heart failure.

The morbid changes seen in lung biopsy specimens from two of the present series accorded with previous descriptions: profuse overgrowth of connective tissue, including smooth muscle and blood-vessels, leading to the formation of numerous small cysts.

REFERENCES

Ackermann, A. J. (1944) *Amer. J. Roentgenol.* **51**, 315.
Addison, T., and Gull, W. (1851) *Guy's Hosp. Rep.* 2nd Series, **7**, 267.
Balzer, F., and Ménétrier, P. (1885) *Arch. de physiol.* **6**, 564.
Berg, G. (1938) *Svenska läkartidn.* **35**, 2174.
—— and Vejlens, G. (1939) *Acta paediat.* **26**, 16.
—— and Nordenskjöld, A. (1946) *Acta med. scand.* **125**, 428.
Bielschowsky, M. (1923–4). *J. Psychol. u. Neurol.* **30**, 167.
—— and Gallus (1913) Ibid. **20**, Ergänz. i, 1.
Board of Control (1935) Annual Report, **22**, 50.
—— (1945) Ibid. **32**, 41.
Borberg, A. (1951) *Clinical and Genetic Investigations into Tuberous Sclerosis and Recklinghausen's Neurofibromatosis*, Copenhagen.
Bourneville, D. M. (1880–1) *Arch. neurol.* **1**, 81.
—— (1900) Ibid. **10**, 29.
Brushfield, T., and Wyatt, W. (1926) *Brit. J. Child. Dis.* **23**, 178.
Buchmann, E. (1911) *Frankfurt. Zts. Path.* **8**, 263.
Buhl, L. (1872) *Lungenentzündung, Tuberkulose und Schwindsucht*, München, p. 58.
Burrell, L. S. T., and Ross, J. M. (1937) *Brit. J. Tuberc.* **31**, 38.
Butterworth, T., and Wilson, M. (1941) *Arch. Dermat. Syph.* **43**, 1.
Church, R. E., and Ellis, A. R. P. (1950) *Lancet*, **1**, 392.
Cockayne, E. A. (1933) *Inherited Abnormalities of the Skin*, Oxford, p. 289.
Critchley, M., and Earl, C. J. C. (1932) *Brain*, **55**, 311.
Cunningham, G. J., and Parkinson, T. (1950) *Thorax*, **5**, 43.
Currens, J. H., and Popp, W. C. (1943) *Amer. J. Med. Sci.* **205**, 780.
Dalsgaard-Nielsen, T. (1935) *Nord. med. tidskr.* **10**, 1541.
Dostrovsky, A. (1947) *Arch. Dermat. Syph.* **55**, 1.
Engel, S., and Newns, G. H. (1939) *J. Path. Bact.* **49**, 381.
Farber, S. (1931) *Amer. J. Path.* **7**, 105.
Feriz, H. (1930) *Virchows Arch.* **278**, 690.
Fowler, J. S., and Dickson, W. E. C. (1910–11) *Quart. J. Med.* **4**, 43.
Fuhs, H. (1925) *Arch. Dermat. Syph.*, Wien, **148**, 509.
Globus, J. H., Strauss, I., and Selinsky, H. (1932) *Zts. ges. Neurol u. Psychiat.* **140**, 1.
Gottlieb, J. S., and Lavine, G. R. (1935) *Arch. Neurol. Psychiat.* **33**, 379.
Gunther, M., and Penrose, L. S. (1935) *J. Genet.* **31**, 413.
Hallopeau, F. H., and Leredde, L. E. (1895) *Ann. dermat. syph.* **6**, 473.
Hand, A. (1921) *Amer. J. Med. Sci.* **162**, 509.
Hartdegen, A. (1881) *Arch. Psychiat. Nervenkr.* **11**, 117.
Hayman, L. D., and Hunt, R. E. (1952) *Dis. of Chest*, **21**, 691.
Hoeve, J. van der (1921) *v. Graefes Arch. Ophthal.* **105**, 880.
Hyman, A. (1922) *J. Urol.* **8**, 317.
Inglis, K. (1950) *Amer. J. Path.* **26**, 521.
Kirpicznik, J. (1910) *Virchows Arch.* **202**, 358.

Kothe, R. (1904) *Arch. Dermat. Syph.*, Wien, **68**, 33 and 359.
Krabbe, K. H. (1922) *Encéphale*, **17**, 281.
Letterer, E. (1924) *Frankfurt. Zts. Path.* **30**, 377.
Licht, E. de F. (1942) *Acta radiol.* **23**, 151.
Loewenstein, A., and Steel, J. (1941) *Amer. J. Ophthal.* **24**, 731.
Lutembacher, R. (1918) *Ann. méd.* **5**, 435.
Madonick, M. J., Savitsky, N., and Hochfeld, L. (1946) *J. Nerv. Ment. Dis.* **103**, 509.
Marcus, H. (1924) *Svenska läk.-sällsk. forh.* 358.
Mittasch, G. (1922) *Münch. med. Woch.* **69**, 571.
Needham, J. (1942) *Biochemistry and Morphogenesis*, Cambridge.
Oecshli, W. R., and Miles, S. H. (1934) *Amer. Rev. Tuberc.* **30**, 239.
Oppenheimer, G. D. (1934) *Ann. Surg.* **100**, 1136.
Orzechowski, K., and Nowicki, W. (1912) *Zts. ges. Neurol. u. Psychiat.* **11**, Orig. 237.
Oswald, N., and Parkinson, T. (1949) *Quart. J. Med.* N.S. **18**, 1.
Otani, S., and Ehrlich, J. C. (1940) *Amer. J. Path.* **16**, 479.
Paliard, Plauchu, Galy, and Papillon (1946) *Poumon*, **2**, 205.
Parr, J. C. (1948) *New Z. Med. J.* **47**, 550.
Pellizi, G. (1901) *Riv. sper. freniat.* **27**, 265.
Penrose, L. S. (1938) Med. Res. Counc. Special Report Series No. 229.
Pratt-Thomas, H. R. (1947) *Amer. J. Path.* **23**, 189.
Pringle, J. J. (1890) *Brit. J. Dermat.* **2**, 1.
Rayer, P. (1835) *Traité des maladies de la peau*, Paris, Pl. 20, Fig. 1.
Recklinghausen, F. von (1862) *Monats. Geburtskunde*, **20**, 1.
Rosendal, T. (1942) *Acta radiol.* **23**, 138.
Sailer, J. (1898) *J. Nerv. Ment. Dis.* **25**, 402.
Samuelsen, E. (1942) *Acta radiol.* **23**, 373.
Santos, R. dos, and Wohlwill, F. (1942) *Lisboa méd.* **19**, 131; quoted by Berg and Nordenskjöld (1946).
Schenck, S. G. (1937) *Arch. Int. Med.* **60**, 1.
Sherlock, E. B. (1911) *The Feeble-minded*, London.
Siwe, S. A. (1933) *Zts. Kinderheilk.* **55**, 212; quoted by Thannhauser (1950).
Spemann, H. (1938) *Embryonic Development and Induction*, New Haven, Conn.
Spillane, J. D. (1952) *Thorax*, **7**, 134.
Stewart, R. M. (1935) *Brit. Med. J.* **2**, 60.
Stossel, E. von (1937) *Beitr. klin. Tuberk.* **90**, 432.
Thannhauser, S. J. (1950) *Lipidoses*, New York.
Vaas, J. (1940) *Arch. Psychiat. Nervenkr.* **111**, 547.
Vejlens, G. (1941) *Acta path. microbiol. scand.* **18**, 317.
Virchow, R. (1864–5) *Die krankhaften Geschwülste*, **2**, 148.
Vogt, H. (1908) *Monats. Psychiat. Neurol.* **24**, 106.
Volland (1909) Quoted by Fowler and Dickson (1910–11).
Warrack, A. J. N. (1950) *Brit. Med. J.* **2**, 1367.
Warren, S., and Warvi, W. N. (1943) *Amer. J. Path.* **19**, 441.
Wright, R. D. (1938) *J. Path. Bact.* **47**, 489.

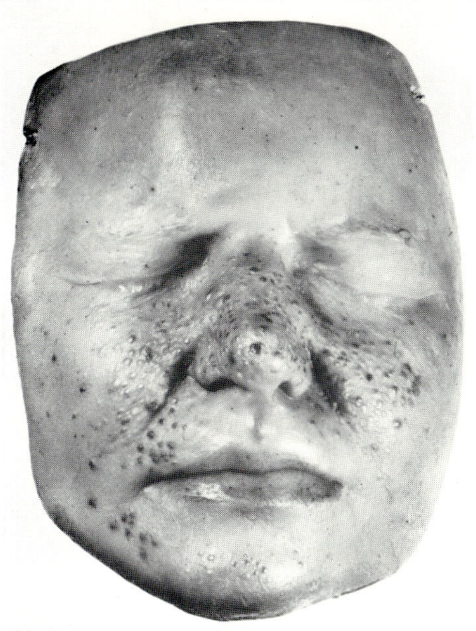

FIG. 1. The moulage of adenoma sebaceum made for Dr. Addison in 1851 (by permission of Dr. Keith Simpson, Curator of the Gordon Museum, Guy's Hospital)

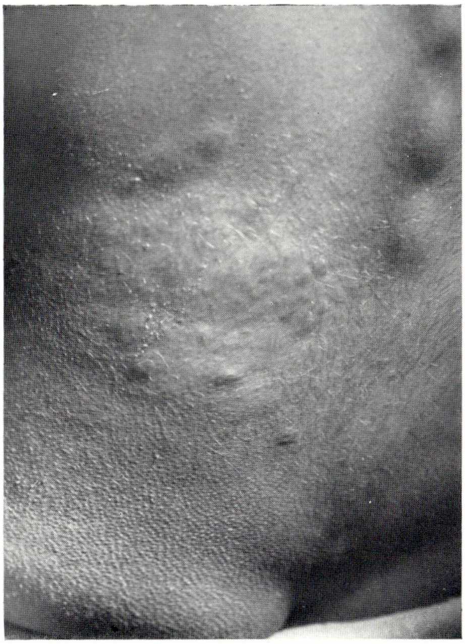

FIG. 2. Case 1. Lumbar peau chagriné

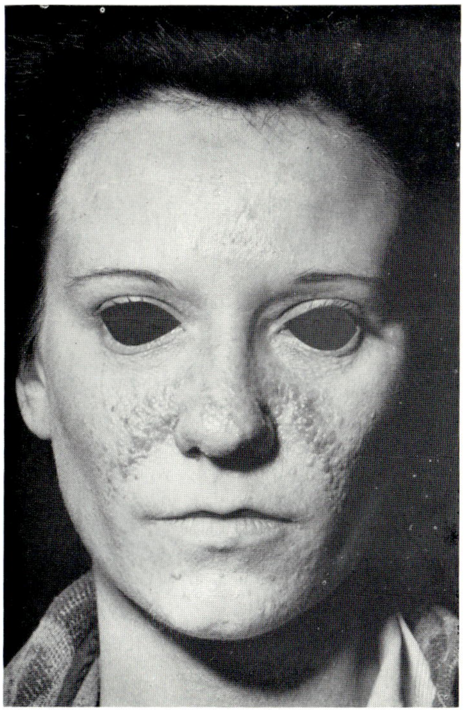

FIG. 3. Case 1. The symmetric eruption of adenoma sebaceum

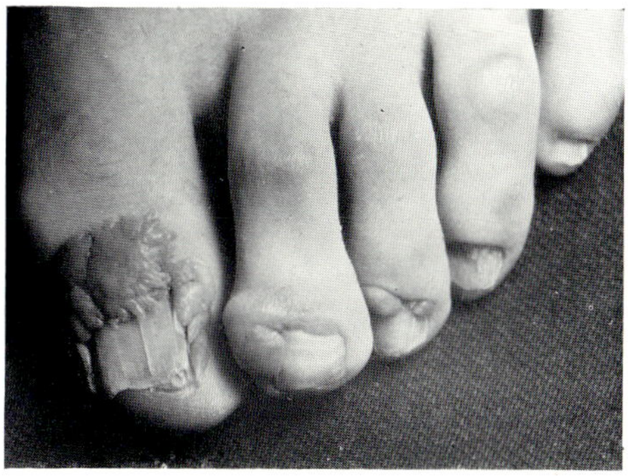

FIG. 4. Case 1. The warty swellings of subungual fibromas, with ridging of the nails

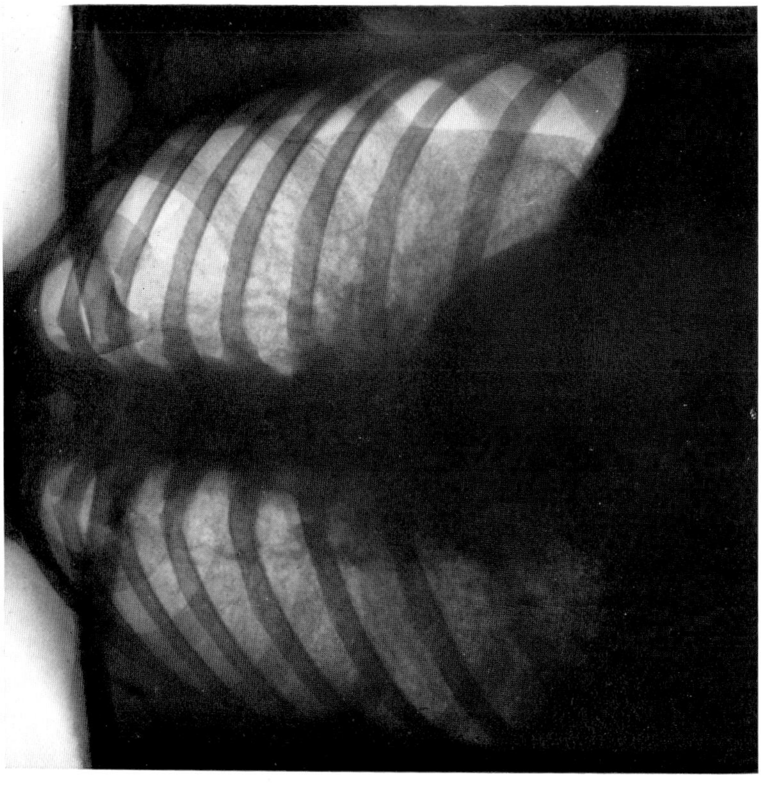

Fig. 5. Case 1. April 1950. Partial left pneumothorax and uniform fine-meshed shadowing, with a small effusion

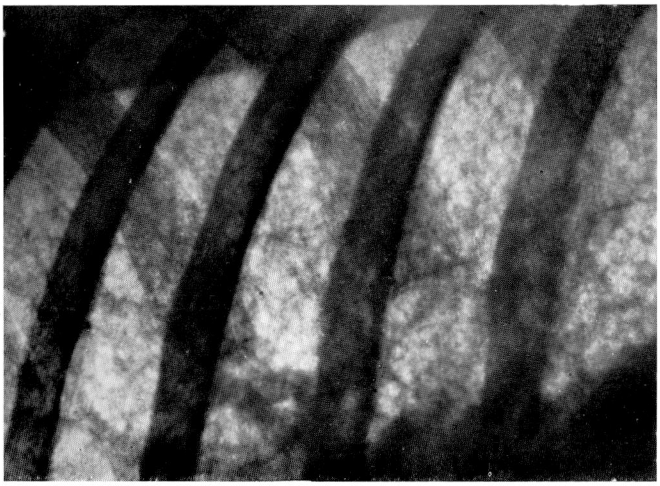

Fig. 6. Case 1. August 1951. An enlarged view of the lung field, showing several small groups of cysts and generalized reticulation

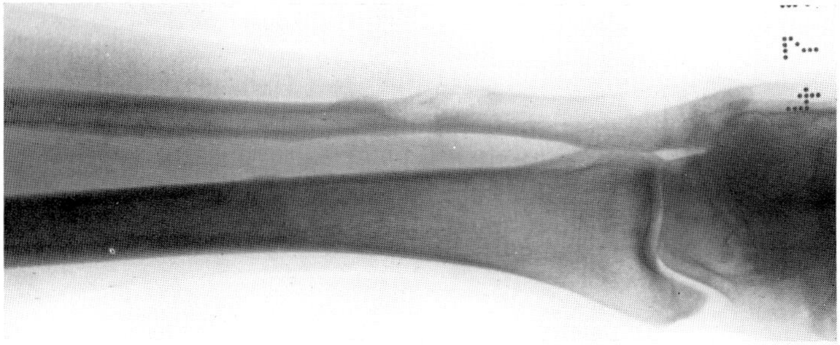

Fig. 7. Case 1. Periosteal thickening and a 'cyst' in the fibula

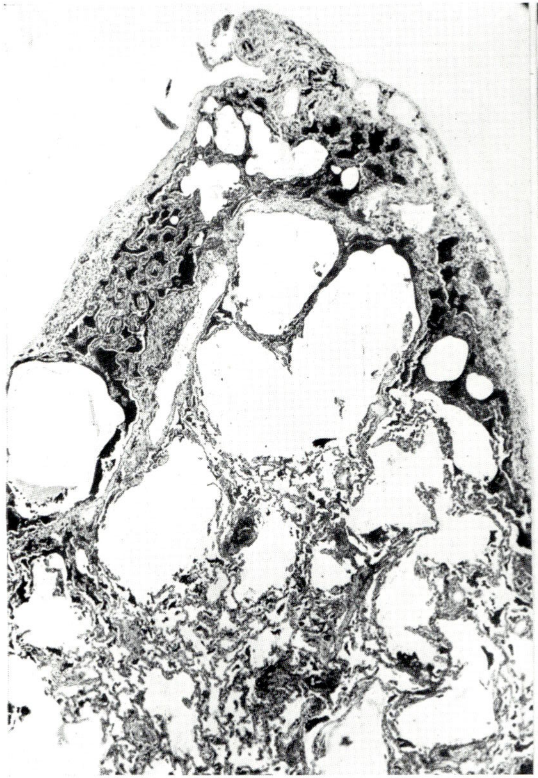

FIG. 8. Case 1. Biopsy specimen from right lung, showing several cyst-like spaces (haematoxylin and eosin, ×25)

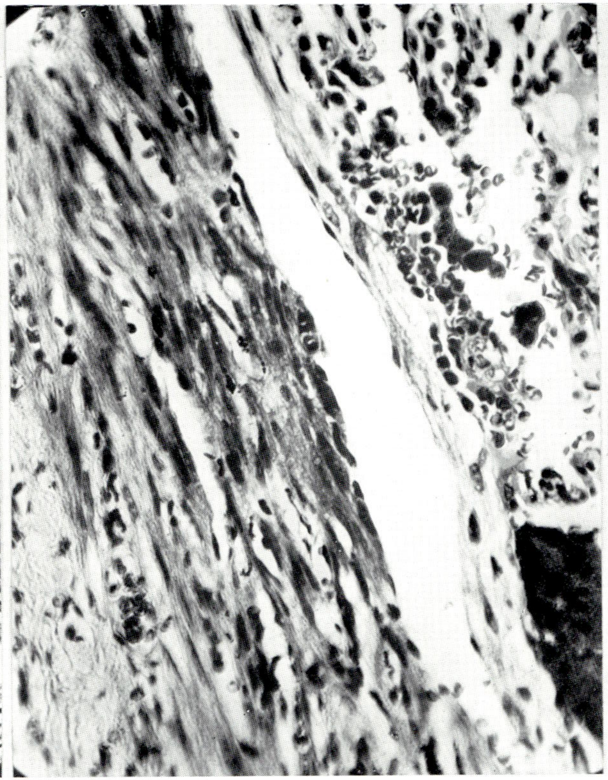

FIG. 9. Case 1. Biopsy specimen from left lung, showing a band of smooth muscle fibres; to the right is a strand of fibroblasts, and a collection of macrophages which are loaded with iron pigments (haematoxylin and eosin, ×320)

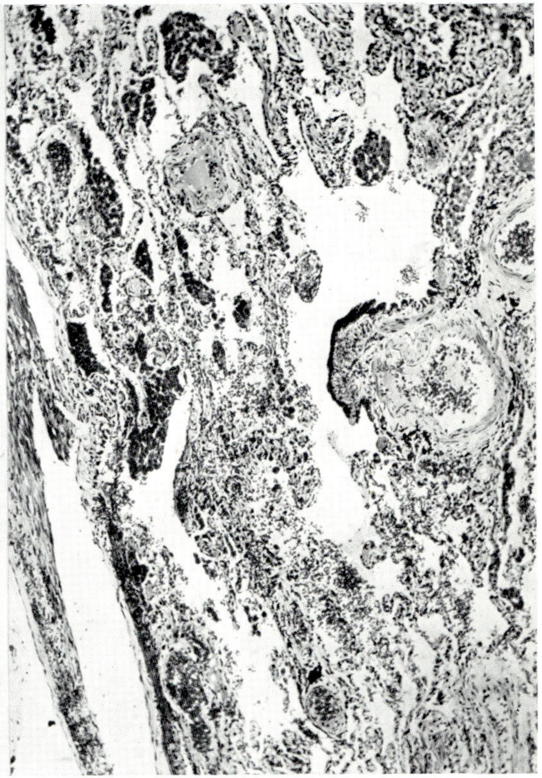

FIG. 10. Case 1. Biopsy specimen of left lung, with numerous collections of iron-bearing macrophages seen as dark groups of cells (haematoxylin and eosin, ×70)

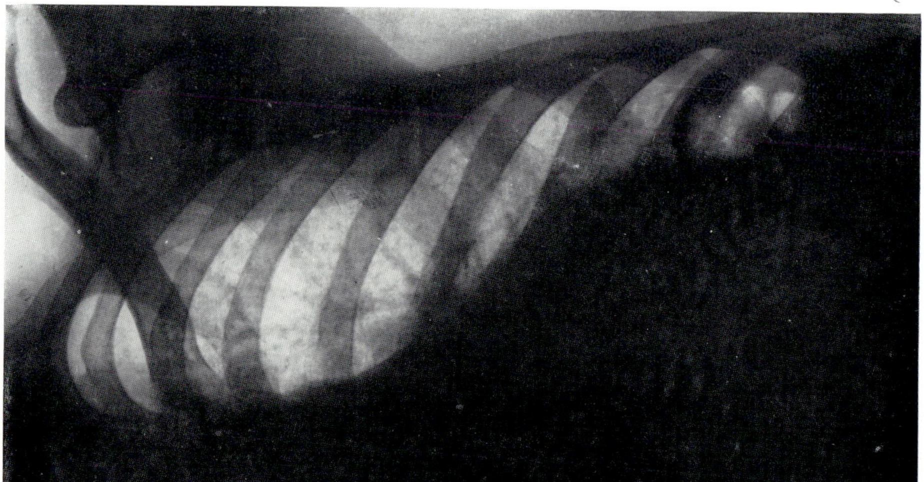

Fig. 11. Case 2. Ill-defined mottling in both lung fields, most conspicuous in the lower half of the right lung

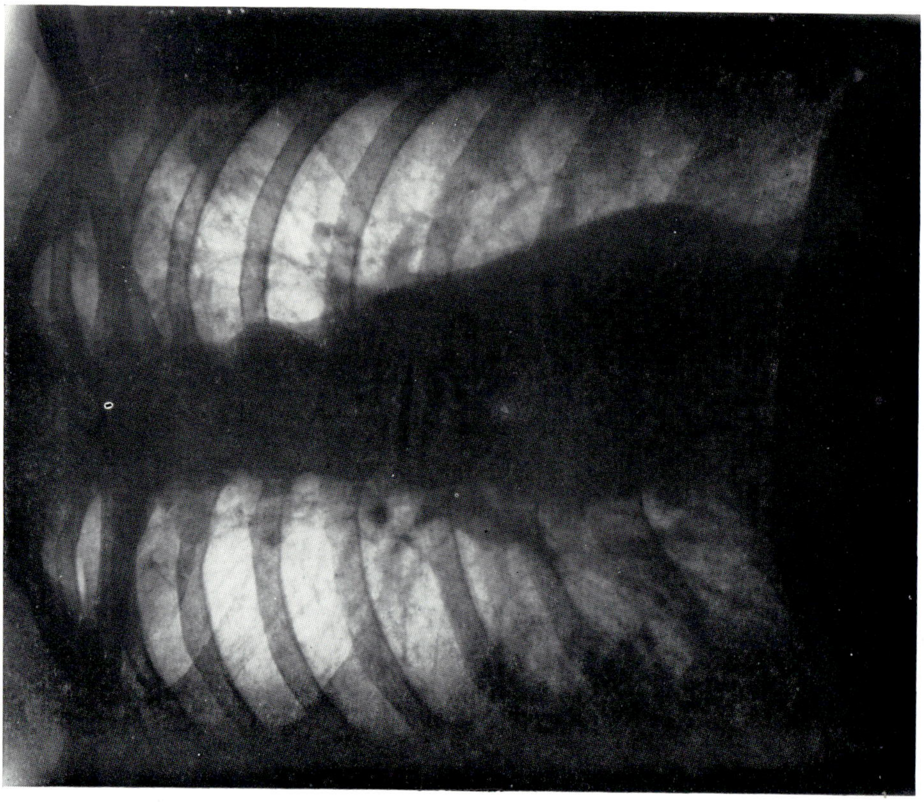

Fig. 12. Case 3. Aug. 1948. Ill-defined patchy mottling in the left upper lobe

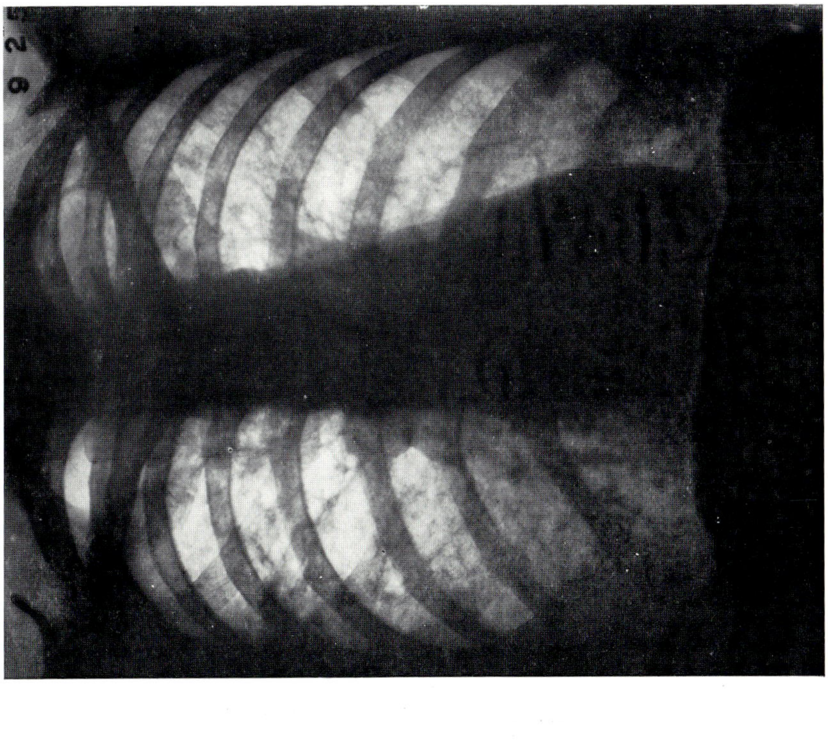

Fig. 13. Case 3. February 1951. Both lungs have become 'transformed by scattered wide-meshed reticulation and intervening cysts'

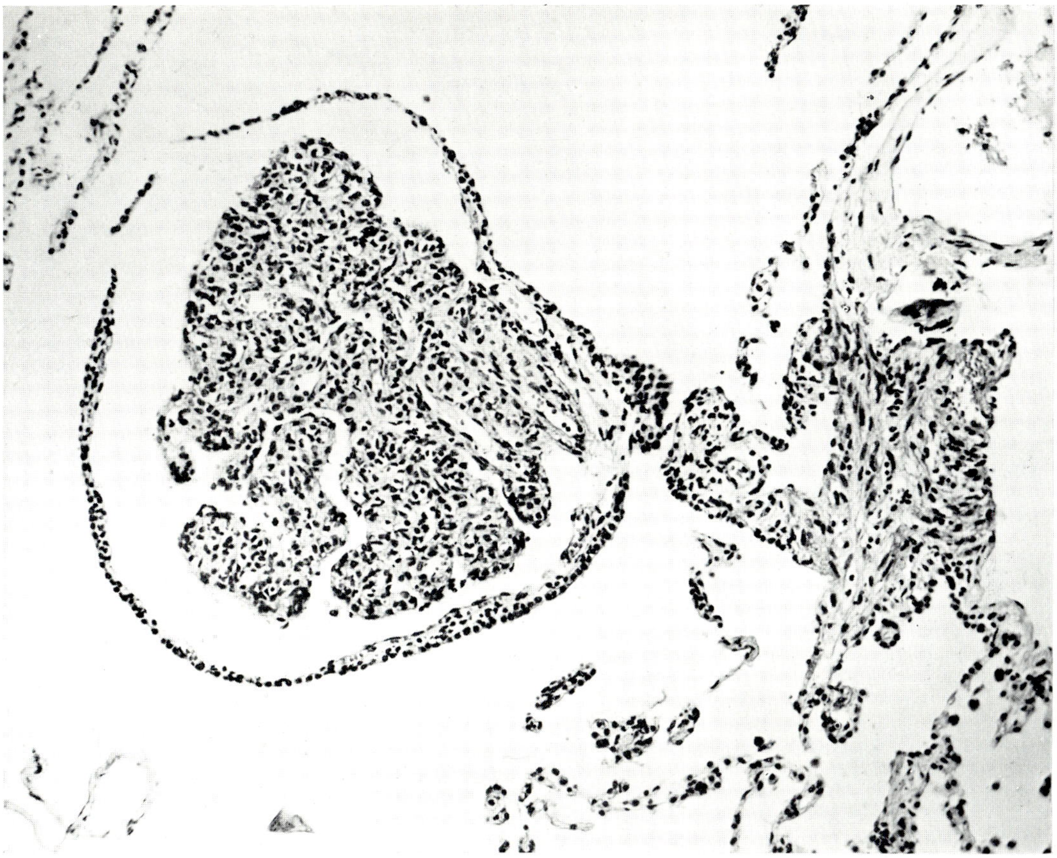

Fig. 14. Case 3. Lung biopsy specimen. The alveolar walls are thickened. This alveolus contains a proliferation of smooth muscle cells (haematoxylin and eosin, ×155)

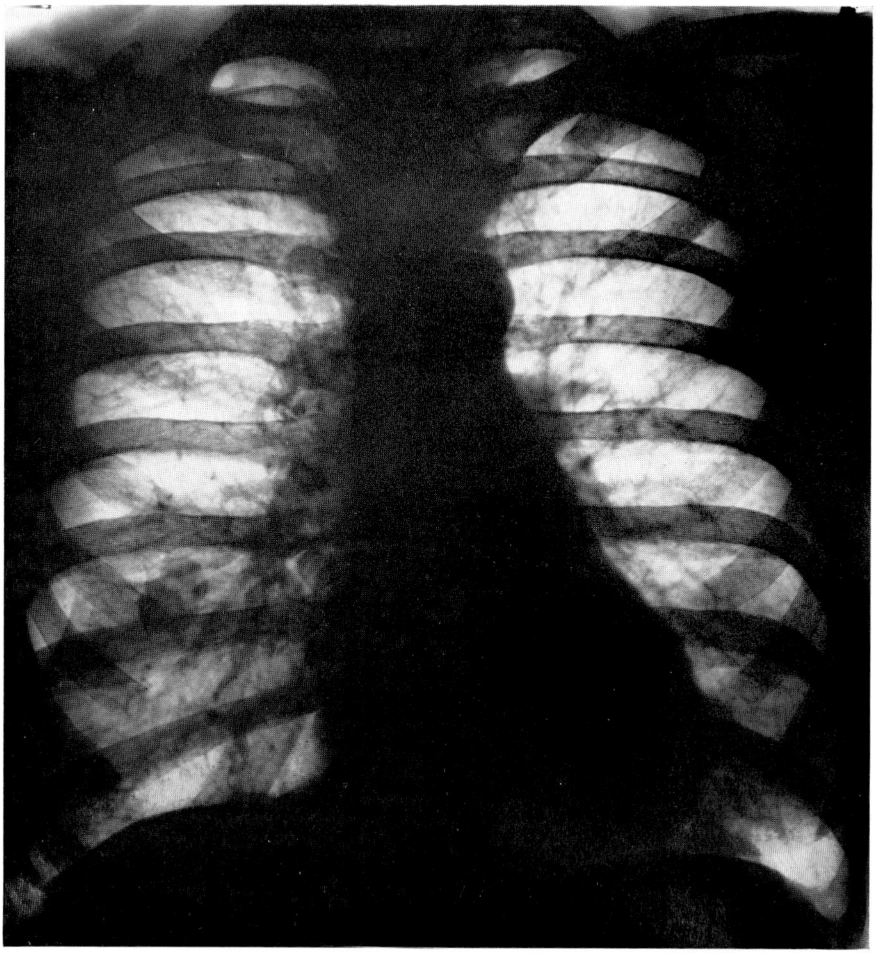

FIG. 15. Case 4. A lobulated shadow due to the adenoma in the right middle lobe

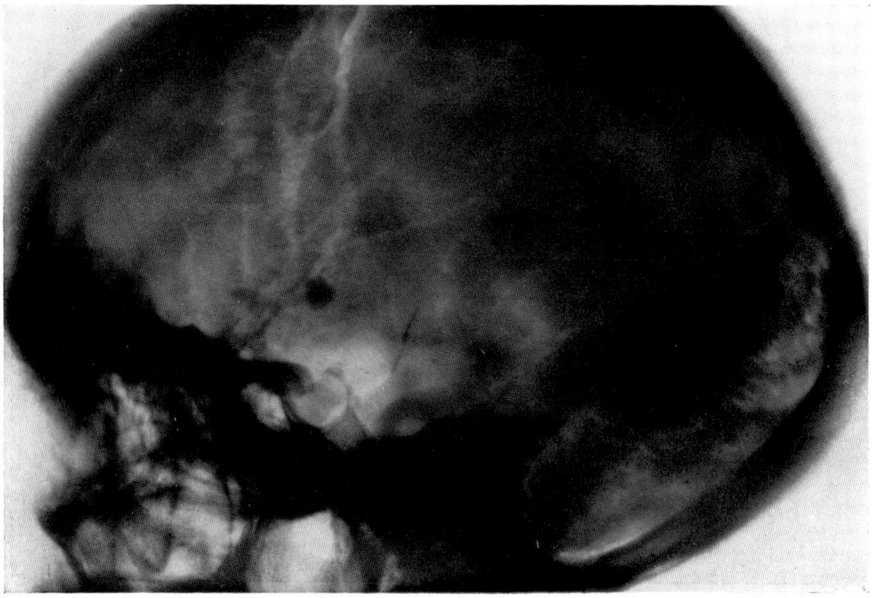

FIG. 16. Case 4. Calcification in the basal ganglia

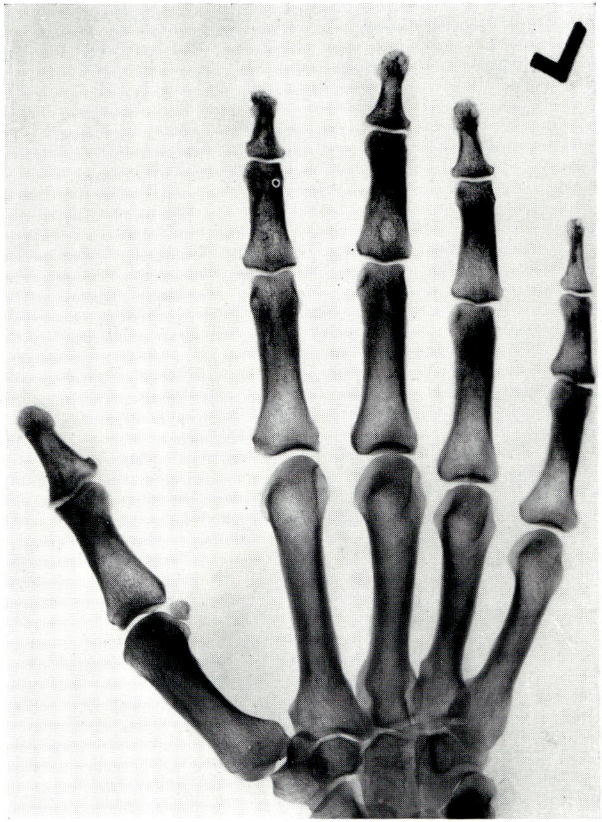

Fig. 17. Case 4. Cystic changes in the phalanges

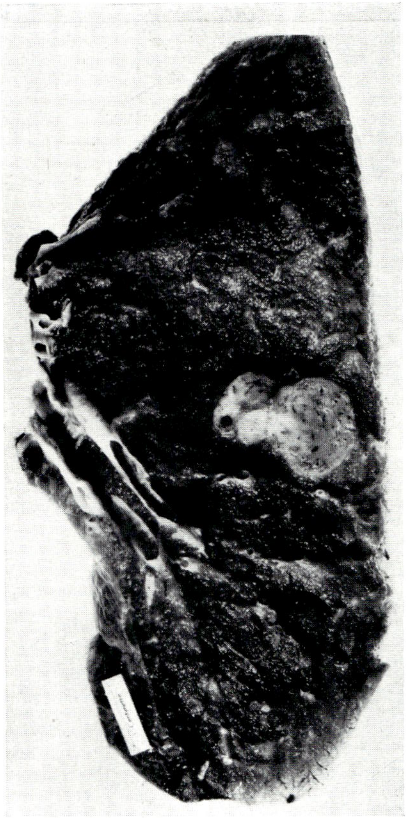

Fig. 18. Case 4. The adenoma in the right middle lobe

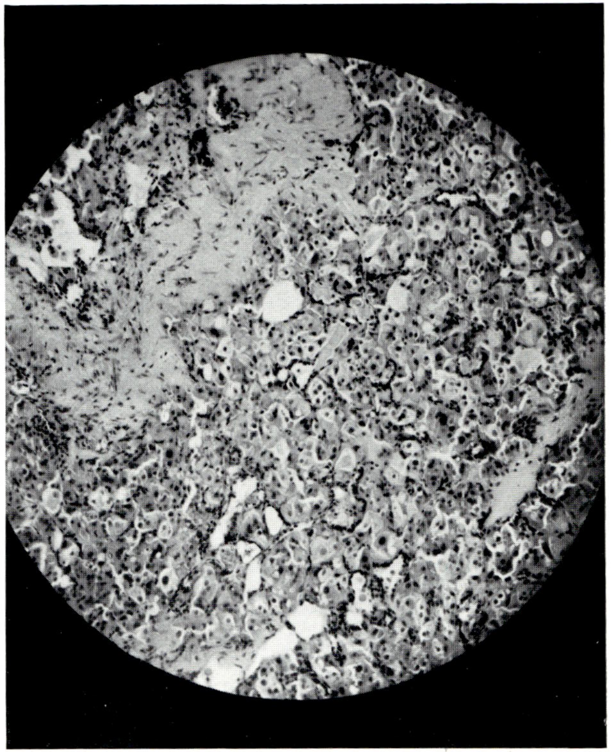

Fig. 19. Case 4. Mucus-secreting adenoma of columnar cells tending to acinar arrangement

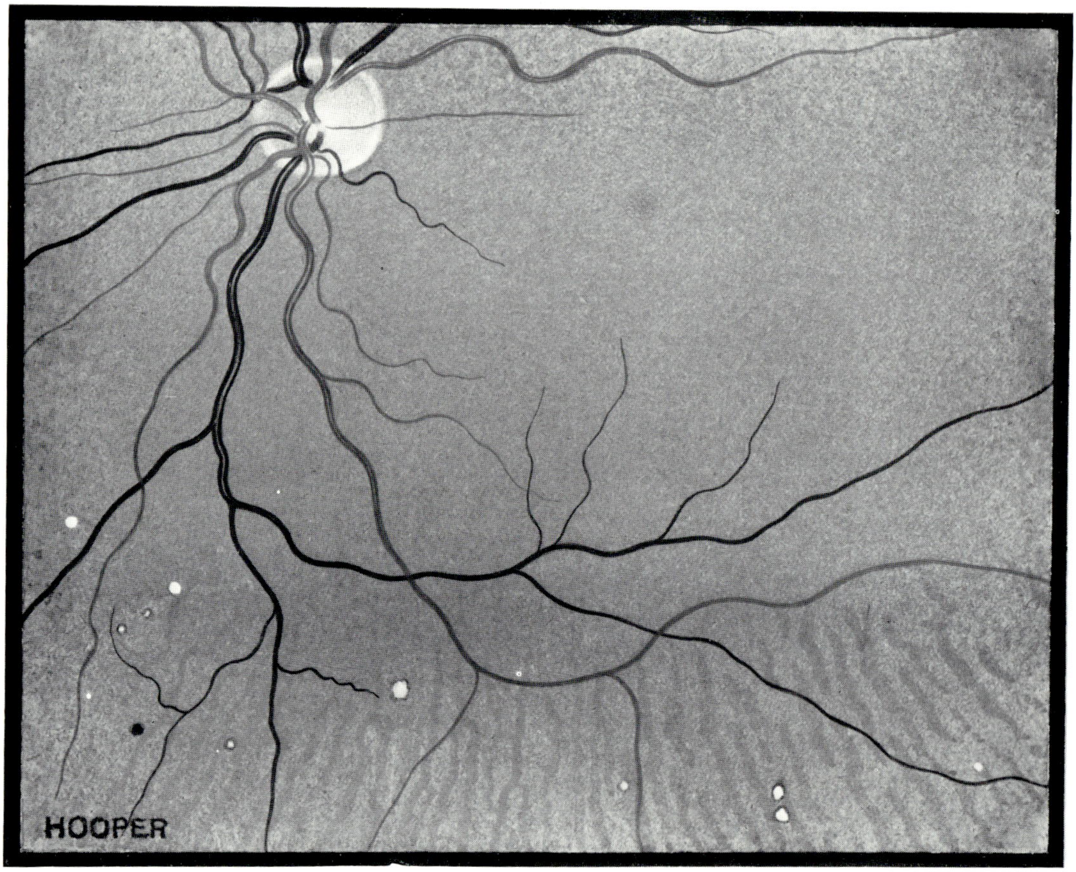

FIG. 20. Case 4. Five white nodules or 'phakomas' and several smaller ones seen in the left eye.

616.612–008

WATER-LOSING NEPHRITIS[1]

A Syndrome Simulating Diabetes Insipidus

By N. J. ROUSSAK and S. OLEESKY
(From Crumpsall Hospital, Manchester)

With Plates 16 and 17

In 1944 Thorn, Koepf, and Clinton first described the syndrome of 'salt-losing nephritis', in which patients with various renal diseases present a clinical picture resembling Addison's disease. This syndrome is attributable to considerable renal loss of sodium, producing a state of sodium depletion, and it has been shown that the renal tubules of such patients are refractory to pitressin, parathyroid extract, and deoxycortone. Platt (1950) has shown that the kidney is usually able to conserve sodium and maintain a normal serum-sodium level even in renal failure, so that the condition of salt-losing nephritis is a rare one; at the most only 11 cases have been described. A few patients with renal failure show an abnormally high excretion of sodium, and it has been suggested that these are possibly the patients who develop the overt salt-losing syndrome (Platt, 1951). In the present paper we describe two patients with renal disease whose initial symptoms were due to failure of renal conservation of water. Both patients were erroneously believed to have diabetes insipidus, particularly because the intravenous injection of hypertonic saline failed to induce antidiuresis. Further investigations, however, showed undoubted evidence of renal disease and resistance to the action of pitressin. It may be mentioned that the present writers, one in Manchester and the other in Sheffield, saw these patients at about the same time and studied them independently.

Case 1. In July 1952 A. W., a male hairdresser aged 50 years, first experienced aching pains in the left arm and the left side of the chest. Later the pain became severe, spreading all over the chest and to the lumbar region. On October 19, quite suddenly after breakfast, he noticed intense thirst, and in the space of a few hours drank six cups of tea, a pint of dandelion and burdock, and several pints of beer. When seen in Dr. Luxton's out-patient clinic at Crumpsall Hospital on November 9, 1952, he was still complaining of pains in the chest and back with intolerable thirst and dryness of the mouth, and painless micturition every 15 to 30 minutes. He appeared ill, and his tongue and buccal cavity were clean but parched. There was a fracture of the left clavicle, with a tender mass at the site, the ribs and sternum were exquisitely sensitive to pressure, and movements of the spine were restricted by pain. The blood-pressure was 205/120, the heart was not enlarged, and there was no oedema. The optic fundi were normal. The urine did not contain sugar, and its specific gravity was 1,000. Carcinomatosis and myelomatosis were considered possible diagnoses, with

[1] Received July 2, 1953.

secondary diabetes insipidus. He was admitted to hospital shortly afterwards; the following investigations were performed, and the diagnosis of myelomatosis established.

Routine investigations. Urine. Bence-Jones protein was constantly present, and albumin initially absent; no formed deposit was found. *Radiological examination.* Multiple small, sharply defined, translucent areas affected the ribs, pelvis, and upper femora. A few similar lesions were seen in the skull, but

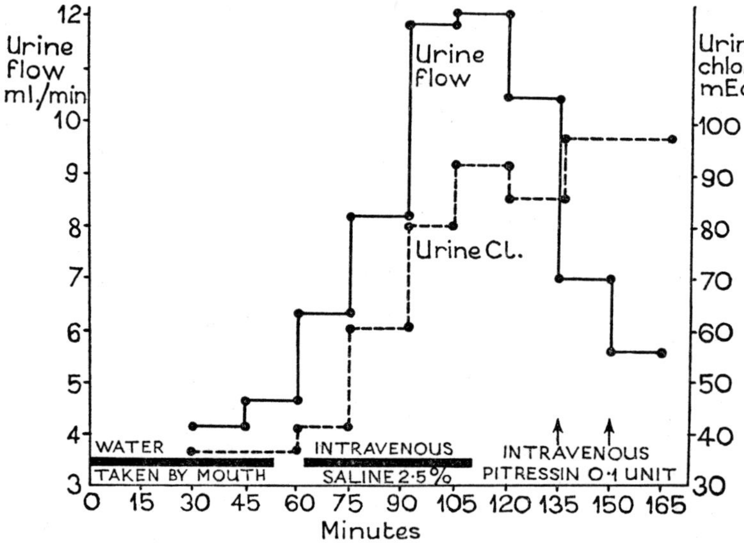

FIG. 1. Case 1. Response to hypertonic saline and pitressin (Table I).

none in the sella turcica. The cervical and lumbar spines were also involved, and there was a pathological fracture of the left clavicle through an expanding lesion. *Sternal marrow examination.* The marrow was replaced by large numbers of myeloma cells. Reticulum cells showed a moderate increase. Erythropoiesis was normoblastic. The changes were those found in myelomatosis. *Blood count*: haemoglobin 13 gm. per 100 ml.; red cells 4,500,000 per c.mm.; white cells 11,600 per c.mm., with normal differential count. *Serum chemistry*: calcium, 13·5 mg. per 100 ml.; inorganic phosphorus, 2·6 mg. per 100 ml.; alkaline phosphatase, 9·6 (later 14·1) King-Armstrong units per 100 ml.; acid phosphatase, 1·6 King-Armstrong units per 100 ml.; urea, 28 mg. per 100 ml.; albumin, 5·3 gm. (later 4·9 gm.) per 100 ml.; globulin, 3·2 gm. (later 2·6 gm.) per 100 ml.

During the first fortnight in hospital the patient's daily urinary output was 3·0 to 5·0 litres, and his fluid intake correspondingly large. At this stage it was thought unlikely that the polyuria was due to renal failure, because he was able to secrete urine with specific gravity as low as 1,000 to 1,004, albuminuria and casts were absent, and the blood-urea was normal.

Further investigations. These were undertaken in order to discover the nature of the polyuria, and to prove or exclude the presence of diabetes insipidus. The results were as follows:

(1) 15.11.52. The urine specific gravity after water deprivation for 11, 12, and 13 hours was 1,004, 1,002, and 1,000 respectively.

(2) 24.11.52. The urine specific gravity after water deprivation for 15 hours was 1,002.

(3) An intravenous hypertonic saline test (Carter and Robbins, 1947, as modified by Cates and Garrod, 1951) showed a failure of antidiuresis as in diabetes insipidus (Fig. 1; Table I). Two intravenous injections each of 0·1 unit pitressin were given, with an interval of 15 minutes, but the rate of urine flow, though slightly reduced, did not fall to the low level normally found after injection of pitressin, nor did the chloride concentration rise. This indicated that the failure to induce antidiuresis with hypertonic

TABLE I

Case 1: Effect of Intravenous 2·5 per cent. Saline on Established Water Diuresis

Period of collection (minutes)	*Urine flow (ml./min.)*	*Urinary chloride concentration (mEq./litre)*
30–44	4·1	35·9
44–60	4·6	35·9
60–75	6·3	41·0
75–91	8·2	60·3
91–105	11·9	80·3
105–120	12·1	92·5
120–135	10·5	85·5
135–150	7·0	97·5
150–165	5·6	97·5

20 ml. of water per kg. of body-weight were taken from 0 to 50 minutes, and 0·25 ml. of 2·5 per cent. saline per kg. was injected per minute from 60 to 105 minutes. 0·1 unit of pitressin was injected intravenously at both 135 and 150 minutes.

saline was due to resistance of the renal tubules to the action of anti-diuretic hormone, rather than failure of the neurohypophyseal mechanism.

(4) During water deprivation for 15 hours, three equally spaced intramuscular injections, each of 20 units of pitressin, were given, and the specific gravity of the urine passed at the end of 14 and 15 hours was 1,008 and 1,006 respectively.

The failure to concentrate the urine under the influence of pitressin was unexpected, and further tests of renal function were performed. These showed impairment of renal function, which became increasingly severe:

(5) 20.11.52. Urea clearance was 11 ml. per minute, the blood-urea being 58 mg. per 100 ml. 5.12.52. Urea clearance was 5·4 ml. per minute, the blood-urea being 124 mg. per 100 ml.

(6) 20.11.52. Endogenous creatinine clearance was 19 ml. per minute.

(7) Serum electrolyte concentrations (mEq. per litre) were as follows: 20.11.52: Na 144, K 4·7, Cl 102; 8.12.52: Na 136, K 5·5, Cl 99.

(8) Radiography of the abdomen did not show calcification in the renal areas.

(9) Chromatography of the urine showed only normal amounts of the usual aminoacids, and glycosuria was never found.

(10) 15.12.52. A urinary acidification test (Lundbaek, 1951) (Table II) was performed when uraemia had already developed and the polyuria had ceased. The urine was acid both before and after the ingestion of ammonium chloride, but the excretion of ammonium ions was very low for the degree of urinary acidity produced, and we cannot offer any explanation for this finding. Reabsorption of sodium was little impaired, about 97 per cent. of the filtered load being reabsorbed; potassium excretion was equivalent to about one-third of the filtered load. The glomerular filtration rate was low.

Further progress in Case 1. The blood-urea showed an almost linear rise, reaching 205 mg. per 100 ml. on 27.12.52, and increasing phosphate retention resulted in depression of the rising serum-calcium level (Fig. 2; Table III). In

TABLE II

Case 1. Urine Acidification Test

Period of collection (minutes)	*Urinary pH*	*Rate of flow (ml./min.)*	Na *excretion (μEq./min.)*	K *excretion (μEq./min.)*	Cl *excretion (μEq./min.)*	NH_4 *excretion (μEq./min.)*	*Endogenous creatinine clearance (ml./min.)*
0–22	5·4	1·2	31	19	14	1·5	6·7
22–84	5·2	1·0	24	17	13	4·0	5·4
84–145	5·0	0·9	19	15	9	3·0	5·1
145–205	5·2	1·0	24	17	15	3·3	5·6
205–264	5·0	1·1	23	17	11	4·2	6·6
264–324	5·0	1·1	26	18	14	2·9	5·9

Four gm. of ammonium chloride were taken at 24 minutes. Serum-creatinine was 9·1 mg. per 100 ml.

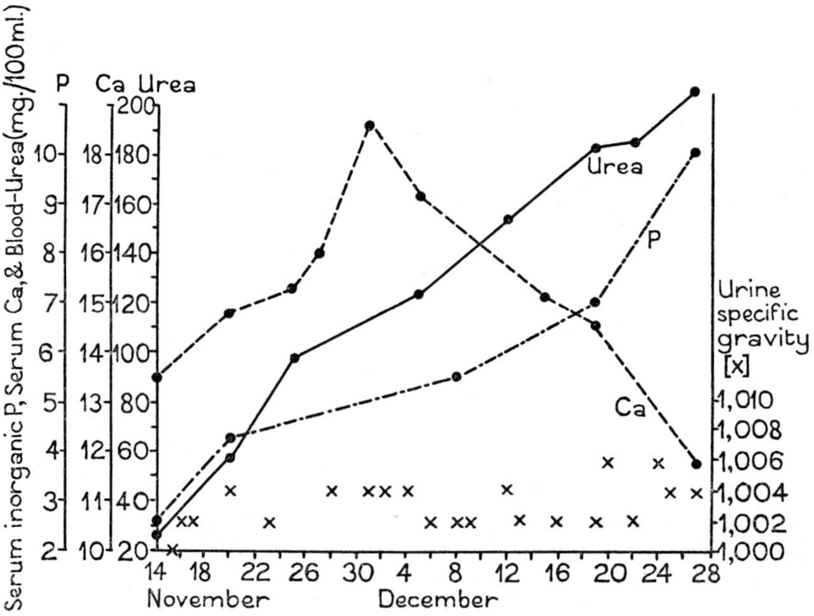

FIG. 2. Case 1. Blood chemistry and urinary specific gravity (Table III).

the last two weeks of life the daily urinary output fell to between 0·5 and 1·0 litre, but even during this period the specific gravity of the pooled 24-hour urine, and of single specimens, was always 1,002 to 1,004, except on two occasions in the last week, when it was 1,006. This low value was found in spite of albuminuria, which was first noted on 3.12.52, and which persisted together with Bence-Jones proteinuria, both of which must have tended to raise the specific gravity. On 5.12.52, when the blood-urea was 124 mg. per 100 ml., the specific gravity after water deprivation was only 1,005. The osmolarity of the urine on 11.12.52 was 186 m.Osmol. per litre, as determined from the depression of the freezing-point. Urethane treatment was given at the end of November, but had to be stopped because of vomiting. The patient died in uraemia on 27.12.52.

Post-mortem examination (Dr. J. Davson). Reddish masses of tumour were present in the ribs, sternum, clavicle, and lumbar spine. There was one such mass in the frontal region of the skull, but the sella turcica was quite normal. The pituitary gland appeared normal. The kidneys each weighed 240 gm., and were pinkish in colour; the cortex was somewhat swollen, with slight loss of cortical pattern, but demarcation from the medulla was clear. Histological examination of the bone-marrow revealed myeloma cells. The pituitary gland was normal, showing no infiltration by myeloma cells. Dr. Davson reported as follows on the histological examination of the kidneys (Plate 16, Fig. 6): 'Glomeruli appear normal apart from occasional ones which show capsulitis. Most convoluted tubules show slight flattening of epithelial cells, and fair numbers contain pink hyaline casts; the epithelium of these tubules shows extreme flattening. Similar casts are present in the collecting tubules. There is slight diffuse intertubular fibrosis in the cortex, and occasional streaks of round-cell infiltration in the boundary zone are present. The appearances are typical of multiple myelomatosis.'

TABLE III

Case 1. Urinary Specific Gravity, Blood-Urea, Serum-Calcium, and Serum Inorganic Phosphorus

Date	*Urinary specific gravity*	*Blood-urea (mg./100 ml.)*	*Serum-calcium (mg./100 ml.)*	*Serum inorganic phosphorus (mg./100 ml.)*
14.11.52	..	28	13·5	2·6
15.11.52	1,000	..	..	..
16.11.52	1,002	..	..	..
17.11.52	1,002	..	..	..
20.11.52	1,004	58	14·8	4·3
23.11.52	1,002	..	..	..
25.11.52	..	98	15·3	..
27.11.52	..	..	16·0	..
28.11.52	1,004	..	..	..
1.12.52	1,004	..	18·6	..
2.12.52	1,004	..	..	..
4.12.52	1,004	..	..	..
5.12.52	..	124	17·1	..
6.12.52	1,002	..	..	..
8.12.52	1,002	..	..	5·5
9.12.52	1,002	..	..	..
12.12.52	1,004	154	..	..
13.12.52	1,002	..	..	..
15.12.52	..	..	15.1	..
16.12.52	1,002	..	..	..
19.12.52	1,002	182	14·5	7·0
20.12.52	1,006	..	..	..
22.12.52	1,002	184	13.5	..
24.12.52	1,006	..	..	..
25.12.52	1,004	..	..	..
27.12.52	1,004	205	11.7	10.0

Summary of Case 1. The patient's symptoms and the results of investigations indicate that the initial diabetes-insipidus-like state, which began so acutely, was due to a defect of renal tubular function occurring in myelomatosis. Thirst and polyuria began before elevation of the blood-urea and, although renal failure later appeared and was the cause of death, the urinary specific gravity remained well below 1,010 throughout.

Case 2. E. S., a 62-year-old pump attendant in a coal mine, attended Professor Wayne's out-patient clinic at the Royal Infirmary, Sheffield, on November 11, 1952, with a three weeks' history of severe thirst and polyuria. There had been a strikingly acute onset while he was down the mine, and since then he had

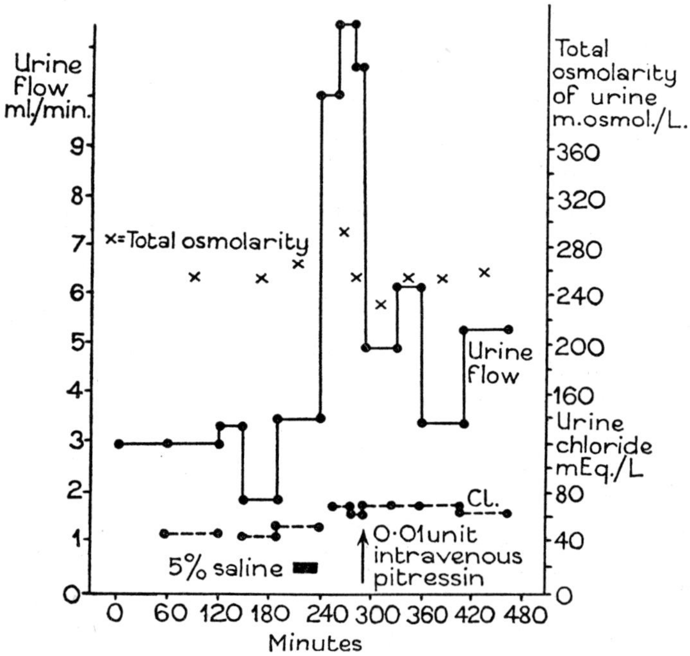

FIG. 3. Case 2. Response to hypertonic saline and pitressin (Table IV).

passed large volumes of pale urine almost hourly, which was found by his general practitioner to be of low specific gravity. There had been marked dryness and soreness of the mouth, tongue, and pharynx, and the patient had drunk seven or eight pints of fluid daily. There were no symptoms of prostatic enlargement, and the patient had felt that he completely emptied his bladder whenever he passed urine. There was no history of head injury or family history suggestive of diabetes insipidus. Physical examination showed a blood-pressure of 220/120 and some prostatic enlargement, but no other abnormalities. The urine was free from albumin, and its specific gravity was 1,000 to 1,002. He was admitted to hospital on November 21, 1952, with a provisional diagnosis of diabetes insipidus.

Routine investigations. In hospital his daily urinary output averaged 3·5 litres. At first albumin could not be detected in the urine, but after the end of November 1952 it was constantly present. The specific gravity of random specimens of urine varied from 1,004 to 1,007. Blood counts, radiological examinations of the skull and chest, and the cerebrospinal fluid were all normal, but the electrocardiogram showed changes indicating left ventricular enlargement. Serum-calcium was 9·6 mg. per 100 ml., and serum alkaline phosphatase was 13 King-Armstrong units per 100 ml. Serum-sodium was 144 mEq. per litre, potassium 4·1 mEq. per litre, and chloride 103 mEq. per litre. The Wassermann reaction was negative. Culture of the urine was sterile, and there was no formed deposit. There was no glycosuria or abnormal aminoaciduria.

Special investigations.

(1) The maximum urinary specific gravity after 18 hours' fasting was 1,008, and ingestion of one litre of water gave a minimum specific gravity of 1,002. This indicated an inability to concentrate but an ability to dilute the urine.

(2) On 25.11.52, 400 ml. of 5 per cent. saline were given intravenously over a period of 20 minutes (Fig. 3; Table IV). The rate of urine flow rose to

TABLE IV

Case 2. Effect of Intravenous Hypertonic Saline

	Urine			
Period of collection (minutes)	*Rate of flow (ml./min.)*	*Total osmolarity (m.Osmol./l.)*	*Chloride concentration (mEq./l.)*	*Urea clearance (ml./min.)*
0–60	2·97	. .	. .	. .
60–120	2·92	253	46	17·4
120–150	3·33	. .	. .	. .
150–190	1·85	253	44	11·2
190–240	3·46	263	52	27
240–260	10·1	. .	. .	. .
260–275	11·6	290	66	80
275–290	10·7	253	64	64
290–330	4·9	231	68	30
330–360	6·2	253	68	42·5
360–410	3·4	253	68	23·4
410–460	5·3	258	66	36

400 ml. of 5 per cent. saline were given intravenously from 215 to 235 minutes. 0·01 unit of pitressin was given intravenously at 295 minutes. Blood-urea was 34 mg. per 100 ml. Total osmolarity was calculated from freezing-point depression.

over 11 ml. per minute, and although 0·01 unit of pitressin given intravenously during the diuresis was associated with a fall in urine flow, the osmolarity and chloride concentration of the urine did not rise. The rise in urine flow with hypertonic saline indicated either a deficient neurohypophyseal mechanism or a resistance of the renal tubules to antidiuretic hormone. The failure to respond to pitressin suggested that the renal tubule cells were insensitive to pitressin. Throughout the test the urine was hypotonic.

(3) On 29.11.52 a much larger dose of pitressin (0·5 unit given intravenously) failed to reduce the rate of urine flow (Fig. 4; Table V), but two days later the same preparation of pitressin, given to a normal subject during water diuresis, produced a typical antidiuresis lasting an hour and a half. These experiments confirmed the view that the renal tubules of the patient were resistant to a potent preparation of pitressin.

(4) On 5.12.52 Dr. D. R. Wood, using the method of Birnie, Jenkins, Eversole, and Gaunt (1949), demonstrated the presence of an antidiuretic substance in the patient's plasma.

(5) Blood-urea was 34 mg. and 37 mg. per 100 ml. on 25.11.52 and 1.12.52 respectively. Urea clearance was low, and rose during the diuresis produced by hypertonic saline (Table IV). This fact suggested a low glomerular filtration rate, which was confirmed by finding on 5.12.52 an endogenous creatinine clearance of 44 ml. per minute with a serum-creatinine of 2·6 mg. per 100 ml., at a urine flow of 5·7 ml. per minute.

(6) On 5.12.52, 3 gm. of ammonium chloride were given by mouth, and the lowest urinary pH reached was 6·0. This finding suggested a moderate degree of failure of the mechanism for urinary acidification.

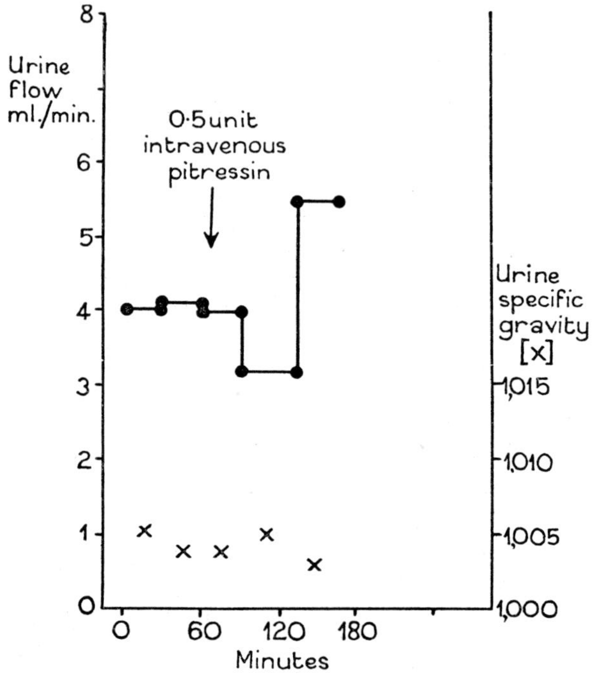

FIG. 4. Case 2. Effect of a large dose of pitressin.

TABLE V

Case 2. Effect of a Large Dose of Pitressin

Period of collection (minutes)	*Urine* *Rate of flow (ml./min.)*	*Specific gravity*
0–30	4·0	1,005
30–60	4·1	1,004
60–90	4·0	1,004
90–135	3·2	1,005
135–165	5·5	1,003

0·5 unit of pitressin was given intravenously at 65 minutes.

(7) An intravenous pyelogram was carried out on 3.12.52, and showed dilatation of the calyces of the kidney, indicating early hydronephrosis (Plate 16, Fig. 7). This result offered a possible anatomical basis for the symptoms and laboratory findings.

Further history of Case 2. The patient was allowed to go home on 9.12.52, to await readmission for cystoscopy and possible prostatectomy. In February 1953 he was readmitted under the care of Mr. Clifford Jones. He still had polyuria with a trace of albuminuria, and on 5.2.53 his blood-urea was 43 mg. per 100 ml. On 9.2.53 the blood-urea had risen to 57 mg. per 100 ml., and the urea clearance had fallen to 11 ml. per minute. The serum acid phosphatase was normal. On 13.2.53 he was operated upon by Mr. Betts, who found a hard, fixed prostate and moderately distended bladder. A wedge resection was performed, and histological examination of the resected portion showed carcinoma of the prostate. After operation stilboestrol therapy was commenced. Since

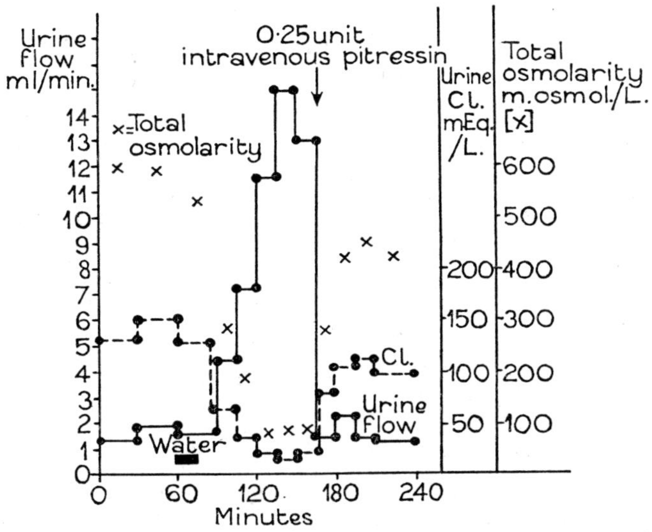

FIG. 5. Case 2. After operation; effect of pitressin on water diuresis.

TABLE VI

Case 2. After Operation. Effect of Pitressin on Water Diuresis

Period of collection (minutes)	*Urine* Rate of flow (ml./min.)	Total osmolarity (m.Osmol./l.)	Chloride concentration (mEq./l.)
0–30	1·4	595	136
30–60	1·9	586	154
60–90	1·7	533	132
90–105	4·5	285	64
105–120	7·3	185	36
120–135	11·6	81	22
135–150	15·0	86	18
150–165	13·0	86	22
165–180	1·5	280	78
180–195	2·27	419	106
195–210	1·5	452	110
210–240	1·4	424	98

1,100 ml. of water were taken from 60 to 75 minutes. 0·25 unit of pitressin was given intravenously at 165 minutes. Total osmolarity was calculated from freezing-point depression.

operation the thirst and polyuria have slowly lessened, so that, when he was seen on 28.5.53, he could go for a whole morning without needing to drink, and only had to pass urine at intervals of five to six hours. There was still slight albuminuria, but the filtration rate as measured by endogenous creatinine clearance was normal (131 ml. per minute with a plasma-creatinine level of 0·67 mg. per 100 ml.). The blood-urea was 24 mg. per 100 ml., with a urea clearance of 74 and 100 ml. per minute. A water diuresis was induced, and during the height of diuresis 0·25 unit of pitressin was given intravenously

(Fig. 5; Table VI). It can be seen that before the diuresis the total osmolarity of the urine was almost twice that of plasma, indicating a return of the ability of the distal tubule to concentrate the urine. Similarly pitressin was now able to inhibit a water diuresis, and to raise the total osmolarity and chloride concentration of the urine.

Summary of Case 2. This patient suddenly developed a diabetes-insipidus-like state, and investigations showed that the inability to concentrate the urine was due to a failure of the renal tubule cells to respond to antidiuretic hormone. The filtration rate was abnormally low during the period of thirst and polyuria, but nitrogen retention only appeared later and was of minor degree. Early hydronephrosis caused by an enlarged prostate gland was demonstrated. After removal of the prostatic obstruction the diabetes-insipidus-like state disappeared and three months later it was found that the distal tubule was able to concentrate the urine. The filtration rate and urea clearance became normal. A difficulty experienced in this study, and in interpreting the results, is doubt as to the completeness with which the patient could empty his bladder, and as to possible variations in the volume of urine held in the dilated renal pelvis and calyces. But the rate of urine flow in all the experiments was so high that the effect of these factors would be reduced to a minimum. The bladder was found at operation to be only moderately dilated, and the patient himself considered that he was able to empty his bladder completely.

Discussion

We have described two patients and the results of studies which we carried out upon them, and it will be seen that, although the renal diseases from which they suffered were quite different in aetiology, each presented the clinical picture of diabetes insipidus. Both conditions, however, differed from classical diabetes insipidus due to a disorder of the neurohypophyseal mechanism, in being resistant to the action of pitressin. This hormone controls the active reabsorption of water, and its failure to act indicates the presence of a lesion of the distal tubules rendering them insensitive to it. For some time this distal tubular lesion was the one which most affected renal function; only later did nitrogen retention occur, and in one patient the mechanism of urinary acidification was affected. In both patients the inability to conserve water, with resulting secretion of dilute urine, persisted, in one case until the patient died. The clinical and laboratory characteristics of the new syndrome, for which we suggest the name 'water-losing nephritis', may be seen in Table VII.

A hereditary form of diabetes insipidus has been described, which in some cases is pitressin-resistant (Forssman, 1945; Waring, Kajdi, and Tappan, 1945; Williams and Henry, 1947; Dancis, Birmingham, and Leslie, 1948; Cates and Garrod, 1951). Renal tubular resistance to the action of pitressin is considered to be the cause of hereditary pitressin-resistant diabetes insipidus. In fact Heller (1952) considered that this syndrome is merely the result of the persistence of the normal neonatal insensitivity to pitressin. It may be, therefore, that congenital and acquired forms of water-losing nephritis exist, but the former, with its familial tendency, commencement in early life, benign course, and absence of other manifestations of renal disease, is clearly different from the acquired conditions described in the present paper. There have also been reports of patients who showed clear evidence of other defects of tubular function, congenital and familial in origin, in association with hereditary pitressin-resistant diabetes insipidus. In fact many of the features of the Fanconi syndrome may be present and dominate the clinical picture. These combined defects of renal tubular

TABLE VII

Characteristics of Water-Losing Nephritis

	Initial symptoms	*Maximum urinary specific gravity*	*Albuminuria*	*Aminoaciduria and glycosuria*	*Uraemia*	*Action of pitressin*	*Serum anti-diuretic substance*	*Glomerular filtration rate*	*Urinary acidification*	Na *or* K *depletion*
Case 1	Polyuria Thirst	1,006	Late	Absent	Late	Absent	Not known	Low	Present	Absent
Case 2	Polyuria Thirst	1,007	Late	Absent	Late	Absent	Normal	Low	Poor	Absent

function have recently been discussed in this journal by Jackson and Linder (1953), but their congenital and familial basis separate them from the acquired water-losing syndrome. Rare cases of non-hereditary diabetes insipidus are resistant to pitressin; such a condition has occurred after head injuries, and also after virus and syphilitic infections of the nervous system (Warkany and Mitchell, 1939). Detailed observations, and the results of the intravenous saline and nicotine tests, are not available; but in view of the causes of diabetes insipidus in such patients it seems highly improbable that the pitressin resistance was due to renal tubular damage. Dyggve and Samsøe-Jensen (1947) described a patient who had non-hereditary diabetes insipidus, resistant to pitressin and of unknown etiology. There was no albuminuria, and the pyelogram was normal, but the filtration rate was low. The authors concluded that the diabetes-insipidus-like state was due to renal disease, so that it is possible that this patient had water-losing nephritis.

The new syndrome must be distinguished from the usual type of renal failure, in which Platt (1952) has suggested that a loss of nephrons gives rise to an osmotic diuresis even before the level of blood-urea rises. It has been shown by Rapoport, Brodsky, West, and Mackler (1949) that, in an osmotic diuresis induced experimentally in man, the total urine osmolarity slowly falls with increasing urine flow, but never falls below that of the plasma. Since their experiments were performed in hydropenic states, each osmolar value represents the maximum urine concentration for that particular rate of urine flow. It is also known that, provided there are no large amounts of abnormal urinary constituents, there is a close relationship between total urine osmolarity and specific gravity (Price, Miller, and Hayman, 1940). These experiments of Rapoport, Brodsky, West, and Mackler (1949) therefore provide a theoretical basis for the known inability of patients in renal failure to form a concentrated urine, but also show that the maximum urinary specific gravity or osmolarity will slowly fall as renal failure progresses, but will not go below the specific gravity or osmolarity of protein-free plasma. Finally the specific gravity becomes fixed at 1,010, that is, isosthenuria develops. All these changes are in sharp contrast to the obligatory hyposthenuria characteristic of the syndrome here described. The term hyposthenuria as used in the present paper means a urinary specific gravity below 1,010. Thus the maximum specific gravity of the urine of our patients was always well below 1,010, and the total osmolarity was always less than that of plasma. It seems that, in the isosthenuric phase of classical renal failure, the distal tubule does not alter the osmolarity of the urine reaching it from the proximal tubule, but that in water-losing nephritis solutes are reabsorbed but not water, so that hyposthenuria results. Further features of water-losing nephritis differentiating it from classical renal failure are a daily urine volume greater than two or three litres, and the late development of albuminuria and uraemia.

Another condition to be differentiated from water-losing nephritis is the diuretic phase occurring during recovery from acute tubular necrosis. During this phase Burnett, Shapiro, Simeone, Beecher, Mallory, and Sullivan (1947) found that the specific gravity of the urine did not fall below 1,010, and Bull, Joekes, and Lowe (1950) found that the urine had the composition of slightly modified glomerular filtrate. This means that the patients did not have hyposthenuria, and so did not show a specific water-losing tendency. The reason is probably that in acute tubular necrosis the tubular lesions are scattered throughout the nephron (Oliver, MacDowell, and Tracy, 1951).

Renal changes in myelomatosis

As the first of our two patients had myelomatosis, it is necessary to consider the structural and functional changes which occur in the kidney in this condition.

Pathological changes in the kidneys in myelomatosis. The most important renal lesion in myelomatosis is widespread tubular obstruction by protein casts (Bell, 1933; Morison, 1941). The casts are unusual in that they become permanently lodged in the tubules where they are formed, and because of the completeness with which they block these channels. They are formed by local coagulation of filtered serum-globulins (Blackman, Barker, Buell, and Davis, 1944) which are perhaps Bence-Jones protein, although no relationship could be found between the presence of casts and either the level of serum-globulin or the presence of Bence-Jones proteinuria (Bell, 1933; Breitenbucher and Hertzog, 1949). Oliver (1945) examined the kidneys from patients with myelomatosis by his microdissection technique, and found 'great stretches of nephron tubule and of the collecting ducts filled with solid occlusions of the protein body', with 'resulting distensions, deformities, and atrophies' of the tubule. He observed that in the commoner types of renal disease with albuminuria proximal tubular casts were not found; but in myelomatosis they sometimes occurred, in addition to casts further along the nephron. The explanation he offered was the predominance of globulins with low isoelectric points, capable of coagulating in less acid conditions than those required for albumin. The other common renal abnormality in myelomatosis is the deposition of calcium in and about the tubules (Perla and Hutner, 1930; Breitenbucher and Hertzog, 1949; Limarzi, 1951), presumably a consequence of hypercalcaemia and hypercalcuria due to skeletal destruction. The nephrocalcinosis of myelomatosis, and its possible functional significance, will be referred to again in the present paper. Glomerular changes have also been described (Bell, 1933), but are usually slight or absent. The mechanism of renal failure in myelomatosis is usually believed to be the progressive intrarenal obstruction to urinary flow, although only one patient has been described in whom the process was carried to the ultimate conclusion of anuria (Holman, 1939).

Renal function in myelomatosis. In those reports of myelomatosis with renal failure in which the specific gravity of the urine is stated, it has been 1,010 or higher (Morison, 1941; Laake, 1949). Such values are presumably the result, as in commoner types of renal disease (Platt, 1952), of an osmotic diuresis through nephrons which are still unobstructed by casts. There have, however, been a few patients with myelomatosis who have had polyuria so considerable as to be construed as indicating the presence of diabetes insipidus. This polyuria has been attributed to the pressure of a myelomatous deposit upon the pituitary or its neural connexions. The reports of such cases may be briefly examined. It is somewhat difficult to accept the case recorded by Aronsohn (1931), although the maximum urinary specific gravity was said to be 1,005; for there is no mention of polyuria, the pituitary gland and sella were normal both macroscopically and histologically, and the histological appearance of the kidney was not described. In the patient of Denker and Brock (1934) the data are inadequate to exclude renal failure as the cause of the polyuria, for renal lesions were found at autopsy, and the pituitary gland was not examined. The patient of Anders and Boston (1903) may have had diabetes insipidus, because his initial symptom was intense thirst, and the urine was hyposthenuric, but no relevant details were given. The evidence for diabetes insipidus was stronger in the case reported by Bach and Middleton (1931), as the daily urinary output was 13·5 litres at home and five litres in hospital, and the specific gravity was 1,005 or less. The output was reduced to less than two litres by treatment with pituitrin, but the effect was inconstant, and usually the negative water balance persisted. Radiological examination, however, did not show myelomatous lesions in the skull, the data as to renal function are inadequate, and autopsy was not reported. It will be seen that the clinical and laboratory findings in none of these cases satisfy the more stringent criteria now required for the diagnosis of diabetes insipidus.

Polyuria in certain other conditions affecting the kidney

It has already been mentioned that in myelomatosis there are obstructive and calcific lesions of the renal tubules, together with hypercalcaemia. Therefore it is pertinent briefly to consider the impairment of renal function which occurs, first in other hypercalcaemic conditions, and secondly in conditions with tubular degeneration and calcification, with or without hypercalcaemia.

A. *Hypercalcaemic states.* (1) *Hyperparathyroidism.* Polyuria and polydipsia are well-recognized symptoms of hyperparathyroidism, but there is no satisfactory explanation of the mechanism of their production. The theory that the polyuria is due to an osmotic diuresis secondary to hypercalcuria, so-called 'calcium-diabetes' (Allan, 1931; Snapper, 1949), is unsatisfactory, because it can easily be calculated that, even with gross hypercalcuria, the amount of calcium present is capable of adding only a small contribution to the total osmolarity of the urine (Törnblom, 1949). There is some evidence that parathyroid hormone may be directly responsible for the diuresis, as it has been shown to increase the glomerular filtration rate (Jacobs and Verbanck, 1953; Klein and Gow, 1953) and the rate of urine flow (Ellsworth and Nicholson, 1935). A third possible cause of the polyuria might be renal failure with isosthenuria; this complication appears to be not uncommon, and is brought about by nephrocalcinosis (Anderson, 1939). But it seems that the common thirst and polyuria are not due to renal failure of this type, and are not necessarily associated with nitrogen retention. In some cases the polyuria has been of the order of six to 13 litres a day (Allan, 1931; Albright and Reifenstein, 1948; Snapper, 1952), and therefore greater than that encountered in the usual osmotic diuresis of renal failure, so that diabetes insipidus has been suspected. Unfortunately most published reports of such patients give little information about renal function, even the levels of urinary specific gravity being omitted in the accounts of Allan and of Snapper; but Snapper's patient had thirst and gross polyuria for seven years without nitrogen retention or polyuria. A similar patient described by Moulonguet and Lièvre (1938) had intense thirst and polyuria, with a urinary specific gravity of 1,005, for three years before the diagnosis of hyperparathyroidism was made. Albright and Reifenstein (1948) thoroughly investigated one such patient, with most interesting results. This was a woman of 59 years, who had had polyuria, with a fluid intake of four to five litres daily, for five years, simulating diabetes insipidus. Random records of urinary specific gravity were 1,001 to 1,010, usually 1,005, and the value did not rise above 1,010 even with pituitrin. There was neither albuminuria nor nitrogen retention. The glomerular filtration rate was about 50 per cent. of normal, renal blood-flow about 60 per cent. of normal, and the maximum capacity of the tubules to secrete diodrast about 66 per cent. of normal. There was no radiological evidence of skeletal involvement, but the serum chemistry was diagnostic of hyperparathyroidism, and a parathyroid adenoma was removed. The ability to concentrate the urine was unchanged one week after operation, but one year later the urinary specific gravity reached 1,018 with pituitrin. This patient therefore had polyuria, pituitrin-resistant hyposthenuria, and normal blood-urea. It will be seen that her condition was strikingly similar to that of our patients.

(2) *Sarcoidosis.* Renal failure is described in this condition (Longcope and Freiman, 1952), usually in association with hypercalcaemia and renal tubular calcification. The specific gravity of the urine in such cases has usually been 1,010 (Klinefelter and Salley, 1946). Thirst, polyuria, and hyposthenuria in a patient with sarcoidosis are usually taken to indicate diabetes insipidus due to

pituitary inolvement. It is not known whether such symptoms have ever been pitressin-resistant, and therefore possibly of renal origin.

(3) *Hypervitaminosis-D, and hypercalcaemic nephrocalcinosis in carcinoma.* Polyuria, thirst, and renal failure are among the symptons of calciferol intoxication, but the urinary specific gravity has usually been 1,010 or above (Adams, 1951; Chaplin, Clark, and Ropes, 1951). There was also isosthenuria in the case of uraemia due to skeletal carcinomatosis reported by Fulton and Paget (1951). In neither of these two renal lesions, therefore, has there been any evidence of a diabetes-insipidus-like state.

(4) *Hypercalcaemia in infants.* Lightwood (1952) recently reported the finding of hypercalcaemia of unknown cause in 10 infants. They had failed to thrive, and had thirst, polyuria, and increased blood-urea, but not renal acidosis. The urinary specific gravities were not given.

B. *Conditions showing tubular calcification, but without hypercalcaemia.* (1) *Hyperchloraemic nephrocalcinosis.* Calcification of the renal tubules in this condition does not seem to interfere with water reabsorption, for the levels of urinary specific gravity in the series of Doxiadis (1952) were all 1,010 or higher. Kelsey, Reinhart, and Fishel (1950) studied an infant who had renal acidosis, and stated that there was polyuria due to a pitressin-resistant diabetes insipidus of renal origin. Nevertheless the urinary specific gravities given in their Table are 1,008 to 1,015, so that hyposthenuria was not present, and there was not really a diabetes-insipidus-like state.

(2) *Alkalosis.* Renal tubular changes, with calcification and associated renal failure, are well-recognized results of alkalosis secondary either to high intestinal obstruction (Brown, Eusterman, Hartman, and Rowntree, 1923; Cooke, 1933) or to ingestion of alkali (Cooke, 1932; Cope, 1936; Sanderson, 1948). It has frequently been observed that the latter group of patients may pass large volumes of urine, sometimes in spite of clinical evidence of dehydration. It is possible that this occurrence is an osmotic diuresis due to the excretion of large amounts of ingested base, as Cope suggested, but unfortunately values for urinary specific gravity were not given in these reports, so that we cannot exclude a 'water-losing' tendency.

Pathogenesis of the syndrome

Having reviewed the above conditions which cause renal tubular lesions, we can see that in only one of them, namely hyperparathyroidism, may the clinical picture be that of the water-losing syndrome. It is clear, therefore, that tubular degeneration, with or without calcification, is usually insufficient to produce this particular abnormality of renal function. Nor does myelomatosis usually produce the water-losing syndrome; and yet, in Case 1, on routine histological examination no extraordinary changes were found. An examination of the nephron by a more searching technique was clearly indicated, and Dr. Darmady kindly carried out microdissection studies.

Report of microdissection of kidney of Case 1 (Dr. E. M. Darmady and Miss Fay Stranack). 'Microdissection of the nephrons showed that the glomerulus, proximal tubules, and loops of Henle were anatomically normal. In some of the distal tubules there is an early precipitation of structureless material which extends to the collecting tubules. In other places, however, the collecting tubules were affected' (Plate 17, Fig. 8). 'Massive precipitation of the structureless protein-like material was most marked in the collecting ducts. Many of the collecting tubules had a patent lumen and flattened epithelium, and they were often distended. In some areas the epithelium in the collecting tubule was completely denuded, although regeneration was not seen. The striking finding was the localization of the lesion to the collecting tubules, which were often surrounded by considerable interstitial reaction and early fibrosis. Histological preparations showed that the normal epithelium of the collecting ducts had been replaced by flattened epithelium. In some areas recanalization of the tubule had been taking place, and had often occurred over the surface of one side of the cast and the denuded tubule wall' (Plate 17, Fig. 9).

The striking abnormality found was therefore the atrophic lesion of the distal and collecting tubules. This part of the nephron is believed to be the site of active reabsorption of water, and it is the failure of this process which is the functional disturbance specific to our syndrome. It appears possible that in obstructive hydronephrosis the raised intrapelvic pressure could cause dilatation and atrophy of the terminal part of the nephron, and so provide an anatomical basis for the water-losing syndrome in Case 2. In support of this hypothesis is the phenomenon of 'pyelotubular backflow', which is sometimes seen in retrograde pyelograms. This phenomenon occurs if the pressure of injection is high enough, and consists in the passage of radio-opaque material into the tubules from the renal pelvis. In addition, neoprene casts of the tubules have been produced by ureteric injection in the cadaver (Ross, 1952). It is therefore possible that similar anatomical changes are responsible for the water-losing syndrome in both cases. We are unable to say why this syndrome does not occur more often in hydronephrosis.

Acknowledgements

We wish to express our gratitude to Dr. R. W. Luxton and to Professor E. J. Wayne for their permission to study these two patients. It is a pleasure to thank Professor Robert Platt for his advice, and for obtaining for us the invaluable assistance of Dr. E. M. Darmady, to whom we are greatly indebted. We also thank Dr. J. Davson for the pathological studies, Dr. M. D. Milne for helpful discussion, Dr. S. W. Stanbury for the biochemical estimations recorded in Table II, and Dr. D. R. Wood for the assay of serum antidiuretic substance. Other biochemical investigations were performed by Mr. H. V. Street and Mr. E. Salvin, and the graphs and illustrations were prepared by Miss J. Perry.

Summary

1. We have described two patients showing a diabetes-insipidus-like syndrome as the initial manifestation of renal disease. Insensitivity of the distal tubules of the kidney to the action of antidiuretic hormone was demonstrated to be the cause of failure of renal conservation of water. The name 'water-losing nephritis' is suggested for this syndrome.

2. In one patient the renal tubular lesion was due to myelomatosis, and post-mortem examination of the kidney revealed an abnormality of the distal tubule. The other patient was found to have hydronephrosis caused by an enlarged prostate gland.

3. The water-losing syndrome has been differentiated from ordinary diabetes insipidus, from pitressin-resistant hereditary diabetes insipidus, and from classical renal failure. In classical renal failure the maximum urinary specific gravity falls, as the renal disease progresses, until the isosthenuric stage is reached; the obligatory hyposthenuria found in water-losing nephritis never develops.

4. It appears from a review of the literature that most acquired renal tubular disorders do not give rise to the water-losing syndrome. Rarely, however, hyperparathyroidism may do so.

REFERENCES

Adams, F. D. (1951) *New Engl. J. Med.* **244**, 590.

Albright, F., and Reifenstein, E. C., Jnr. (1948) *The Parathyroid Glands and Metabolic Bone Disease*, London.

Allan, F. N. (1931) *Proc. Staff M. Mayo Clin.* **6**, 684.

Anders, J. M., and Boston, L. N. (1903) *Lancet*, **1**, 93.

Anderson, W. A. D. (1939) *Arch. Path.* **27**, 753.

Aronsohn, H. G. (1931) *Virchows Arch.* **281**, 78.

Bach, M. J., and Middleton, W. S. (1931) *J. Amer. Med. Ass.* **97**, 306.

Bell, E. T. (1933) *Amer. J. Path.* **9**, 393.

Birnie, J. H., Jenkins, R., Eversole, W. J., and Gaunt, R. (1949) *Proc. Soc. Exp. Biol. Med.* **70**, 83.

Blackman, S. S., Jnr., Barker, W. H., Buell, M. V., and Davis, B. D. (1944) *J. Clin. Invest.* **23**, 163.

Breitenbucher, R. B., and Hertzog, A. J. (1949) *Minnesota Med.* **32**, 986.

Brown, G. E., Eusterman, G. B., Hartman, H. R., and Rowntree, L. G. (1923) *Arch. Int. Med.* **32**, 425.

Bull, G. M., Joekes, A. M., and Lowe, K. G. (1950) *Clin. Sci.* **9**, 379.

Burnett, C. H., Shapiro, S. L., Simeone, F. A., Beecher, H. K., Mallory, T. B., and Sullivan, E. R. (1947) *Surgery*, **22**, 994.

Carter, A. C., and Robbins, J. (1947) *J. Clin. Endocrin.* **7**, 753.

Cates, J. E., and Garrod, O. (1951) *Clin. Sci.* **10**, 145.

Chaplin, H., Clark, L. D., and Ropes, M. W. (1951) *Amer. J. Med. Sci.* **221**, 369.

Cooke, A. M. (1932) *Quart. J. Med.* N.S. **1**, 527.

—— (1933) Ibid. **2**, 539.

Cope, C. L. (1936) *Clin. Sci.* **2**, 287.

Dancis, J., Birmingham, J. R., and Leslie, S. H. (1948) *Amer. J. Dis. Child.* **75**, 316.

Denker, P. G., and Brock, S. (1934) *Brain*, **57**, 291.

Doxiadis, S. A. (1952) *Arch. Dis. Childh.* **27**, 409.

Dyggve, H., and Samsøe-Jensen, T. (1947) *Acta paediat.* **34**, 174.

Ellsworth, R., and Nicholson, W. M. (1935) *J. Clin. Invest.* **14**, 823.

Forssman, H. (1945) *Acta med. scand.* Suppl. **159**.

Fulton, R. M., and Paget, G. E. (1951) *Lancet*, **1**, 886.

Heller, H. (1952) *Ciba Foundation Colloquia on Endocrinology*, Vol. 4, London, p. 476.

Holman, R. L. (1939) *Arch. Path.* **27**, 748.

Jackson, W. P. U., and Linder, G. C. (1953) *Quart. J. Med.* N.S. **22**, 133.

Jacobs, E., and Verbanck, M. (1953) *Acta med. scand.* **145**, 143.

Kelsey, W. M., Reinhart, J. B., and Fishel, J. (1950) *Pediatrics*, **5**, 689.
Klein, R., and Gow, R. C. (1953) *J. Clin. Endocrin.* **13**, 271.
Klinefelter, H. F., Jnr., and Salley, S. M. (1946) *Bull. Johns Hopkins Hosp.* **79**, **333.**
Laake, H. (1949) *Acta. med. scand.* **132**, 440.
Lightwood, R. (1952) *Arch. Dis. Childh.* **27**, 302.
Limarzi, L. R. (1951) *Med. Clin. N. America*, **35**, 189.
Longcope, W. T., and Freiman, D. G. (1952) *Medicine*, **31**, 1.
Lundbaek, K. (1951) *Lancet*, **2**, 419.
Morison, J. E. (1941) *J. Path. Bact.* **53**, 403.
Moulonguet, P., and Lièvre, J.-A. (1938) *Bull. mém. Soc. méd. hôp. Paris*, **54**, 764.
Oliver, J. (1945) *Harvey Lectures*, **40**, 102.
—— MacDowell, M., and Tracy, A. (1951) *J. Clin. Invest.* **30**, 1307.
Perla, D., and Hutner, L. (1930) *Amer. J. Path.* **6**, 285.
Platt, R. (1950) *Clin. Sci.* **9**, 367.
—— (1951) *Lancet*, **1**, 1239.
—— (1952) *Brit. Med. J.* **1**, 1313.
Price, J. W., Miller, M., and Hayman, J. M., Jnr. (1940) *J. Clin. Invest.* **19**, 537.
Rapoport, S., Brodsky, W. A., West, C. D., and Mackler, B. (1949) *Amer. J. Physiol.* **156**, 433.
Ross, J. A. (1952) *Brit. J. Urol.* **24**, 27.
Sanderson, P. H. (1948) *Clin. Sci.* **6**, 207.
Snapper, I. (1949) *Medical Clinics on Bone Diseases*, New York.
—— (1952) *Rare Manifestations of Metabolic Bone Disease*, Springfield, Ill.
Thorn, G. W, Koepf, G. F., and Clinton, M., Jnr. (1944) *New Engl. J. Med.* **231**, 76.
Törnblom, N. (1949) *Acta endocrin.* **2**, 178.
Waring, A. J., Kajdi, L., and Tappan, V. (1945) *Amer. J. Dis. Child.* **69**, 323.
Warkany, J., and Mitchell, A. G. (1939) Ibid. **57**, 603.
Williams, R. H., and Henry, C. (1947) *Ann. Int. Med.* **27**, 84.

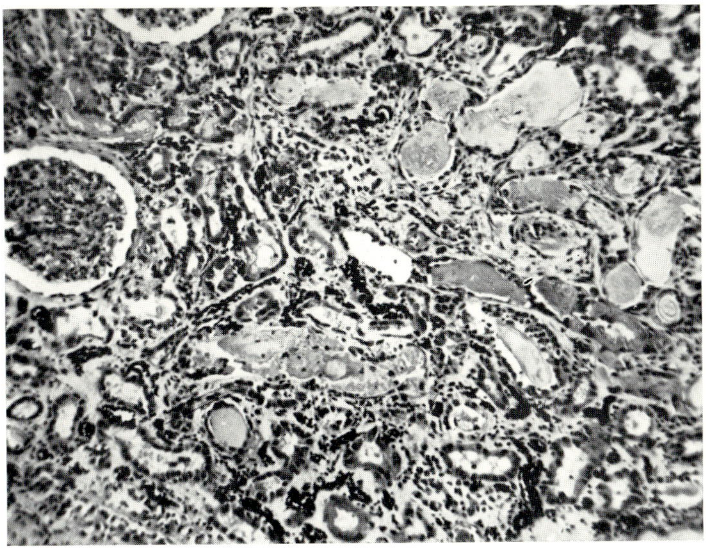

FIG. 6. Kidney of Case 1. Cortex, showing a normal glomerulus with a group of dilated tubules containing pale-staining casts. Adjacent tubules show flattening of epithelium but no casts. Intertubular fibrosis is present

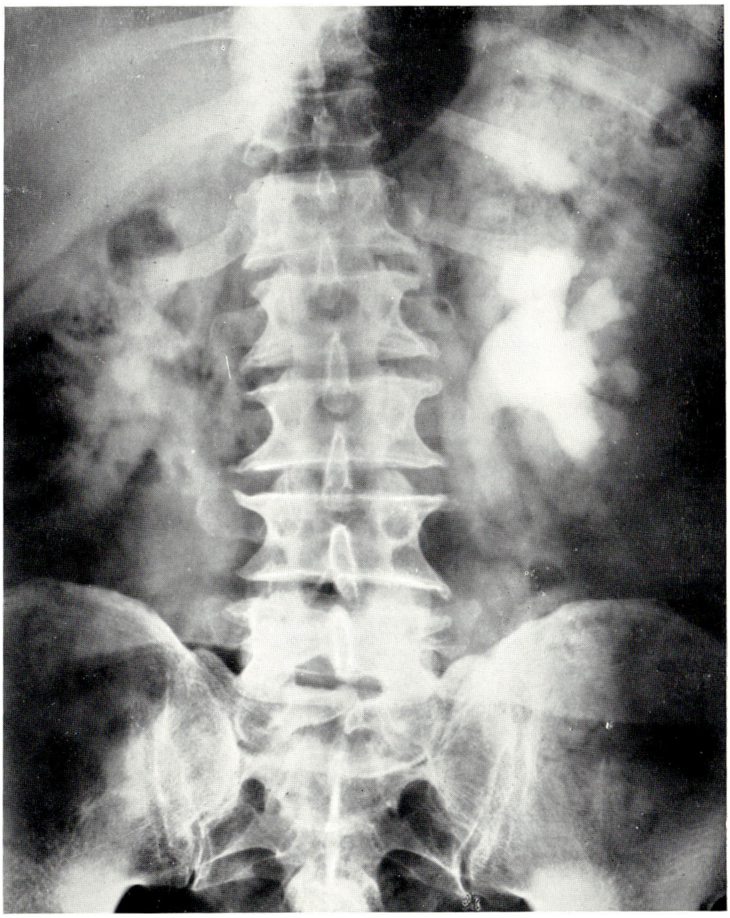

FIG. 7. Case 2. Intravenous pyelogram showing hydronephrosis. The outline of the right kidney showed more clearly in other films

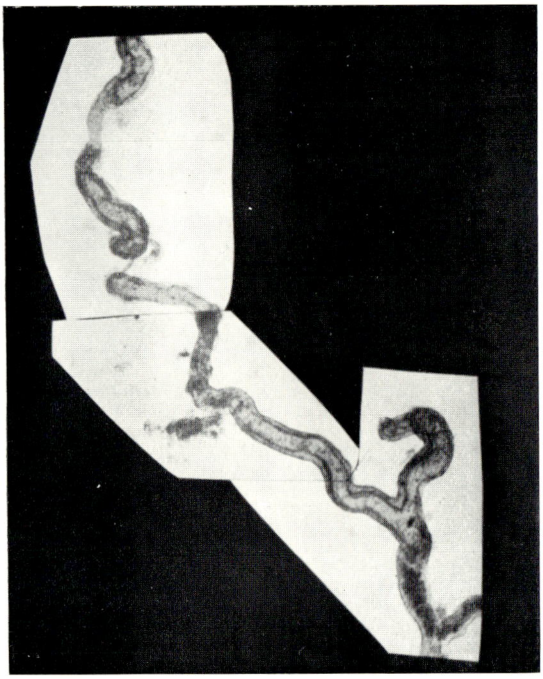

FIG. 8. Case 1. Microdissection of a portion of a collecting tubule (×50). Note the casts and epithelial atrophy

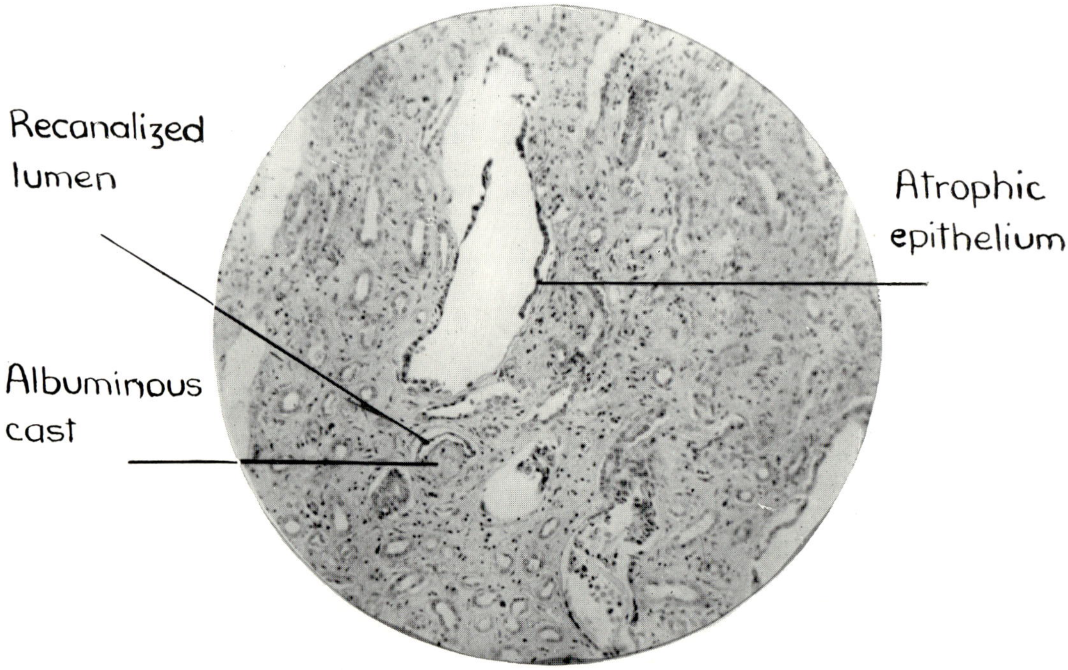

FIG. 9. Case 1. Section of pyramidal area of the kidney, showing flattening of the epithelium of the collecting tubules, with recanalization of a tubule to one side of an albuminous cast

616.34–008.337:616.71

OSTEOMALACIA IN STEATORRHOEA[1]

By JOHN BADENOCH and PAUL FOURMAN

(From the Nuffield Department of Clinical Medicine, The Radcliffe Infirmary, Oxford)

Deficiency of calcium in adults leads to osteomalacia. In osteomalacia the bones are decalcified, spontaneous fractures may occur, and narrow bands of decalcified bone or 'pseudo-fractures' appear where an artery is in contact with bone (Le May and Blunt, 1949). Chemical analysis of the serum reveals characteristic changes: the level of calcium is normal or low, the phosphate level is usually found to be low if the blood is taken from the fasting patient, and the phosphatase is increased (Albright and Reifenstein, 1948). In this country osteomalacia is most often a complication of steatorrhoea, and the deficiency of calcium is the result of a failure to absorb it. Many workers have studied the absorption of calcium in the sprue syndrome. In 1919 Findlay and Sharpe found that calcium was poorly absorbed by patients with steatorrhoea, and a year later Barach and Murray confirmed this finding, and attributed the faecal loss of calcium to the high content of fat in the stools. But Linder and Harris (1929) thought that the failure to absorb calcium was the result of a diminished absorption of the fat-soluble vitamin D, because vitamin D improved the osteomalacia in their patients. Marble and Bauer (1931) believed that the poor absorption of calcium could not be due to a deficiency of vitamin D, because improvement could be brought about by treatment with liver alone. The experiments of Bassett, Keutmann, Hyde, Van Alstine, and Russ (1939) and Bassett, Keutmann, Hyde, and Van Alstine (1939) supported the hypothesis put forward by Linder and Harris. They showed that a moderately high intake of calcium and phosphorus did not produce consistently positive balances of these elements in osteomalacia. When large doses of vitamin D were added the absorption of calcium and phosphorus from the gut increased, and the excretion of phosphorus in the urine increased. Fourman and Spray (1948) found that a moderate dose of vitamin D was not effective when given by mouth, but the same dose was effective when given parenterally. Thus the absorption of vitamin D is impaired in the osteomalacia of steatorrhoea, and the resulting deficiency of vitamin D is at least partly responsible for the failure to absorb calcium. It is not clear whether there is also a primary failure to absorb calcium in these patients (Bodansky and Bodansky, 1952).

The present report concerns six patients with osteomalacia and steatorrhoea. In three of them osteomalacia developed while they were receiving 1,500 units of vitamin D daily by mouth, calcium lactate 2 gm. daily, and folic acid 20 mg.

[1] Received August 1, 1953.

daily. We have investigated the fault in calcium absorption in two ways: by measuring the absorption of calcium with different doses of calcium and vitamin D, and by following the effect of treatment for osteomalacia in these patients. The clinical histories are summarized in the Appendix.

Experimental Procedure

Calcium balances were measured in periods of four or six days, and the experiment lasted for 12 or 16 days for each treatment tested. The patients' diets were prepared in the hospital diet kitchen, and were as far as possible constant during each experiment. Water for cooking and drinking was distilled, and the diets contained relatively little calcium. A day's diet was analysed for calcium in the course of each experiment. In addition the patients received black-currant juice (Ribena) containing 0·41 mg. of calcium per ml. and, to ensure regular bowel action, one or two drachms daily of vegetable mucilage (Normacol) containing 10·8 mg. of calcium per gm. In one experiment agar was given containing 5·5 mg. of calcium per gm. The fruit juice and the laxative were accurately measured. Added calcium was given in the form of lactate, in doses of 2, 4, or 25 gm. daily, which was accurately weighed. Thus errors in the intake of calcium arose only from minor variations in the diet, which contained little calcium. Urine and faeces were collected, and faecal collections were separated with carmine markers (0·4 gm.). The method used for determining calcium was that of Shohl and Pedly for urine and that of McCrudden for diets and faeces (Hawk, Oser, and Summerson, 1947). In the determination of urinary calcium we introduced a simplification which made it unnecessary to oxidize the uric acid. The urine was acidified with 2 per cent. of hydrochloric acid, and left in the refrigerator for a week or more until the uric acid had settled out. The supernatant fluid was taken for the determination of calcium.

Results of the Balance Studies

The results of six balance studies (experiments 1 to 6) of two patients are shown in Tables I and III. The experiments to be described first were carried out while the patients took 70 to 80 gm. of fat in the diet daily.

Patient I, experiment 1 (Table I). Without vitamin D the calcium balance was negative. The calcium intake during this experiment was 0·8 gm. daily and included 4 gm. daily of calcium lactate. The faecal loss of calcium exceeded the dietary intake, and largely accounted for the negative balance of 2·3 gm. of calcium incurred during 12 days. The urinary loss was about 20 mg. daily.

Patient I, experiment 2 (Table I). When vitamin D was added to the treatment in a dose of 10,000 units daily by mouth, the negative balance persisted. The urinary loss of calcium was 37 mg. daily. There was no rise in the levels of serum-calcium or serum-phosphate.

Patient I, experiment 3 (Table I). Vitamin D was then given intramuscularly in the same dose, 10,000 units daily. The negative balance of calcium still persisted. The average urinary loss of calcium was 48 mg. daily; this was not significantly different from the previous values. The data for the serum values were incomplete.

Patient I, experiment 4 (Table I). Two months later the intake of calcium was increased to 3·5 gm. daily, while the vitamin D was again given intramuscularly in a dose of 10,000 units daily. The negative balance of calcium was

TABLE I

The Effect of Calcium and Vitamin D on the Calcium Balance in Steatorrhoea

Experiments lasted twelve days. The values are for the total duration of each experiment.

	Experiment	*Fat intake (gm./day)*	*Vitamin D (units/day)*	*Total calcium intake (gm.)*	*Faecal calcium (gm.)*	*Urinary calcium (gm.)*	*Balance (gm.)*
Patient I	1 17–28 July 1951	80	None	10·0	12·1	0·2	−2·3
	2 29 July–9 Aug. 1951	80	10,000 by mouth	9·1	10·9	0·4	−2·2
	3 10–21 Aug. 1951	80	10,000 intramuscular	8·6	10·6	0·6	−2·6
	4 9–21 Nov. 1951	73	10,000 intramuscular	42·4	39·4	0·7	+2·3

TABLE II

Patient I. Effect of Varying Calcium Intake: the Amount of Calcium in the Diet Compared with the Amount of Calcium which could Combine with the Faecal Fat as Soap in the Four Balance Experiments

Experiment	*Faecal fat (gm.)*	*Equivalent amount of calcium (gm.)*	*Calcium intake (gm.)*	*Balance (see Table I)*
1	288	21·3	10·0	Negative
2	200	14·8	9·1	Negative
3	239	17·7	8·6	Negative
4	324	24·0	42·4	Positive

abolished; in fact a positive balance of 2·3 gm. in 12 days occurred. A positive balance of this magnitude is not significant against an intake of 42·4 gm. in the same period; but it may be noted that in this experiment the faecal loss of calcium was less than the dietary intake, although the weight of the faeces and their content of fat and nitrogen were greater than in the previous experiments, in which the faecal calcium exceeded the dietary calcium. The apparent improvement in calcium absorption in this experiment is therefore not likely to have been an effect of error in separating the faecal collections. The urinary excretion of calcium rose to 59 mg. daily. The serum-calcium level remained low, but the serum-phosphate increased. There was a clinical improvement (see page 169).

It seems that in this patient a negative calcium balance was reversed when a high calcium intake was added to the treatment with parenteral vitamin D. In an earlier experiment with another patient (Fourman and Spray, 1948) a high

TABLE III

Effect of Change in Fat Intake on the Calcium Balance in Steatorrhoea

Experiment 5 lasted 16 days, and experiment 6 12 days. The values are for the total duration of each experiment.

	Experiment	*Fat intake (gm./day)*	*Vitamin D (units/day)*	*Total calcium intake (gm.)*	*Faecal calcium (gm.)*	*Urinary calcium (gm.)*	*Balance (gm.)*
Patient II	5 14–30 April 1950	40	50,000 by mouth	5·9	4·8	0·1	+1·0
Patient II	6 13–25 Feb. 1952	80	50,000 by mouth	5·2	7·4	0·5	−2·7

calcium intake itself was not effective, but calcium was absorbed when vitamin D was given parenterally. Theoretically calcium may combine with fatty acid in the proportion of 74 mg. of calcium to 1 gm. of fatty acid. Table II shows the output of fat in the faeces in each of these four experiments with Patient I, and the amount of calcium that would combine with this fat if it were entirely in the form of calcium soaps. In the experiments in which there was a loss of calcium from the body, the intake of calcium was less than the amount which might combine as calcium soap; in the experiment in which there was a gain of calcium, the intake of calcium was greater than the amount which might combine as soap. The fact that calcium and fat are present together in the intestine does not mean that they are combined as soap. Nevertheless it seemed possible that the relation between calcium intake and faecal fat might be more important than the absolute amount of calcium in the diet, and we sought to obtain further evidence on this point in Patient II.

Patient II, experiment 5 (Table III). In this experiment, which lasted 16 days, the intake of fat was only 40 gm. daily, and the output of fat in the faeces was lower than in the experiments on Patient I. With vitamin D, 50,000 units daily by mouth, and a calcium intake of 0·37 gm. daily (total 5·9 gm. in 16 days), there was a positive balance of 1 gm. of calcium. The urinary output of calcium was less than 10 mg. daily. The serum-calcium level rose from 5 mg. to 9·1 mg. per 100 ml., and a positive Chvostek's sign disappeared. This experiment showed that calcium could be absorbed when vitamin D was given by mouth if the dose of vitamin D was large.

Patient II, experiment 6 (Table III). Another balance experiment was carried out two years later on the same patient with a fat intake of 80 gm. daily, so that the amount of fat in the faeces was increased. The patient was again receiving 50,000 units of vitamin D daily by mouth, and 0·43 gm. daily of calcium. There was now a negative calcium balance of 2·7 gm. in 12 days. The faecal calcium exceeded the dietary intake. The urinary excretion of calcium was 39 mg. daily. There are no balance data for the succeeding period, when the

TABLE IV

Patient II. Effect of Varying Fat Intake: the amount of Calcium in the Diet Compared with the Amount of Calcium which could Combine with the Faecal Fat as Soap in the Two Balance Experiments

Experiment	*Faecal fat (gm.)*	*Equivalent amount of calcium (gm.)*	*Calcium intake (gm.)*	*Balance (see Table I)*
5	73	5·4	5·9	Positive
6	146	10·8	5·2	Negative

intake of calcium was increased to 3·7 gm. daily, because the patient suffered from faecal impaction; but the urinary calcium now increased to 103 mg. daily, suggesting that with the higher dose of calcium more calcium may have been absorbed, in spite of the increased amount of fat in the faeces.

Table IV shows the output of fat in the faeces in these two experiments with Patient II, together with the theoretical amount of calcium that could combine as soap. When the amount of faecal fat was low, the equivalent amount of calcium was smaller than the intake of calcium; when the amount of faecal fat was high, the equivalent amount of calcium was greater than the intake of calcium. In the first instance the balance of calcium was positive, and in the second it was negative. Thus in this patient the absorption of calcium depended in part on the amount of fat remaining in the bowel.

Clinical Effects of Different Treatments

Effective treatment with parenteral vitamin D and large doses of calcium, but not with small doses of calcium. Patient I, the subject of balance experiments 1 to 4, was a married woman of 51 years, who had suffered from coeliac disease in childhood; she developed severe pain in the back and shoulders at the age of 48. A fat balance showed that she was excreting 25 per cent. of the fat in her diet. The bones were decalcified. The serum-calcium was 8·2 mg. per 100 ml., serum-phosphate 3·4 mg. per 100 ml., and serum alkaline phosphatase 46 King-Armstrong units. In hospital she was given a high-protein diet, with vitamin D 10,000 i.u. daily by mouth and calcium lactate 4 gm. daily. She did not improve, and after two weeks the vitamin D was given parenterally in the same dose. The dose of calcium was not changed. When the vitamin was given parenterally she improved slightly, and the serum-calcium level rose to 9·2 mg. per 100 ml., but nine weeks later, when she was discharged from hospital, she was still complaining of pain in the back and limbs. At home the vitamin was given in a dose of 50,000 i.u. daily by mouth, and within four weeks she had suffered a relapse, with an increase in the pain in the back and limbs. The serum-calcium had fallen to 7·9 mg. per 100 ml. She was readmitted to hospital where, after another balance experiment, the vitamin was given in a dose of 40,000 i.u. weekly by intramuscular injection, with 25 gm. of calcium lactate daily. She improved rapidly, and three months later all her pain had gone and the serum-calcium had increased to 9·5 mg. per 100 ml. The serum alkaline phosphatase had fallen to 19 King-Armstrong units.

Effective treatment with a low-fat diet, vitamin D 50,000 i.u. daily by mouth, and calcium lactate in smaller doses. Patient II, an unmarried woman of 52 years (the subject of balance experiments 5 and 6), developed osteomalacia while under treatment for steatorrhoea, although her treatment had included vitamin D 1,500 i.u. daily by mouth and calcium lactate 2 gm. daily. She complained of pain in the back. Chvostek's and Trousseau's signs were positive. X-rays revealed decalcification of the bones. The serum-calcium was 5·0 mg. per 100 ml., the serum-phosphate 3·8 mg. per 100 ml., and the serum alkaline phosphatase 10 King-Armstrong units. She was given a diet containing about 40 gm. of fat daily, with vitamin D 50,000 i.u. daily by mouth, and the calcium lactate was continued in a dose of 2 gm. daily. Within six weeks the pain in the back had gone, there was no evidence of tetany, and the serum-calcium had increased to 9·1 mg. per 100 ml. She has remained well on this régime, but two years later it proved possible to induce a negative calcium balance by increasing the amount of fat in her diet; this fact suggested that the small dose of calcium was effective because there was little fat in her diet.

Calcium lactate 25 gm. daily ineffective without vitamin D in available form. Patient III, a nun aged 65 years, was previously reported by Fourman and Spray (1948). She had severe osteomalacia, with spontaneous fractures. She received calcium lactate 25 gm. daily, with vitamin D 12,000 i.u. daily by mouth, but her symptoms persisted, and a strongly positive calcium balance was not achieved until the same dose of the vitamin was given parenterally. A month after that all her pain had gone, and she could walk unaided. In spite of the clinical improvement, however, chemical evidence of osteomalacia could still be found one year later, and the bones were still decalcified 18 months after treatment had been started.

Vitamin D in available form ineffective without large doses of calcium. Patient IV, a nun aged 75 years who had tropical sprue, developed osteomalacia of such severity that every movement caused pain. The bones were grossly decalcified. The serum-calcium was 9·4 mg. per 100 ml., serum-phosphate 2·4 mg. per 100 ml., and serum alkaline phosphatase 60 King-Armstrong units. She was given a high-protein, low-fat diet, with folic acid 10 mg. daily, vitamin D 10,000 i.u. daily by intramuscular injection, and calcium lactate 2 gm. daily. Her general condition improved, but the pain in the bones persisted. Three months later the serum-calcium was 6·4 mg. per 100 ml., lower than before treatment was started. The dose of calcium lactate was increased to 30 gm. daily, and the dose of vitamin D was not changed; she rapidly became free from pain. After five months the serum-calcium had increased to 9·2 mg. per 100 ml., and the serum-phosphate to 4·7 mg. per 100 ml., while the serum alkaline phosphatase had fallen to 12 King-Armstrong units, but there was still no change in the radiological appearance of the bones.

Effective treatment with vitamin D, 10,000 i.u. daily by intramuscular injection, together with calcium lactate in large doses. Patient V, a married woman of 44 years, developed severe osteomalacia while under treatment for steatorrhoea, although her treatment had included vitamin D 1,500 units by mouth with calcium lactate 2 gm. daily. On her admission the serum-calcium was 7·4 mg. per 100 ml., serum-phosphate 4·7 mg. per 100 ml., and serum alkaline phosphatase 10 King-Armstrong units. X-rays of the bones showed advanced generalized decalcification. Treatment with intramuscular vitamin D 10,000 i.u. daily and calcium lactate 15 gm. daily produced rapid improvement, and six months later she was not only free from pain but could walk for half a mile without fatigue. But one year after treatment was started the serum-calcium level had risen only to 8·7 mg. per 100 ml.

Effective treatment with vitamin D 10,000 i.u. daily by mouth together with calcium lactate in large doses. Patient VI, a girl of 17 years who had steatorrhoea and a resistant anaemia, developed pain in the back and limbs, and walking was painful. X-rays of the bones revealed gross decalcification, with a pseudo-fracture of the neck of the left femur. The serum-calcium was 6·6 mg. per 100 ml., serum-phosphate 3·4 mg. per 100 ml., and serum alkaline phosphatase 58 King-Armstrong units. Treatment with vitamin D 10,000 i.u. daily by mouth, with calcium lactate 20 gm. daily, produced a steady improvement in her symptoms. She remained well, and two years later the serum-calcium was 10·6 mg. per 100 ml., serum-phosphate 5.7 mg. per 100 ml., and serum alkaline phosphatase 9 King-Armstrong units. The radiological appearance of the bones had become normal.

Discussion

The above results confirm the view that in patients with osteomalacia secondary to steatorrhoea there is a failure to absorb vitamin D. The results also suggest that there may be a failure to absorb calcium because it combines with unabsorbed fat in the small intestine to form soaps. These two faults may be overcome by giving vitamin D parenterally, or in large doses by mouth, and by giving large doses of calcium. All the patients so treated became cured of their osteomalacia; nevertheless the amount of calcium retained by them was never large and, though their pain usually remitted quickly, the cure of the osteomalacia was slow. When vitamin D is given to patients with primary osteomalacia incurred through dietary deficiency, the retention of calcium is greater than in our patients (Liu, Hannon, Chu, Chen, Chou, and Wang, 1935); it is reasonable to infer that in steatorrhoea the absorption of calcium is defective even with optimum amounts of calcium and vitamin D. According to Frazer (1949) steatorrhoea is associated with an excessive production of intestinal mucus. Some calcium may combine with the mucus and thus become unavailable, but the amount bound in this way cannot be large, and it is possible that calcium is in some way more directly involved in the absorption defect of steatorrhoea.

These results have important therapeutic implications. Three of our patients developed osteomalacia while they were receiving 1,500 units of vitamin D and 2 gm. of calcium lactate daily; much larger doses are needed in the treatment of this condition. If the vitamin D is given parenterally, the equivalent of 10,000 units daily is certainly effective, and less may suffice; the discomfort of injections can be reduced by giving an appropriate dose at weekly or monthly intervals. Froehlich (1952) has given as much as 15 mg. (600,000 units) of calciferol in one injection. If the vitamin D is given orally it is not possible to know how much is absorbed. One of our patients responded to 10,000 units daily by mouth, but in others this dose has had little effect. A daily dose of 50,000 units may safely be given if the patient lacks calcium. There is no risk of overdosage so long as the urinary output of calcium continues to be low, and a rough estimate of the urinary calcium is easily obtained by the Sulkowitch test.

Acknowledgements

We are indebted to our colleagues of the Biochemistry Department of the United Oxford Hospitals for the serum values included in this paper, and to Miss Beryl Brinkhurst, Miss Barbara Hunt, and Miss Barbara Siebert for technical assistance. We are grateful to Professor L. J. Witts for his help and criticism, and to the Medical Research Council and the Haematology Research Fund for grants which made it possible to carry out this study.

APPENDIX

Patient I. Radcliffe Infirmary No.143814. Mary D., a married woman, born 1901. She had suffered from attacks of diarrhoea since childhood. At the age of 27 years, after the birth of her first child, she suffered from soreness of the mouth, flatulence, and indigestion. In 1949, when aged 48, she had a recurrence of ulcers in the mouth. In October 1949 she developed low back pain, which grew steadily worse. In January 1951 she had pain in the upper back and shoulders, and began to lose weight. In June 1951 she was admitted to the Radcliffe Infirmary. Her tongue appeared raw, her fingers clubbed, and her abdomen normal. Movement caused pain over the lower chest. The haemoglobin was 82 per cent., and the mean cell-diameter $8{\cdot}2\,\mu$; the blood film showed mixed liver and iron deficiency. The serum-calcium was 8·2 mg. per 100 ml., serum-phosphate 3·2 mg. per 100 ml., and serum alkaline phosphatase 46 King-Armstrong units. X-rays of the bones showed generalized decalcification. A histamine test meal gave a normal acid curve. The oral glucose-tolerance curve was flat. Fat balance (12 days): 75 per cent. of dietary fat absorbed. Treatment with vitamin D in large doses by mouth, and later parenterally, proved ineffective until she was given calcium lactate 25 gm. daily, when rapid improvement occurred.

Patient II. Radcliffe Infirmary No. 7143. Lilian C., an unmarried woman, born 1900. She was diagnosed as a case of pernicious anaemia in 1934. She did not respond to treatment, and became very anaemic. In 1939 she was admitted to the Radcliffe Infirmary complaining of lassitude, breathlessness, poor appetite, and diarrhoea. She was pale and oedematous. The skin was dry and pigmented, the tongue smooth, and the abdomen distended. There was a moderate macrocytic anaemia: haemoglobin 8·3 gm. per 100 ml., red cells 2,280,000 per c.mm., colour index 1·2, and white cells 3,000 per c.mm. The bone-marrow was partially megaloblastic. X-rays showed calcified mesenteric glands. Fat-content of faeces: 52 per cent. of dry weight. The serum-calcium was 8·4 mg. per 100 ml., serum-phosphate 5·4 mg. per 100 ml. (not fasting), and serum alkaline phosphatase 5 King-Armstrong units. The anaemia failed to respond to parenteral liver extract, and between 1940 and 1943 she was admitted 14 times for blood transfusions. In September 1942 yeast, 1 oz. by mouth daily, was added to the treatment, and the need for blood transfusion became less. She was given a high-protein, low-fat diet, with vitamin supplements including one capsule of vitamins A and D thrice daily. Since 1944 the anaemia has been controlled with proteolysed liver, folic acid, and iron by mouth. The steatorrhoea was confirmed in 1950, when a 12-day fat balance showed that only 83 per cent. of the fat in the diet was being absorbed. From the beginning of 1942 she complained of pain in the legs and back, which became more severe when she required a blood transfusion. Little notice was taken of the symptom at the time, but the pain persisted, and in 1950 Chvostek's and Trousseau's signs were found to be positive. The serum-calcium was 5 mg. per 100 ml., serum-phosphate 3·8 mg. per 100 ml., and serum alkaline phosphatase 10 King-Armstrong units. X-rays showed rarefaction of the bones. She was given vitamin D, 50,000 i.u. daily by mouth, with calcium lactate 2 gm. daily, in addition to the haematinics, and within six weeks the pain in the legs had gone and the serum-calcium had increased to 9·1 mg. per 100 ml. She has since remained well.

Patient III. Radcliffe Infirmary No. 29353/44. Sister L. M., an unmarried woman; born 1886, died 1951. In 1938, when 52 years of age, she had a right hemicolectomy, with resection of the terminal four inches of the ileum, for suspected carcinoma of the colon. During convalescence she developed diarrhoea, and when she was admitted six years later, in 1944, for investigation of anaemia, she was found to be suffering from steatorrhoea. Fat balance (12 days): 73 per cent. of dietary fat absorbed. The anaemia was severe: haemoglobin 5·5 gm. per 100 ml., red cells 2,060,000 per c.mm., and colour index 0·95. The marrow was megaloblastic. Treatment was begun with a high-protein, low-fat diet, vitamin D 1,500 units daily by mouth, and weekly injections of liver. Two years later she developed severe pain in the lower back, with twitching of the muscles of the abdomen and legs, and had to pull herself up with the aid of the bedclothes. On examination she was thin and wasted. The ribs were tender, and the abdomen distended. Chvostek's sign was positive. X-rays of the bones revealed advanced decalcification, with multiple pathological fractures of the ribs. The serum-calcium was 8·8 mg. per 100 ml., serum-phosphate 2·9 mg. per 100 ml., and serum alkaline phosphatase 58 King-Armstrong units. Treatment with calcium lactate 25 gm. with vitamin D 12,000 i.u. daily by mouth proved ineffective, but improvement occurred when the same dose of the vitamin was given parenterally.

Patient IV. Radcliffe Infirmary No. 3792/43. Sister F., an unmarried woman, born 1875. She was in India from 1916 to 1919 and from 1923 to 1930. Ten years after her return to this country, in 1940, she developed a bulky diarrhoea. Three years later she was admitted to hospital, where a diagnosis of tropical sprue was made. She was treated with a low-fat diet and liver by injection, and improved. She remained well for two years, and then relapsed. The diarrhoea returned, she lost weight, and at the end of 1947 she began to complain of aching pains in the bones, especially at night. She was admitted to the

Radcliffe Infirmary in February 1948. She was pale, with a dry, pigmented skin. The tongue was smooth, and the abdomen distended. There was koilonychia. Movement caused pain in the arms, legs, and lower back, and there was tenderness on pressure over the bones of the forearms and lower ribs. The haemoglobin was 9·7 gm. per 100 ml., red cells 3,689,000 per c.mm., and colour index 1·0. The sternal marrow was cellular and predominantly normoblastic, but the cells of the myeloid series showed changes typical of liver-factor deficiency. X-rays of the bones showed generalized decalcification. The serum-calcium was 9·4 mg. per 100 ml., serum-phosphate 2·4 mg. per 100 ml., and serum alkaline phosphatase 60 King-Armstrong units. Fat balance (12 days): 80 per cent. of dietary fat absorbed. Treatment with vitamin D 10,000 i.u. daily by intramuscular injection, with calcium lactate 2 gm. daily, produced little improvement, but she responded rapidly when the dose of calcium lactate was increased to 30 gm. daily.

Patient V. Radcliffe Infirmary No. 70551/47. Mary D., a married woman, born 1908. In 1939, at the age of 31 years, she began to suffer from flatulence and diarrhoea. She lost weight, and her mouth became sore. In 1945 she developed pain in the back and legs, with breathlessness and increasing lassitude. In 1946 she was investigated in another hospital, and found to have steatorrhoea and hypochromic anaemia. The serum-calcium was normal. She was treated with a low-fat diet, liver, iron, and capsules of vitamins A and D, one thrice daily, with calcium lactate 2 gm. daily. The diarrhoea improved, but the pain in the back grew worse In April 1947 she was admitted to the Radcliffe Infirmary. On examination she was pale and slightly pigmented. There was tenderness over the back, no tetany, and slight oedema of the ankles. The abdomen was normal. The haemoglobin was 9·2 gm. per 100 ml., and red cells 4,300,000 per c.mm. The serum-calcium was 7·4 mg. per 100 ml., and serum alkaline phosphatase 10 King-Armstrong units. X-rays of the bones showed advanced generalized decalcification. A histamine test meal showed achlorhydria. Fat balance (12 days): 77 per cent. of dietary fat absorbed. The oral glucose-tolerance curve was flat. She was discharged taking a high-protein, low-fat diet with calcium lactate 15 gm. daily, vitamin D 15,000 i.u. intramuscularly each day, folic acid 20 mg. daily, and ferrous sulphate 0·2 gm. thrice daily. This treatment produced a rapid improvement in her general condition. At the time of her admission to hospital she was so crippled that she could walk only with the aid of two sticks, but within six months she could walk half a mile with ease. She has continued to take 15 gm. of calcium lactate daily, with 40,000 i.u. of vitamin D intramuscularly every two weeks, and has remained quite free from symptoms; but one year after treatment was started the serum-calcium had increased only to 8·7 mg. per 100 ml.

Patient VI. Radcliffe Infirmary No. 78650/47. Gaynor M., a girl born in 1930. In 1947 she developed a progressive and severe anaemia, with breathlessness, drowsiness, dyspepsia, and ulceration of the tongue and lips. On admission she was underdeveloped, and was febrile. The fingers were clubbed, and the ankles oedematous. The haemoglobin was 2·55 gm. per 100 ml., red cells 770,000 per c.mm., and white cells 2,000 per c.mm. The marrow was very acellular. The serum-protein was 6·7 gm. per 100 ml.; albumin 4·2 per 100 ml. She was treated with ferrous sulphate 0·2 gm. thrice daily, liver extract 4 ml. intramuscularly twice weekly, and blood transfusions. She received 25 pints of blood between October 1947 and June 1948. In December 1948, although she felt better and had begun to grow, she complained of pain in the back and legs. She was admitted in February 1949, having survived without a blood transfusion for eight months. On review, an occasional megaloblast was seen in the marrow films made in 1947. A histamine test meal showed free acid to be present. Fat balance (12 days): 78 per cent. of dietary fat absorbed. X-rays of the bones revealed generalized decalcification, and a pathological fracture of the neck of the left femur. The serum-calcium was 6·6 mg. per 100 ml., serum-phosphate 3·4 mg. per 100 ml., and serum alkaline phosphatase 58 King-Armstrong units. She was treated with a high-protein, low-fat diet, vitamin D 10,000 i.u. and vitamin A 4,000 i.u. daily by mouth, calcium lactate 20 gm. daily, and folic acid 20 mg. daily, and improved steadily.

Summary

Six patients with steatorrhoea and osteomalacia were observed for periods of two to ten years. Three of these patients developed osteomalacia while receiving vitamin D, 1,500 i.u. daily by mouth, and calcium lactate 2 gm. daily. Six calcium balance experiments, lasting 12 to 16 days, were carried out on two of the patients. The output of fat in the faeces was also measured.

Vitamin D in a dose of 10,000 units daily by mouth did not improve the absorption of calcium. Vitamin D given in the same dose parenterally, or in a dose of 50,000 units by mouth, improved the absorption of calcium if the intake of calcium was high. It did not improve absorption if the intake of calcium was only moderate, unless the excretion of fat in the faeces was diminished at the same time by reducing the fat in the diet. With parenteral vitamin D and large doses of calcium by mouth (15 to 30 gm. of calcium lactate daily) these patients became cured of their osteomalacia; but the amount of calcium that they retained was small, and the cure was slow.

These facts are explained as follows. In patients with osteomalacia secondary to steatorrhoea there is a failure to absorb vitamin D. The resulting deficiency of vitamin D is partly responsible for a failure to absorb calcium. In addition there is a failure to absorb calcium because calcium may combine with unabsorbed fat in the intestine to form soaps. Lastly, when these two faults are overcome, it is seen that calcium is also directly involved in the absorption defect of steatorrhoea.

REFERENCES

Albright, F., and Reifenstein, E. C. (1948) *The Parathyroid Glands and Metabolic Bone Disease*, London.

Barach, A. L., and Murray, H. A., Jnr. (1920) *J. Amer. Med. Ass.* **74,** 786.

Bassett, S. H., Keutmann, E. H., Hyde, H. van Z., Van Alstine, H. E., and Russ, E. (1939) *J. Clin. Invest.* **18,** 101.

— — — and Van Alstine, H. E. (1939) Ibid. **18,** 121.

Bodansky, M., and Bodansky, O. (1952) *Biochemistry of Disease*, 2nd ed., New York.

Findlay, L., and Sharpe, J. S. (1919–20) *Quart. J. Med.* **13,** 433.

Fourman, L. P. R., and Spray, G. H. (1948) *Brit. Med J.* **1,** 142.

Frazer, A. C. (1949) Ibid. **2,** 769.

Froehlich, A. L. (1952) *Proceedings of Second International Congress of Internal Medicine*, London.

Hawk, P. B., Oser, B. L., and Summerson, W. H. (1947) *Practical Physiological Chemistry*, 12th ed., Philad., p. 897.

Le May, M., and Blunt, J. W. (1949) *J. Clin. Invest.* **28**, 521.
Linder, G. C., and Harris, C. F. (1929) *Quart. J. Med.* **23**, 195.
Liu, S. H., Hannon, R. R., Chu, H. I., Chen, K. C., Chou, S. K., and Wang, S. H. (1935) *Chin. Med. J.* **49**, 1.
Marble, A., and Bauer, W. (1931) *Arch. Int. Med.* **48**, 515.

616.72–002.771 : 615.752.2

SALICYLATES IN RHEUMATIC FEVER: AN ATTEMPT TO ASSESS THEIR VALUE[1]

By R. S. ILLINGWORTH, J. BURKE, S. A. DOXIADIS, J. LORBER, M. G. PHILPOTT, and D. G. H. STONE
(From the Department of Child Health, University of Sheffield, and the Children's Hospital Unit, United Sheffield Hospitals)

With statistical assistance by J. F. SCOTT
(Department of Mathematics, University of Sheffield)

With the introduction of cortisone and corticotrophin it seemed possible that salicylates would no longer be the treatment of choice in rheumatic fever. Early enthusiasm for the use of cortisone has now somewhat waned, and it seems likely that attention will once more be focused on salicylates. There is a wide difference of opinion about the value of salicylates in rheumatic fever, and early in 1948 we decided to attempt to determine their value by means of a controlled experiment. The investigation is a long-term one, and is continuing, but we now feel that we should present our preliminary findings. In an extensive survey of the literature concerning the subject we were unable to find any critical review which would satisfy modern scientific demands. We shall therefore attempt to review the most important and most frequently quoted of the relevant papers, selected from over 170 papers studied.

Review of the Literature

The use of salicylates in rheumatic fever was popularized by Maclagan (1876) and Stricker (1876). Maclagan tried salicin because nature seemed to him to produce remedies under climatic conditions similar to those which give rise to disease. He therefore looked for a remedy for rheumatism in plants whose habitat is low-lying damp places which favour the development of rheumatism. Since then a large number of papers have been written about salicylates. In 1926 Hanzlik wrote a review of the literature, and in 1948 Gross and Greenberg published their book on salicylates, with over 300 references concerning their use in rheumatic fever. These reviews were more descriptive than analytical. The use of large doses in the treatment of rheumatic fever is no recent innovation. Lees (1903) recommended that doses of 20 grains of sodium salicylate should be given two-hourly by day and four-hourly by night. Since then there have been numerous papers advocating large doses. Danielopolu, Dimitriu, and Cimino-Beranger (1934) used up to 25 gm. per day. Goodman and Gilman (1941), in their textbook of pharmacology and therapeutics, advocated high doses.

[1] Received August 10, 1953.

Coburn (1943*a*, *b*) described the results of treatment with massive doses, and revived interest in this form of therapy.

Among the papers in favour of salicylates are those by Finlay and Lucas (1879), Levy and Turner (1927–8), and Murray-Lyon (1936). Finlay and Lucas treated 60 of 120 cases of rheumatic fever with sodium salicylate, and 60 others with alkalies. In the salicylate group the duration of fever averaged 5·7 days, in the alkali group 10·3 days. The duration of joint swellings averaged 5·0 days in the salicylate group, compared with 12·2 in the alkali group. Yet 11·6 per cent. of the salicylate group and 6·6 per cent. of the other patients developed carditis or pericarditis during treatment. 26·6 per cent. of the salicylate group and 8·3 per cent. of the alkali group had relapses. Ten per cent. of the salicylate group had a return of pain when the drug was stopped, compared with 6·6 per cent. of the patients treated with alkalies. Much has been learnt in recent years about the application of the scientific method to the assessment of drugs, and it is only to be expected that the paper by Finlay and Lucas does not enable us to form any conclusion. The authors did not supply the necessary data for comparing the two groups, and they did not state the dose of the drugs used, or the method of selecting cases. The paper by Levy and Turner (1927–8) has been frequently quoted as evidence of the value of salicylates in rheumatic carditis. They described three cases in which the electrocardiograph showed a long PR interval (0·23 to 0·24 second). Salicylates (in doses not stated) were said to cause a reduction of the PR interval to 0·2 second or less. The interval increased when the drug was stopped, and decreased when it was restarted. It is impossible, however, to form conclusions on three cases, and Wyckoff, DeGraff, and Parent (1929-30) showed that similar fluctuations in the PR interval occurred in untreated cases. Murray-Lyon (1936) studied the records of 40 male and 60 female patients, aged seven to 56 years, who had been treated with large doses of salicylates, and assessed the average duration of fever and pain and the incidence of pericarditis. He then compared the average duration of fever in his cases with that in cases collected from the literature by Hood in 1881, and the incidence of pericarditis in the patients with that found in cases described by several writers between 1845 and 1847. Murray-Lyon found that the duration of pain and fever was shorter in his patients, but there was no difference in the incidence of pericarditis and other cardiac complications. He concluded that 'the salicylate is effective in shortening the acute stage of the disease'. This method of comparison is not satisfactory, for diseases change in type and severity, and the management of disease varies from place to place and from time to time. It is not possible, therefore, to draw any firm conclusions from his work.

Wyckoff, DeGraff, and Parent (1929–30) investigated the effect of sodium salicylate on the atrioventricular conduction time. By performing electrocardiograms twice weekly on all their patients suffering from rheumatic fever, they found 16 patients with a PR interval of 0·2 second or more. Alternate patients were then given 8 gm. of sodium salicylate daily after one week of observation, and the rest served as controls. Daily electrocardiograms were done in all these 16 patients. The authors showed that considerable daily fluctuations occurred in the PR interval in both groups, and that both decreases and increases were noted during salicylate treatment, as well as in patients receiving no therapy. There was no relationship between the trend of the PR interval and the clinical response in the treated patients, symptomatic response being excellent in all. The authors concluded that there is no proof that salicylate therapy influences the atrioventricular conduction time, and their data justified their conclusions at the time. In their days serum-salicylate estimations could not be done, but it may be said by some that the daily dose (8 gm.) given to their patients was not quite sufficient to give an adequate plasma-salicylate level. Only one of their patients responded in the way described by Levy and Turner (1927–8).

Master and Romanoff (1932) criticized the existing evidence of the value of salicylates in rheumatic fever. They investigated 63 patients, aged 13 to 53 years, treating alternate patients with 8 to 12 gm. of sodium salicylate per day, and control patients with sedatives alone. The criteria for diagnosis are not given. They assessed their results by the average length of stay in hospital, the number of deaths (one in each group), the complications, and the electrocardiographic findings. They concluded: 'There is no evidence that salicylates prevent cardiac complications or shorten the duration of hospital stay, although they are at present the most efficient antipyretics and analgesics for the treatment of rheumatic fever.' The incidence of complications was approximately the same in each group, but it is not stated whether they were present on admission or developed later. The comparison would clearly be invalidated if they were present before the experiment began. They included the usual complications, such as pericarditis, but also surprising ones such as pulmonary infarction, glomerulonephritis, chronic otitis media, thrombophlebitis, diarrhoea, toxic psychosis, and urticaria. The authors stated: 'There was a 100 per cent. involvement of the heart in both the control and the salicylate group. Not a patient's myocardium escaped damage, no matter whether or not salicylates were administered.' They supplied a list of 25 changes in the electrocardiogram which they considered to be criteria for the diagnosis of myocardial involvement in rheumatic fever; these changes include tachycardia, sinus arrhythmia, extrasystoles, and 'change P waves', and other findings which are hardly acceptable criteria. The authors did not state whether these changes were present on admission, before the experiment started, or appeared later. The duration of stay in hospital is an unreliable criterion for the assessment of the value of a drug, because so many variables are concerned. It was about the same in each group, varying from nine to 108 days. No mention was made of erythrocyte sedimentation rates. For these reasons the investigation was inconclusive.

Coburn (1943*a*) revived interest in massive salicylate dosage, and introduced a method for the estimation of salicylate in the plasma (Brodie, Udenfriend, and Coburn, 1944). He claimed that in order to obtain the best results a plasma-salicylate level of 35 to 50 mg. per 100 ml. must be maintained, and that to achieve this intravenous therapy was essential, in doses of 10 gm. or more per day. For an intense reaction at the height of an attack, a plasma level of 60 mg. might be required, but maintenance levels of 36·8 mg. per 100 ml. appeared to be adequate for subsequent continued suppression of the rheumatic reaction. He selected 40 patients from a group of 58 adults with rheumatic fever, '20 of them having proven polycyclic attacks, and 20 others with attacks so severe that it seemed unlikely that they would be monocyclic'. He divided them into three groups. The first consisted of 20 cases in which activity had been prolonged for an average period of 49 days. The range was not given. These patients had already been treated with doses of 6 gm. daily or less, and were already symptom-free when large oral doses of 10 gm. daily were given. The erythrocyte sedimentation rate then fell to normal in 14 days or less. In the second group, consisting of 14 patients in their first attack, the dose was 10 gm. daily by mouth. The erythrocyte sedimentation rate fell to normal in an average of 17 days. All escaped valvular heart disease. The third group consisted of six severely ill patients, who were given 10 gm. of salicylate daily by intravenous infusion. They became 'symptom-free in four hours, afebrile in 24 hours, and the erythrocyte sedimentation rate of all became normal in two weeks'. Coburn's charts show, however, that in three of these six the erythrocyte sedimentation rate was over 20 mm. in an hour at the end of treatment. A Group 4 is then unexpectedly described, consisting of three patients who relapsed after discontinuation of salicylates, and who responded well to a second course with high dosage. This group had not been mentioned before, and does not appear to be included in the 40 cases selected for study. Coburn described another series of 64 patients mentioned in an earlier paper (Coburn, 1943*b*) in which 43 adults were given 3 to 6 gm. of sodium salicylate daily, and compared them with seven adults who had 10 gm. daily by mouth, and 12 others who were given intravenous infusions of 10 gm. daily for two weeks. He claimed that the erythrocyte sedimentation rate fell more rapidly and clinical recovery was quicker in those who had large doses, and that the incidence of carditis was less. He claimed that, in the 12 patients who had intravenous infusions of salicylates, 'without exception these sedimentation rates fell progressively and were normal or approaching normal after 14 infusions'. His Table shows, however, that the sedimentation rates on the 12th to the 14th day were 20, 28, 20, 25, 19, 55, 24, 30, 56, 42, 9, and 55 mm. in an hour. Most of these values could hardly be called normal. In no case was the rate recorded after the drug had been stopped.

Much importance was attached by subsequent workers to Coburn's papers. They are difficult to interpret, because four groups of patients were treated with different therapeutic régimes, several of which were altered during the course of treatment. His cases were selected, but the method of selection was not stated, and some patients remained unaccounted for. The number of patients in the various groups was grossly unequal, and no evidence is presented that the groups were comparable; the only evidence available suggests that the reverse was the case. The charts do not support the claims made in the text. The patients were observed only until the completion of treatment (a few weeks), and the claim that intravenous therapy with the dosage recommended prevents the development of valvulitis is unwarranted. The possibility of a direct action of the drug on the erythrocyte sedimentation rate is not mentioned. Although Coburn has provided suggestive evidence that there was a good response to large doses of salicylates, proof is lacking. The evidence that intravenous therapy is more effective than oral medication is inconclusive, and its dangers are not emphasized.

Many subsequent workers attempted to confirm Coburn's results. Taran and Jacobs (1945), Manchester (1946*a*), and Reid (1948) were convinced of the value of large doses of salicylates, not necessarily given intravenously. Taran and Jacobs treated 64 children, aged six to 14 years. All were kept in hospital until all signs of rheumatic activity disappeared. The children were divided into eight groups. In the first two groups were children with acute rheumatic polyarthritis without carditis, and in the other six groups were children with active carditis but without other rheumatic manifestations. Carditis was defined as follows: 'tumultuous cardiac action, changing cardiac murmurs, significant electrocardiographic findings' (not specified), 'a low haemic component which failed to improve with a normal, well-balanced diet, failure to gain weight continuously, and a low vital capacity'. These definitions are not universally acceptable. All 14 children with acute polyarthritis received massive salicylate therapy. In Group 1 (seven cases) it was given intravenously at first, and then by mouth. In Group 2 (seven cases) it was given by mouth alone. Plasma-salicylate levels of 30 to 45 mg. per 100 ml. were maintained. The clinical response was good in all patients, though toxic manifestations were encountered in the intravenously treated group. The erythrocyte sedimentation rate returned to normal in an average of four weeks (11 to 49 days) in Group 1, and in three to 23 weeks in Group 2. No progressive cardiac damage was detected in these children. In Group 3 two children with severe carditis were treated with intravenous salicylates, and both died with symptoms of severe salicylate poisoning. In Group 4 six children with early carditis were treated with massive oral doses. Their erythrocyte sedimentation rate returned to normal in an average of nine weeks, and no evidence was found of progression of cardiac damage. In Group 5 six other children were similarly treated. They had a history of rheumatic activity of several weeks' duration. In these children the erythrocyte sedimentation rate returned to normal after an average of 28 weeks. In Group 6 five children with recent carditis, and in Group 7 ten children with a longer history of carditis, were treated 'with the usual doses of salicylate' by mouth (exact dose not stated). The erythrocyte sedimentation rate in Group 6 returned to normal almost as quickly (average 10·9 weeks) as in the comparable Group 4, but four of the five children continued to present evidence of active carditis, as defined above, in spite of a normal sedimentation rate. Similar observations were made in Group 7, in which only small doses of salicylate were given after several weeks of rest in bed. The average period of elevation of the erythrocyte sedimentation rate was 28 weeks, which was the same as in the comparable Group 5. Finally, in Group 8, 21 children received no salicylate. They all had carditis, and the erythrocyte sedimentation rate returned to normal after an average of 25·8 weeks, a period similar to that found in comparable patients who were treated with massive or small doses of salicylate. Taran and Jacobs concluded that massive doses of salicylate cause a 'prompt and effective subsidence of all clinical and laboratory evidence of rheumatic activity in children having rheumatic polyarthritis'. 'Massive doses in acute rheumatic carditis are equally effective, in promptly suppressing all clinical and laboratory evidence of rheumatic activity.' 'The usual small doses of salicylates have no therapeutic value in rheumatic carditis in children.' These conclusions could not be drawn legitimately from their data. It was not a controlled experiment. The children were treated in different ways without an apparent previous plan, and after an unspecified time the authors attempted to analyse the results. This attempt was bound to fail, because in seven of the eight groups the numbers were too small, ranging from two to 10 patients. There was no evidence that the cases were successive or unselected, and no criteria were given for the allocation of patients to the various groups. No controls were included among the patients with polyarthritis. We can detect no difference between the fate of the children with carditis in more or less comparable groups who received massive doses, small doses, or nothing at all. It is noteworthy, however, that the only two deaths in the series occurred in patients treated by the intravenous route. No information was given about the patients, or their erythrocyte sedimentation rates, after discontinuing treatment. From the evidence provided no conclusion is possible.

Manchester (1946*a*) treated 54 men with large doses of sodium salicylate or acetylsalicylic acid with two-thirds of the amount of sodium bicarbonate, according to Coburn's (1943*a*) recommendation, until the erythrocyte sedimentation rate had been normal for two weeks. Thirty-five of them had intravenous treatment for up to 10 days, followed by oral therapy, and 19 had oral therapy throughout. Twenty-three control patients were given unspecified small quantities of salicylate to relieve acute symptoms, but those who exhibited prolonged infection received intensive therapy later. The average period of observation was only 66 days (range 27 to 284 days). It appears from another paper (Manchester 1946*b*) that the range of serum-salicylate levels was 25 to 35 mg. per 100 ml. The following table summarizes his findings:

	Treated patients	*Controls*
Average duration of fever . . .	2·6 days	15 days
Average duration of elevated sedimentation rate	20 days	42 days
Objective articular manifestations (duration)	2·8 days	26 days
Carditis present at start of treatment .	15%	9%
No cardiac signs at end of treatment .	71%	48%
Active carditis at end of treatment .	7·4%	13%
Deaths	2	0

He concluded that 'intensive salicylate therapy suppresses rheumatic infection in the acute stages occurring in young adults, when treatment is started within 25 days after inception of the acute infection. Acute articular and toxic manifestations are dramatically relieved. Significant cardiac residua are prevented if therapy is instituted before signs of significant carditis have appeared. Already existing acute carditis is favourably influenced. The period of active infection is materially shortened and relapses and residual chronic infection, although not prevented, occur less frequently in patients receiving intensive salicylate therapy than in those receiving symptomatic therapy.' He found no difference in the duration of electrocardiographic changes between the treated and control groups, nor was there any difference in response between the orally and intravenously treated patients. These conclusions do not seem to be justifiable. Manchester's cases were arbitrarily chosen for the treated and control groups, and patients with milder disease were selected for the control groups. Further, less severe and spontaneously subsiding infections have for the most part been excluded. He gave no figures for the erythrocyte sedimentation rate before, during, or after treatment, and it is surprising that it was said to be raised in only one of the four patients in the 'high salicylate' group who relapsed. He stated that the relapse rate was less in treated patients, but, as the period of observation was very short and different for each case, such a comparison is unjustified. Nevertheless Manchester produced suggestive evidence that high salicylate dosage is of benefit.

Reid (1948) described the effect of treating nine adults with daily oral doses of 10 gm. and three children with doses of 6·6 gm. of sodium salicylate. Seven of the adults and two of the children also received sodium bicarbonate in equal amounts. Treatment was continued 'until complete recovery'. He stated that 'the return of the erythrocyte sedimentation rate to normal was used as the index of cure of an attack of the disease'. The criteria for diagnosis were adequate. He set the figure for a normal erythrocyte sedimentation rate at 20 mm. per hour, but it is seen in his Table II that the final rates, in the seven cases for which he gave figures, were 10, 20, 30, 40, 50, 65, and 125 mm. per hour. In the last case there had been no change in the erythrocyte sedimentation rate in three weeks' treatment, but it rapidly fell to 20 mm. when the dose was doubled. He did not add that this could well have happened without treatment. He gave no figures for the final sedimentation rate in the remaining five cases. He estimated the serum-salicylate level in his patients, and found that the peak was reached between the third and eighth days, and varied from 20 to 46 mg. per 100 ml., and that the level later fell to between 11 and 31 mg. per 100 ml. without the dose being altered. In six of the 10 cases in which it is given, the salicylate level fell to below 20 mg. per 100 ml. In some of his patients the serum-salicylate level did not reach 35 mg. per 100 ml., as advocated by Coburn (1943*a*), and in most of the remainder the level was not maintained. In one of his patients joint pain and swelling persisted more or less continuously throughout the first three weeks of treatment. The dose of sodium salicylate was then doubled, and three days later all symptoms had disappeared. Two other patients had relapses associated with a drop in the salicylate level. In one child pericarditis cleared in two days, at a time when there was a high salicylate level, and returned when the level fell. The friction disappeared when the level rose, but when the level fell again there was no return of friction. This fact admittedly suggests that salicylates had some therapeutic action, but the same waxing and waning of symptoms and signs, such as arthritis and pericarditis, occurs without any salicylate treatment. Reid did not include controls in his series, and did not say how the cases were selected. Carditis was not considered. His patients were observed for only three weeks after treatment was stopped. His conclusion that salicylates 'cure' rheumatic fever is unwarranted.

Other workers (Keith and Ross, 1945; Jager and Alway, 1946; Watkinson, 1949) were not quite so enthusiastic about the value of large doses of salicylates. Keith and Ross treated 70 adults with 10 to 13·3 gm. doses of sodium salicylate or acetylsalicylic acid per day, with equal quantities of sodium bicarbonate. Thirty-three control patients were given up to 2·0 gm. daily. Treatment was continued in most cases for two to four weeks after the erythrocyte sedimentation rate had fallen to normal. Eighteen additional cases had been studied, but were taken out of the series on account of streptococcal infections, inadequate dosage, or intolerance of salicylates. The authors concluded that salicylates in high dosage control joint symptoms and keep the temperature and pulse-rate down, but have no effect on the duration of the elevation of the erythrocyte sedimentation rate (which was above 15 mm. in an hour for an average of 4·0 weeks in the treated patients and 4·5 weeks in the controls), and no effect on the development of carditis. Of 57 treated patients who had a normal heart on admission, five developed cardiac signs; of 29 controls, three developed heart disease. No information was provided about the method of allocation of cases to the treated and the control groups, nor was it stated to which group the 18 excluded cases had belonged. The dosage system was unsatisfactory. No salicylates were given between 10 p.m. and 7 a.m. Plasma-salicylate levels were estimated in 26 cases. The levels, nine hours after the first dose, ranged from 19 to 39 mg. per 100 ml. Levels had probably, therefore, been higher during the daytime. They said: 'At times those large doses of salicylates were associated with an increased force and intensity of heart beat. It is possible that the cases that respond in this fashion may sometimes have harm done to their mitral valve from the added force of impact, in the same way that too early exercise may damage the valve.' The result of the investigation was inconclusive, because no evidence was presented that the two groups were comparable and selected without bias.

Jager and Alway (1946) attempted to confirm Coburn's (1943*a*) findings. They treated 18 adults, aged 16 to 46 years, and eight children, aged nine to 15 years, with large doses of sodium salicylate. Some of the patients were in their first attack, but others had established valvular lesions from previous attacks. In 19 patients the first day's treatment was given intravenously. In five adults and an unspecified number of children the drug was given intravenously for a further three to 14 days. In all these cases the drug was then given by mouth. The remaining patients were treated by mouth from the beginning. Serum-salicylate levels were estimated on at least six occasions in 19 of the 26 patients, and an effort was made to maintain the level at between 30 and 40 mg. per 100 ml., but these values were often exceeded. Wide variations in the serum levels were observed with the same dose, and very different doses were required in different patients to maintain similar levels. The addition of sodium bicarbonate made it necessary to use high doses, which were mostly of the order of 0·20 to 0·25 gm. per kg. body-weight. Treatment was continued for four to 14 weeks in adults, but information on this point was not given for children. One adult died on the eighth day of the treatment from heart failure, and two others died during second courses from salicylate poisoning. The serum-salicylate level in one of these patients reached 81·2 mg. per 100 ml. before death, showing the danger of intravenous therapy without the most rigid control. Lesser toxic symptoms occurred in most patients on intravenous therapy. Abnormalities of the electrocardiogram did not always disappear during treatment, and in two patients appeared for the first time. In only five of 17 patients did the erythrocyte sedimentation rate return to normal within four weeks. Relapse after stopping treatment was frequent. The authors concluded that 'treatment with large doses of salicylate appeared to be effective in the five patients with initial attacks and in four of the seven patients with recurrent attacks who could be followed for short periods after medication had stopped'. They added: 'It is probable that the results would not appear so favourable if every patient could have been followed. Several of those who did not return for examination had evidence suggestive of persistent rheumatic activity at the time of discharge from the hospital.' As there were no controls, the effectiveness of the treatment could not be assessed. It is clear that the treatment was not continued long enough. The period of subsequent observation was inadequate, varying from 0 to 20 months. No conclusions can be drawn from their paper, except that intravenous therapy is dangerous.

Watkinson (1949) divided 80 young adults into three groups, but the total number in the three groups only adds up to 75 patients. Of 25 in the first group, 14 had no drugs, and 11 had small doses of salicylates not exceeding 100 gr. (6·7 gm.) per day. The 29 in the second group were given 200 gr. (13 gm.) daily, 10 of them with half that quantity of sodium bicarbonate. Serum-salicylate levels were not estimated. The third group consisted of 21 patients in whom dosage was dependent on the serum levels, which were maintained at over 30 mg. per 100 ml. In all groups the drug was stopped when the erythrocyte sedimentation rate had been normal on three successive weekly occasions. The average sedimentation rate in the three groups was comparable on admission. The criteria for diagnosis were adequate. The following are extracts from his results:

	Average duration (in days) of		
	Fever	*Pain*	*Elevated sedimentation rate*
Group 1	22·7	22·7	73·6
Group 2	5·1	6·1	37·0
Group 3	1·9	1·9	16·6

He concluded: 'A significant reduction in the period of fever, arthralgia and active infection was demonstrated in the group receiving massive therapy. No reduction in the relapse rate or in the incidence of carditis was seen.' Unfortunately the three groups were studied at three different Royal Air Force Station hospitals. Although all groups were comparable in numbers, in the severity of the disease, and in the incidence of previous rheumatic attacks, the method of control is not perfect, for there may be differences in management in different hospitals. It is not clear whether any cases were excluded, but five remain unaccounted for. Nevertheless the paper affords strongly suggestive evidence of the short-term value of high salicylate dosage in young adults.

Finally, Wégria and Smull (1945), Wright (1945), Murphy (1945), and Warren, Higley, and Coombs (1946*a*) thought that salicylates were of very little value. Wégria and Smull treated 21 patients, almost all adults, with large doses of sodium salicylate (without sodium bicarbonate) by the oral or intravenous route or both, and attempted to maintain serum levels of 35 to 45 mg. per 100 ml. until the erythrocyte sedimentation rate had been below 20 mm. in an hour (Westergren) for two weeks. Patients were discharged the following week. There were 19 control patients. The following are the words of the writers: 'Nine of these were patients under our own observation, and were not adequately treated for various reasons; in two of those nine patients optimal levels were never reached; in the other seven patients optimal levels were obtained only for short periods. The remaining 10 patients of the control group had acute rheumatic fever and were admitted to the Presbyterian Hospital in 1943; none of these patients received consistently more than 3·6 gm. per day of sodium salicylate, and most of them received equal doses of sodium bicarbonate.' Serum-salicylate levels were not determined in these 10 cases. The authors assessed progress entirely by the erythrocyte sedimentation rate. They concluded that 'the course of an attack of acute rheumatic fever is not shortened by adequate salicylate therapy. It is possible, however, that the course of the attack might be shortened by early institution of adequate salicylate therapy, i.e. within one week of the onset of symptoms of acute rheumatic fever.' They found no benefit from intravenous as opposed to oral treatment. The writers did not say how the patients were selected for treatment, or what were the criteria for diagnosis. They used patients as controls because adequate serum levels were not reached. This is clearly inadmissible. It is not stated what the various reasons were for inadequate treatment of nine of the controls. The erythrocyte sedimentation rate was not recorded after the salicylates were stopped, and the patients were discharged a week later. For these reasons no conclusions can be drawn from their study.

Wright (1945) reviewed his experience with rheumatic fever in the United States Army. He found that in a comparable series of 58 patients, half of whom had massive intravenous therapy and the other half massive oral treatment, no advantage was seen in those treated intravenously. Four patients having intravenous therapy developed pericarditis, and altogether 20 developed significant cardiac lesions, which in five cases were considered to be permanent. The orally treated patients fared much the same way, although blood levels of 35 mg. per 100 ml. were achieved. The response of the erythrocyte sedimentation rate was 'disappointingly slow'. These figures are in sharp contrast with Coburn's (1943*a*, *b*) claims, and show that massive salicylate therapy is not the final solution to the problem of the treatment of rheumatic fever. As, however, Wright's series did not include untreated patients or those receiving a smaller dosage of salicylates, it cannot be concluded from his data whether massive salicylates are better than small doses or nothing at all.

Murphy (1945) conducted a careful study of 12 specially selected patients with severe rheumatic fever receiving high salicylate dosage which maintained adequate serum levels. He measured the size of involved joints, and in six of them recorded the skin temperature. In other cases biopsy specimens of fresh lesions were examined. He showed that in several patients rheumatic lesions developed during treatment. Two joints became involved 15 days after the beginning of treatment. Two patients developed tendon-sheath nodules, one developed a fatal rheumatic pneumonitis, and another an episcleral nodule. Histological examination of biopsy material from these lesions, which developed during treatment, did not support the contention of other authors that salicylates effect the absorption of rheumatic inflammatory exudate and cause the subsidence of rheumatic activity. This is a valuable and thorough paper, from which certain limited conclusions may be justifiably drawn. It shows that salicylates, even in optimal dosage, are not always capable of arresting rheumatic activity. It does not show that they are valueless, or that large doses are preferable to small ones, for there were no controls.

Warren, Higley, and Coombs (1946*a*, *b*) treated 98 men with salicylates, 10 to 16 gm. daily by the oral or intravenous route, to maintain a serum level of 35 to 45 mg. per 100 ml. until the erythrocyte sedimentation rate had been normal for two weeks. The treatment was repeated if the sedimentation rate rose. They compared them with 88 control patients who were given doses of 2 to 7 gm. per day with equal quantities of sodium bicarbonate. The criteria for diagnosis, definition of fever, elevation of the erythrocyte sedimentation rate, and heart disease were adequately defined, but the duration of illness before treatment was not stated. They concluded that 'large doses will not prevent the development of cardiac damage or stop the progression of pre-existing heart disease'. They 'will not serve to shorten the period of rheumatic activity any more than small amounts'. They 'will not prevent the development of polycyclic attacks'. 'It appears that the use of large amounts of salicylate may offer some advantage in the first weeks of therapy, and may bring about a rapid reduction of the fever and alleviation of the symptoms: but the continued administration of large amounts of this drug until the erythrocyte sedimentation rate is normal is of questionable value.' They thought that the use of the intravenous route is not warranted. They divided their patients into 'severe' cases, with an erythrocyte sedimentation rate of over 60 mm. in an hour, and 'mild' cases with a rate of below 60 mm. in an hour. Eighty-five per cent. of the mild cases were controls, and in 70·4 per cent. of the severe cases high doses of salicylate were given. In addition, the control patients were treated at a different time (1942 to 1944) from the 'high salicylate' patients, who were treated from 1944 onwards. The cases are therefore not fully comparable, as the authors recognized. Their conclusions were based on a short period of observation. Had the selection of patients for the two groups been unbiased, this large, adequately studied series might have provided conclusive evidence about the value of salicylates in the treatment of rheumatic fever. As it is, the only possible conclusion is that mild cases do as well on small doses as severe cases do on massive doses.

The effect of salicylates on the erythrocyte sedimentation rate. Nearly all the papers referred to record the figure for the sedimentation rate only while the patient was still having salicylates. If salicylates have a direct action on the sedimentation rate, this would introduce an error. A survey of the literature has failed to elucidate this problem. Bendien, Neuberg, and Snapper (1932) noted a slowing of the erythrocyte sedimentation rate *in vitro* when the concentration of sodium salicylate in the blood was 90 to 120 mg. per 100 ml. Homburger (1945) found that reduction of the sedimentation rate occurred when the concentration of sodium salicylate was about 90 mg. per 100 ml., but it also occurred when the level was 25 to 30 mg. per 100 ml. if the drug was left in contact with fresh plasma for 24 hours. In a further paper (1946) he showed that the erythrocyte sedimentation rate fell in three cases of carcinomatosis when the patients were given salicylates. The paper does not give figures, but a graph shows that in two cases a fall did occur. Rapoport and Guest (1946) gave salicylates to 15 patients, aged two to 14 years, who had an elevated erythrocyte sedimentation rate. Some had nephritis, others rheumatic fever, osteitis, and other conditions. (The description of the cases in the text differs from that given in the Table.) In 10 of the 15 cases the sedimentation rate (and plasma fibrinogen) decreased. It is not stated how long the sedimentation rate had been observed before the drug was given, and the extent of its fall is not easy to see from the Table. Harris (1947) gave salicylates to six patients with pulmonary tuberculosis and to four with rheumatoid arthritis. In all but one there was a fall of the erythrocyte sedimentation rate. In only two of the 10 cases did the rate fall below 20 mm. in an hour. In clinical studies of the effect of salicylates on rheumatic fever there is a difference of opinion whether salicylates cause any fall in the erythrocyte sedimentation rate. Lichty and Hooker (1941) noted that in seven rheumatic patients there was a rise of the sedimentation rate when salicylates were stopped. This rise was occasionally associated with an elevation of the temperature and a return of symptoms, or both. One would have thought that the rise of the rate *in vivo* might be due merely to stopping the drug too soon, just as the temperature may rise in pneumonia or any other infection when an antibiotic is stopped too soon. Wégria and Smull (1945), Warren, Higley, and Coombs (1946*a*), and Keith and Ross (1945) found that the sedimentation rate was unaffected by salicylates. Jager and Alway (1946) reached the same conclusion, except that in the first two to four weeks after instituting treatment there was actually a rise in the sedimentation rate in two-thirds of their cases. The rise was often considerable. Some of the fallacies in these four papers have already been mentioned.

The Present Investigation

Fifty-nine children, aged three to 14 years, suffering from rheumatic fever, were admitted to the investigation. Four of these patients were subsequently excluded. Of the 55 remaining children 44 were in their first attack ('new cases'), and 11 had had previous attacks ('relapse cases'). Twenty-seven were given salicylates, and 28 served as controls (Table I). They were admitted to the Professorial Unit at the Children's Hospital, Sheffield, between February 1949 and February 1953. All cases in the investigation satisfied the criteria for diagnosis suggested by Jones (1944), and no cases which satisfied those criteria were excluded, except those in the M.R.C. series mentioned below. No case of uncomplicated chorea was admitted to the investigation. There was no selection of cases for the Children's Hospital, and no child with rheumatic fever requiring hospital treatment was refused admission. Admission to the Professorial Unit was by alternation with another unit. All children admitted to the investigation had an erythrocyte sedimentation rate (henceforward termed 'E.S.R.') of more than 20 mm. in the first hour (Westergren or Wintrobe).

TABLE I

Patients Investigated

	Salicylate group			*Control group*			*Total*		
	New cases	*Relapse cases*	*Total*	*New cases*	*Relapse cases*	*Total*	*New cases*	*Relapse cases*	*Total*
Admitted to the investigation . .	22	7	29	24	6	30	46	13	59
Subsequently excluded .	2	2	4	..	..	..	2	2	4
Transfers in the first week	..	..	..	2	..	2	2	..	2
Final composition of series	22*	5	27	22	6	28	44	11	55

* Including two transferred cases.

Method of study

1. *Allocation to 'control' and 'salicylate' groups.* Once the diagnosis was established, the treatment to be given was decided throughout by the random sampling method. Late in 1950 we accepted an invitation from the Medical Research Council to take part in the joint Anglo-American investigation into the use of cortisone and ACTH in rheumatic fever. Our own investigation continued, however, and the random sampling envelopes were accordingly modified by the Medical Research Council to include five groups: cortisone (M.R.C.), ACTH (M.R.C.), low salicylate dosage (M.R.C.), and our own two groups, namely controls (no salicylates) and cases of high salicylate dosage. The first three groups are not considered in the present paper. No further cases were admitted to the M.R.C. series after October 1952, when we reverted to the two original groups. Some of the children in both groups had been given small doses of salicylates for a short time at home. In all cases the dosage was such

that only low serum-salicylate levels would be achieved. There was no difference between the two groups in this respect.

2. *Exclusion of four cases after allocation.* Three patients did not fully satisfy the criteria for diagnosis suggested by Jones (1944). They were allocated to the salicylate group in error, and were excluded from the subsequent analysis. One was admitted for treatment because of a raised E.S.R., there being a previous history of rheumatic fever. The heart was normal, and the E.S.R. rapidly fell to normal. Another child was admitted with a history of 10 months' persistent rheumatic activity, as indicated by a raised E.S.R., with an established cardiac lesion. There were no other criteria. A third child was referred to us because of a persistently raised E.S.R. of many months' duration, with a history of a first attack of rheumatic fever four years previously. He died in hospital, and necropsy revealed the usual lesions of old-standing inactive rheumatic infection. A fourth child was allocated to the salicylate group, but was withdrawn on the ninth day and given ACTH on account of a severe deterioration in his condition, with bilateral consolidation of the lung, delirium, and Cheynes-Stokes breathing. He was moribund, but made an unexpected recovery, with residual cardiac damage. This boy will be mentioned later.

3. *Transfers after allocation.* It was only after the most careful consideration and discussion with senior members of the profession that we embarked on the investigation, for we were determined not to allow any child to suffer if he was allocated to the control group and subsequently it was felt that his progress was unsatisfactory. These ethical considerations inevitably raised difficulties in the final analysis. In all, four 'new cases' and one 'relapse case' were eventually given salicylates, although allocated to the control group. Two of the new cases (Nos. 43 and 44) were transferred on the seventh and fourth days[2] respectively, because they were seriously ill with pericarditis. After transfer these two patients were regarded as belonging entirely to the salicylate group. As a result the salicylate group was weighted with two severe cases; but we felt that if subsequent analysis showed that there was any difference between the two groups in favour of salicylates, that difference would then be all the more significant. Case 3 was transferred to the salicylate group on the 44th day, because of a persistently high E.S.R. and sleeping pulse-rate. Case 5 was transferred on the 28th day, because of recurrent arthritis and a persistently high E.S.R. and temperature. The progress of these two patients after transfer is described below. All relevant data concerning these two transferred patients, such as the pulse-rate, temperature, and E.S.R., were included in the control group up to the time of their transfer. Thereafter none of their records were used in either group, except for the final assessment, which was recorded separately from that of the other children. It would be inadvisable to insert data for these children in both groups, for in that case they would be counted twice. One other new case (No. 18) received salicylates, for five days only, from the 23rd day in error; it was felt that this should be ignored. Of the

[2] In the text and tables 'day' denotes the number of days from admission: day 1 means the day of admission.

children seen during a relapse, Case 46 was transferred to the salicylate group 300 days after admission because of a persistently high E.S.R., a recurrence of arthritis on the 290th day, and severe cardiac damage. The data for this child were treated in the same way as those of Cases 3 and 5 mentioned above.

4. *Relapses.* It is doubtful whether it is profitable or possible to distinguish 'relapses' from 'exacerbations'. A child was considered to have relapsed if he satisfied the criteria of Jones (1944) for the diagnosis of active rheumatic fever, and was known to have had an earlier attack of the disease. Eleven children were admitted to the investigation for the first time in relapses. Data concerning subsequent relapses, in either new cases or children admitted to the investigation in a relapse, are not analysed in this paper.

General treatment and supervision. Rheumatic fever is notifiable in Sheffield, and the great majority of the patients notified during the period of the investigation were brought to the Children's Hospital for confirmation of the diagnosis, and if necessary for admission. When they were admitted to the Professorial Unit, and therefore to the investigation, supervision by the same team was continuous. After discharge from the Children's Hospital they were sent to the Rheumatic Fever Hospital School, under the medical care of one of the team, and stayed there as long as was considered necessary. After discharge they were followed up in the School Heart Clinic by the same physicians for an indefinite number of years. It would not be profitable to calculate the average duration of stay in hospital, because of the wide scatter. One child, for instance, died after seven days in hospital, while another was in hospital for over three years. Four children were taken home by their mothers against advice. Of the 50 children admitted in the first three and a half years of the investigation, 14 were in the hospital or hospital school for 200 to 299 days, 13 for 300 to 399 days, and 15 for 400 days or longer. These figures include some children still in hospital at the time of writing (February 1953); they do not include the duration of stay in hospital, in their initial attacks, of those who were first admitted to the investigation in relapses. The treatment of all patients, apart from salicylate therapy, was the same. They were kept in bed until all signs of activity had disappeared, except when there was a persistently high E.S.R. over a prolonged period without other signs of activity. At the hospital school they were given carefully graduated activity according to their physical condition. In the acute stage analgesics, other than salicylates, were given in either group for painful arthritis. No placebos were given. All children during their stay in hospital or hospital school were given 200,000 units of penicillin daily by mouth in tablet form, in two doses, or daily prophylactic sulphonamides. The prophylactic treatment was continued for an indefinite period after discharge from the hospital school.

Salicylate dosage. Patients in the salicylate group were given sodium salicylate in large doses, with the aim of maintaining the serum-salicylate level at 30 to 40 mg. per 100 ml. The initial dose was $1\frac{1}{2}$ gr. (0·1 gm.) per lb. (455 gm.) body-weight per day, with an equal quantity of sodium bicarbonate. Salicylate levels were determined at frequent intervals, and the dose of sodium salicylate was adjusted accordingly. If a dose of 2 gr. per lb. did not give a satisfactory level, the sodium bicarbonate was reduced or omitted. The aim was to administer the drug until the E.S.R. had been normal for two consecutive weeks. (In fact the E.S.R. was normal in 19 of 22 new cases when the drug was stopped.) The average duration of salicylate treatment was 65 days. The variations are shown

TABLE II

Children Treated with Salicylates: Duration of Treatment with Serum Levels

			Serum-salicylate readings (mg. per 100 ml.)				
				Number of instances			
Case number	*Duration of salicylate therapy in days*	*Number of serum-salicylate estimations*	*Average level*	*Below 20*	*20–24*	*25–29*	*30 or over*
23	40	12	29·5	..	3	5	4
24	63	12	30·0	..	1	5	6
25	69	15	31·2	..	3	3	9
26	31	4	22·0	2	1	..	1
27 D	5	1	29·0	..	..	1	..
28	49	9	31·2	..	..	5	4
29	28	3	25·1	..	1	2	..
30	44	5	22·8	1	3	..	1
31	139	18	31·3	1	..	3	14
32	158	27	30·0	2	2	8	15
33	29	6	29·6	1	2	1	2
34	83	15	31·1	..	2	6	7
35	58	10	33·7	..	1	2	7
36	44	9	31·7	..	2	1	6
37	66	11	27·0	1	4	4	2
38	34	6	30·6	..	2	1	3
39	35	9	30·1	..	1	3	5
40	60	9	32·7	..	..	1	8
41	24	5	28·7	..	..	4	1
42	46	7	31·3	1	1	..	5
43	70	17	30·4	2	2	5	8
44	154	25	36·8	..	3	..	22
51 R	131	18	32·4	2	..	1	15
52 R	50	4	32·9	..	2	..	2
53 R	48	8	27·5	1	1	3	3
54 R	86	17	30·0	2	2	4	9
55 R	56	4	31·0	..	1	2	1
3 T	56	10	22·2	2	6	2	..
5 T	133	29	33·3	4	3	3	19
46 T R	76	10	31·3	..	1	3	6
Percentages of total	.	.	. .	6·6	14·9	23·3	55·2

D = Died. R = Relapse cases. T = Transferred cases.

in Table II. It is probable that the drug was discontinued too soon in two patients (Cases 52 and 53), for the E.S.R. was not normal at the time, and that in five others (Cases 24, 35, 42, 43, and 3), a second course should have been given, for there was a considerable rise of the E.S.R. (the rebound phenomenon), without a rapid return to normal. In six children (Cases 31, 32, 44, 51, 54, and 55) a second course was given when the rebound phenomenon occurred, but in three of them (Cases 31, 44, and 51) there was a further considerable rebound after the drug was stopped, and it is probable that a third course should have been given. It was difficult to maintain an adequate serum-salicylate level. It will be seen that the average level reached in 18 of the 27 children was 30 mg. per 100 ml. or higher (Table II; the three transferred cases are excluded). Toxic symptoms were frequent. In all children who developed hyperpnoea the drug was omitted for two or three days and then restarted. It was largely the development of toxic symptoms which made the maintenance of a high level difficult. A total of 335 serum-salicylate determinations were made in the 30 children treated. The levels were determined by the method described by Brodie, Udenfriend, and Coburn (1944) in blood taken two hours after the last dose. Several tests were made of the strength of the salicylate solution in the bottles provided by the dispensary, in order to check the accuracy of the doses given. The sodium bicarbonate was given from a separate bottle, because of the precipitation which occurs on standing when the two drugs are mixed.

Other investigations. The sleeping pulse-rate was recorded once or twice every 24 hours. When there were two readings in the day, the highest figure alone was used for analysis. In the majority of children the temperature was recorded four-hourly. The figure used in all analyses was the highest temperature recorded in the 24 hours. The temperature was regarded as normal if it was 98·4° F. (37° C.) or below throughout the 24 hours. It was intended that daily records should be made of the degree of swelling of joints and the presence or absence of pain, but there were a few omissions, and our records are therefore not complete. The presence of nodules on admission, and the development of new nodules, were also recorded. Systolic murmurs were graded 1 to 6, as in the classification of Levine and Harvey (1949), and every effort was made to record changes in the murmurs and especially their appearance or disappearance. It is so much a matter of individual opinion whether a murmur has increased or decreased in intensity, that we have only considered a change of two grades or more to be of significance for the purposes of analysis. We decided to carry out E.S.R. estimations weekly in the first three months, thereafter fortnightly, and later monthly. The estimations were continued until discharge, and in many cases were carried out during the subsequent period of observation in the school clinic. Subsequent analysis showed that some records were lacking, either because the test was not carried out or because the result was not recorded. Although a total of 1,145 E.S.R. estimations were made on the 55 patients during their stay in hospital or hospital school, more frequent estimations would have been desirable in some cases. Rises of the E.S.R. due to infections were disregarded. In one girl monthly rises of the E.S.R. in association with menstruation were similarly disregarded. It was intended that the micro-modification of the Westergren method (uncorrected) should be used for estimating the E.S.R. This method gives a possible maximum reading of about 75 to 80 mm. in the first hour. Later, as the Anglo-American investigation demanded the use of the Wintrobe method, this method was also used in five of our salicylate cases and in six of the controls. This change introduced a difficulty in the analysis. In Tables III and IV the cases in which the Wintrobe method was used are marked 'W'. There is, however, a fairly close relationship between the results obtained by the two methods, and statistical analysis (Table XIII) showed that in our cases the results obtained by the two methods were strictly comparable. We have regarded an E.S.R. of 10 mm. or less in the

Table III

Controls : Data on Admission

Case number	*Sex*	*Age (years and months)*	*Duration of symptoms before admission (days)*	*Highest temperature in first week (°F.)*	*Highest sleeping pulse-rate in first week*	*Apical systolic murmur (Grade)*	*Apical diastolic murmur*	*Aortic diastolic murmur*	*Pericarditis*	*Chorea*	*Highest of first two E.S.R. readings (mm. per hr.)*	*Erythema marginatum*
1	F	6·11	7	N	84	3	+	..	..	..	46	..
2	M	9·7	17	N	90	1	..	..	..	+	40	..
3	M	6·4	4	100·7	116	1	..	..	..	..	55	..
4	F	11·0	3	102·2	112	1	..	..	..	..	62	..
5	F	10·7	2	104·2	140	..	..	..	..	..	56 W	..
6	F	5·8	11	N	90	3	..	..	..	..	70	..
7	F	7·4	2	102·0	100	2	..	..	..	..	55	..
8	M	12·3	2	100·0	100	..	..	..	..	..	46	..
9	F	14·1	42	N	88	3	..	..	..	..	26	..
10	F	10·10	21*	100·6	130	3	+	+	..	..	50	..
11	F	8·1	10	N	85	3	+	..	..	+	22	..
12	F	8·11	7	99·8	126	3	..	..	..	..	65	..
13	F	6·4	70	N	108	3	+	..	..	..	43	..
14	F	8·11	35	100·6	126	2	..	..	..	..	67	..
15	F	8·8	63	N	92	1	..	..	..	+	25 W	..
16	F	12·8	2	101·6	100	1	..	..	..	..	62	..
17	M	7·7	7	100·0	110	..	..	..	..	..	47	..
18	M	9·7	4	102·0	118	2	..	..	..	..	57 W	..
19	F	9·7	10	N	88	3	..	..	..	..	53	..
20	F	10·10	2	104·2	114	2	..	..	..	..	56 W	..
21	M	7·11	14	102·2	114	1	..	..	..	..	64	..
22	M	7·5	14	100·2	98	..	..	..	..	..	55	..
45 R	F	10·0	14	100·4	120	3	+	..	..	+	52 W	..
46 R	M	12·2	7	99·6	82	1	..	..	..	..	49	..
47 R	F	9·3	7	N	84	3	+	..	..	+	38	..
48 R	F	7·4	35	N	120	3	+	..	..	..	46	..
49 R	M	9·9	90	N	..	3	+	..	..	..	66	+
50 R	M	10·10	5	100·0	76	2	..	..	..	..	51 W	..

W = Wintrobe method. * = Possibly only 2 days. R = Relapse cases. N = Normal.

Table IV

Salicylate Group: Data on Admission

Case number	*Sex*	*Age (years and months)*	*Duration of symptoms before admission (days)*	*Highest temperature in first week (°F.)*	*Highest sleeping pulse-rate in first week*	*Apical systolic murmur (Grade)*	*Apical diastolic murmur*	*Aortic diastolic murmur*	*Pericarditis*	*Chorea*	*Highest of first two E.S.R. readings (mm. per hr.)*	*Erythema marginatum*
23	F	9·2	3	102·6	95	2	..	..	..	..	55	+
24	F	11·9	28	N	76	1	..	..	..	..	42	..
25	M	11·7	14	N	96	1	..	..	..	..	45	..
26	F	11·6	13	99·2	106	..	..	..	..	..	54	..
27	M	3·11	3	99·0	120	3	..	..	..	..	46	..
28	M	6·10	5	104·6	92	3	..	..	..	..	53 W	..
29	M	10·0	4	103·4	112	..	..	..	..	..	30	..
30	F	6·4	14	100·0	120	3	+	..	+	..	55	..
31	M	7·5	90	99·0	100	4	..	..	..	..	31	..
32	F	12·10	49	100·4	134	3	..	..	..	+	52	..
33	M	4·8	56	101·4	112	..	..	..	..	..	51	..
34	F	5·1	7	99·8	100	1	..	..	..	..	60	..
35	M	6·11	21	99·8	108	3	..	..	..	..	40 W	..
36	M	5·6	4	99·4	88	3	..	..	..	..	44	..
37	M	12·1	28	99·0	90	3	..	..	..	..	35	..
38	M	7·4	28	100·8	84	3	..	..	..	..	37	..
39	M	8·0	2	101·0	92	1	..	..	..	..	47	..
40	M	12·9	10	99·0	80	..	..	..	..	..	44 W	..
41	M	6·5	56	N	118	3	..	..	..	..	43	..
42	F	7·7	1	102·5	116	..	..	..	..	..	42	..
43 T	M	10·1	30*	102·6	120	1	+	..	+	..	60	..
44 T	F	12·11	3	105·0	120	3	+	..	+	..	56 W	..
51 R	F	10·3	60	N	104	4	..	..	..	..	50	..
52 R	M	8·1	30	102·2	108	2	+	..	+	..	36	..
53 R	M	11·6	28	101·0	..	1	..	..	..	..	57	+
54 R	F	10·10	5	101·0	120	4	+	..	+	+	61 W	..
55 R	F	11·0	5	100·2	84	3	+	..	..	..	62	..

W = Wintrobe method. * = Possibly only 4 days. T = Transferred from controls. N = Normal. R = Relapse cases.

first hour (uncorrected) as normal in the micromethod, and 20 mm. or less in the first hour (uncorrected) as normal in the Wintrobe method. Other investigations included routine tuberculin tests and throat swabs in all cases, blood counts, and radiological and electrocardiographic studies. These are not analysed in the present paper.

Observation and assessment. All children were kept under continuous observation from the time of the first admission. For the purpose of the analysis, however, a special examination was arranged for all new cases which had been observed for a year or more (average 32 months; range 12 to 48 months). This assessment was carried out by a member of the team (J. B.) who joined it at the time when the analysis of results was being made, and by the consultant radiologist to the Children's Hospital, Dr. J. Wilkie. Neither knew to which group any of the children belonged. The clinical findings agreed with those of other members of the team, who did know to which group the children belonged. It would not have been useful to analyse the findings in the relapse cases, because these children, when admitted to the investigation, all had established valvular disease from the first attack. It was inevitable that in some cases there should be an element of doubt concerning the presence or absence of cardiac damage. When there was a Grade 1 or 2 systolic murmur, or the radiological examination showed a possible slight enlargement of the left auricle, which might be within normal limits, the final conclusion was inevitably a matter of judgement, after careful discussion, based on both clinical and radiological findings.

Comparability of the Two Groups

Data concerning the comparability of the two groups are given in Tables III to V. Among the new cases, the average age in the control series was nine years and one month, and in the salicylate group eight years and eight months. Twelve children in each group were below the age of nine years. There was no significant difference in the duration of symptoms before admission. This was 14 days or less in 16 of the new cases in the control series, and in 13 of the new cases in the salicylate group. In two or three cases it was difficult to assess the duration of symptoms. One patient (Case 10), for instance, had tonsillitis six weeks before admission, and although she returned to school she was easily tired. Three weeks before admission there were vague aching pains between the scapulae, not related to movement. Two weeks before admission she again developed tonsillitis. She recovered quickly, but remained tired, and two days before admission developed polyarthritis. The duration of the rheumatic fever may have been two days, three weeks, or six weeks. The average of the maximum sleeping pulse-rate recorded in the first week, in the new cases, was 106 per minute in the control group and 104 per minute in the salicylate group. The average E.S.R. on admission was 51 mm. per hour in the controls (new cases) and 46 mm. in the salicylate group. In 14 of the 22 controls and 19 of the 22 salicylate cases the temperature was 99°F. or higher in the first week. It is of interest that in the two severest cases, the child who died (Case 27), and the child who became moribund and was given ACTH, the temperature was normal on admission. Table V shows that, when new and relapse cases were considered together, the E.S.R., temperature, and a sleeping pulse-rate on admission were similarly comparable. There was a slightly higher incidence of unquestionable carditis in the salicylate group. Many feel that Grade 1 or 2 apical systolic murmurs may be functional or organic, but there is little doubt that a Grade 3 or 4 apical systolic murmur in a case of rheumatic fever is

TABLE V

Comparability of the Two Groups on Admission (New and Relapse Cases Combined)

	Erythrocyte sedimentation rate				*Temperature*				*Sleeping pulse-rate*			
Group	*Number of cases*	*Mean (mm. per hour)*	*Student's t*	*Degrees of freedom*	*Number of cases*	*Mean (°F.)*	*Student's t*	*Degrees of freedom*	*Number of cases*	*Mean*	*Student's t*	*Degrees of freedom*
Control	28	50·9	1·06	53	28	100·1	1·04	53	27	104·7	0·10	51
Salicylate	27	47·7			27	100·6			26	103·7		

organic. In the control group there were 14 new cases with no murmur, or with a Grade 1 or 2 apical systolic murmur, on admission, compared with 11 in the salicylate group. In the control group there were eight children with a Grade 3 or 4 systolic apical murmur, compared with 11 in the salicylate group. One new case and two relapse cases in the salicylate group had pericarditis on admission to the investigation. Two of the control cases, both new (Nos. 43 and 44), had pericarditis, but were transferred at the onset to the salicylate group. The salicylate group, therefore, was weighted with five cases of pericarditis, while, after transfer of the two children mentioned above, there were no cases of pericarditis in the control group. It will be seen that the two groups were comparable on admission, apart from a higher incidence of severe cardiac changes in the salicylate group.

Analysis of Results

The extraction of data from the records and their analysis was made by one of us (R. S. I.) with statistical help by J. F. S.

1. *The effect on arthritis.* We found it difficult to determine whether sodium salicylate had any effect on the arthritis, because in many children arthritis subsided very quickly with mere rest in bed. The figures given below are based on all the children who at some stage of their rheumatic fever had arthritis; there were 22 such children in the control group, and 27 in the salicylate group. Tables VI and VII show the relevant data. In eight of the 22 control cases and 11 of the 27 salicylate cases the arthritis had already disappeared before admission to the hospital. In a further three of the control cases and eight of the salicylate cases the arthritis disappeared after admission to hospital, during the period in which the diagnosis was being established, and therefore, in the case of the salicylate group, before sodium salicylate had been given. In one patient of the salicylate group, in whom the arthritis had subsided before admission to

hospital, there was a recurrence of arthritis on the fifth day, the day on which sodium salicylate was first given; there remain for study, therefore, this child and eight others in the salicylate group, and 11 in the control group. The average duration of arthritis in the 11 children in the control group was 5·8 days after allocation to the group, compared with 4·0 days in the nine children in

TABLE VI

Course of Arthritis: Control Group

Case number	*Arthritis better before admission to hospital*	*Arthritis when admitted to hospital; better before admission to investigation (day after admission to hospital by which arthritis had disappeared)*	*Arthritis when admitted to investigation. Loss of pain and swelling (day after admission to investigation)*	*Relapse of arthritis (day after admission to investigation. Second figure indicates day on which arthritis subsided)*
1	..	..	2	..
2	+	..	..	..
3	..	..	5	12–17
4	..	..	12	..
5 T	..	..	27 T	T
6	+	..	..	..
7	..	..	2	..
8	..	..	1	..
9	+	..	..	..
10	..	1	..	..
14	..	..	2	15–17
15	+	..	..	..
16	+	..	..	5–14
17	..	2	..	..
18	+	..	..	8–20
19	+	..	..	..
20	..	..	6	10–11; 30–31
21	..	..	2	..
22	..	..	4	..
45	+	..	..	25–31
46	..	..	1	..
50	..	1	..	..

Cases 11, 12, 13, 47, 48, and 49 did not have arthritis.

T = Transferred to salicylate group on day 28.

the salicylate group. This difference is not significant, especially in view of the fact that the control group was weighted with one child (Case 5) who had continuing arthritis for 27 days after allocation to her group. She was then transferred to the salicylate group, and it is interesting to note that the arthritis was not controlled by sodium salicylate, although a high serum-salicylate level was maintained; for she developed a recurrence of arthritis on the 90th day, when the level was 36 mg. per 100 ml., and on the 121st day, when the level was between 36 and 42 mg. per 100 ml. There was a recurrence of arthritis in six of the 22 control cases, one child suffering two recurrences. In the salicylate group one child had two short recurrences shortly after commencing treatment, and one child had a recurrence when the salicylate was discontinued, when a rebound phenomenon occurred. Although the figures suggest that the arthritis settled down more quickly in the salicylate group, the difference is not of

TABLE VII

Course of Arthritis: Salicylate Group

Case number	Arthritis better before admission to hospital	Arthritis when admitted to hospital; better before salicylates were given (day after admission to hospital by which arthritis had disappeared)	Arthritis when admitted to investigation. Loss of pain and swelling (day after admission to investigation)	Relapse of arthritis (day after salicylates were started. Second figure indicates day on which arthritis subsided)
23	..	..	1	..
24	..	2	..	..
25	..	..	2	..
26	+	..	7*	..
27 D	+	..	..	..
28	..	..	2	..
29	..	..	8	..
30	+	..	..	..
31	+	..	..	..
32	+	..	..	..
33	..	1	..	..
34	..	2	..	..
35	+	..	..	..
36	..	3	..	..
37	..	2	..	..
38	..	..	7	..
39	..	1	..	..
40	+	..	..	..
41	+	..	..	..
42	..	..	4	..
43	..	..	2	..
44	..	..	3	5–6; 11–12
51	+	..	..	..
52	+	..	..	..
53	..	1	..	48–55†
54	+	..	..	..
55	..	5	..	..

* This patient had no arthritis on admission, but it recurred on the 5th day, and salicylates were started on that day. It was better on the 12th day after admission, 7 days after the drug was started.

D = Died on the 7th day.

† After salicylates were stopped.

TABLE VIII

Comparison of Temperatures

Group	Number of children	Highest temperature in first 7 days (°F.) (mean)	First day (from admission) on which the temperature became normal	First day (from admission) on which the temperature became normal and remained so for 3 days
Control . .	15	101·4	9·5*	14·0*
Salicylate . .	15	101·9	5·2	6·8

* The temperature of one child (Case 18) had not fallen to normal by the 23rd day, when he was in error given sodium salicylate for 5 days. For the purpose of calculating the mean day on which the temperature first became normal for one day and for three days, the figure of 23 was used for this child. Subsequent figures had to be disregarded. Another child (Case 5) had a normal temperature on the 15th day, but did not have a normal temperature for 3 days before her transfer to the salicylate group on the 28th day. For the purpose of calculating the mean day on which the temperature first fell to normal for 3 days, the figure of 28 was used for this child.

Table IX

Mean Sleeping Pulse-Rate

Group	*Highest in first 7 days*	*Days from admission*							
		1–7	8–14	15–21	22–28	60–66	90–96	120–126	180–186
Control . (28 children)	104	92	86	88	86	83	84	87	82
Salicylate . (26 children)*	100	93	84	86	81	83	80	82	83

* One child (Case 27) died on the 7th day.

statistical significance. The results give a definite impression, however, that recurrences of arthritis were less likely in children receiving the drug.

2. *The effect on the temperature.* In most of the control cases the temperature fell rapidly after admission to hospital, and in many of the salicylate cases it had already fallen or begun to fall before the drug was started, in the period between admission and the establishment of the diagnosis. For purposes of comparison we have studied the 30 children, 15 in each group, in whom the

TABLE X

Changes in Apical Systolic Murmurs

	Control group		*Salicylate group*	
	Number of cases at risk	*Number in which change occurred*	*Number of cases at risk*	*Number in which change occurred*
Increase by 2 grades or more, or change from no murmur to Grade 2	22 N	2	21 N	0
	6 R	1	5 R	0
Reduction by 2 grades or more	12 N	4	11 N	6
	5 R	0	4 R	1

N = New cases. R = Relapse cases.

TABLE XI

Changes in Apical Diastolic Murmurs

	Control group		*Salicylate group*	
	Number of cases	*Disappearance of murmur in hospital*	*Number of cases*	*Disappearance of murmur in hospital*
Apical diastolic murmur on admission	4 N	2 N	3 N	3 N
	4 R	1 R	3 R	2 R
Apical diastolic murmur developed in hospital	2 N	2 N	1 N	1 N
	1 R	..	1 R	1 R
Total	11	5	8	7

N = New cases. R = Relapse cases.

temperature was 100° F. or over at any time in the first seven days after admission to hospital. We calculated the mean day on which the temperature first remained normal for one day, and the mean day on which it first remained normal for three consecutive days (Table VIII). It will be seen that, although the initial temperature was slightly higher in the salicylate group, its fall was significantly quicker than in the control group.

3. *The effect on the sleeping pulse-rate.* The assessment of the effect of salicylates was complicated by the frequent occurrence of sinus bradycardia just after the acute stage. This bradycardia, however, was of short duration, and had no effect on the figures after the first month or two. Table IX shows the mean sleeping pulse-rate in the two groups at varying periods after admission. It will be seen that there is no significant difference in the two groups.

4. *Changes in cardiac murmurs.* Tables X and XI show the data concerning significant changes in cardiac murmurs. In the case of apical systolic murmurs,

17 children in the control group and 16 in the salicylate group had a murmur of Grade 2 or more on admission. One of the children in the salicylate group died on the seventh day. Excluding this child, there was a reduction of two grades or more in the intensity of the murmur before discharge in four of the 17 children at risk in the control group, compared with seven of the 15 children at risk in the salicylate group. This reduction involved complete disappearance of the murmur in three of the control group and two of the salicylate group.

TABLE XII

Development of Certain Rheumatic Manifestations

Case number	*Day after admission on which the manifestations developed* — *Nodules*	*Erythema marginatum*	*Pneumonia*	*Chorea*	*Heart failure*	*Years and months after admission* — *Relapses*
Control group:						
1	..	..	..	..	..	1
3	..	..	..	28	35	1·4 T
4	..	..	..	..	..	1·4
7	36	..	..	..	..	..
13	..	..	..	..	120	3·9
14	90	..	..	..	..	2·5
46 R	..	..	..	120	..	0·8
47 R	..	..	..	260	..	2·1
48 R	..	..	..	..	..	3·1 D
49 R	64	180	..	..	..	1·5+2·7
50 R	..	18	..	..	..	..
Salicylate group:						
30	..	..	14	..	..	3·4
37	12+40	..	..	43	..	1·2
41	..	103	..	..	..	..
51 R	84+126	..	..	..	..	..
52 R	..	..	..	..	..	2·4
53 R	..	38+97	..	..	..	..

R = Relapse case. T = After transfer to salicylate group. D = Died.

Three of the control group, and none of the salicylate group, had an increase of two or more grades in the intensity of the murmur. In the case of apical diastolic murmurs, four new cases and four relapse cases in the control series had diastolic murmurs on admission; three of these eight children lost the murmurs before discharge. Three other children developed apical diastolic murmurs during their stay in hospital, and in two the murmurs disappeared before discharge. Three new cases and three relapse cases in the salicylate series had apical murmurs on admission; five of these six lost their diastolic murmur before discharge. Two children developed diastolic murmurs during their stay in hospital, and both lost them before discharge. In no case was the development of an aortic diastolic murmur observed after admission. None of these differences are significant, but they give the impression that the salicylate group fared better than the control group.

5. *The development of other rheumatic manifestations in hospital, and relapses.* Thirteen children, eight in the control group and five in the salicylate group,

developed fresh manifestations of rheumatic fever while in hospital. These manifestations consisted of new rheumatic nodules, erythema marginatum, rheumatic pneumonia, chorea, and heart failure in the course of active rheumatic fever. The child who was excluded from the investigation and given ACTH has already been mentioned. It is of interest that eight of the nine episodes in the five patients in the salicylate group occurred while they were still receiving the drug, and in six out of seven of these episodes the serum-salicylate level was adequate (over 30 mg. per 100 ml.) at the time. There was a relapse of rheumatic fever in eight patients in the control group; one relapse was fatal. One child had two relapses. Four of these patients were new cases and four were relapse cases when admitted to the investigation. In the salicylate group three patients relapsed, two new cases and one relapse case. In addition one child (Case 3), who was transferred from the control group, relapsed after a course of salicylate treatment. The findings are summarized in Table XII. These data give the impression that patients receiving salicylates were less likely to develop fresh rheumatic manifestations, and to suffer relapses, than those who were not given the drug. The numbers, however, are small, and the differences are not of statistical significance.

6. *The effect on the erythrocyte sedimentation rate.* It was difficult to analyse the changes because, in 29 out of 49 children in whom the E.S.R. fell to normal before discharge, it rose again and remained raised for two or more consecutive readings after the first normal result, and in several children it subsequently remained above normal for many weeks. In 18 out of 43 children it rose above normal, and remained so for two or more consecutive readings, after two consecutive normal figures. Eventually, however, the E.S.R. returned to normal in all survivors, though in some cases only after they had gone home. Another difficulty in the analysis was the 'rebound phenomenon' when salicylates were stopped. In 11 out of 25 children[3] in the salicylate series the E.S.R. rose when the drug was discontinued. Of the six children who received a second course of salicylates, four and possibly five had a further 'rebound'. It is interesting to note that one of these children (Case 53) had a recurrence of arthritis in the rebound as soon as the drug was stopped, while another (Case 54) had a recurrence of her pericarditis. These recurrences may have been coincidental, but it is possible that they indicate that salicylates had been exerting a suppressive effect on the rheumatic manifestations. A normal E.S.R. does not absolutely exclude rheumatic activity. It is commonly normal in heart failure. It was normal in two of our patients (Cases 43 and 51) at a time when erythema marginatum developed, and in one of these (Case 51) when new rheumatic nodules developed, but these cases are exceptional.

As a preliminary step to analysis of the data, the statistician compared the figures obtained by the Wintrobe and Westergren methods (Table XIII). In neither group was the difference in the fall of the E.S.R., as recorded by the two methods, significantly different, the 'Student's *t*' for control and salicylate

[3] The two patients excluded were one who died (Case 27) and one who was taken home against advice (Case 26).

groups being 1·36 and 1·03 respectively. An attempt was then made to determine whether the E.S.R. fell more quickly in one group than in the other. Since the initial E.S.R. varied quite considerably (from 21 to 70 mm. in an hour), some allowance must be made for this initial value. The figures for each child were plotted as a time-series, and it appeared that the E.S.R. fell fairly steadily in most cases, varying about what looks like a decreasing exponential curve. It is reasonable to take the estimated time the E.S.R. takes to fall to half its initial value as a measure of the rate of fall. This has been called

TABLE XIII

The Wintrobe and Westergren Methods

	Control group		*Salicylate group*	
Method	*Mean log half-time*	*Number of cases*	*Mean log half-time*	*Number of cases*
Wintrobe	1·902	5	1·510	5
Westergren	1·672	20	1·384	21

the 'half-time'. A short half-time means that the E.S.R. falls quickly, and a long one means that it falls more slowly. The half-time was estimated from the graphs by eye by two independent observers, and their results were quite consistent. The use of this half-time avoids the difficulty of dealing with the figures for children whose E.S.R. is still above normal on discharge. The distribution of half-times was decidedly skew, however, both for the control and salicylate groups, there being one or two abnormally high values. Since the t test is theoretically applicable only to normally distributed variables, it is necessary to transform the half-times to give a more symmetrical distribution. The use of a logarithmic transformation would achieve this, and this procedure is supported by the fact that the standard deviation of half-times rises in proportion with the mean, as various groups and sub-groups of children are considered. Taking the logarithms of half-times, in effect, avoids giving undue weight to the one or two abnormally high values mentioned above. In three children of the control group it was impossible to obtain reliable half-times: two of these (Cases 3 and 5) were transferred to the salicylate group, and one (Case 11) was discharged against advice before sufficient figures could be obtained. One child of the salicylate group (Case 27) died after only one E.S.R. measurement. This leaves a total of 25 control and 26 salicylate cases.

There is some evidence to show that the E.S.R. takes longer to fall in relapse cases than in new cases. A comparison of the mean log half-times for relapse and new cases gives $t = 1{\cdot}86$ (on 23 degrees of freedom) for controls, and $t = 2{\cdot}23$ (on 24 degrees of freedom) for salicylate cases. The second figure is significant, and the first approaches significance. Among the relapse cases, however, the readings in the salicylate group fell much more quickly than those in the control group. Comparing new cases, the mean log half-time for the salicylate group is 1·36 (corresponding to about 23 days), and for the control group 1·65 (corresponding to about 45 days). This gives $t = 3{\cdot}26$ (on 38 degrees of freedom), which is significant at the 1 per cent. level. Comparison of the relapse cases gives $t = 1{\cdot}82$ (on 9 degrees of freedom), and even this approaches significance. There is thus strong evidence that salicylates cause the E.S.R. to fall more quickly. As a confirmatory test the first day on which the E.S.R. became normal was recorded, and for reasons similar to those given above a logarithmic transformation was made. This gave $t = 3{\cdot}36$ (on 39 degrees of freedom), which is significant at the 1 per cent. level (new cases only). There were two control children who were discharged without ever reaching a normal E.S.R. In these cases the E.S.R. was assumed to become normal immediately on leaving hospital. This approximation only strengthens the conclusion that the E.S.R. in the salicylate group reached normal sooner than in the control group. The more rapid fall of the E.S.R. in the salicylate group is also shown by a study of those children in whom the E.S.R. was 40 mm. or more per hour

TABLE XIV

Percentage of Children with Normal Erythrocyte Sedimentation Rate at Intervals after Admission

	Months after admission		
	3	4	5
Control group:			
Percentage with normal E.S.R. . . .	43	48	50
Salicylate group:			
Percentage with normal E.S.R. . . .	76	65	60
Number of patients still receiving salicylate .	4	4	2

The following were excluded from the Table: *Control group*: two children who were discharged against advice (both with a raised E.S.R.), and two transfer cases (Nos. 3 and 5). *Salicylate group*: three children who were discharged against advice (two with a raised E.S.R.), and one who died (Case 27).

TABLE XV

Relationship of Duration of Attack Before Admission to Fall of E.S.R.

Group	*Short duration (less than 21 days); log half-time*	*Long duration (21 days or more); log half-time*	*t*	*Degrees of freedom*
Control	1·542	1·882	2·39*	17
Salicylate	1·321	1·411	1·09	19

* Significant at the 5 per cent. level.

at the time of admission. There were 22 such children in the salicylate group and 24 in the control group. Of the 22 children in the salicylate group, one was discharged against advice on the 35th day with a slightly raised E.S.R., and one died; in 19 of the remaining 20 children the E.S.R. had returned to normal for the first time in under 50 days. By the 62nd day the E.S.R. had returned to normal in all children in the salicylate group, but in the control group it was still raised in 13 children after 100 days, and in four children after 200 days.

We then set out to determine whether the more rapid fall of the E.S.R. in the salicylate group was due merely to a direct chemical action of the salicylate on the blood. For this purpose we calculated the percentage of children in each group who had a normal E.S.R. three months, four months, and five months after admission (Table XIV). It will be seen that three months after admission, at a time when only four patients were still receiving salicylates, 76 per cent. of the children in the salicylate group had a normal E.S.R., compared with 43 per cent. in the control group. This difference is of statistical significance. The other differences give the impression that the E.S.R. was lower in the salicylate group, but they are not of statistical significance.

The next question was whether the duration of the attack before admission had any bearing on the rate of fall of the E.S.R. The children were divided into two classes; those with a short duration (less than 21 days), and those with a longer one (21 days or more). The mean log half-times for the two classes, in both control and salicylate groups, were then calculated (new cases only). The difference between the 'short' and 'long-duration' patients was significant in the control group, but not in the salicylate group. Table XV shows the results.

The findings may be summarized as follows:

(1) There was no significant difference in the rate of fall of the E.S.R. when the Wintrobe and Westergren methods were used.

(2) The rate of fall was significantly quicker in the salicylate group than in the control group. The E.S.R. reached normal much sooner in the salicylate group.

(3) The more rapid fall of the E.S.R. in the salicylate group was not due merely to a direct action on the blood, for after the drug had been discontinued the E.S.R. remained at a lower figure than in the control group.

(4) In the control group the rate of fall was significantly quicker in cases of short duration than in those of long duration; in the salicylate group the rate of fall was unrelated to the duration of the attack.

7. *The effect of salicylates on the patients transferred to the salicylate group.* Five patients originally belonging to the control group were given salicylates, as already mentioned. The transfer of two patients (Cases 43 and 44) took place so soon after admission (on the ninth and third days respectively) that they were regarded as belonging to the salicylate group from the beginning. The course of the illness in the other three requires separate consideration.

Case 3. This six-year-old boy was transferred to the salicylate group on the 44th day on account of a persistently high E.S.R. and sleeping pulse-rate, and the development of an apical diastolic murmur and heart failure. He had no fever at the time of transfer. It was not possible to maintain a satisfactory serum-salicylate level, the average reading being only 22·2 mg. per 100 ml. Fig. 1 shows the course of the E.S.R. in graphic form, and Table XVI shows the sleeping pulse-rate. The boy recovered from his heart failure, and his diastolic murmur disappeared. The E.S.R. fell rapidly after transfer, but the fall of the sleeping pulse-rate was not accelerated.

Case 5. This 10-year-old girl was transferred on the 28th day to the salicylate group on account of recurrent attacks of arthritis, with persistent fever and a high E.S.R. She was treated with sodium salicylate for 133 days, and the average serum level was 33·3 mg. per 100 ml. Fig. 2 shows the course of the E.S.R. Table XVI shows that the sleeping pulse-rate and temperature had begun to fall before the drug was started. The E.S.R. fell, but rose again, and remained above normal. Recurrent attacks of arthritis continued in spite of a good serum-salicylate level. Salicylates in this case apparently had no effect.

Case 46. This 12-year-old boy was transferred to the salicylate group on the 300th day on account of continued rheumatic activity and a recurrence of arthritis. He had developed chorea on the 120th day after admission, and a mitral diastolic murmur on the 245th day. Fig. 3 shows that there was a fairly rapid fall in the E.S.R. Unfortunately a page of the sleeping-pulse records was lost, and figures respecting them cannot be given. He had no fever. The

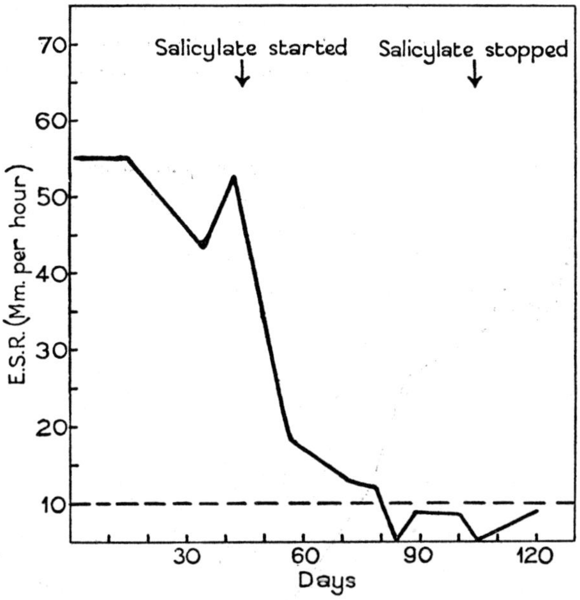

FIG. 1. Course of erythrocyte sedimentation rate in Case 3. The dotted line indicates the upper limit of normal (micromethod).

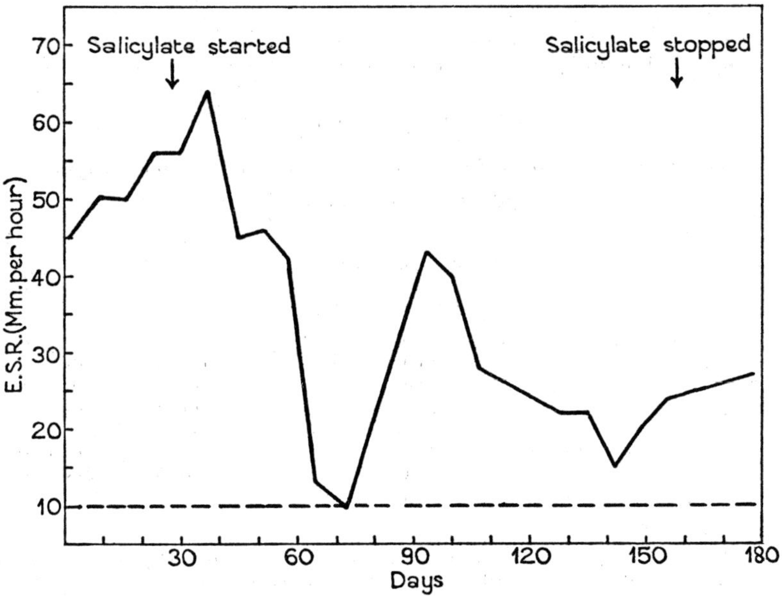

FIG. 2. Course of erythrocyte sedimentation rate in Case 5. The dotted line indicates the upper limit of normal (micromethod).

average serum-salicylate level was 31·3 mg. per 100 ml. There was no apparent improvement in his clinical condition, and it is uncertain whether the drug helped.

The above data leave one uncertain whether these three children were benefited by being given salicylates.

8. *Findings on the last examination of new cases.* Table XVII summarizes the results of the clinical and radiological studies at the time of the last examination. Cases 3 and 5 are placed at the foot of the Table, and cannot be used

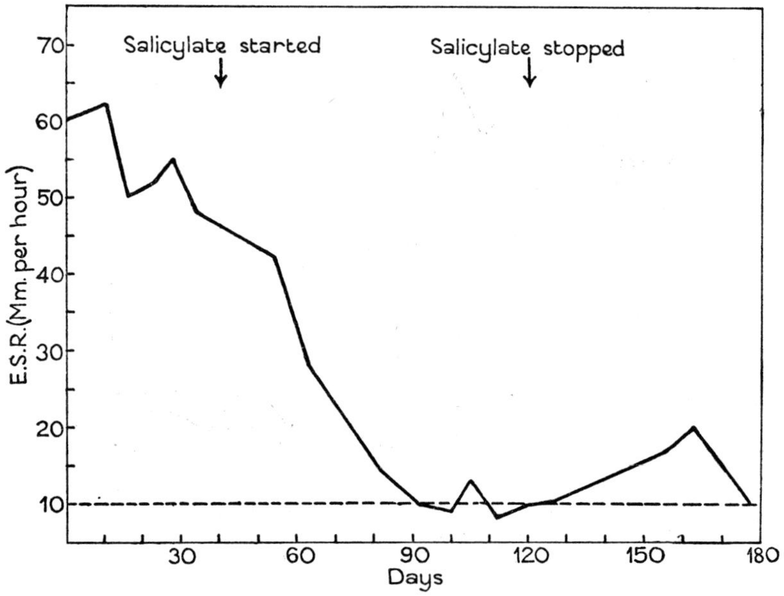

FIG. 3. Course of erythrocyte sedimentation rate in Case 46. The dotted line indicates the upper limit of normal (micromethod).

TABLE XVI

Sleeping Pulse-Rate and Temperature in Transfer Cases Before and After Starting Salicylate Therapy

	Average sleeping pulse-rate		*Temperature (°F.) Case 5*	
	Case 3	*Case 5*	*Average*	*Range*
4 weeks before starting drug	110	120	101·3	99·0–104·2
3 ,, ,, ,,	119	104	100·3	99·2–101·2
2 ,, ,, ,,	118	96	100·1	98·4–103·5
1 week ,, ,,	118	87	100·4	99·4–102·0
1st week after starting drug	116	81	99·7	98·4–102·0
2nd ,, ,, ,,	94	84	98·8	98·4–100·6
3rd ,, ,, ,,	96	84	..	..
4th ,, ,, ,,	..	87	..	..

The average sleeping pulse-rate and temperature is calculated from the maximum in each 24 hours. Case 46 is not included in the Table because some figures were incomplete.

for comparison, as they were transferred to the salicylate group on the 44th and 28th days respectively. The average duration of observation from the date of admission in the control cases was 32·2 months, and in the salicylate cases 31·0 months. These figures exclude the two transferred cases, Nos. 3 and 5.

Of the 17 new control cases left for study, nine were considered to have escaped cardiac damage, one had mitral and aortic disease, three had mitral disease alone, and the remaining four children had doubtful, though probable, clinical

TABLE XVII

Results of Last Examination

The children not included in this Table are Case 27, who died, and those in whom the period of observation was less than one year.

Group	Case number	Duration of observation (years and months)	Condition of heart: Normal	Condition of heart: Mitral disease	Condition of heart: Mitral and aortic disease
Control group	1	4·0	+	..	..
	2	3·2	+	..	..
	4	3·11	..	±	..
	6	2·9	..	±	..
	9	3·2	+	..	..
	10	2·3	..	..	+
	11	2·10	..	+	..
	13	4·0	..	+	..
	14	2·10	..	±	..
	15	1·4	+	..	..
	16	3·3	+	..	..
	17	3·4	+	..	..
	18	1·1	+	..	..
	19	1·0	..	±	..
	20	1·1	..	+	..
	21	2·8	+	..	..
	22	2·11	+	..	..
	3 T	2·9	..	+	..
	5 T	1·4	+	..	..
Salicylate group	24	2·9	+	..	..
	25	2·11	+	..	..
	26	3·2	+	..	..
	28	1·1	..	±	..
	29	3·1	+	..	..
	30	3·4	..	..	+
	31	2·2	..	+	..
	32	2·3	+	..	..
	33	3·0	+	..	..
	34	2·10	+	..	..
	35	1·1	+	..	..
	36	2·8	+	..	..
	37	2·11	..	+	..
	38	2·9	+	..	..
	39	2·5	+	..	..
	41	3·3	..	+	..
	42	3·5	+	..	..
	43 T	2·7	+	..	..
	44 T	1·3	+	..	..

T = Transferred from control group.

± = Doubtful but probable mitral disease.

and radiological signs of valvular disease. One child (Case 13) had lost a diastolic murmur since discharge, and in one child (Case 16) there had been a reduction of three grades in the systolic apical murmur since he left hospital. Of the 19 children in the salicylate group, 14 were considered to have escaped cardiac damage, one had mitral and aortic disease, three had mitral disease alone, and one had doubtful, though probable, signs of valvular disease. It should be noted that of the three children who had had pericarditis, two (Cases 43 and 44), who had been transferred from the control group because of their grave illness, were considered to have no evidence of cardiac damage. In one child (Case 32) there had been a reduction of two grades in the apical systolic murmur. In one child (Case 30) an apical diastolic murmur had reappeared since her discharge from hospital. These differences are not of statistical significance.

Discussion

The present study amply shows the difficulty of assessing the value of a drug by strict statistical methods in a disease which has such great variations in its natural history. We approached the investigation with no preconceived ideas concerning the value of salicylates, and a detailed analysis had to be made before we could reach any conclusion. The number of cases is small, and the period of observation has not yet been concluded. Ethical considerations make an investigation of this kind difficult, and it is likely to be impossible to determine how patients with severe rheumatic fever would fare without salicylates, because one is forced to give them the benefit of the doubt and treat them. The severity of diseases of infective origin changes from time to time, and it may well be that the cases which we see now are less severe than those seen 50 years ago. The differences between the two groups might have been more obvious if the disease had been more severe, if we had given salicylates for a longer period, or if we had achieved higher serum-salicylate levels. Nevertheless the present investigation provides some evidence that salicylates as we gave them, and in large doses, are of value in the treatment of rheumatic fever.

The salicylate group was loaded with two severe cases transferred from the control group, and by chance contained more children with pericarditis and definite carditis on admission. In spite of that, the salicylate group gave the impression of faring better in all the manifestations of rheumatic fever which we studied, although the differences were usually small and most of them were not of statistical significance. It must be remembered that one patient in the salicylate group died on the seventh day after admission,[4] and that another was withdrawn in order to be treated with ACTH. In the salicylate group the temperature and erythrocyte sedimentation rate fell more quickly, and it was shown that the more rapid fall was not merely due to a direct action of salicylate on the blood. It was of special interest to note that, whereas the duration of symptoms before treatment began had no effect on the speed of fall of the erythrocyte sedimentation rate in the salicylate cases, there was a considerable effect in the control cases, the rate falling more slowly in those of long duration. This fact is not in keeping with the idea, so often expressed, that salicylates are of value only if they are given early. Other differences were not

[4] There was one other death during the period of observation: No. 48, a relapse case in the control series.

of statistical significance, but in every aspect of the disease analysed the differences were in favour of salicylates. The arthritis settled down a little more quickly in the salicylate group, and there were fewer relapses of arthritis. Fewer children in the salicylate group developed new rheumatic manifestations, such as nodules; fewer had relapses of their rheumatic fever; fewer developed apical diastolic murmurs, and more lost them; fewer showed an increase in the grade of apical systolic murmurs, and more showed a decrease; and the impression gained in the last examination was that the salicylate group had escaped with less cardiac damage. There was practically no difference in the sleeping pulse-rate between the two groups; what difference there was favoured salicylates. As none of these manifestations are interdependent, it seems reasonable to suggest that, even though only a few differences were of statistical significance, the overall picture indicates that salicylates were of value in treatment. It is of special interest that we were unable to detect a significantly more rapid subsidence of arthritis in the children who were treated with salicylates. The children had arthritis of varying degrees of severity, but it is possible that we should have been able to demonstrate a greater effect if the arthritis had been more severe. The results also demonstrate the inadequacy of using the erythrocyte sedimentation rate as a sign of 'cure' of rheumatic fever: its frequent rise when salicylates were stopped indicates that only long-term studies are of real value.

In conclusion, though we feel that salicylates are of value in rheumatic fever, we do not know what dose should be given, or for how long the drug should be continued. We do not know whether the drug should be restarted when a rebound phenomenon occurs. All these are matters for future study. It seems especially important to determine whether children treated with salicylates in high dosage fare as well as those treated with low dosage, such as is commonly used in general practice; and this we propose to try to determine. From our experience of toxic complications, which are very frequent with the dosage used by us, we feel that this dosage should not be used in general practice, because of the lack of constant supervision and of adequate biochemical assistance.

Acknowledgements

Our thanks are due to Dr. John Wilkie for the radiological studies, to Miss Ethel Finch for the biochemical studies, to Mr. G. H. Jowett for statistical advice, and to Miss W. M. Gibson for help with calculations. We wish to thank Dr. J. Knowelden, of the London School of Hygiene and Tropical Medicine, and Professor E. J. Wayne, of the University of Sheffield, for reading through the paper. We owe a particular debt to all the house physicians, nurses, and sisters who were responsible for the day-to-day care of the children. We would also like to thank the numerous family doctors who sent us their cases.

Summary

1. We have presented a preliminary report of a controlled investigation into the value of salicylates in rheumatic fever. The natural history of rheumatic

fever in children receiving high doses of salicylates was compared with that seen in children not receiving the drug. The treatment was chosen by random sampling. Fifty-five cases were studied, including 22 new cases treated with the drug and 22 new cases treated as controls. All the children were observed continuously for an average period of nearly three years. The observation of these children is continuing.

2. The fall of temperature was significantly quicker in the salicylate group than in the control group.

3. The fall of the erythrocyte sedimentation rate was significantly quicker in the salicylate group, and the rate reached normal sooner. It was shown that this difference was not merely due to a direct action of the drug on the blood. In the control group the fall of the erythrocyte sedimentation rate was significantly quicker in cases of short duration than in those of long duration; in the salicylate group its rate of fall was unrelated to the duration of the attack.

4. Other differences between the two groups were not of statistical significance. The results all gave the impression, however, that the salicylate group fared better than the control group. Fewer children in the salicylate group developed rheumatic manifestations, such as nodules, while in hospital; fewer suffered relapses; fewer had recurrences of arthritis; fewer developed apical diastolic murmurs, and more lost them; fewer had an increase in the intensity of apical systolic murmurs, and more had a decrease in the intensity of those murmurs; more were apparently free from cardiac involvement at the time of the last examination.

REFERENCES

Bendien, W. M., Neuberg, J., and Snapper, I. (1932) *Biochem. Zts.* **247**, 306. Quoted by Homburger (1945).
Brodie, B. B., Udenfriend, S., and Coburn, A. F. (1944) *J. Pharmacol. Exp. Therap.* **80**, 114.
Coburn, A. F. (1943*a*) *Bull. Johns Hopkins Hosp.* **73**, 435.
—— (1943*b*) *U.S. Nav. M. Bull.* **41**, 1324.
Danielopolu, D., Dimitriu, C., and Mme Cimino-Beranger (1934) *Acta rheumatol.* **6**, 42.
Finlay, D. W., and Lucas, R. H. (1879) *Lancet*, **2**, 420.
Goodman, L., and Gilman, A. (1941) *The Pharmacological Basis of Therapeutics*, New York.
Gross, M., and Greenberg, L. A. (1948) *The Salicylates*, New Haven, Conn.
Hanzlik, P. J. (1926) *Medicine*, **5**, 197.
Harris, T. N. (1947) *Amer. J. Med. Sci.* **213**, 482.
Homburger, F. (1945) Ibid. **210**, 168.
—— (1946) Ibid. **211**, 346.
Hood, D. W. C. (1881) *Lancet*, **2**, 1119.
Jager, B. V., and Alway, R. (1946) *Amer. J. Med. Sci.* **211**, 273.
Jones, T. D. (1944) *J. Amer. Med. Ass.* **126**, 481.
Keith, J. D., and Ross, A. (1945) *Canad. Med. Ass. J.* **52**, 554.
Lees, D. B. (1903) *Brit. Med. J.* **2**, 1318.
Levine, S. A., and Harvey, W. P. (1949) *Clinical Auscultation of the Heart*, London.
Levy, R. L., and Turner, K. B. (1927–8) *Proc. Soc. Exper. Biol. Med.* **25**, 64.
Lichty, J. A., and Hooker, S. P. (1941) Ibid. **48**, 69.
Maclagan, T. (1876) *Lancet*, **1**, 342.
Manchester, R. C. (1946*a*) *Arch. Int. Med.* **78**, 170.

Manchester, R. C. (1946*b*) *J. Amer. Med. Ass.* **131**, 209.
Master, A. M., and Romanoff, A. (1932) Ibid. **98**, 1978.
Murphy, G. E. (1945) *Bull. Johns Hopkins Hosp.* **77**, 1.
Murray-Lyon, R. M. (1936) *Edin. Med. J.* **43**, 84.
Rapoport, S., and Guest, G. M. (1946) *Proc. Soc. Exper. Biol. Med.* **61**, 43.
Reid, J. (1948) *Quart. J. Med.* N.S. **17**, 139.
Stricker, S. (1876) *Berl. klin. Woch.* **13**, 15, 99. Quoted by Murphy (1945).
Taran, L. M., and Jacobs, M. H. (1945) *J. Pediat.* **27**, 59.
Warren, H. A., Higley, C. S., and Coombs, F. S. (1946*a*) *Amer. Heart J.* **32**, 311.
—— —— —— (1946*b*) *J. Lab. Clin. Med.* **31**, 485.
Watkinson, G. (1949) *Ann. Rheum. Dis.* **8**, 120.
Wégria, R., and Smull, K. (1945) *J. Amer. Med. Ass.* **129**, 485.
Wright, I. S. (1945) *Bull. New York Acad. Med.* **21**, 419.
Wyckoff, J., DeGraff, A. C., and Parent, S. (1929–30) *Amer. Heart J.* **5**, 568.

616.8–009.7–031.59

PINK DISEASE: THE AUTONOMIC DISORDER AND ITS TREATMENT WITH GANGLION-BLOCKING AGENTS[1]

By B. D. BOWER

(From the Department of Paediatrics and Child Health, University of Birmingham, and the Children's Hospital, Birmingham)

With Plate 18

In the earliest description of pink disease (Selter, 1903) signs suggesting a disorder of autonomic function are mentioned, and ever since the term 'vegetative neurosis' was invented (Feer, 1925; Selter, 1927) attention has been directed to the autonomic nervous system in discussions on the pathogenesis of this disease. It is therefore curious that little experimental work designed to delineate more clearly the nature of the autonomic disorder has been published. During an investigation into peripheral vasomotor control in children at various ages, it was discovered that patients suffering from pink disease reacted quite differently from normal children of the same age. The purpose of the present paper is to demonstrate this difference, and to show how the two ganglion-blocking agents, hexamethonium bromide and pentapyrrolidinium bitartrate ('M. and B. 2050A'), can both experimentally and clinically restore vasomotor and other autonomic disturbances to normal.

Method of Investigation

When a part of the body is heated so that warmed blood, and possibly also afferent nervous impulses, reach the hypothalamus, the result in the normal adult is vasodilatation (Duthie and Mackay, 1940; Fulton, 1943), which is most marked at the extremities. Arteriolar tone is inhibited, and possibly vasodilator fibres are stimulated (Lewis and Pickering, 1931; Duthie and Mackay, 1940); but, whatever the precise nature of the peripheral mechanism, the efferent pathway is the sympathetic nervous system (Lewis and Pickering, 1931; Richards, 1946). The classical method of estimating the degree of vasodilatation is to measure acral skin temperatures and, although the relationship between blood-flow and skin temperature is not simple, this method gives useful information when comparisons are made between patients subjected to similar conditions. Recent criticism of the method as being of no value because large increases in blood-flow only produce small increases in skin temperature (McPherson, 1953) is surely unjustified. Lewis (1946) regarded it as 'perhaps the most reliable method of gauging the state of blood-flow to a resting limb clinically'. Cooper, Cross, Greenfield, Hamilton, and Scarborough (1949), in comparing the results of skin thermometry, plethysmography, and calorimetry, found that skin thermometry reflected increases in blood-flow fairly well, although the relationship

[1] Received August 18, 1953.

was not linear. The apparatus is fairly simple, and the method requires little co-operation from the patient, and is therefore suitable for children.

The 'limb-immersion' method (Gibbon and Landis, 1932; Richards, 1946) was modified for infants and used throughout the investigation. (In older children no modification was needed. The child sat in a chair with one arm in a basin of warmed water.) The apparatus is shown in Plate 18, Fig. 5. The baby lay on his right side, with his right arm passing through a hole in the canvas sheet *A* into a heat-lagged can containing water (not shown), which throughout the experiment was maintained at 42° to 44° C. by frequent partial replacement of cool water with hot through the hole *B*. He was naked except for a napkin, and was kept in position by canvas bands *C*, attached to the canvas sheet *A*, which secured his trunk, left arm, and if necessary his legs. Temperatures were recorded at three- to six-minute intervals with a Cambridge Instrument Co. skin-temperature measuring apparatus, and copper-constantan thermocouples attached to the three non-immersed limbs with strips of zinc oxide plaster. The sites of attachment were, in the feet, on the dorsum between the bases of the first and second toes, and in the non-immersed hand on the dorsum between the index and middle fingers. Two further leads recorded the temperature of the water in the immersion can and that of the air above the cot. Room temperature did not vary by more than 1° C. in any experiment. Since a constant-temperature room was not available, it varied from day to day, but the range was not extreme (18° to 23° C.), and it was felt that this factor could be ignored, as had been done in adults (Gibbon and Landis, 1932; Richards, 1946), provided no conclusions were drawn from initial temperatures, which would partly depend upon room temperature. The arm was immersed throughout the experiment, which was discontinued either when the temperature of the other three limbs had reached its maximum, or when it was clear that no rise would occur. Graphs were plotted, and from them the following values were selected for comparison (Fig. 1*a*).

T_R: the time in minutes after immersion of the arm before the temperature of the feet started to rise (mean value for the two feet).

$T_{max.}$: the time in minutes from immersion of the arm to attainment of the maximum temperature in the feet (mean value for the two feet).

m.t.: the maximum temperature of the feet (degrees Centigrade) (mean value for the two feet).

The effect of a low initial temperature in increasing the value of $T_{max.}$ was considered to be negligible, since once the rise started it was completed fairly quickly (Fig. 1*a*) except in the infants of under two weeks (see below). The values for $T_{max.}$ in the latter patients were also thought to be comparable, since all their initial temperatures happened to be similar. It was soon seen that the curves for the hand were similar to those for the feet, except that the temperature of the hand started to rise more quickly, and the maximum temperature was achieved more quickly, than in the feet. Values for the hand have therefore been omitted for simplicity, unless there was an atypical response not shown in the results for the feet.

The Normal Response in relation to Age

Although there is adequate information in the literature concerning the normal vasomotor response in adults (Gibbon and Landis, 1932; Richards, 1946; Brattgård, Lindqvist, and Sigroth, 1951) no reference could be found to the

TABLE I

Effect of Arm Immersion on Skin Temperature in Normal Children

Name	*Age*	T_R (*minutes*)	$T_{max.}$ (*minutes*)	*Maximum temperature* (°*C.*)
N. K.	13 years	10	30	34·5
M. W.	12 years	5	30	34·2
J. L.	2 years, 3 months	3	26	34·0
C. T.	1 year, 11 months	4	26	34·8
A. H.	1 year, 2 months	14	33	34·5
S. C.	1 year	4	22	34·8
M. H.	1 ,,	5	27	36·0
D. B.	11 months	4	34	36·2
R. S.	11 ,,	14	33	34·5
D. H.	10 ,,	4	13	34·3
P. L.	10 ,,	< 2	9	35·7
G. W.	8 ,,	8	23	34·5
A. R.	4 ,,	10	38	34·4
J. C.	4 ,,	4	32	34·8
L. H.	3¼ ,,	6	20	35·3
W. W.	2½ ,,	18	58	36·0
A. T.	1¾ ,,	9	34	36·2
H. L.	1½ ,,	25	60	36·2
P. H.	1¼ ,,	17	51	35·4
K. E.	1¼ ,,	6	33	35·7
E. T.	1 month	23	65	36·1
J. H.	1 ,,	12	32	35·5
Baby Ta.	12 days	37	95	35·6 (R) 30·8 (L)
Baby B.	9 ,,	44	98	36·5
Baby To.	8 ,,	20	83	32·8
Baby D.	7 ,,	27	49	32·7 (R) 30·0 (L)
Baby Q.	7 ,,	19	80+	32·2+
Baby Ca.	6 ,,	30	64	35·4
Baby McC.	6 ,,	17	60	36·2
Baby Wr.	5 ,,	20	57+	33·0
Baby Ch.	3 ,,	15	64	36·2
Baby W.	2 ,,	30	102	35·0
Baby K.	2 ,,	13	65	36·3
Baby Cr.	2 ,,	16	60	34·6

response in children. The initial investigation was therefore designed to ascertain the normal response at various ages, and to discover at what age the adult type of response develops. Table I shows these values in 34 healthy children whose ages ranged from 13 years to two days. All the 12 infants under two weeks old were full-term normal babies. It will be seen that the 15 children over the age of three months all gave a similar response (T_R less than 15 minutes, $T_{max.}$ less than 40 minutes, *m.t.* over 34° C.) (Fig. 1*a*). This response approximates to

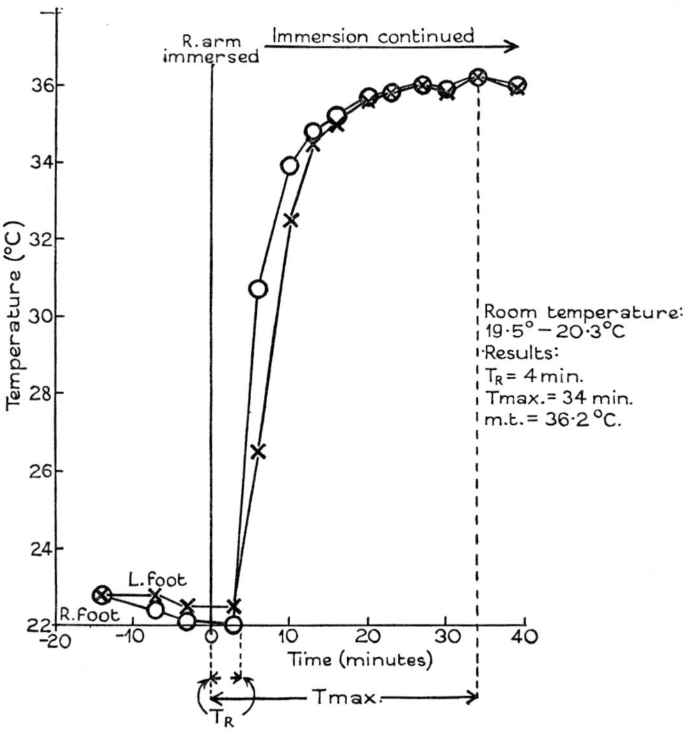

FIG. 1*a*. D. B., aged 11 months. Normal child.

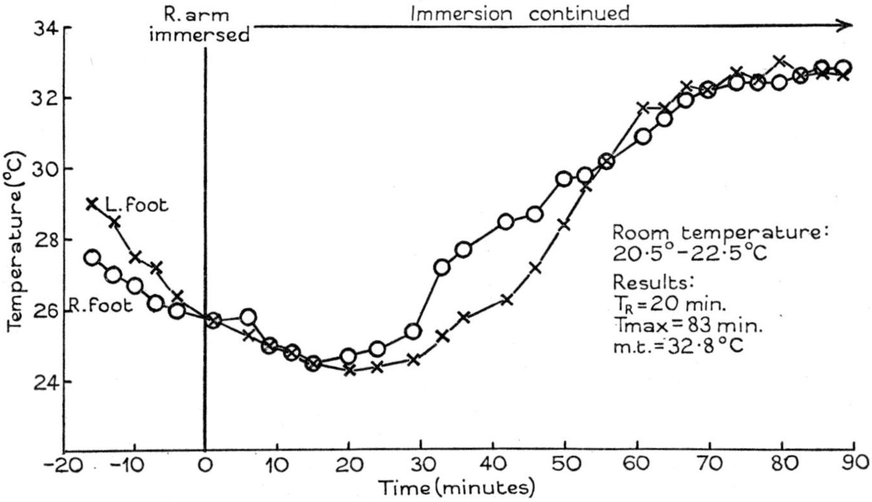

FIG. 1*b*. Baby To., aged eight days. Normal child.

T_R = time in minutes from immersion to first rise in temperature.
$T_{max.}$ = time in minutes from immersion to maximum temperature attained.
m.t. = maximum temperature attained (°C.).
} (mean value for the two feet)

that found in normal adults (Gibbon and Landis, 1932; Richards, 1946), although in the latter the maximum temperatures are often lower (30·5–32° C.). The 12 children in the first fortnight of life gave a much more sluggish response, for only one attained the maximum temperature in under one hour, and some took far longer (Fig. 1*b*). In some the temperature did not reach 34·0° C. at any

TABLE II

Effect of Arm Immersion on Skin Temperature in Pink Disease

Patient	*Age (months)*	T_R *(minutes)*	$T_{max.}$ *(minutes)*	*Maximum temperature (°C.)*	*Duration of test (minutes)*
Marie P.	11	15	44	30·1	54
Muriel P.	11	No rise	..	..	36
L. R.	11	No rise in one foot, slight in other to 27·3°	..	..	44
A. D.	11	No rise	..	..	47
A. H.	11	No rise	..	..	55
S. M.	10	No rise	..	..	50
P. G.	10	No rise in feet (late in hand)	..	..	70
J. H.	9	3	11	30·2	21
T. W.	8	No rise in one foot, slight in other. Late rise in hand	..	..	65
J. C.	8	No rise in one foot and hand, slight in other foot to 29·4°	..	..	47
M. D.	7	No rise	..	..	51
L. S.	7	No rise	..	..	43
M. S.	6	No rise	..	..	73

stage. The age group between two weeks and three months contains seven patients, three of whom gave an adult type of response and four a more sluggish response, although all eventually reached a maximum temperature of more than 34·0° C. It seems likely, therefore, that the adult type of response develops in normal children between the ages of two weeks and three months, an assumption which accords with clinical observation as regards the age at which a stable body temperature is attained. Investigation is being continued along these lines, but for the present comparison the figures suffice to demonstrate the normal response of children over the age of six months.

The Response in Cases of Pink Disease

Thirteen typical patients, aged six to twelve months, were tested. The results are shown in Table II. In all cases the responses were quite abnormal. In seven cases there was no rise of temperature in any of the three limbs over periods ranging from 36 to 73 minutes (Fig. 2). In four others there was a late rise in one or two of the three limbs to a maximum below 34·0° C., and in the remaining two there was a small rise in all three limbs, but the maximum was well below 34·0° C.

These results show that there is a clear difference in the field of vasomotor control between sufferers from pink disease and normal children of the same age. Since the main, if not sole, stimulus for peripheral vasodilatation is the action of warmed blood on the hypothalamus, the only sites of disorder which can bring about this particular disturbance of function in pink disease are the hypothalamus, the sympathetic nervous system, the vessels themselves, and possibly the cerebral cortex. It will be shown in a subsequent section that the vessels can dilate normally after ganglion blockage. Because the sympathetic

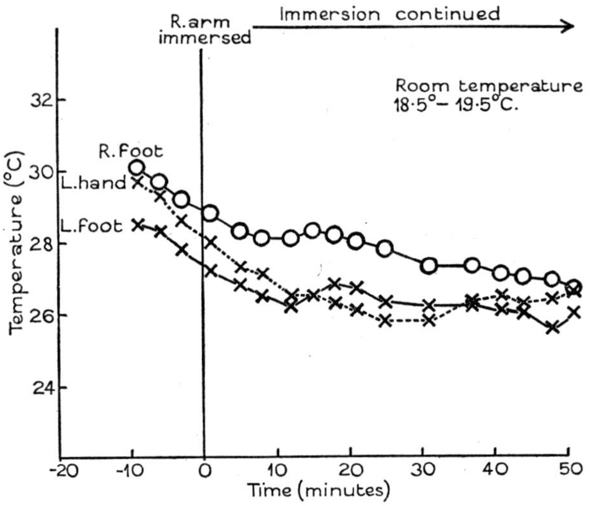

FIG. 2. A. H., aged 11 months. Pink disease.

overactivity is widespread, and parasympathetic overactivity, as shown by the excessive salivation, is also present, a disturbance of the hypothalamus has seemed likely, and the term 'diencephalopathy' proposed (Leys, 1950). Vulliamy (1952) has suggested a humoral mechanism as an alternative explanation. Yet neither of these hypotheses wholly explains the functional disorder, since it has been obvious from the first descriptions that the disease may involve other regions. The occurrence of such features as hypotonia, anaesthesia, and signs of upper and lower motor neurone lesions, makes it clear that most regions of the central and peripheral nervous systems can be affected. The nature of the fundamental disorder remains unknown, in spite of the many explanations which have been put forward, and little further can be deduced from the above results concerning aetiology. The results demonstrate, however, that sympathetic overaction is a constant feature of pink disease. Vulliamy, whose paper appeared during the course of the present investigation, came to the same conclusion. Using a different method (heating the trunk and legs with an electric blanket) he found that in 10 of his 11 patients there was no reflex vasodilatation in the hand, and in the other patient it was delayed. The fact that all 24 patients in his and the present series showed an abnormal response suggests that this may be a useful diagnostic test in atypical cases. The plethora of signs and symptoms which have been described in pink disease sometimes makes diagnosis difficult, especially in the mild case, when only one set of symptoms may be evident. The present form of test has been applied in one or two cases where signs of autonomic disorder such as excessive sweating, cold extremities, or hypertension have not been obvious, and the results have been abnormal. The apparatus is more cumbersome than that of Vulliamy, but this method has the advantage, which is a real one in doubtful cases, of testing three limbs instead

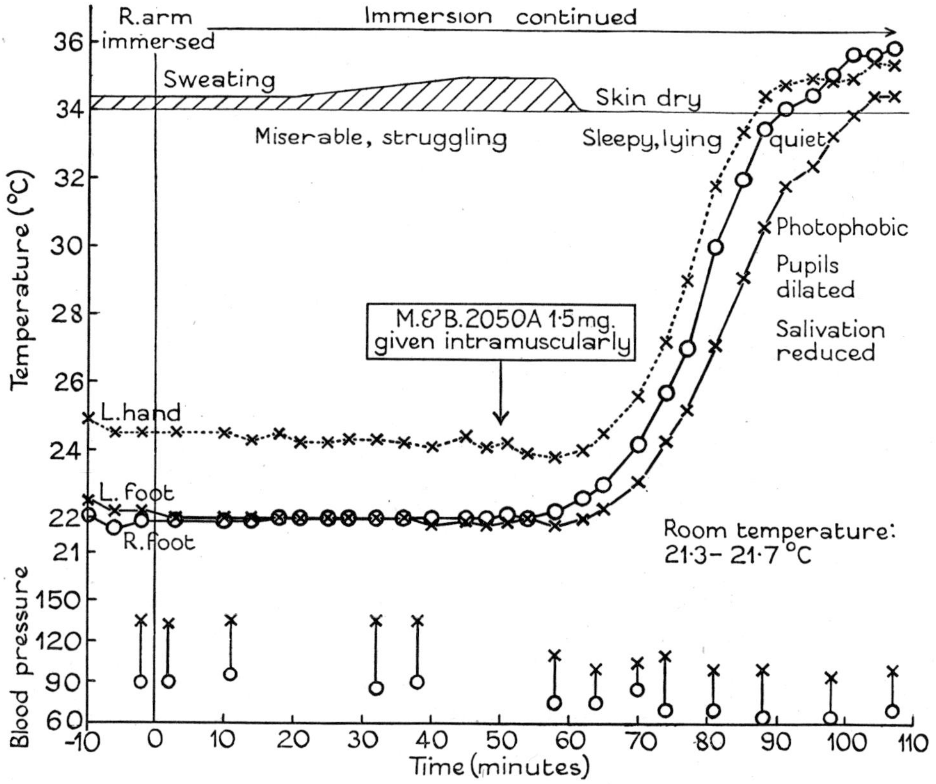

FIG. 3. S. M., aged 10 months. Pink disease.

of one. One limb may show a rise in temperature, albeit inadequate, while the others show none, so that the results in one limb may be doubtful, while those in all three considered together will be more definite. Another reason for preferring a method which records the temperature of the legs as well as an arm is that it was found, in contrast to Vulliamy's results, that often the hands were initially quite warm (in several cases over 30° C.) (Fig. 4*a*), making demonstration of vasodilatation difficult, whereas the feet were nearly always colder.

Sweating was excessive in nine of the 13 cases, and made the patients very uncomfortable (Figs. 3 and 4*a*). It might be argued that this could be responsible for the failure of the temperature to rise. As Vulliamy has said, this is unlikely, for there was no relationship between the amount of sweating and the temperature. In the patient Muriel P., for instance, sweating was less than that seen in some of the normal children, and yet there was no rise of temperature in any of the limbs.

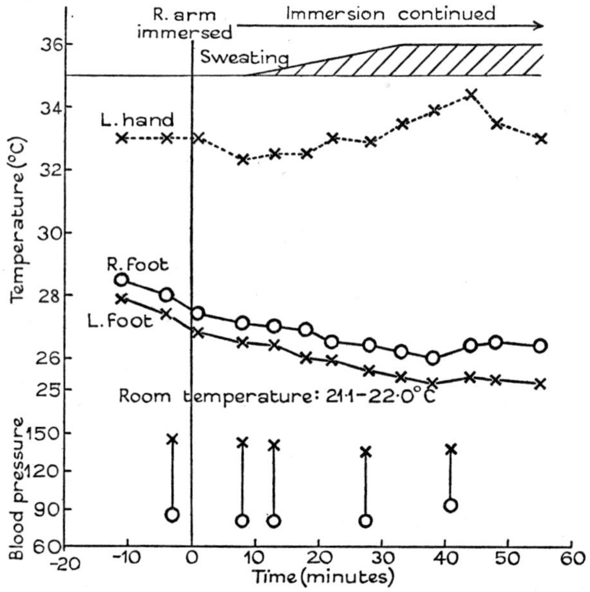

FIG. 4*a*. L. S., aged 7 months. Pink disease. May 5, 1953.

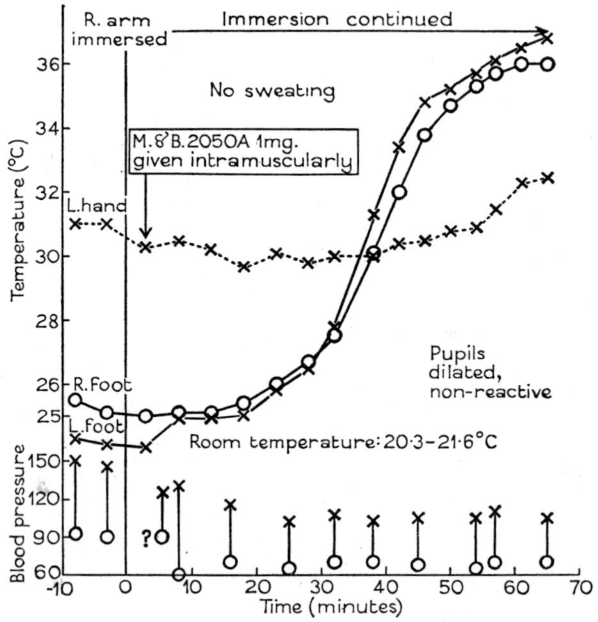

FIG. 4*b*. L. S., aged 7 months. Pink disease. May 7, 1953.

Ganglion-Blocking Agents in Pink Disease

It seemed reasonable in the light of these observations to try the effect of drugs which have been shown in adults to reduce sweating, salivation, hypertension, and peripheral vasoconstriction. Accordingly hexamethonium bromide and pentapyrrolidinium bitartrate ('M. and B. 2050A') were given by intramuscular injection to 11 of the 13 patients while subjected to the heating test. It was felt that, if sweating and the resulting discomfort could be abolished in patients subjected to this severe stimulus, the drugs would be worth a therapeutic trial, which would be still further indicated if the normal temperature response could be established in the limbs. In five cases the drug was injected after an adequate period of arm immersion had shown a complete or partial failure of peripheral vasodilatation, the arm remaining immersed while further temperature measurements were made (Fig. 3), and in the other six cases it was given at the start of the test, when the arm was first immersed, a previous test without the drug having shown the abnormal response discussed above (Fig. 4).

Table III

Pink Disease: Dose and Blood-Pressure Before and After Injection

Patient	*Drug*	*Dose (mg.)*	*Blood-pressure* *Before*	*After (minimum)*
A. H.	H.M.B.	2·5	130/70	104/60
L. R.	H.M.B.	10	140/75	100/75
Muriel P.	H.M.B.	5	130/90	110/75
Marie P.	H.M.B.	10	140/90	80/50
T. W.	H.M.B.	15	125/80	80/65
M. D.	2050A	1	110/80	105/60
L. S.	2050A	1	145/90	100/65
P. G.	2050A	2	155/100	100/75
M. S.	2050A	2	140/90	95/65
S. M.	2050A	1·5	135/90	90/70
J. C.	2050A	1·5	Not measured	

H.M.B. = hexamethonium bromide. 2050A = pentapyrrolidinium bitartrate.

Results. No real difference in action was noticed between the two drugs except in relation to dosage, and they will therefore be discussed together.

1. *Sweating.* The effect was striking. In four of the five patients in the first group the skin became quite dry within 12 minutes of the injection, and remained so for the remainder of the test, and in the fifth sweating was greatly reduced (Fig. 3). In the six cases in the second group no sweating occurred at any time (Fig. 4). This effect seemed to be more pronounced than any other, for in three patients the dose of hexamethonium bromide or 'M. and B. 2050A' which was given initially proved to be too small to produce any peripheral vasodilatation or much hypotension, yet complete suppression of sweating occurred.

2. *Vasoconstriction.* In all cases except one (A. H.) a satisfactory rise in foot temperature (to over 34° C.) was produced, although the dosage required to bring this about varied from patient to patient (Table III). There was no opportunity to test again the one failure (where the maximum foot temperature was only 31° C.) with a larger dose, but there is little doubt that this patient

also would have shown a normal rise, since the temperature of her feet had risen 5° after the small dose. The results for the hand were less satisfactory, as might be expected from investigations in adults (Burt and Graham, 1950). In all except two patients, however, the maximum temperature attained was over 32° C.

3. *Hypertension.* This was reduced in the 10 cases in which blood-pressure was measured. The time at which maximum hypotension occurred was usually between 20 and 45 minutes, and the systolic pressure fell more than the diastolic (Table III). Measurements were all made personally, using the same mercury-column sphygmomanometer and a $2\frac{1}{2}$-inch-wide cuff. In spite of the difficulties inherent in taking the blood-pressure in babies, it was felt that readings were accurate to 5 mm.

4. *Demeanour.* In the tests without drug injection, nine of the 11 children whimpered or cried outright, and were obviously uncomfortable. All these patients either fell asleep, or lay awake without making a sound, during the test after the drug was given. Somnolence occurs in adults (Morrison and Paton, 1953), presumably owing to reduction in cerebral blood-flow, and the improvement in our patients was probably due partly to this factor and partly to the reduction in sweating and peripheral vasospasm.

After these encouraging results, nine of these patients were treated with the drugs, three being given hexamethonium bromide, five being given 'M. and B. 2050A', and one receiving a course of each drug.

Case 1. L. R., aged 11 months, with four months' history of irritability, difficulty in feeding, photophobia, and loss of weight. On admission she was a miserable, photophobic, hypotonic baby, lying in the typical genupectoral position. The hands and feet were cold, pink, and peeling. A slight sweat rash was present on the trunk. The blood-pressure varied between 115/70 and 140/75.

Progress and treatment. After observation for 10 days, during which there was no change in her clinical condition, hexamethonium bromide 10 mg. was given subcutaneously four times daily half an hour before feeds. Sweating was noticed to be much less, and she became less peevish, in the first two days. On the third day she smiled for the first time since admission, and started to sit up. The photophobia also improved during the first week. Hypertension was only reduced for about one or two hours after an injection. After 10 days of this treatment hexamethonium was stopped. On the following day she was very miserable, with hyperhidrosis, and once more lay in the genupectoral position, rubbing her nose on the mattress. This deterioration seemed to be in part a rebound phenomenon, since there was some improvement during the next few days. She was then discharged, and when seen a week later, although still a little miserable and hypotonic, was on the whole very well. After a further two weeks she was quite normal, and has remained so for three months.

Case 2. Marie P., aged 11 months, with two months' history of loss of weight, irritability, and hypotonia. She had ceased to sit up. There was one week's history of nasal discharge and cough. On admission she was an ill, apathetic child, with bronchopneumonia, hypotonia, pink scaling hands, and a generalized sweat rash. The blood-pressure was 140/90.

Progress and treatment. The pneumonia slowly cleared with systemic penicillin and sulphadiazine, and three weeks after admission she was well enough to undergo a heating test. Hexamethonium bromide was then started in doses of 10 mg. six-hourly, and there was an immediate improvement in appetite and demeanour; sweating was reduced. Reduction in hypertension lasted only one to two hours after each dose. A gradual return of symptoms necessitated an increase of dose to 15 mg. after one week, and again to 20 mg. after a further week. After each increase in dose she became less peevish, but the photophobia increased. After 19 days treatment was stopped and, although she became more irritable and difficult with feeds, there was no striking deterioration, as in Case 1. A further week's course of 20 mg. four times daily was accompanied by improvement in her demeanour, hyperhidrosis, hypertension, and hypotonia. Treatment was then stopped, and she was discharged. Ten days later she had improved still further, and three weeks later there were no signs of pink disease.

Case 3. Muriel P., aged 11 months, with six weeks' history of irritability, excessive sweating, listlessness, anorexia, dribbling, and photophobia. For three weeks her hands had been peeling. All her symptoms had become exaggerated during the previous week, and she had lost one pound in weight. On admission she was a miserable, very hypotonic infant, with hyperhidrosis and pink, peeling hands. The blood-pressure was 130/100.

Progress and treatment. Hexamethonium bromide was started in subcutaneous doses of 5 mg. six-hourly and increased to 10 mg. during the next four days. There was an improvement in appetite and demeanour, and her extremities became warm and the skin of her hands normal. Hypertension was abolished for one or two hours after a dose. After six days the treatment was stopped, and she became miserable and more difficult to feed, and started to chew her cot, as she had done before treatment was started. Her extremities became colder. Her blood-pressure, which during treatment had varied between 145/105 and 120/95, rose to 170/110 on the day after cessation, and then gradually diminished in the next five days to 125/100. The drug was then tried orally, in doses of 50 mg. six-hourly, for six days, but no effect was seen. It was then given subcutaneously again for a week, in doses of 15 mg. four times daily before feeds, with the same results as on the previous subcutaneous course. There was no deterioration on cessation this time. She was then discharged, and when seen two weeks later had further improved, although still hypotonic. Further follow-up has not been possible.

Case 4. M. D., aged seven months, with three months' history of peevishness, insomnia, and photophobia, following pertussis. A rash had been noticed on the day of admission. She was a very miserable, very photophobic child, with a red, puffy face. Salivation was excessive. A fine macular rash was present on the trunk and forearms. The extremities were cold, but not red or oedematous. She had a blood-pressure of 125/100 (whimpering).

Progress and treatment. For the first six days she was treated with sedation, and showed no improvement except that her rash disappeared. 'M. and B. 2050A', 1 mg. subcutaneously six-hourly, was then started. Within two days she was much less miserable and her extremities were warmer. The dose was increased to 2 mg., and the photophobia improved, the puffiness and redness of her face also disappearing as she ceased to rub her eyes. After a week's treatment she was so much better that injections were stopped. There was no deterioration, and she was discharged six days later. Her mother described her improvement as a 'miracle'. When reviewed two weeks and six weeks later she was a normal child apart from some sweating.

Case 5. L. S., aged seven months, with 10 weeks' history of lassitude, inability to sit up, anorexia, excessive sweating, and salivation. She had had a rash from time to time, and her fingers had been peeling. On admission she was a very hypotonic, lifeless infant, with hyperhidrosis, excessive salivation, and pink, warm hands and cold feet. She was very slow in reacting to pin-prick. The blood-pressure was 180/120.

Progress and treatment. After observation for 10 days, during which she was so apathetic that she was thought to have encephalitis, 'M. and B. 2050A' was started in doses of 1 mg. eight-hourly. There was no great change in the apathy, but sweating and salivation were controlled, her feet became warm, and her blood-pressure fell to 110/85. The sweat rash disappeared, but a few pustules appeared on her trunk at the same time. These subsided with oral penicillin. The dose was increased to 3 mg. eight-hourly by the 14th day, but no improvement in the apathy occurred, although the autonomic symptoms, except photophobia, remained under control. At this stage she became a little less inert, and this improvement continued after cessation of the drug on the 25th day. There was an increase in salivation and sweating, and her feet became cold, after stopping the drug; but this change was less obvious a few days later. Her slow improvement has been maintained since discharge, but she is still not normal two months after the treatment was stopped.

Case 6. T. W., aged eight months. He had a history of apathy, loss of weight, and anorexia for three months following a respiratory infection, and excessive sweating, redness of the extremities, and a macular rash for about three weeks. On admission he was an apathetic, ill-looking, febrile baby, with bronchitis, hypotonia, pink peeling extremities, a macular rash, and slight photophobia.

Progress and treatment. He remained apathetic and febrile for two weeks. His chest X-ray was normal. Antibiotics failed to control his fever, and on the 11th day hexamethonium bromide, 10 mg. six-hourly, was started. There was an improvement in demeanour in the next 48 hours, and the temperature fell from 103° to 99° F. Sweating was greatly diminished, and the extremities became warm. Reduction of hypertension was transient, as in the other patients, lasting about two hours after an injection, and photophobia increased. The dose was increased to 15 mg. on the third day, and the improvement continued. After cessation of the drug on the fifth day he became more miserable, and sweating increased, but his fever did not return. Five days later the drug was again given in 15-mg. doses, and during the next week he became more cheerful, laughing and gurgling occasionally. He again became miserable when the drug was stopped, and his extremities became cold and blue, although the day was hot. 'M. and B. 2050A' was then started in 0·5-mg. doses eight-hourly, but no improvement occurred until the dose reached 2·5 mg., when he again improved, and after five days was well enough to be sent home without treatment. He remained fairly well at home for a month, and then had an attack of vomiting and was admitted in a very dehydrated state. He responded quickly to oral fluid feeding, but was still apathetic. No sign of autonomic disorder could be found at this time, and no ganglion-blocking drugs were given. He went home after 10 days, and is still under observation.

Case 7. P. G., aged 10 months, with three weeks' history of peevishness, photophobia, anorexia, excessive sweating, and head-banging. His hands had been cold and pink for this period. On admission he was a moderately irritable baby, with pinkish-blue feet and hands, the latter being extremely cold moist. Hypotonia and photophobia were slight. The blood-pressure was 105.

Progress and treatment. For the first eight days he was not treated, and his condition remained unchanged. His blood-pressure was 185/120 on two occasions, and his hands remained cold and moist. 'M. and B. 2050A' was then started in doses of 2 mg. eight-hourly. His hands became warm and dry, his blood-pressure was reduced, and he became less irritable. After five days the treatment was stopped because his mother wanted him home. His blood-pressure rose after cessation of treatment, but his hands did not revert to the state found before treatment. When seen a month later he was improved, but was still not eating well.

Case 8. M. S., aged six months, with seven weeks' history of irritability following stomatitis and otitis media; irritability had been worse for the past week, with hyperhidrosis and a sweat rash. He had recently lost weight. On admission he was a fretful, somewhat hypotonic baby, with a generalized sudaminal rash, pink peeling extremities, the hands being warm and the feet cold, and mild photophobia. He was constantly scratching his trunk, and rubbing his feet together. The blood-pressure was 145/90.

Progress and treatment. He was observed for four days, during which his condition remained unchanged. He was then given 'M. and B. 2050A', 2 mg. eight-hourly, and the dose was gradually increased to 3 mg. during the next week. It was stopped after eight days. During this time his rash had disappeared, his sweating had been controlled, and the peeling of the extremities was much less obvious. His feet were warm, and his irritability and pruritus less.

He then had an attack of infective gastroenteritis of moderate severity, and after recovery the return of sweating and peevishness made a second course of 'M. and B. 2050A' desirable. This treatment caused a temporary improvement, but was interrupted by a second and more severe attack of gastroenteritis. During this illness the signs of autonomic overaction were in abeyance, and when he recovered three weeks later there were no signs of pink disease apart from hypotonia. He was a normal child when examined after a further month.

Case 9. J. C., aged eight months. She had six weeks' history of photophobia, anorexia, and peevishness, with a sweat rash. On admission she was a wasted, hypotonic, apathetic, and miserable baby, with very cold, moist, bluish-red hands and feet, slight photophobia, but no rash. The blood-pressure was 135/90.

Progress and treatment. After observation for two weeks, during which there was no change, 'M. and B. 2050A' was given eight-hourly in 1·5-mg. doses. Her extremities became warm, pink, and dry, and the blood-pressure was reduced to 85/65. The photophobia was increased. Her demeanour did not change as had been anticipated. During the next two weeks the dose was increased to 3 mg. eight-hourly, but no change in demeanour was noticed, although the hyperhidrosis, vasospasm, and hypertension were still absent. Cessation of the drug, however, at that time caused an increase in irritability, as well as the recurrence of the other features. It may be, therefore, that the disease was becoming more severe during this period, and that without the drug she would have become more irritable. The drug was resumed 24 hours later, and hypertension, hyperhidrosis, and vasospasm were again abolished within a few minutes. Three days later she showed an improvement in demeanour, and sat up in her cot for two hours. This improvement was maintained for the next week. She is still under treatment.

Comment. Assessment of the effect of a drug whose action is relatively short and to which patients become resistant is difficult, especially in a disease in which the recognition of improvement or deterioration depends partly upon subjective impressions, the duration varies from patient to patient, and nursing care and sedation alone can bring about improvement. The method used, that is the administration of the drug in short courses, increasing the dose when thought necessary, with observation of symptoms in the phases with and without treatment, was thought the most suitable, but its limitations are recognized. Nevertheless it was clear that certain beneficial effects resulted from the administration of these two drugs.

1. Hyperhidrosis was probably affected most. In fact, if sweating was not abolished, the dose was increased. This result is obviously very valuable, for not only is discomfort largely relieved, but any sweat rash which is present rapidly disappears, as in Cases 5 and 8.

2. Peripheral vasospasm was also relieved, although to a greater extent in the feet than in the hands. This effect is very useful in patients with cold hands or feet, and in most cases either the hands or the feet are affected to some extent. Although no patient in the present series had ulceration of the extremities, the drug should be very useful in this type of case, since peeling, oedema, and ulceration are probably, at least in part, the result of arteriolar spasm. Whether the paraesthesiae of pink disease are due to hyperhidrosis, arteriolar spasm, or peripheral neuritis, or to a combination of two or three of these factors, it is difficult to say, but since the first two factors can be removed by ganglion-blocking agents, amelioration of irritation might be expected to occur. In fact, scratching was reduced in Case 8, the only child who initially had a distressing pruritus, but it was not completely abolished, in spite of the cessation of sweating and disappearance of the rash. A typical feature of this disease is the waving of the hands in front of the body, with alternating pronation and supination. This was noticed in two patients, and was abolished by the drug.

3. Demeanour improved in seven of the nine patients, the change being very obvious in Cases 1 and 4. In Case 5, one of the failures, the patient probably had encephalitis.

4. Hypertension was temporarily reduced in all cases. It was thought that 'M. and B. 2050A' had the longer effect, but no other difference in action between the two drugs was noted, although no systematic attempt to compare them was made. It is difficult to know what effect, if any, hypertension has upon the patient in this disease, and the reduction of blood-pressure has been regarded solely as a sign that vasodilatation has occurred.

5. Excessive salivation was checked in Case 3, the only case in which it was a prominent feature, and it returned on cessation of treatment.

6. Photophobia was the only symptom which was aggravated. Dilatation of the pupil often occurred, but the two effects did not run parallel, as had been shown in adults (Morrison and Paton, 1953). Neither sign gave a constant indication of the degree of ganglion blockage at a particular time. In Cases 1 and 4 photophobia appeared to improve after administration of the drug.

7. Other effects: hypotonia was unaffected in all cases, as might be expected. It is uncertain whether the reduction of fever which occurred in Case 6 was a consequence of the drug or coincidental.

Dosage. The initial dose chosen was that which produced a rise of temperature in the feet to over 34° C. during the heating test. The doses are shown in Table III. It seems that a suitable initial dose of hexamethonium bromide is 10 mg., and of 'M. and B. 2050A' 1 mg. By comparison with the doses given to adults (Smirk, 1953), infants appear to be relatively more tolerant. Administration was theoretically too infrequent, since in adults hexamethonium bromide is usually given four-hourly by day, and it is recommended by Smirk that 'M. and B. 2050A' should be given five-hourly by day, with the proviso that the doses after the first of each day may need to be reduced. It was felt, however, that in infants the frequency of injections should be reduced if possible, and not more than four doses of hexamethonium bromide or three doses of 'M. and B. 2050A' were given in the 24 hours. This scheme also seemed safer. It may be that better results would accrue with more frequent doses. A longer-acting preparation is now under trial. Oral administration was tried only once, and it seemed that the inconstancy of absorption precluded its use at the present stage of investigation. Tolerance developed more rapidly in some patients than in others, and the dose of hexamethonium bromide was increased by increments of 5 mg., and of 'M. and B. 2050A' by 0·5 mg., when a return of symptoms indicated it. Because of the shortness of the courses a stable dose was not attained, except in Case 9 in which administration was continued for a longer period.

Conclusions

Hexamethonium bromide and pentapyrrolidinium bitartrate are theoretically very suitable for the symptomatic treatment of pink disease. A therapeutic trial in nine cases has had some success, and it is hoped that other observers will report similar trials. It does not seem that all cases of pink disease require a treatment which necessitates injections, especially since the child must be in hospital under close supervision, with the inherent risk of superimposed infection. It is suggested, however, that patients with manifestations of autonomic overaction and its sequelae (that is, irritability, skin rashes, and ulceration of the extremities) should be given the benefit of a trial with one of the drugs. It is interesting that Case 9 was the only case of a child who, after treatment had been stopped, experienced autonomic symptoms as severely as before treatment, and it was the impression of the nursing staff that the drugs 'started them off towards recovery'. One cannot on present evidence discount the results of good nursing and the passage of time, and attribute a permanent therapeutic effect to the drugs, nor would this be expected on theoretical grounds. They appear, however, to offer a promising symptomatic treatment in this distressing disease.

I wish to thank Professor J. M. Smellie for his encouragement and help during this investigation. I am indebted to the consultant physicians of the Children's Hospital, Birmingham, and to Dr. V. Mary Crosse, for permission to investigate and treat patients under their care, and to Mr. J. G. Williamson for the photograph. Messrs. May and Baker supplied the hexamethonium bromide and 'M. and B. 2050A'.

Summary

In an investigation of 34 normal children between the ages of two days and 13 years, reflex vasodilatation of the other three limbs during immersion of one limb in warmed water was much slower and less complete in infants under two weeks old than in older children. The adult type of response, however, was present in children over the age of three months.

In 13 cases of pink disease which were tested the response was either late and incomplete or non-existent.

When hexamethonium bromide or pentapyrrolidinium bitartrate was given to these patients by injection while a limb was heated, peripheral vasodilatation occurred, and sweating, hypertension, and irritability were abolished.

A therapeutic trial of these drugs administered subcutaneously in nine cases gave similar results, abolishing sweating, coldness of the extremities, hypertension, and in one case excessive salivation, clearing up sweat rashes, and with one exception improving demeanour. Photophobia was aggravated in seven cases. Details of the dosage schemes are given.

It is suggested that this treatment is well worth a trial in those cases of pink disease in which autonomic symptoms predominate.

REFERENCES

Brattgård, S.-O., Lindqvist, T., and Sigroth, K. (1951) *Acta med. scand.* **140**, 220.
Burt, C. C., and Graham, A. J. P. (1950) *Brit. Med. J.* **1**, 455.
Cooper, K. E., Cross, K. W., Greenfield, A. D. M., Hamilton, D. McK., and Scarborough, H. (1949) *Clin. Sci.* **8**, 217.
Duthie, J. J. R., and Mackay, R. M. I. (1940) *Brain*, **63**, 295.
Feer, E. (1925) *Jb. Kinderheilk.* **108**, 267.
Fulton, J. F. (1943) *Physiology of the Nervous System*, 2nd ed., London.
Gibbon, J. H., Jnr., and Landis, E. M. (1932) *J. Clin. Invest.* **11**, 1019.
Lewis, T. (1946) *Vascular Disorders of the Limbs*, 2nd ed., London.
—— and Pickering, G. W. (1931) *Heart*, **16**, 33.
Leys, D. (1950) *Arch. Dis. Childh.* **25**, 302.
McPherson, A. (1953) *Lancet*, **1**, 648.
Morrison, B., and Paton, W. D. M. (1953) *Brit. Med. J.* **1**, 1299.
Richards, R. L. (1946) *The Peripheral Circulation in Health and Disease*, Edinburgh.
Selter, P. (1903) *Arch. Kinderheilk.* **37**, 468.
—— (1927) Ibid. **80**, 244.
Smirk, F. H. (1953) *Lancet*, **1**, 457.
Vulliamy, D. G. (1952) Ibid. **2**, 1248.

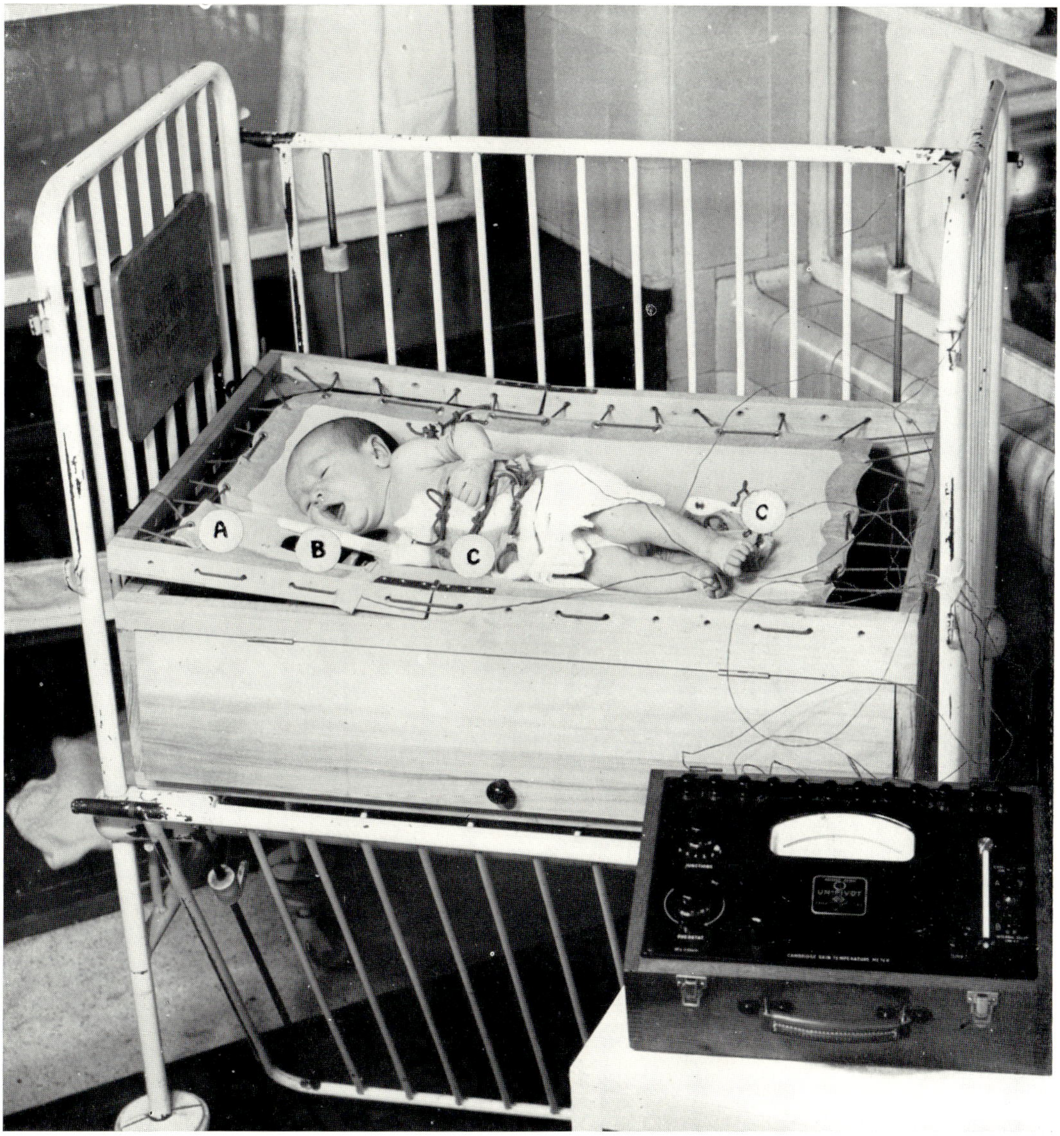

Fig. 5. Arm-immersion apparatus

615.7 : 547.233.3–222

BIOLOGICAL ACTIONS AND THERAPEUTIC APPLICATIONS OF NITROGEN MUSTARD[1]

By J. W. BEATTIE and LEONARD H. HOWELLS
(From the Cardiff Royal Infirmary)

Introduction

The nitrogen mustards are amine derivatives of mustard gas, and contain two β-chloroethyl groups, but linked by a nitrogen instead of a sulphur atom. Although known since before 1935, when Ward discussed the preparation of 'the chlorinated ethylamines—a new type of vesicant', they aroused little interest until the exigencies of the recent war compelled a thorough investigation into their properties and actions. At the same time a review of the earlier knowledge of mustard gas showed that observations had been made regarding the following properties: systemic intoxication both in man (Pappenheimer, 1919) and in dogs (Lynch, Smith, and Marshall, 1918–19); a direct toxic action on the lympho-reticular system, with impairment of regeneration of blood cellular elements both in man (Stewart, 1918; Krumbhaar, 1919 *a*, *b*; Krumbhaar and Krumbhaar, 1919) and in rabbits (Pappenheimer, 1918–19; Pappenheimer and Vance, 1920), and depression of the formation of antibodies in animals (Hektoen and Corper, 1921); an interference with cell division, consisting of inhibition or delayed rate of cleavage of fertilized starfish eggs, with the production of irregular or abnormal larval forms (Lillie, Clowes, and Chambers, 1919–20), and a depressant effect on the multiplication of yeast cells (Magne and Rémy, 1937); mitotic alterations in *Hordeum distichum* similar to those obtained with colchicine and aniline dyes (Favorsky, 1939); an interference with certain enzymatic reactions (Berenblum, Kendal, and Orr, 1936; Peters, 1936); and a direct action, under physiological conditions of pH and temperature, on serum-proteins, with immunological specificity of the resulting product (Berenblum and Wormall, 1939). Perhaps the most interesting property, however, was the ability to inhibit the induction by tar of mouse skin tumours, an effect which was local and of limited duration, and was first observed by Berenblum (1929, 1931). Subsequently, experimental tumour-destructive effects were observed by Kabelik (1932) and by Visser and de Vos (1935), the latter authors using systemic and local administration. Therapeutic applications of these important properties were undertaken by Adair and Bagg (1931), who treated 13 patients suffering from superficial cancers, 12 by local application and one by intra-tumour injection. With the previous pertinent information about mustard gas available in various degrees, war-time studies of the actions of sulphur and nitrogen mustards were undertaken, especially along three lines indicated by Rhoads (1947): (1) the chemical changes undergone by the agents in the course

[1] Received October 10, 1953.

of their metabolism, (2) the effects upon essential bodily constituents of each one of the metabolites of the poison, and (3) the general pharmacological effects of the compounds. In general, the results confirmed the great biological similarity between nitrogen and sulphur mustards.

Chemical Reactions

The nitrogen mustard compounds most intensively studied were methyl-bis-(β-chloroethyl)amine (2,2′-dichlorodiethylmethylamine) and tris(β-chloroethyl)-amine (2,2′,2″-trichlorotriethylamine). Methyl-bis(β-chloroethyl)amine—the more important compound—as the free base, is an oily volatile liquid sparingly soluble in water and actively vesicant, while as the hydrochloride it exists as a stable white powder very soluble in water. It was appreciated early that the activity of the mustards might be due to the well-known property of halo-alkylamines of forming cyclic onium cations (Gibbs and Marvel, 1935). It was shown kinetically by Bartlett, Ross, and Swain (1947, 1949) and Bartlett, Davis, Ross, and Swain (1947) that cyclic ethyleneimonium ions of the type

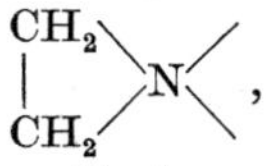

, formed by an intramolecular transformation at the chloroethyl radical, were involved in hydrolysis, dimerization, and all replacement reactions of the tertiary β-chloroethylamines. Hanby and Rydon (1947) and Hanby, Hartley, Powell, and Rydon (1947) found that the free base in dilute aqueous solution undergoes a rapid first stage—transformation to the quaternary ethyleneimonium chloride

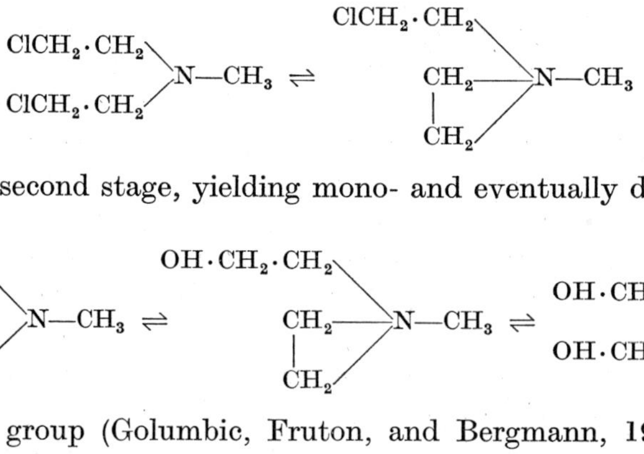

—and a slower second stage, yielding mono- and eventually di-hydroxy compounds

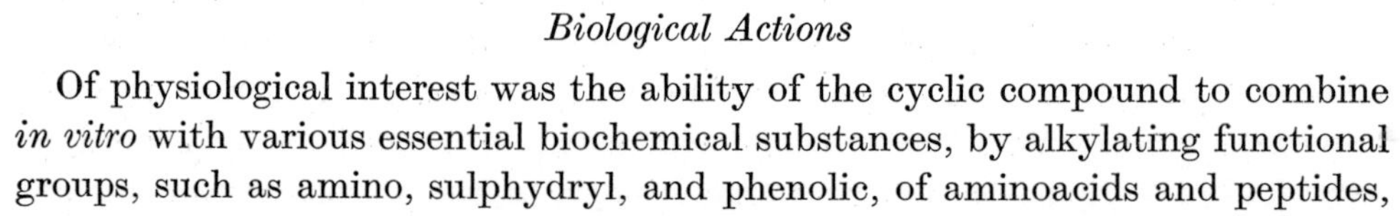

The Bergmann group (Golumbic, Fruton, and Bergmann, 1946) isolated in crystalline form these successive transformation products, and studied their properties.

Biological Actions

Of physiological interest was the ability of the cyclic compound to combine *in vitro* with various essential biochemical substances, by alkylating functional groups, such as amino, sulphydryl, and phenolic, of aminoacids and peptides, inorganic phosphates as well as glycerophosphate and hexose phosphate, and the amino groups of adenosine and theamine (Gilman and Philips, 1946). Numerous proteins were also found reactive through the carboxylic and amino groups, for example haemoglobin, insulin, and tobacco mosaic virus. The Bergmann group were active in these studies (Fruton, Stein, and Bergmann, 1946; Fruton, Stein, Stahmann, and Golumbic, 1946). Several other groups carried out similar chemical investigations, mainly with mustard gas. Inhibition of certain enzyme systems by the nitrogen mustards has also been observed. Barron, Bartlett, and Miller (1948) found inactivation of acetylcholine esterase, choline acetylase, and choline oxidase, and Cori (1943) and other workers found inactivation of phosphokinases, inorganic pyrophosphatases, and pyruvate oxidase. Barron, Bartlett, and Miller (1948) considered the former reactions to be due to the structural similarity between the ethyleneimonium derivatives and choline or acetylcholine, and the latter reactions to result from the interaction of certain groups of the protein (NH_2, carboxyl, or SH) with the highly reactive halogen groups of the mustard. Special enzymatic investigations started earlier in this country by Dixon and Needham (1946), Thompson (1946–7), and Adams and Thompson (1948) had produced similar results with mustard gas. Moreover, other enzyme systems were studied by Herriott, Anson, and Northrop (1946–7). It became apparent, however, that the mustards were not general enzyme poisons, and that there were numerous difficulties in the way of the concept of a primary enzymatic attack (Peters, 1947). Studies of tissue metabolism by Barron, Bartlett, Miller, Meyer, and Seegmiller (1948) showed inhibition of respiration in bone-marrow, lymphoid tissue, spleen, and liver, partial inhibition of urea synthesis in the liver, and strong inhibition of pyruvate oxidation and complete inhibition of choline oxidation in the kidney. The value of the enzymatic-inactivation hypothesis still remains undefined. Peters has recently (1951) stated that we have still to learn which is the actual cell-component with which activated mustard combines most easily. Nevertheless these studies offer explanation for the parasympathomimetic (cholinergic), paralytic, and nicotinic actions of the mustard compounds alluded to by Rhoads (1947).

Among the most important effects of nitrogen mustard from the standpoint of potential utility were those observed by Cameron, Courtice, and Jones (1947) and Graef and his colleagues (1946, 1948). These systemic pathological lesions consisted of the occurrence, within a few hours, of progressive necrosis of the germinal centres of the lymph-nodes and spleen, and congestion of the marrow sinusoids, followed one to three days later by rapid depletion of the myeloid tissue, resulting in an early decrease of all white-cell elements. The decrease in these cells was greatest on the third or fourth day, with a return to normal in about a week. Repeated administration of the mustards for four weeks caused progressive depletion in the red cells, but single doses did not cause anaemia. These quantitative changes occurring in the leucocytes of the peripheral blood and the histological changes in the haemopoietic organs of animals have been serially analysed by Kindred (1947, 1949). Apart from these necro-toxic effects, a diminution in production of the cellular elements was also demonstrated by Cameron, Courtice, and Jones (1947). When recovery occurred it was rapid for all blood-cell types, indicating the remarkable reparative and regenerative power of the haemopoietic tissues. Karnofsky, Graef, and Smith (1948) and Bass and Feigelson (1948) showed that these effects were not mediated through the alarm reaction of Selye; Karnofsky and his colleagues also demonstrated that the bone-marrow damage was directly caused via the circulation, and was rapidly completed. Boursnell, Francis, and Wormall (1946), from studies with radioactive mustard gas, found that marrow tissue, which suffered the greatest damage, had the lowest mustard content, while other tissues such as that of the lung and liver, which were practically undamaged, had the highest content. This result may possibly be due to the excreting function of these organs, or they may concentrate degradation products rather than take part in direct reactions. Somewhat similar results were obtained with nitrogen mustard by Seligman, Rutenburg, and Friedman (1949). Dixon and Needham (1946) suggested as an explanation that the agent might be fixed by a substance in the tissues to a varying extent, and correspondingly diverted from the enzyme systems. In explanation of the cytotoxic action, Anslow, Karnofsky, Jager, and Smith (1947) suggested that the reactivity of the imonium ion was such that chloride competed with organic radicals subject to alkylation, and with water, for any imonium ion present; thus the greater amount of chloride in extracellular fluid would favour the accumulation there of re-formed free amine, and of imonium ion secondarily in the intracellular fluid, in which therefore conditions would be favourable for alkylating reactions. This suggestion is of considerable importance, since cell membranes are considered relatively impermeable to ionic substances, though, of course, these membranes might be damaged by the mustard compounds.

There seems no doubt that proliferative activity determines the susceptibility of the tissues to the cytotoxic effect (Karnofsky, Burchenal, Ormsbee, Cornman, and Rhoads, 1947). Proliferating tissues would presumably be specially susceptible to substances which disturb the nuclear components concerned with cell division. Friedenwald, Buschke, Scholz, and Moses (1947) found that the lowest threshold effect on the mammalian corneal epithelium was an inhibition of mitosis, apparently selective for the excitatory premitotic phase. Greater local concentrations of the nitrogen mustard resulted in nuclear fragmentation, and finally karyolysis of stroma cells, and pyknosis of all cell types. After systemic administration they found inhibition of mitosis in the bone-marrow and in the intestinal mucosa. With sulphur mustard Marshak (1946) noted in the rat a diminution in the mitotic rate of regenerating liver cells after partial hepatectomy, but normal tissues showed no visible changes with similar dosage. Kinsey and Grant (1947) noted an immediate reduction in the rate of cell division of yeast cultures, which could be sustained at lower levels by several succeeding generations. Bodenstein (1947) proved that nitrogen mustard, acting on embryonic tissues of *Amblystoma punctatum*, selectively affected centres of proliferation, leaving differentiating regions unaffected. Auerbach, Robson, and Carr (1947) demonstrated the ability of the mustard compounds to produce gene mutations and chromosome rearrangements, while Auerbach and Robson (1946) found a higher proportion of sex-linked lethal factors in treated than in untreated fruit flies. They concluded that the mutagenic action was on the chromosomes and not by way of a cytoplasmic change, for the mutation rate was not increased when untreated spermatozoa were introduced into treated eggs. Similar results were found with *Neurospora crassa* by Tatum (1947–8) and McElroy, Cushing, and Miller (1947), and in *Penicillium notatum* by Stahmann and Stauffer (1947). Koller (1947) found breakage and translocations of the chromosomes, and delays in mitosis, in the pollen grains of *Tradescantia* exposed to mustard gas. The work of Ford (1948) and of Loveless and Revell (1949) showed that the nitrogen-mustard-induced chromosome breaks were much increased towards regions of demonstrable heterochromatin, if not actually in them; it is of interest that heterochromatin has a high nucleic-acid charge in the resting nucleus. Gjessing and Chanutin (1946) and Butler, Gilbert, and Smith (1950) found that the nitrogen mustards produced a decrease in viscosity of deoxyribonucleic acid, which may be regarded as representative of the characteristic nucleic acid of the chromosome. Mitchell (1942, 1943) considered that the reaction, involving the synthesis of deoxyribonucleic acid at the expense of ribonucleic acid, found in embryonic cells, occurred also in tumour cells, and was inhibited by X-radiation and γ-radiation. Nitrogen mustard was found by Bodenstein and Kondritzer (1948) to prevent the synthesis of deoxyribonucleic acid during the development of *Amblystoma punctatum*, though not interfering with the production of ribonucleic acid.

It is an attractive hypothesis that the main effect of the mustard compounds should be on the nucleic acids and nucleoprotein substances, which, as Stowell (1947) has indicated, play an important role in the transfer of genetic characteristics, in cellular division, in the synthesis of proteins, and probably on the function or action of certain enzymes. In spite of the general similarity of the actions of nitrogen mustards and X-rays, Schreck (1948–50) has been able to detect certain differences in the nuclear structural effects of these agents. The work of Fell and Allsopp (1948), however, indicated that the mustards are not entirely nucleotoxic in their action. The compounds infiltrated the cell via the fat-globules, and caused distortion of cell outline and disintegration of protoplasm. Both nuclear and cytoplasmic changes could be explained by the observations of Berenblum and Schoental (1947) concerning the rapid attack on nucleoprotein and its coagulation by mustard gas—ribonucleic acid being a component of the cytoplasm, as well as occurring with deoxyribonucleic acid in the nucleus.

Therapeutic Applications

The depressant effect of halogenated alkylamines on the leucopoietic tissues of those exposed to them suggested to Wilkinson a possible therapeutic application (Wilkinson and Fletcher, 1947). In 1942 he had made clinical trials of 2,2′-dichlorodiethylmethylamine in cases of chronic myeloid leukaemia and chronic lymphatic leukaemia, and almost immediately, in America, clinical trials with 2,2′,2″-trichlorotriethylamine were carried out by Gilman, Goodman, Lindskog, and Dougherty (1942–3) on six patients suffering from terminal neoplastic conditions. These authors were already familiar with the toxic effects of the mustard compounds on lymphoid and haemopoietic tissues and the marked vulnerability of proliferating tissue, and with the experimental work of Dougherty, Gilman, Goodman, and Dougherty (1942–3), which indicated that disappearance of the tumour tissues of transplanted mouse lymphosarcoma could be effected by mustard compounds. The results obtained in these trials suggested that further clinical trials were justified. After the official statement concerning clinical possibilities by Rhoads (1946), the clinical results were published by Goodman, Wintrobe, Dameshek, Goodman, Gilman, and McLennan (1946), Jacobson, Spurr, Barron, Smith, Lushbaugh, and Dick (1946), Karnofsky, Craver, Rhoads, and Abels (1947), Wilkinson and Fletcher (1947), and ApThomas and Cullumbine (1947). Further justification of the clinical applications was afforded by the beneficial effects of the mustard compounds on experimental neoplasms noted by several authors. Johnson (1948) found that nine out of 33 chickens suffering from fowl leucosis, a leukaemia-like disease transmitted by a filterable virus, showed clinical recovery after only one treatment; it seemed that the chemical agent also had a lethal effect on the virus, as the disease could not be transmitted by blood drawn from treated birds. Karnofsky, Parisette, and Patterson (1948) reported the consistent chemotherapeutic activity of 2,2′-dichlorodiethylmethylamine, 2,2′,2″-trichlorotriethylamine, and various homologues (as well as X-rays and di(β-chloroethyl)sulphide) on sarcoma 180 grown on the chorio-allantoic membranes of the chick embryo. Boyland, Koller, and Warwick (1948–50) obtained complete inhibition of Walker rat carcinoma and partial inhibition of spontaneous mammary tumours in mice; the inhibition was of a temporary nature. Burchenal, Riley, and Lester (1948, 1948–50) found, in studies of transmitted mouse leukaemia, that groups of mice treated with methyl-bis(β-chloroethyl)amine or the newer compound (Sk 137), 1:3-propanediamine-2-chloro-NNN′N′-tetrakis(2-chloroethyl), usually showed an average increase in survival time of about 100 per cent. over untreated controls. Therapeutic activity appeared to be related to the presence of at least two β-haloalkyl groups (Burchenal and Riley, 1949).

Personal Experience

Our study of nitrogen mustard therapy began in July 1948, and, for the purposes of the present analysis, was terminated in June 1952. Altogether 51 patients were treated. As little success was obtained in cases of chronic lymphatic leukaemia, acute leukaemia, polycythaemia vera, and carcinoma of the lung, it was decided at an early stage not to treat any more patients suffering from these conditions with nitrogen mustard. None of our patients had any previous radiotherapy.

Administration and dosage. The preparation used in our series has been 'mustine hydrochloride' (Boots)—2,2′-dichlorodiethylmethylamine hydrochloride (Howells, 1953). The solution is prepared for intravenous injection by adding 10 ml. of normal saline solution to the vial containing 10 mg. of the nitrogen mustard hydrochloride, withdrawing 5 ml. of the resulting solution

Results of Nitrogen Mustard Therapy

		Patients dead							Patients living						
			Survival after therapy							Duration after therapy					
Disease	*Effect*	*Number*	*1–3 mths.*	*3–6 mths.*	*6–12 mths.*	*1–2 yrs.*	*2–3 yrs.*	*over 3 yrs.*	*Number*	*1–3 mths.*	*3–6 mths.*	*6–12 mths.*	*1–2 yrs.*	*2–3 yrs.*	*over 3 yrs.*
Hodgkin's disease 27 patients	No response	21	5	..	..	..	..	..	6	..	..	..	..	..	..
	Improvement		1	6	2	4	2	1		1	..	..	2	..	3
Lymphosarcoma 8 patients	No response	6	3	..	..	..	..	..	2	..	..	..	..	..	..
	Improvement		..	1	..	1	1	..		..	..	..	1	1	..
Myeloid leukaemia 8 patients	No response	6	2	..	..	..	..	..	2	..	..	..	..	..	..
	Improvement		..	1	3	..	..	..		..	1	..	..	1	..
Chronic lymphatic leukaemia 3 patients	No response	3	1	..	..	..	..	..	..						
	Improvement		..	..	2	..	..	..							
Acute leukaemia 2 patients	No response	2	1	..	..	..	..	..	..						
	Improvement		1	..	..	..	..	..							
Carcinoma of lung 2 patients	No response	2	..	..	..	..	..	..	..						
	Improvement		1	1	..	..	..	..							

into a 20 ml. syringe, and then filling the syringe to the 20 ml. mark with more saline solution, thus obtaining a concentration of 5 mg. of nitrogen mustard hydrochloride in 20 ml. of saline. This concentration has proved satisfactory, and with reasonable care in the technique of intravenous injection a greater dilution has not proved necessary. The solution should be freshly prepared, and the injection given slowly with repeated withdrawals of blood into the syringe, taking great care to avoid extravasation. The operator is advised to wear rubber gloves, because the solution has vesicant properties which may damage the skin if contact occurs, causing blistering or dermatitis. Although the recommended dose is 0·1 mg. per kg. of body-weight, it has been found in practice that a dose of 5 mg. is suitable for most patients, and this should not be exceeded except on rare occasions. The average course consists of six injections, one being given daily or on alternate days. More than one course may be given, but it is advisable to allow at least four weeks between courses. A close watch should be kept on the total white-cell count, and especially on the proportion of granular white cells. In Hodgkin's disease and lymphosarcoma the depression of the white cells is seldom serious enough to cause concern, even when there is an initial leucopenia, but in the case of leukaemia the fall in the white-cell count may be sudden and severe, and accordingly it is not wise to use this form of therapy in any case of leukaemia with a white-cell count of less than 30,000 per c.mm. A rare complication is the development of gynaecomastia in male patients, but, although painful, it is not serious and need not interfere with the continuance of treatment.

Hodgkin's disease. Of the 27 patients treated 21 have died, and only six are still living. In 15 of the 21 who have died, a careful clinical assessment indicated a favourable response to initial treatment. All the six still living are considered to have shown a favourable response for a substantial period.

Twenty-one patients who have died. Six were female and 15 were male. The youngest was 26 years of age, and the oldest 74 years. When first seen the general condition was poor in 12, fair in seven, and good in two patients. The lymph-nodes were enlarged in the cervical region in all patients, in the axillae and also in the groins in all except four, and in the mediastinum in 12. There was splenomegaly in 10 patients, and hepatomegaly in nine. The number of courses of nitrogen mustard was one in eight patients, two in six patients, three in one patient, four in two patients, five in two patients, and six in two patients.

Six patients who are living. All these are male, the youngest being 25 years of age and the oldest 60 years. When first seen the general condition was considered to be fair in two and good in four patients. The lymph-nodes were enlarged in the cervical region in six patients, in the axillae in five, in the groins in three, and in the mediastinum in one; the spleen was enlarged in one patient and the liver in one patient. The number of treatment courses was one in three patients, three in two patients, and five in one patient. The following is a brief account of the six patients who are still alive.

E. P., a man aged 49 years, was admitted to hospital with histologically proved Hodgkin's disease confined to the right side of the neck. One course of nitrogen mustard therapy produced a good clinical response, and there was no evidence of extension of the disease three and a half years later.

W. J., a man aged 25 years, was admitted to hospital with three months' history of asthenia, loss of weight, and Hodgkin's lymphadenopathy in the neck, axillae, and groins; the haemoglobin was 69 per cent. He received five courses of treatment, each producing a favourable remission lasting six to eight months, and at the end of two years there was no sign of extension of the disease.

J. A. G. B., a man aged 36 years, had a recent history of Hodgkin's lymphadenopathy confined to the neck and axillae. Three courses of treatment were administered over a period of three years and four months, each being followed by a favourable response, with no clinical evidence of extension of the disease.

E. Y., a man aged 39 years, was admitted to hospital with 20 months' history of cervical lymphadenopathy. Hodgkin's lymphadenopathy was present in the neck and one axilla, and the liver was enlarged. He received three courses of treatment, each followed by a remission lasting up to 18 months, and at the end of three years and one month there was no evidence of spread of the disease.

A. P., a man aged 36 years, was admitted with three years' history of cervical lymph-node enlargement, proved histologically to be Hodgkin's disease. There was no other evidence of the disease 13 months after a course of treatment.

D. McK., a man aged 60 years, received one course of treatment for Hodgkin's lymphadenoma confined to the neck, axillae, and groins; there was a good immediate response, which had been maintained when he was seen two months later.

The following brief account of three patients who responded for a time, but died later, will illustrate some important features.

E. H. W., a married woman aged 34 years, was admitted to hospital with enormous enlargement of the cervical lymph-nodes due to Hodgkin's disease. Her general condition was extremely poor; the haemoglobin was 47 per cent.; minor lymphadenopathy was present in the groins and mediastinum. She had six courses of nitrogen mustard therapy, each followed by striking symptomatic improvement which, however, was of short duration, the results being less favourable with later courses. Death occurred after two and a half years.

F. W., a man aged 56 years, was admitted with a recent history of swelling in the neck and constitutional disturbance. There was extensive involvement of the lymph-nodes in the neck, axillae, and groins, with enlargement of the liver and spleen, anasarca, and bilateral pleural effusion. Death seemed imminent, but after the first few injections of nitrogen mustard the response was striking. His dyspnoea was relieved, and most of the aforementioned signs disappeared. Each of two further courses also evoked a good remission with relief of mediastinal obstruction, the remissions lasting 20 months and 10 months respectively. Later the disease progressed rapidly, a fourth and final course had no effect, and he died at the end of two years and seven months.

W. B., a man aged 53 years, was admitted to hospital with 16 months' history of enlargement of lymph-nodes and constitutional disturbance. Hodgkin's disease was present in the neck, axillae, and groins, and there was hepatic and splenic enlargement, ascites, and a right pleural effusion, his general condition being very poor. After nitrogen mustard therapy there was a rapid and marked improvement in symptoms and signs, and for more than three years he was able to work as a clerk. He received a total of five courses of treatment, each resulting in a remission lasting six months or more, but eventually treatment had to be discontinued on account of thrombophlebitis. He died three years and four months after the first course of injections.

Lymphosarcoma. Eight patients with lymphosarcoma were treated, the diagnosis being confirmed by histological examination of biopsy material, and in some patients of autopsy material as well. Six were male and two female; the youngest was 40 years of age, and the oldest 76 years. When first seen the general condition was considered to be poor in four patients and fair in four. The lymph-nodes were enlarged in the cervical region in all patients, in the axillae in all except two, in the groins in all except three, and in the mediastinum in three patients. The spleen was enlarged in three and the liver in one patient. The number of courses of treatment administered was one in five patients, two in two patients, and six in one patient. Of the six patients who have died, three showed temporary improvement and survived for a total period of four months, 34 months, and 49 months respectively. Of the two who are still living, one has survived one year and the other two years, each having shown a good response after one course of treatment. The following case history of one patient who died will serve to illustrate the type of response seen in these cases, and will support the claim that, although not curative, this form of treatment will effect temporary symptomatic improvement in some cases.

W. N., a man aged 71 years, was found to have multiple lymph-node enlargement in the neck, axillae, and groins, considerable splenomegaly, and moderate anaemia, and also radiological evidence of mediastinal and hilar lymph-node enlargement. The first course of treatment was followed by a good remission lasting eight months, and a second course by one lasting five months. Further courses, of which six were given, evoked a diminishing response, and he died 22 months after commencing treatment, the diagnosis of lymphosarcoma being confirmed at autopsy.

Myeloid leukaemia. Eight patients with myeloid leukaemia are included in the series, all except one being male, and the ages ranging from 26 to 74 years. The number of courses of treatment administered was one in five patients, three in two patients, and seven in one patient. Of these patients six died within 12 months of treatment, some of them having shown some temporary improvement. One, who is still alive after five months, has shown a good initial response, but the only patient in the series for whom success can reasonably be claimed is still alive after 29 months. His case history is as follows:

J. W. M., a man aged 40 years, was admitted to hospital with enormous splenomegaly, axillary lymphadenopathy, and blood and bone-marrow films typical of myeloid leukaemia. During the next 29 months he received seven courses of nitrogen mustard therapy, each being followed by a good remission, but the response diminishing in degree towards the end of the period. Nevertheless he was able to continue at work, and is still alive. A typical blood count showed white cells 610,000 per c.mm. before a course of injections, and 103,000 per c.mm. immediately afterwards.

Other cases. These include polycythaemia vera (one patient), acute leukaemia (two patients), chronic lymphatic leukaemia (three patients), and carcinoma of the lung (two patients). In all these cases treatment was without effect, with the possible exception of one young man with carcinoma of the lung, who showed a striking initial response by the relief of mediastinal obstruction, only to relapse very quickly and die six months later.

Discussion

It is difficult to assess the significance of apparent changes in the course of diseases such as the reticuloses, which vary in severity and duration in different individuals. Karnofsky and Burchenal (1948) and Burchenal, Karnofsky, Ersler, Craver, and Rhoads (1948) have discussed the important points in such an evaluation in the chemotherapy of neoplastic and leukaemic states, and we agree that there should be a clear distinction between the removal or abatement of the patient's symptoms, caused by some disturbance of function, and the cessation or otherwise of the underlying pathological process. These principles have been applied in our evaluation of nitrogen mustard therapy in the following groups of diseases.

Hodgkin's disease. Although the results based on the survival rates might suggest that this form of therapy is disappointing, such results do not give a true picture of its value, because when cases are studied in greater detail it will be seen that a number of patients responded favourably at first, with improvement in general health, and diminution in the size of lymph-nodes and spleen. The relief of distressing symptoms caused by mediastinal lymphadenopathy has sometimes been striking. Most other investigators have also noticed the striking improvement in the patients' general condition—the relief of night sweats and other toxic symptoms, the rapid drop in fever, the return of appetite, the gain in weight, and the shrinkage of granulomatous masses and infiltrations. In a series of 27 cases ApThomas (1948) noted an improvement of the general condition in every patient in whom it was affected (18 cases), of mediastinal lymphadenopathy in seven patients, of enlargement of the abdomen in seven patients, of splenomegaly in four patients, of skin rash in two patients, and of pain in five patients. Dameshek, Weisfuse, and Stein (1949) found a variable response in the relief of particular manifestations of the disease. None of their six patients with osseous involvement showed any radiological improvement. Karnofsky, Craver, Rhoads, and Abels (1947) have also commented on bone involvement being unaffected, although relief of pain might be obtained. Wintrobe and Huguley (1948), however, observed healing in some instances of spinal involvement, and relief of backache in other cases without radiological evidence of vertebral lesions. They also reported relief of severe pruritus in some cases. In spite of the possibility of toxic effects upon the bone-marrow, improvement in anaemia has been noted in a few patients by Karnofsky, Craver, Rhoads, and Abels (1947), Wintrobe and Huguley (1948), and Brown and Davis (1949).

Although Goodman, Wintrobe, Dameshek, Goodman, Gilman, and McLennan (1946) found that in most patients some benefit was obtained, other investigators, including ourselves, have noticed that certain patients, for no obvious reason, do not respond with remissions. In the opinion of many workers, nitrogen mustard therapy is not definitely superior to deep X-ray therapy, in that the remissions obtained are often of shorter duration (Karnofsky, Craver, Rhoads, and Abels, 1947; Spurr, Smith, and Jacobson, 1948; Wintrobe and Huguley, 1948; Dameshek, Weisfuse, and Stein, 1949). The length of remissions very often diminishes as further courses of nitrogen mustard are given, so that eventually a state of resistance is reached. Diamond (1953) has pointed out that, while remissions may vary from a few weeks to many months, six weeks is a common period. He suggested that patients with local lymphadenopathy and without constitutional symptoms (Class I) should be treated always with X-rays; nitrogen mustard would be beneficial in some patients with regional involvement of lymph-nodes, whether accompanied by constitutional symptoms or not (Class II), and in most of those who show generalization of the disease with toxic symptoms (Class III). Wintrobe and Huguley (1948) would not exclude the use of nitrogen mustard in Class I, in view of the difficulty of determining the true extent of the disease in any case, and from personal experience of remissions obtained by nitrogen mustard when radiotherapy had been ineffective; they also suggested the possibility of increased benefit from a combination of the two modes of therapy. ApThomas (1948) and Dameshek, Weisfuse, and Stein (1949) favoured drastic X-ray therapy for the early cases. Craver (1948), from experience of 102 patients, considered nitrogen mustard contra-indicated in early localized lymphadenopathy, and in patients with regional involvement and without marked constitutional symptoms. Even in the patients of Class III he considered X-rays to have a place, either in conjunction with mustard or as interim treatment of bulky residual nodal masses or bone lesions. Nitrogen mustard has definitely had a great effect—at times dramatic—in the treatment of many patients in serious and apparently terminal illness, with generalized involvement and marked constitutional symptoms (Jacobson, Spurr, Barron, Smith, Lushbaugh, and Dick, 1946; Brown and Davis, 1949). Further, its use is essential under two conditions—when the skin is no longer able to tolerate radiotherapy, and when lymph-nodes remain enlarged and toxic symptoms persist in spite of intensive courses of X-rays (ApThomas and Cullumbine, 1947; Karnofsky, Craver, Rhoads, and Abels, 1947; Dameshek, Weisfuse, and Stein, 1949; Reinhard, Good, and Martin, 1950). In a few cases in which neither radiotherapy nor nitrogen mustard alone was effective, a combined course was beneficial. Bethell, Andrews, Neligh, and Meyers (1950) considered that alternating irradiation and nitrogen mustard showed promise in the treatment of Hodgkin's disease. In some other patients sensitivity to X-rays has apparently been restored after the mustard treatment, whether or not benefit accrued from the latter (Jacobson, Spurr, Barron, Smith, Lushbaugh, and Dick, 1946; Zanes, Doan, and Hoster, 1948; Dameshek, Weisfuse, and Stein, 1949). Karnofsky and Burchenal (1950), Reinhard, Good, and Martin (1950), and Boland (1951) have suggested that nitrogen mustard should be utilized in cases such as the mediastinal syndrome and compression paraplegia, in which the initial radiotherapy reaction may cause an aggravation of the symptoms.

A review of 37 reports comprising 832 patients, of whom about 10 to 15 per cent. had received only nitrogen mustard therapy, revealed that poor results were obtained in about 20 per cent. of all cases. The average duration of the remissions was found by Wintrobe and Huguley (1948) to be three months (range 1 to 26 months), and by Spurr, Smith, Block, and Jacobson (1950) to be 2·7 months (range ½ to 18 months); nearly half of the 50 patients of Dameshek, Weisfuse, and Stein (1949) obtained remissions of less than two months. The average duration of the disease in the 13 living patients of Wintrobe and Huguley (1948) was 36 months in all, and 15 months after the onset of nitrogen mustard therapy; in the 19 dead the times were 32 months and eight months respectively. Spurr, Smith, Block, and Jacobson (1950) found that the average duration of the disease in their 17 living patients was 65·1 months in all and 22·4 months after the onset of therapy; the average duration of the disease in the 40 dead was 39·7 months. In a critical examination of a combined régime of X-rays and nitrogen mustard in 67 patients, Gellhorn and Collins (1951) found that the four-year survival rate from the time of onset of symptoms, the time of biopsy diagnosis, or the time of evident generalization of the disease, was not significantly different from that of 65 patients treated with radiotherapy alone; but the amount of time necessary for radiation therapy appeared to be reduced by one-half. Boland (1951) found a slight improvement (from 33 per cent. to 40 per cent.) in the three-year survival rate since the addition of nitrogen mustard, and in the case of patients dying within the three years an improvement from 11 months to 14 months in the average duration of life. It is of interest here that Boden (1951) noted that a crude five-year survival rate of 26 per cent. in X-ray treated patients was distributed as follows: localized disease 53 per cent. (20 in 38), generalized disease 12 per cent. (nine in 74). Some Continental experience has been indicated by di Guglielmo (1949) and Justin-Besançon and his colleagues (1948 *b*).

Lymphosarcoma group. The results have been qualitatively similar to those described in Hodgkin's disease, but nitrogen mustard has been much more frequently unsuccessful (Jacobson, Spurr, Barron, Smith, Lushbaugh, and Dick, 1946; Karnofsky, Craver, Rhoads, and Abels, 1947; Wintrobe and Huguley, 1948). When obtained, the remissions lasted variable times, but again repeated courses were less successful. Goldman, Egeberg, Ware, Evans, and Fishkin (1948) reported that of the 25 patients listed in reports, improvement occurred in 14 (56 per cent.) with remissions lasting from ½ to 18 months. Many patients were unresponsive without obvious reason. From experience of 66 patients, Craver (1948) thought that while nitrogen mustard might be life-saving, in general the remissions were incomplete and temporary, and in the most aggressive forms of the disease a rapid relapse was usual, while continued growth of the neoplastic tissue might occur in spite of very large doses; in some of the less acute or aggressive lymphosarcomas and in some lympholeukosarcomas large doses had produced remissions lasting from a few months to a year or more. Perusal of 23 reports, involving 194 patients, of whom about 20 per cent. were initially treated with nitrogen mustard, showed that poor results were obtained in about 20 to 25 per cent. of all cases. The longest average remission—three and a half months—was reported by Spurr, Smith, Block, and Jacobson (1950) in nine out of ten patients. The average duration of the disease in their six living patients was 51·3 months, and in the four dead 41½ months. The average duration of the disease reported by Wintrobe and Huguley (1948) was 34 months in the nine patients who died from lymphosarcoma and 11 months in the five who died from reticulum-cell sarcoma.

Leukaemia. All authors are agreed that the acute leukaemias are not responsive to nitrogen mustard, though temporary remissions lasting a few weeks may be obtained (Craver, 1948; Wintrobe and Huguley, 1948; Gardikas and Wilkinson, 1952). Our experience has been similar. Craver (1948) considered that the remissions in cases of chronic leukaemia (17 lymphatic and 30 myeloid) were of short duration—a month or so—with, as a rule, little alteration in the differential count. He believed that in the myeloid variety longer remissions, with greater reduction in the splenomegaly, could be produced by X-rays, with more prospect of improvement in the anaemia. Wintrobe and Huguley (1948) were impressed with the results in chronic myeloid leukaemia, controlling seven out of 11 patients by using maintenance therapy with frequently repeated small courses of nitrogen mustard. They divided their lymphatic leukaemia patients into two groups: (*a*) those really not ill, in whom the characteristic blood findings were more or less incidental; favourable responses occurred here; and (*b*) those with marked lymphadenopathy, splenomegaly, thrombocytopenia, and anaemia; these patients usually were refractory. Burchenal, Myers, Craver, and Karnofsky (1949), reviewing the reports of 127 cases of leukaemia including 38 of their own, found in acute leukaemias no consistent clinical remissions; in chronic myelocytic leukaemia results similar to, but generally no better than, those obtained with irradiation or radiophosphorus; and in chronic lymphocytic leukaemia very variable results, depending largely on the general condition of the patient before therapy. About half of the 107 patients with chronic lymphatic leukaemia reported in 15 articles showed a poor response to nitrogen mustard; of 80 patients with chronic myeloid leukaemia, a poor response was obtained in one-third to one-half. Gardikas and Wilkinson (1952) used small courses, carefully and strictly supervised, as often as required, in 50 patients with chronic myeloid and 32 with chronic lymphatic leukaemia, all of whom had progressing and advanced symptoms and signs. In myeloid leukaemia 42, and in lymphatic leukaemia 26, showed a satisfactory remission after the first course. Using Bethell's (1943) criteria the comparable results in the series of Gardikas and Wilkinson, treated with nitrogen mustard, and Bethell's (1943) series, treated by irradiation, were respectively: excellent response in 24·0 per cent. and 12·5 per cent.; very good in 22·0 per cent. and 41·3 per cent.; good in 36·0 per cent. and 36·5 per cent.; fair in 12·0 per cent. and 7·7 per cent.; and no effect in 6·0 per cent. and 1·9 per cent. Gardikas and Wilkinson found that the average times of survival from the onset of the disease and from the start of nitrogen mustard therapy were 3·7 and 2·25 years respectively in chronic myeloid leukaemia, and 3·6 and 2·1 years respectively in chronic lymphatic leukaemia. They believed, from an analysis of published reports, that nitrogen mustard was at least as effective as X-rays and radioactive phosphorus.

Carcinoma of the lung. We have not proceeded with nitrogen mustard therapy in inoperable carcinoma of the lung, in view of the unfavourable responses obtained. Boyland, Clegg, Koller, Rhoden, and Warwick (1948) and Karnofsky, Abelman, Craver, and Burchenal (1948) considered that nitrogen mustard was valuable in the prolongation of useful life for a short time, and in relieving discomfort or distressing symptoms. Brown and Davis (1949) considered that it offered no significant therapeutic advance in this condition. Craver (1948) thought that a combination of nitrogen mustard with subsequent X-ray therapy was a useful means of palliation in anaplastic cancer of the lung. Skinner, Carr, and Denman (1948) felt that the majority of their patients gained in weight and strength, being able to continue working nearly until the terminal stages of the disease. They observed that the end usually came rather rapidly, narcotics being required only rarely in their patients previously treated with nitrogen mustard.

Histological changes. It is of interest to consider the histological effects of nitrogen mustard on the neoplastic masses. During the week following treatment (Spitz, 1948) cytological changes observed in Hodgkin's disease included striking enlargement of the reticular cells and the Sternberg-Reed cells, principally due to fat; nuclear changes consisted mainly of swelling, with loss of chromatin pattern, and occasionally pyknosis was present. Not all cells were equally affected, and mitoses in the unaltered cells were apparent even during the destructive phase. The nuclear and cytoplasmic changes were not evident in the cases of Hodgkin's disease after an interval of eight days. In most cases there was a definite transformation of the tumour into a cellular and more pleomorphic one, in which multinucleated giant cells were present. In lymphosarcoma, in spite of the less striking results observed clinically, the histological changes were more widespread and of longer duration. Cytological alterations consisted of ballooning of the cytoplasm by fat, and nuclear fragmentation which persisted as long as three weeks after therapy. Even after this period large numbers of macrophages remained within the tumour nodules. During the steady destruction of tumour cells there was at the same time growth of the unaltered cells, as indicated by easily demonstrable mitoses and an increasing pleomorphism of the residual cells of the tumour. Cytological alterations were not seen in chronic lymphatic leukaemia or the lymphocytic type of lymphosarcoma; there seemed simply to be a reduction in the number of cells comprising the infiltrates, restricted to those cases in which the peripheral blood count had been lowered. Dameshek, Weisfuse, and Stein (1949) noted that the lymph-nodes in Hodgkin's disease, within 24 hours of starting therapy, showed a decrease in cellularity, with pyknosis and smudging of lymphocytic cells; four days later these findings were more marked; polymorphonuclears showed vacuolation and hypersegmentation, and reticulum cells were bizarre and degenerate and showed frequent vacuolation. On the other hand, Cornell and Blauw (1949), after studying 17 cases, reported that the criteria noted in treated tissues were not found consistently in the series, and might even be observed in untreated cases.

Toxic effects. The toxic effects of the nitrogen mustards fall into three groups: local, alimentary, and haematological. Locally thrombophlebitis may occur, while extravasation outside the vein may cause necrosis of tissue. A patient of Goldman, Egeberg, Ware, Evans, and Fishkin (1948) developed vesiculation of the skin where a drop of the solution fell, and one of our operators developed a contact dermatitis. Almost all patients suffer some epigastric discomfort, nausea, and anorexia, but vomiting is less common. Sedatives and a gastric sedative mixture have been very effective in our hands; Wintrobe, Huguley, McLennan, and Lima (1947) and Goldman, Egeberg, Ware, Evans, and Fishkin (1948) found that a satisfactory procedure was to administer the nitrogen mustard in the evening after a sedative. Ulceration in the alimentary canal has been reported by Zanes, Doan, and Hoster (1948) and Bauer and Erf (1950) and severe haematemesis has occurred in patients of Dameshek, Weisfuse, and Stein (1949), Videbaek (1949), and Bauer and Erf (1950). Diarrhoea is infrequent, and has not been troublesome (Spurr, Jacobson, Smith, and Barron, 1947; Wilkinson and Fletcher, 1947; Boyland, Clegg, Koller, Rhoden, and Warwick, 1948; Ariel and Kanter, 1949). Haematological studies have been carried out by several investigators. Depression of the cellular elements of the blood, and various degrees of hypoplasia of the bone-marrow, are potentially the most serious toxic effects. Jacobson, Spurr, Barron, Smith, Lushbaugh, and Dick (1946) found that the initial change in the peripheral blood was a diminution in the lymphocytes within 24 hours, progressing for about a week; degenerating forms also appeared. The lymphocyte values usually began to tend towards normal about two weeks after the last injection, that is in the third week. The monocytes followed the same course, and atypical forms were again common in the first week. The total leucocyte count diminished progressively for about two to three weeks, owing largely to the severe neutropenia. The duration of the leucopenia was usually relatively short. Recovery tended to begin within two weeks after the maximum reduction, and with its onset a marked shift to the left occurred in the granular series. Dameshek, Weisfuse, and Stein (1949) found the maximum cytopenic levels on the 21st to 25th days. Wintrobe and Huguley (1948) confirmed the observation that granulocytopenia occurred in about 14 days (from four to 37 days); recovery took place four to five weeks after the injections (11 to 90 days). They noted that a leucopenia below 4,000 per c.mm. developed after 51 per cent. of 126 injections when the drug was given to patients with normal or high white-cell counts. Leucopenia was seldom severe in cases in which there had been none prior to therapy. With a dose per course of approximately 25 mg., Jacobson, Spurr, Barron, Smith, Lushbaugh, and Dick (1946) found that 60 per cent. of 42 courses produced a leucopenia below 3,000 per c.mm. Both groups of workers observed a thrombocytopenia, usually in the third week (8 to 39 days); recovery occurred in about six to seven weeks (21 to 105 days). As a result prolonged bleeding times and delayed clot-retraction occurred, but no significant changes were found in the prothrombin level or clotting time. A defect in the blood coagulation, associated with the presence of a heparin-like substance in the plasma, has been observed by Smith, Jacobson, Spurr, Allen, and Block (1948). Haemorrhages—petechial, purpuric, and mucosal—have been reported, though almost always without fatalities.

The reticulocytes in the peripheral blood have been found reduced to less than 0·1 per cent. during the first week. Evidence of regeneration was seen occasionally in the second and third weeks, but recovery was not complete until the fourth or fifth week. Anaemia occurred in the first few weeks of treatment. Wintrobe and Huguley (1948) found that the volume of the packed red cells dropped below 40 ml. after 29 per cent. of courses, the lowest level being reached usually in 15 days (seven to 31 days). A tendency towards macrocytosis was seen in the fifth week, and recovery occurred in seven to eight weeks (20 to 75 days). Zanes, Doan, and Hoster (1948) found that the most marked anaemia occurred three to four weeks after therapy; the maximum depression of the peripheral white blood-cells was noted on an average on the 20th day after therapy. There has been some indication that, with each of the three cellular elements, depression was more frequent the larger the dose per course. Studies of urobilinogen excretion performed by Jacobson, Spurr, Barron, Smith, Lushbaugh, and Dick (1946) showed a definite increase in haemolysis after nitrogen mustard.

The events shown in the peripheral blood ran closely parallel in time to those in the bone-marrow. Block, Spurr, Jacobson, and Smith (1948) observed a very slight increase in degeneration in the bone-marrow within 24 hours after an injection. Spurr, Jacobson, Smith, and Barron (1947) observed a prompt destruction of haemopoietic cells, occurring initially at the level of the immature cells, which might proceed to a stage in which only reticulum cells, plasma cells, atypical blast forms, and megakaryocytes remained. The total nucleated cell count in the marrow was reduced to 17 per cent. by the end of the third week, with a sharp rise to 65 per cent. at the end of the fourth week. Three weeks after treatment the counts had increased to levels observed before treatment. The total erythroblasts declined from a normal level of 25 to 30 per cent. to about 3 per cent. in the weeks following therapy, increasing to about 40 to 48 per cent. in the fourth week. Myelocytes were reduced in the first and second weeks, with a spectacular regeneration to 20 per cent. in the third week; metamyelocytes fell to a minimum in the third week, with regeneration in the fourth week. The polymorphonuclears were lowest in the third and fourth weeks, regenerating in the fifth week. The peaks of the different cell regeneration phases followed chronologically according to the developmental history of the cell types. Brown and Davis (1950) also reported degeneration and hypoplasia of the marrow in the second and third weeks, with hyperplasia in the fourth. Dameshek, Weisfuse, and Stein (1949) also noted the hypoplasia of the marrow, with a return to normality in six to eight weeks. Notwithstanding the obvious haematological damage, the great majority of patients show a prompt reversion to a relatively normal equilibrium within a few weeks of therapy. Spurr,

Jacobson, Smith, and Barron (1947), unlike Roswit and Kaplan (1949), found no conclusive evidence of cumulative injury to the bone-marrow, provided the white-cell count was permitted to return to normal before further treatment. In spite of the severity of the leucopenia at times, the development of the complete agranulocytic syndrome has occurred very infrequently. Jacobson, Spurr, Barron, Smith, Lushbaugh, and Dick (1946) found that recovery from the leucopenia was not influenced by the administration of adequate amounts of pentnucleotide, iron, leucocytic extract, or folic acid, nor did blood transfusions appear to alter the spontaneous recovery observed in all their patients. Nevertheless the aplasia has been so complete that fatalities have occurred from agranulocytosis (Kurnick, Paley, Fieber, and Adler, 1949; Videbaek, 1949). Recently we have obtained a favourable response by using cortisone and corticotrophin in a patient who developed agranulocytosis after nitrogen mustard therapy. Skin reactions following treatment have been reported: a maculopapular pruritic rash (Zanes, Doan, and Hoster, 1948); a varicelliform eruption (Justin-Besançon, Lamotte-Barrillon, and Polonovski, 1948 *a*); exfoliative dermatitis (Alpert, Greenspan, and Peterson, 1950); and morbilliform and copper-coloured macular eruptions (Goldman, Egeberg, Ware, Evans, and Fishkin, 1948).

Supralethal doses of the nitrogen mustards have produced in animals acute neurological disturbances with convulsions and coma (Boyland, 1946; Anslow, Karnofsky, Jager, and Smith, 1947). In the doses used such effects have not been observed in patients. There have been reported, however, lightheadedness and drowsiness (Boyland, Clegg, Koller, Rhoden, and Warwick, 1948), toxic psychosis (Roswit and Kaplan, 1949) and encephalopathy (Bierman, Shimkin, Mettier, Weaver, Berry, and Wise, 1949).

Biochemical investigations carried out before and after nitrogen mustard therapy have not revealed any changes (Jacobson, Spurr, Barron, Smith, Lushbaugh, and Dick, 1946; Kurnick, Paley, Fieber, and Adler, 1949). This result might be expected, since histological examination of non-haemopoietic organs, other than the gonads, has revealed no consistent or significant injury which might contribute to the toxic effects of nitrogen mustards (Graef, Karnofsky, Jager, Krichesky, and Smith, 1948; Spitz, 1948). Indeed, Jacobson, Spurr, Barron, Smith, Lushbaugh, and Dick (1946) treated patients showing definite damage to the liver and kidneys with repeated courses, without untoward effect on the measurable functions of the organs. Landing, Seed, and Banfield (1949) showed experimentally an apparent immunity of normal liver-cells to the mustards, not altered even in rapidly dividing cells after partial hepatectomy, when mitosis was inhibited. It is of interest that Spitz found no demonstrable changes in the mucosa of the stomach and intestine, or in the adrenals. An effect on the gonads, with reduction in active spermatogenesis, has been reported both in animals (Landing, Goldin, and Noe, 1949) and in man (Spitz, 1948; Gaensler, McKay, Ware, and Lynch, 1948; Justin-Besançon, Lamotte-Barrillon, and Polonovski, 1948 *a*).

It has been hoped that other compounds more specifically toxic for the neoplastic cells would be elaborated from the haloalkylamine series. Screening techniques, such as those of Karnofsky, Burchenal, Ormsbee, Cornman, and Rhoads (1947) and Shapiro, Goldin, Landing, Bergner, Faiman, and Goldberg (1949), have been applied to various derivatives. Reports by Burchenal, Lester, Riley, and Rhoads (1948) and Burchenal, Burchenal, and Johnston (1951) have not revealed any compounds superior to ordinary nitrogen mustard against transmitted mouse leukaemia. In the experimental examination of a number of mustard compounds, Landing and Eisenberg (1949) found no instance of greater damage to tumour cells (sarcoma 180) than to susceptible normal cells of mice. In a series of haloalkylamines administered to mice, Landing, Goldin, Noe, Goldberg, and Shapiro (1949) found that bis- or poly-2-chloroethylamines produced the most severe lymphoid destruction, but also, unfortunately, caused the greatest bone-marrow damage. Skipper (1949), however, found some indication of synergistic action between nitrogen mustard and urethane against transmitted mouse leukaemia, while Brandt and Griffin (1951) obtained in rats a protective effect or reduction of toxicity, without loss of the mustard activity, by the previous administration of cysteine. The clinical results of four new derivatives (Burchenal, 1948; Burchenal, Myers, Craver, and Karnofsky, 1949) showed no definite therapeutic superiority, except that one (Sk 136), 1:3-propanediamine-NNN′N′-tetrakis(2-chloroethyl) hydrochloride, was better tolerated by some patients. Some therapeutic advance has been made by Klopp, Alford, Bateman, Berry, and Winship (1950) in their attempt to obtain more satisfactory regional effects by fractionated intra-arterial administration of the agent. A series of aromatic nitrogen mustards was prepared by Haddow, Kon, and Ross (1948), including the aniline (R74), *m*-toluidine (R50), and β-naphthylamine (R48) analogues and β-naphthylamine-bis(2-chloropropyl)-amine (R151). The reports by Matthews (1950), McWhirter (1951), Galton (1951), Nabarro (1951), and Gardikas and Wilkinson (1951) on R48 (the least toxic) and on R151 (of intermediate toxicity) indicated that these aromatic mustards were less active than the ordinary compounds; they acted more slowly, and remissions were less frequent, less complete, and of shorter duration; on the other hand, nausea and vomiting did not occur. The advantage of relatively low toxicity was counterbalanced by feeble therapeutic action. A new compound allied to the nitrogen mustards, and containing the active ethylene-imonium grouping—triethylene melamine (2,4,6-triethyleneimino-5-triazine)—has recently been used (Karnofsky, Burchenal, Armistead, Southam, Bernstein, Craver, and Rhoads, 1951; Meyer, Schwartz, Sawitsky, Beyers, Ritz, Brahin, Diefenbach, Kleinschmidt, and Friedmann, 1952). It has been found to be similar in activity to ordinary nitrogen mustard both experimentally and clinically, and suitable for oral and intravenous administration, producing only slight nausea and occasional vomiting. The authors considered the compound to have a definite place in the treatment of the leukaemias.

Summary

1. The biological actions of the nitrogen mustards are reviewed.

2. These actions, including interference with some enzyme systems, interactions with certain essential biochemical substances such as nucleic acids and nucleoproteins, inhibition of mitosis, induction of gene mutations, chromosomal alterations and fragmentation, cytoplasmic changes, and destruction of proliferating tissues, suggested during the 1939–45 war the possibility of therapeutic application.

3. Our experiences with 51 patients, including 27 with Hodgkin's disease, eight with lymphosarcoma, and eight with chronic myeloid leukaemia, are recorded.

4. Results obtained by various authors are discussed.

5. The role of nitrogen mustard in the treatment of diseases of the lymphoreticular system is discussed.

6. The toxic effects of nitrogen mustard are reviewed.

REFERENCES

Adair, F. E., and Bagg, H. J. (1931) *Ann. Surg.* **93,** 190.
Adams, D. H., and Thompson, R. H. S. (1948) *Biochem. J.* **42,** 170.
Alpert, L. K., Greenspan, E. M., and Peterson, S. S. (1950) *Ann. Int. Med.* **32,** 393.
Anslow, W. P., Jnr., Karnofsky, D. A., Jager, B. V., and Smith, H. W. (1947) *J. Pharmacol. Exp. Therap.* **91,** 224.
ApThomas, M. I. R. (1948) *Proc. R. Soc. Med.* **41,** 47.
—— and Cullumbine, H. (1947) *Lancet,* **1,** 899.
Ariel, I. M., and Kanter, L. (1949) *Amer. J. Surg.* **77,** 509.
Auerbach C., and Robson, J. M. (1946) *Nature,* **157,** 302.
—— —— and Carr, J. G. (1947) *Science,* **105,** 243.
Barron, E. S. G., Bartlett, G. R., and Miller, Z. B. (1948) *J. Exp. Med.* **87,** 489.
—— —— —— Meyer, J., and Seegmiller, J. E. (1948) Ibid. **87,** 503.
Bartlett, P. D., Davis, J. W., Ross, S. D., and Swain, C. G. (1947) *J. Amer. Chem. Soc.* **69,** 2977.
—— Ross, S. D., and Swain, C. G. (1947) Ibid. **69,** 2971.
—— —— —— (1949), Ibid. **71,** 1415.
Bass, A. D., and Feigelson, M. (1948) *Cancer Research,* **8,** 503.
Bauer, R. D., and Erf, L. A. (1950) *Amer. J. Med. Sci.* **219,** 16.
Berenblum, I. (1929) *J. Path. Bact.* **32,** 425.
—— (1931) Ibid. **34,** 731.
—— Kendal, L. P., and Orr, J. W. (1936) *Biochem. J.* **30,** 709.
—— and Schoental, R. (1947) *Nature,* **159,** 727.
—— and Wormall, A. (1939) *Biochem. J.* **33,** 75.
Bethell, F. H. (1943) *Ann. Int. Med.* **18,** 757.
—— Andrews, G. A., Neligh, R. B., and Meyers, M. C. (1950) *Amer. J. Roentgenol.* **64,** 61.
Bierman, H. R., Shimkin, M. B., Mettier, S. R., Weaver, J., Berry, W. C., and Wise, S. P. (1949) *Calif. Med.* **71,** 117.
Block, M., Spurr, C. L., Jacobson, L. O., and Smith, T. R. (1948) *Amer. J. Clin. Path.* **18,** 671.
Boden, G. (1951) *Brit. J. Radiol.* **24,** 494.
Bodenstein, D. (1947) *J. Exp. Zool.* **104,** 311.
—— and Kondritzer, A. A. (1948) Ibid. **107,** 109.
Boland, J. (1951) *Brit. J. Radiol.* **24,** 513.

Boursnell, J. C., Francis, G. E., and Wormall, A. (1946) *Biochem. J.* **40,** 737; and subsequent papers.
Boyland, E. (1946) *Brit. J. Pharmacol.* **1,** 247.
—— Clegg, J. W., Koller, P. C., Rhoden, E., and Warwick, O. H. (1948) *Brit. J. Cancer,* **2,** 17.
—— Koller, P. C., and Warwick, O. H. (1948–50) *Acta un. internat. contra cancrum,* **6,** 435.
Brandt, E. L., and Griffin, A. C. (1951) *Cancer,* **4,** 1030.
Brown, A., and Davis, L. J. (1949) *Glasgow Med. J.* **30,** 197.
—— —— (1950) Ibid. **31,** 93.
Burchenal, J. H. (1948) *Radiology,* **50,** 494.
—— Burchenal, J. R., and Johnston, S. F. (1951) *Cancer,* **4,** 353.
—— Karnofsky, D. A., Ersler, A. J., Craver, L. F., and Rhoads, C. P. (1948) *Cancer Research,* **8,** 387.
—— Lester, R. A., Riley, J. B., and Rhoads, C. P. (1948) *Cancer,* **1,** 399.
—— Myers, W. P. L., Craver, L. F., and Karnofsky, D. A. (1949) Ibid. **2,** 1.
—— and Riley, J. B. (1949) *Cancer Research,* **9,** 553.
—— —— and Lester, R. A. (1948) Ibid. **8,** 385.
—— —— —— (1948–50) *Acta un. internat. contra cancrum,* **6,** 448.
Butler, J. A. V., Gilbert, L. A., and Smith, K. A. (1950) *Nature,* **165,** 714.
Cameron, G. R., Courtice, F. C., and Jones, R. P. (1947) *J. Path. Bact.* **59,** 425.
Cori, C. F. (1943) quoted by Barron, Bartlett, and Miller (1948) and Dixon and Needham (1946).
Cornell, V. H., and Blauw, A. S. (1949) *Amer. J. Path.* **25,** 233.
Craver, L. F. (1948) *Radiology,* **50,** 486.
Dameshek, W., Weisfuse, L., and Stein, T. (1949) *Blood,* **4,** 338.
Diamond, H. D. (1953) *Med. Clin. N. America,* **37,** 843.
Dixon, M., and Needham, D. M. (1946) *Nature,* **158,** 432.
Dougherty, T., Gilman, A., Goodman, L., and Dougherty, J. (1942–3) quoted by Gilman and Philips (1946).
Favorsky, M. V. (1939) *Compt. rend. Acad. sci. U.R.S.S.* **25,** 71. Abstracted in *Chem. Abst.* (1940) **34,** 3285.
Fell, H. B., and Allsopp, C. B. (1948) *Cancer Research,* **8,** 145, 177.
Ford, C. E. (1948) *Proc. 8th Internat. Cong. Genet.* p. 570.
Friedenwald, J. S., Buschke, W., Scholz, R. O., and Moses, S. G. (1947) *Approaches to Tumour Chemotherapy,* p. 358. Amer. Assoc. Adv. Science.
Fruton, J. S., Stein, W. H., and Bergmann, M. (1946) *J. Organ. Chem.* **11,** 559.
—— —— Stahmann, M. A., and Golumbic, C. (1946) Ibid. **11,** 571.
Gaensler, E. A., McKay, D. G., Ware, P. F., and Lynch, J. P. (1948) *Arch. Path.* **46,** 503.
Galton, D. A. G. (1951) *Brit. J. Radiol.* **24,** 511.
Gardikas, C., and Wilkinson, J. F. (1951) *Lancet,* **1,** 137.
—— —— (1952) Ibid. **2,** 161.
Gellhorn, A., and Collins, V. P. (1951) *Ann. Int. Med.* **35,** 1250.
Gibbs, C. F., and Marvel, C. S. (1935) *J. Amer. Chem. Soc.* **57,** 1137.
Gilman, A., Goodman, L., Lindskog, G. E., and Dougherty, J. (1942–3) quoted by Gilman and Philips (1946).
—— and Philips, F. S. (1946) *Science,* **103,** 409.
Gjessing, E. C., and Chanutin, A. (1946) *Cancer Research,* **6,** 593.
Goldman, R., Egeberg, R. O., Ware, E. R., Evans, E. R., and Fishkin, B. G. (1948) *Arch. Int. Med.* **82,** 125.
Golumbic, C., Fruton, J. S., and Bergmann, M. (1946) *J. Organ. Chem.* **11,** 518, and subsequent papers.
Goodman, L. S., Wintrobe, M. M., Dameshek, W., Goodman, M. J., Gilman, A., and McLennan, M. T. (1946) *J. Amer. Med. Ass.* **132,** 126.
Graef, I., Karnofsky, D. A., Jager, B. V., and Smith, H. W. (1946) *Federation Proc.* **5,** 221.
—— —— —— Krichesky, B., and Smith, H. W. (1948) *Amer. J. Path.* **24,** 1.
Guglielmo, G. di (1949) *Minerva med.* **2,** 277.

Haddow, A., Kon, G. A. R., and Ross, W. C. J. (1948) *Nature,* **162,** 824.
Hanby, W. E., Hartley, G. S., Powell, E. O., and Rydon, H. N. (1947) *J. Chem. Soc.,* p. 519.
—— and Rydon, H. N. (1947) Ibid., p. 513.
Hektoen, L., and Corper, H. J. (1921) *J. Inf. Dis.* **28,** 279.
Herriott, R. M., Anson, M. L., and Northrop, J. H. (1946–7) *J. Gen. Physiol.* **30,** 185.
Howells, L. (1953) *Medical Press,* **230,** 87.
Jacobson, L. O., Spurr, C. L., Barron, E. S. G., Smith, T., Lushbaugh, C., and Dick, G. F. (1946) *J. Amer. Med. Ass.* **132,** 263.
Johnson, E. P. (1948) *Science,* **107,** 40.
Justin-Besançon, L., Lamotte-Barrillon, S., and Polonovski, G. (1948 *a*) *Sem. hôp. Paris,* **24,** 1518.
—— —— —— (1948 *b*) *Bull. mém. Soc. méd. hôp. Paris,* **18–19,** 576, 582.
Kabelik, J. (1932) *Compt. rend. Soc. biol.* **110,** 394. Abstracted in *Chem. Abst.* (1932) **26,** 4869.
Karnofsky, D. A., Abelman, W. H., Craver, L. F., and Burchenal, J. H. (1948) *Cancer,* **1,** 634.
—— and Burchenal, J. H. (1948) *Cancer Research,* **8,** 388.
—— —— (1950) *Amer. J. Med.* **8,** 767.
—— —— Armistead, G. C., Southam, C. M., Bernstein, J. L., Craver, L. F., and Rhoads, C.P. (1951) *Arch. Int. Med.* **87,** 477.
—— —— Ormsbee, R. A., Cornman, I., and Rhoads, C. P. (1947) *Approaches to Tumour Chemotherapy,* p. 293. Amer. Assoc. Adv. Science.
—— Craver, L. F., Rhoads, C. P., and Abels, J. C. (1947) Ibid. p. 319.
—— Graef, I., and Smith, H. W. (1948) *Amer. J. Path.* **24,** 275.
—— Parisette, L. M., and Patterson, P. A. (1948) *Cancer Research,* **8,** 389.
Kindred, J. E. (1947) *Arch. Path.* **43,** 253.
—— (1949) Ibid. **47,** 378.
Kinsey, V. E., and Grant, W. M. (1947) *J. Cell. Comp. Physiol.* **29,** 51.
Klopp, C. T., Alford, T. C., Bateman, J., Berry, G. N., and Winship, T. (1950) *Ann. Surg.* **132,** 811.
Koller, P. C. (1947) *Symposia Soc. Exp. Biol.* **1,** 270.
Krumbhaar, E. B. (1919*a*) *J. Amer. Med. Ass.* **72,** 39.
—— (1919*b*) Ibid. **73,** 715.
—— and Krumbhaar, H. D. (1919) *J. Med. Research,* **40,** 497.
Kurnick, N. B., Paley, K. R., Fieber, M. H., and Adler, D. K. (1949) *Ann. Int. Med.* **30,** 974.
Landing, B. H., and Eisenberg, F. F. (1949) *Cancer,* **2,** 1083.
—— Goldin, A., and Noe, H. A. (1949) Ibid. **2,** 1075.
—— —— —— Goldberg, B., and Shapiro, D. M. (1949) Ibid. **2,** 1055.
—— Seed, J. C., and Banfield, W. G. (1949) Ibid. **2,** 1067.
Lillie, R. S., Clowes, G. H. A., and Chambers, R. (1919–20) *J. Pharmacol. Exp. Therap.* **14,** 75.
Loveless, A., and Revell, S. (1949) *Nature,* **164,** 938.
Lynch, V., Smith, H. W., and Marshall, E. K., Jnr. (1918–19) *J. Pharmacol. Exp. Therap.* **12,** 265.
McElroy, W. D., Cushing, J. E., and Miller, H. (1947) *J. Cell. Comp. Physiol.* **30,** 331.
McWhirter, R. (1951) *Brit. J. Radiol.* **24,** 503.
Magne, H., and Rémy, P. (1937) *Bull. Soc. chim. biol.* **19,** 1092. Abstracted in *Chem. Abstr.* (1937) **31,** 8589.
Marshak, A. (1946) *Proc. Soc. Exp. Biol. Med.* **63,** 118.
Matthews, W. B. (1950) *Lancet,* **1,** 896.
Meyer, L. M., Schwartz, S. O., Sawitsky, A., Beyers, M. R., Ritz, N. D., Brahin, C., Diefenbach, W., Kleinschmidt, W., and Friedmann, I. (1952) *Acta med. scand.* Suppl. **272,** 1.
Mitchell, J. S. (1942) *Brit. J. Exp. Path.* **23,** 285, 296, 309.

Mitchell, J. S. (1943) *Brit. J. Radiol.* **16,** 339.
Nabarro, J. D. N. (1951) Ibid. **24,** 507.
Pappenheimer, A. M. (1918–19) *Proc. Soc. Exp. Biol. Med.* **16,** 92.
—— (1919) *J. Amer. Med. Ass.* **73,** 690.
—— and Vance, M. (1920) *J. Exp. Med.* **31,** 71.
Peters, R. A. (1936) *Nature,* **138,** 327.
—— (1947) Ibid. **159,** 149.
—— (1951) *Edin. Med. J.* **58,** 197.
Reinhard, E. H., Good, J. T., and Martin, E. (1950) *J. Amer. Med. Ass.* **142,** 383.
Rhoads, C. P. (1946) Ibid. **131,** 656.
—— (1947) *J. Mt. Sinai Hosp.* **13,** 299.
Roswit, B., and Kaplan, G. (1949) *Amer. J. Roentgenol.* **61,** 626.
Schreck, R. (1948–50) *Acta un. internat. contra cancrum,* **6,** 848.
Seligman, A. M., Rutenburg, A. M., and Friedman, O. M. (1949) *Cancer Research,* **9,** 624.
Shapiro, D. M., Goldin, A., Landing, B. H., Bergner, A. D., Faiman, F., and Goldberg, B. (1949) *Cancer,* **2,** 100.
Skinner, E. F., Carr, D., and Denman, W. E. (1948) *J. Thoracic. Surg.* **17,** 428.
Skipper, H. E. (1949) *Cancer,* **2,** 475.
Smith, T. R., Jacobson, L. O., Spurr, C. L., Allen, J. G., and Block, M. H. (1948) *Science,* **107,** 474.
Spitz, S. (1948) *Cancer,* **1,** 383.
Spurr, C. L., Jacobson, L. O., Smith, T. R., and Barron, E. S. G. (1947) *Approaches to Tumour Chemotherapy,* p. 306. Amer. Assoc. Adv. Science.
—— Smith, T. R., Block, M., and Jacobson, L. O. (1950) *Amer. J. Med.* **8,** 710.
—— —— and Jacobson, L. O. (1948) *Radiology,* **50,** 387.
Stahmann, M. A., and Stauffer, J. F. (1947) *Science,* **106,** 35.
Stewart, M. J. (1918) *Chemical Warfare Medical Committee Rep.* No. 12, H.M.S.O.
Stowell, R. E. (1947) *Symposia Soc. Exp. Biol.* **1,** 190.
Tatum, E. L. (1947–8) *Ann. New York Acad. Sci.* **49,** 87.
Thompson, R. H. S. (1946–7) *J. Physiol.* **105,** 370.
Videbaek, A. (1949) *Acta med. scand.* **135,** 47.
Visser, J., and de Vos, J. J. T. (1935) *Geneesk. tijdschr. v. Nederl.-Indië,* **75,** 1363. Abstracted in *Chem. Abst.* (1935) **29,** 7485.
Ward, K., Jnr. (1935) *J. Amer. Chem. Soc.* **57,** 914.
Wilkinson, J. F., and Fletcher, F. (1947) *Lancet,* **2,** 540.
Wintrobe, M. M., and Huguley, C. M., Jnr. (1948) *Cancer,* **1,** 357.
—— Huguley, C. M., Jnr., McLennan, M. T., and Lima, L. P. de C. (1947) *Ann. Int. Med.* **27,** 529.
Zanes, R. J., Jnr., Doan, C. A., and Hoster, H. A. (1948) *J. Lab. Clin. Med.* **33,** 1002.

ADDITIONAL SOURCES CONSULTED, OR INDIRECTLY REFERRED TO IN THE TEXT

Alpert, L. K., and Peterson, S. S. (1947) *Bull. U.S. Army Med. Dep.* **7,** 187.
Ben-Asher, S. (1949) *Amer. J. Med. Sci.* **217,** 162.
Bortz, D. W., and Haden, R. L. (1947) *Cleveland Clin. Quart.* **14,** 218.
Erf, L. A., and Bauer, R. D. (1949) *Amer. J. Clin. Path.* **19,** 372.
Falcon, W. W., and Gorham, L. W. (1948) *New York St. J. Med.* **48,** 612.
Greenwalt, T. J., and Grueninger, A. J. (1948) *J. Lab. Clin. Med.* **33,** 1648.
Hettig, R. A. (1947) Ibid. **32,** 1431.
Hofmeyer, H. O. (1947) *South Afr. Med. J.* **21,** 195.
Mayo, J. (1949) *Med. J. Aust.* **2,** 47.
Meyer, A. H., and Overmiller, W. C. (1949) *Ann. Int. Med.* **30,** 381.
Nabarro, J. D. N. (1949) *Brit. Med. J.* **2,** 622.
Scott, R. B. (1948) *Quart. J. Med.* N.S. **17,** 329.
Sherry, M. (1948) *South. Med. J.* **41,** 118.

Shullenberger, C. C., Watkins, C. H., and Kierland, R. R. (1949) *J. Amer. Med. Ass.* **139**, 733.
Taffel, M. (1947) *Yale J. Biol. Med.* **19**, 971.
Talbott, J. H. (1947) *New York St. J. Med.* **47**, 1883.
Watson, D. C., and Pemberton, H. S. (1948) *Quart. J. Med.* N.S. **17**, 328.
Wawro, N. W. (1948) *Connecticut St. Med. J.* **12**, 625.

519.2:615

SEQUENTIAL TESTS IN PROPHYLACTIC AND THERAPEUTIC TRIALS[1]

By P. ARMITAGE

(From the Statistical Research Unit of the Medical Research Council, London School of Hygiene and Tropical Medicine)

A STRIKING aspect of post-war research in clinical and preventive medicine is the extent to which new drugs and vaccines have been tested by controlled trials. The essential feature of these trials has been the random allocation of subjects to groups receiving different treatments, a principle of experimentation due to Sir Ronald Fisher, and now regarded as fundamental in many fields of scientific research. In a survey of the aims and methods of the clinical trial, Hill (1950–1) has emphasized the difficulties in interpreting the results of trials in which the precaution of randomization has not been followed. The statistical methods for testing the significance of observed differences between groups, normally applied at the end of such a trial, assume that the number of subjects included was determined either before the start of the trial, or at least by some circumstance independent of the results themselves. For instance, the customary test for an observed difference between two fatality rates is based on an enumeration of the probabilities, on the initial hypothesis that two treatments do not differ in their effects (the 'null hypothesis'), of all the various results which would occur if the trial were repeated indefinitely with different random samples *of the same size as those actually used*. If a trial is brought to a close at a certain point because, at that point, the results for the different treatments are either sufficiently alike or sufficiently distinct, then the traditional tests of significance are, strictly speaking, inapplicable. In prophylactic and therapeutic trials, however, there are strong ethical reasons why the results should, whenever possible, be subject to continuous analysis as they become available; it is clearly desirable that a trial should be discontinued as soon as it can safely be concluded that one treatment is more effective than another. Furthermore, quite apart from ethical considerations, this 'sequential' method of experimentation can be defended on grounds of economy, since it leads to a reduction in the average number of subjects required. Sequential experimentation should, however, be associated with appropriate methods of statistical analysis; some of these methods are described in the present paper.

The fact that classical significance tests are inapplicable when a trial is analysed sequentially is illustrated in Fig. 1. Suppose that, in order to assess the relative effects of two treatments on some measured characteristic such as temperature, we take patients in pairs and allot the members of each pair

[1] Received November 4, 1953.

randomly to the two treatments. The customary method of analysis at the end of such a trial would be to record the change in temperature for each patient, take the difference in temperature-change for each pair, calculate the mean difference for all pairs, and (provided that the differences are approximately normally distributed) test whether this mean differs significantly from zero (by the 't'-test). If, on the other hand, we wished to examine the results continuously, we might

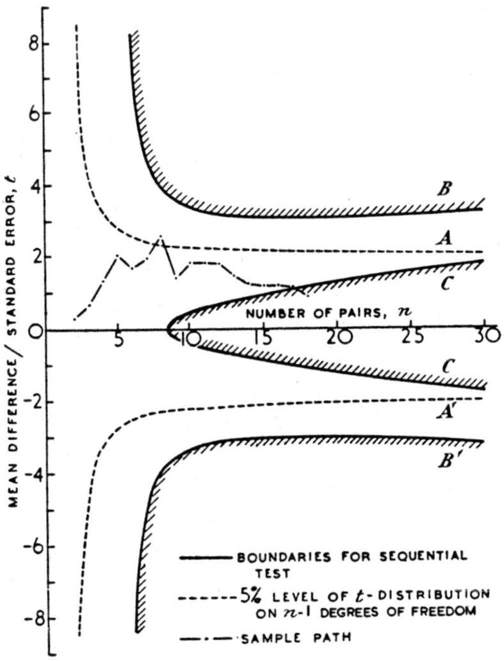

FIG. 1. Boundaries for a sequential t-test, showing the false boundaries based on the t-distribution, and a sample path based on the data of Table V.

be tempted to perform such a t-test when each pair of results was obtained, using at each stage all the results so far obtained. In Fig. 1 (dotted lines A and A') the '$P = 0{\cdot}05$' points for the t-distribution on $n-1$ degrees of freedom have been plotted against the number of pairs, n; thus with any five pairs of observations the value of t must reach $\pm 2{\cdot}776$ before the difference becomes significant at the 5 per cent. level, with 10 pairs it must reach $\pm 2{\cdot}262$, and so on. The procedure in such a continuous test could be followed graphically by plotting the value of t obtained after the entry of each pair of patients. One such 'sample path' (based on the data shown in Table V) is shown as a semi-dotted line in Fig. 1. This path crosses the boundary A at the eighth pair, and we should be tempted to stop the trial at this stage, concluding that a significant difference had been found. It must, however, be noted that with this method of continuous analysis the probability that one of these boundaries, A or A', will eventually be crossed, on the null hypothesis that the two treatments are equally effective, is considerably greater than the nominal $0{\cdot}05$ level of significance. In fact, if the trial were to continue indefinitely, the sample path would be certain to cross one of these lines. For an adequate test of the sequential t we require the boundaries B and B' in Fig. 1. These, calculated by methods described below, have the required probability, 0·05, of being crossed on the null hypothesis, and lie entirely outside the false boundaries A and A'. If, in performing a trial sequentially, we used the customary boundaries A and A', we should be working at a much less stringent level of significance than the nominal figure of 5 per cent. would lead us to believe.

The new methods for sequential tests which are described in the present paper spring largely from the war-time researches of the late A. Wald (Wald, 1947). Other methods, perhaps more suitable for medical trials, may eventually be discovered, but Wald's methods are more adaptable than any others available at the present time. In this paper I shall discuss the principles of sequential analysis and their applications to prophylactic and therapeutic trials. For simplicity I shall consider only trials in which one new treatment is being tested against a control treatment, and in which subjects are paired as they enter the trial, one member of each pair (chosen randomly) receiving the 'new treatment' and the other the 'control treatment'. The criterion by which the success of the treatment is to be measured may be either a proportion, such as a fatality rate, or the mean value of some measurements, such as change in temperature. The application of Wald's sequential methods to controlled trials (for proportions only) has previously been discussed briefly in a mathematical paper by Armitage (1950), and in more detail by Bross (1952).

Suitability of sequential approach. Whatever the advantages of the sequential approach in prophylactic and therapeutic trials, there will frequently be situations in which, for various reasons, it is impracticable, and for which the classical statistical methods are quite suitable. Three conditions must usually be satisfied in order that a trial may be carried out sequentially. First, there must usually be some single characteristic by which the success or failure of a treatment is to be judged, and which is very much more important than other possible measurements of success. In many clinical trials the conclusions must rest upon the effect of different treatments on a number of different characteristics—reduction of temperature, gain of weight, X-ray assessment, subjective impression of improvement, and so on. Clearly, it will be of little use to stop the trial as soon as a conclusion can be made about the effect on one of these characteristics, only to find that the trial has been so short that no useful statement can be made about the others. (It would perhaps be possible, however, to set up a sequential scheme for each characteristic separately, and stop the trial when a conclusion could safely be reached about some defined combination of measurements.) In some trials, on the other hand, one characteristic may be of overwhelming importance; the obvious instance is death or survival. Here we may be willing to follow a sequential scheme based on this characteristic, ignoring any other measurements until the final analysis at the end of the trial.

The second condition is that it should be administratively possible to run a trial without previously deciding its ultimate length. The sequential approach may be impracticable in large-scale collaborative trials involving a great deal of organization and perhaps special medical staff. In such a trial it may be necessary to decide the ultimate length in advance, in order both to assess its cost and to ensure reasonable security for the specially engaged staff.

Finally, a sequential approach is unlikely to be of value if the time required to assess the response of a subject to treatment is long in comparison with the period during which subjects enter the trial. Thus, in the preventive field, it would not be suitable for a trial comparing a vaccine with a placebo, if the period of entry of persons into the trial was of the order of a few months, whereas the period during which each subject was exposed to infection was two or three years. This might be the situation, for instance, in a trial to determine the efficiency of an anti-tuberculosis vaccine in preventing infection in children during the first few years after leaving school. In some prophylactic trials with highly infectious diseases, on the other hand, it might be possible to define a relatively short period of exposure. In such trials the preventive treatment might be given immediately before the short period of exposure, as in the Medical Research Council's trial of gamma globulin in the prevention of measles (Medical Research Council, 1950); or it might be possible to inoculate a large number of subjects within a short period of time, to follow up all the inoculated subjects, but to count in the final assessment only those subjects who were known to be exposed to an appreciable risk. The latter procedure was followed, for instance, in the trials of pertussis vaccine (Medical Research Council, 1951), where the final assessment was based mainly on children exposed to infection in the home. In either of these situations sequential methods would appear to be applicable. In trials like those of pertussis vaccine, for instance, even with a fixed number of subjects initially brought into the trial, the follow-up could be stopped as soon as a sufficient number of home exposures had been observed. In the clinical field, the sequential approach might be admirably suited to a long-term investigation, perhaps in a single hospital, of the treatment of some acute disease, where the recovery of any particular patient is decided in a few days, but where cases are seen so infrequently that the trial might go on for months or years.

Methods

Fixed-sample-size tests and sequential tests. Before discussing sequential methods it will be useful to consider certain features of the classical significance tests which assume a fixed sample size. The rules to be followed in applying these tests are determined by (*a*) the sample size, and (*b*) the significance level adopted (the probability of rejecting, when it is true, the null hypothesis that the two treatments are equally effective). The significance level is usually taken to be 0·05 (in other words, when the two treatments are equally effective, five times in 100 one will erroneously conclude that they differ). When (*a*) and (*b*) have been decided upon, any observed contrast between the two treatments can be classified as either (*A*) a significant difference in favour of the new treatment, (*B*) a significant difference in favour of the control treatment, or (*C*) a non-significant difference. Of these results, (A) and (B) would usually lead us to recommend, respectively, the adoption or abandonment of the new treatment, for the type of subject used in the trial; when (C) occurs we should normally suspend judgement, which in practice would mean that we should act as though the null hypothesis were true until reliable evidence to the contrary was produced.

As Hogben and Wrighton (1952) have recently emphasized, a small clinical trial may be so insensitive that real and important differences between the two treatments may go undetected. They recommend the use of confidence limits for the true difference. Clearly, if the trial is extensive, the only differences which are likely to remain undetected are small ones; the confidence limits may then be so narrow that further attempts to disprove the null hypothesis for this particular new treatment are not worth while. A reasonable way, then, of choosing the sample size in a classical trial would be to decide in advance what difference between the *true* effects of the treatments one wishes to be fairly certain to detect, if there really is such a difference ('to be fairly certain' might conveniently be interpreted as meaning 'with a probability of 0·95'; we shall regard a true difference as being 'detected' if the observed contrast is significant at the 0·05 level). The required sample size can then be determined mathematically. The phrase 'true difference' has been used here in a rather general sense, and the units in which it is measured will depend on the particular type of significance test which is being applied. In considering the t-test performed on differences, for instance, it is convenient to measure the 'true difference' not simply by the arithmetic mean difference, but by the ratio of the mean to the standard deviation of the differences.

In planning a sequential test we must decide, before the trial starts, how small a true difference (measured in suitable units) we wish to detect, if it exists. This decision will then determine the rules for carrying out the sequential scheme, which will have the properties that (a) if the true difference is zero, a significant result will be obtained only once in 20 times, and (b) if the true difference reaches the critical value chosen in advance, a significant result will be obtained 19 times out of 20. If the true difference is greater than the critical value, a significant result is even more likely to be obtained.

For a given choice of the critical value of the true difference, then, we can use either (1) a fixed-sample-size scheme, determining in advance the required number of pairs, n, or (2) a sequential scheme, determining in advance the rules for deciding at each stage whether or not to stop the trial. Each of these schemes will perform, with equal probabilities of success, the same function of detecting true differences between the effects of the treatments, of the order of magnitude in which we are interested, and we can refer to them as 'equivalent'. In the fixed-sample-size test, as the critical value chosen for the true difference decreases, the sample size required increases. In the sequential method the sample size varies from trial to trial, and the *average* sample size depends on what the true difference really is, but as the critical value chosen for the true difference decreases the maximum value of the *average* sample size required increases. If, therefore, we wish to compare the two methods for economy in the long run, we may compare the sample size required by the classical test with the maximum average sample size required by the sequential test. The advantage lies usually with the sequential method. In some situations the equivalent fixed sample size may be slightly lower than the maximum average sample size in the sequential test, but it is invariably higher than the average required when the null hypothesis is true, or that required when the true difference is in fact equal to the critical value chosen in advance.

The sequential test for the difference between two proportions. When the criterion by which the treatments are to be compared is, for an individual patient, an all-or-none event rather than a continuous measurement, different treatment groups are normally compared by examining the proportions of subjects in each group which exhibit the characteristic in question. In a trial for the efficacy of a pertussis vaccine, for example, we might compare the attack rates among the children in each group who are known to have been exposed at home to a case of pertussis. The classical, fixed-sample-size, method of testing the significance of the difference between two such proportions would be to compare the difference with its standard error; an equivalent procedure is to arrange the data in a 2×2 contingency table, and use the χ^2 test.

In the sequential method the subjects are arranged in pairs as they enter the trial, one member of each pair being allocated to each treatment group. (The method of pairing is discussed more fully at the end of this paper.) If we call the result for an individual subject a 'success' (S) or a 'failure' (F), then the results for each pair will be one of the four types SS, SF, FS, and FF, the first letter representing the subject in the control group, the second representing the subject in the 'new treatment' group. Of these four types of pairs, SS and FF might be called 'tied' pairs, because the comparison of the two treatments in that pair has resulted in a tie. It so happens that the sequential test makes use only of the 'untied' pairs, FS and SF. If the new treatment is appreciably better than the standard, most of the untied pairs will be of the type FS. If the standard is appreciably the better treatment, most will be SF. If the two treatments are equally effective, we should expect in the long run just as many untied pairs of type FS as of type SF. As a measure of the true difference between the effects of the two treatments, then, we shall take the expected proportion of untied pairs which are of type FS; this we shall denote by θ. If the success-rates for the control and new treatments are respectively p_1 and p_2, and if there are no systematic differences in response from one pair to another, then

$$\theta = \frac{p_2(1-p_1)}{p_1(1-p_2)+p_2(1-p_1)}.$$

On the null hypothesis that $p_1 = p_2$, it is easily verified that $\theta = \frac{1}{2}$. If p_2 is greater than p_1 (that is, the new treatment is better than the standard), θ is greater than $\frac{1}{2}$; and if p_2 is less than p_1 (new treatment worse than standard), θ is less than $\frac{1}{2}$. It should be noted that the quantities p_1 and p_2 denote the 'true' success-rates in a long series of subjects from which the subjects used in the trial may be regarded as a sample; the observed success-rates in the completed trial will in general differ somewhat from p_1 and p_2 owing to sampling fluctuations. For given values of p_1 and p_2, the value of θ may be read from Fig. 2.

Following the procedure outlined in the preceding section, we should, in setting up a sequential test, choose critical values of θ, corresponding to whatever differences (in each direction) between p_1 and p_2 we wish to be fairly

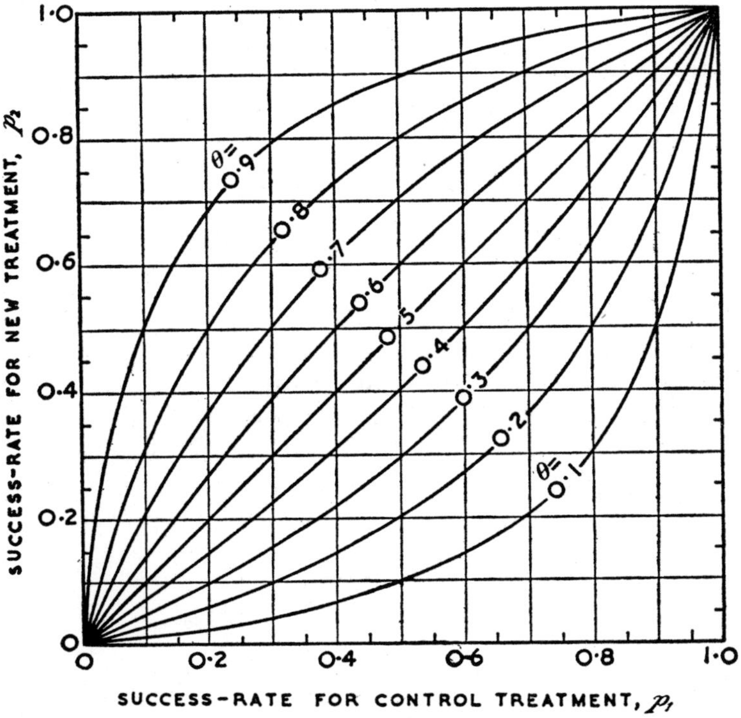

FIG. 2. Chart for θ in terms of the success-rates for the two treatments.

certain ($P = 0{\cdot}95$) of detecting. One critical value, θ_0 say, will be less than $\frac{1}{2}$, representing an advantage in using the control treatment; the other critical value, θ_1, will be greater than $\frac{1}{2}$, representing an advantage in the new treatment. We shall consider here only schemes in which $\theta_0+\theta_1 = 1$. Suppose, for instance, that we know that the attack rate amongst uninoculated children exposed to some infectious disease in the home is about 80 per cent. We wish to plan a sequential trial for a proposed vaccine, such that if the vaccine really reduces the home-exposure attack rate, in the long run, from 80 per cent. to 50 per cent., we shall have a fairly high chance ($P = 0{\cdot}95$) of detecting its value. Taking as a measure of success the home-exposure 'escape' rate (one minus the attack rate), we should have, for the critical difference, $p_1 = 1-0{\cdot}8 = 0{\cdot}2$, and $p_2 = 1-0{\cdot}5 = 0{\cdot}5$. Entering these values in Fig. 2, we find $\theta = 0{\cdot}8$. We shall therefore select, for the critical values of θ, $\theta_1 = 0{\cdot}8$ and $\theta_0 = 1-\theta_1 = 0{\cdot}2$. The test to be described below will have a probability of 0·95 of detecting an advantage in the vaccine such that $\theta = 0{\cdot}8$, and exactly the same probability of detecting a disadvantage such that $\theta = 0{\cdot}2$. To see what this choice of θ_0 implies in terms of the attack rates, we may refer again to Fig. 2. Entering $p_1 = 0{\cdot}2$ and $\theta = 0{\cdot}2$, we find $p_2 = 0{\cdot}05$ (which corresponds to an attack rate of 95 per cent.). If, then, the vaccine should for some reason increase the home-exposure attack rate from 80 per cent. to 95 per cent., we should be very likely to detect the fact. Such an effect is perhaps unlikely in the case of a vaccine

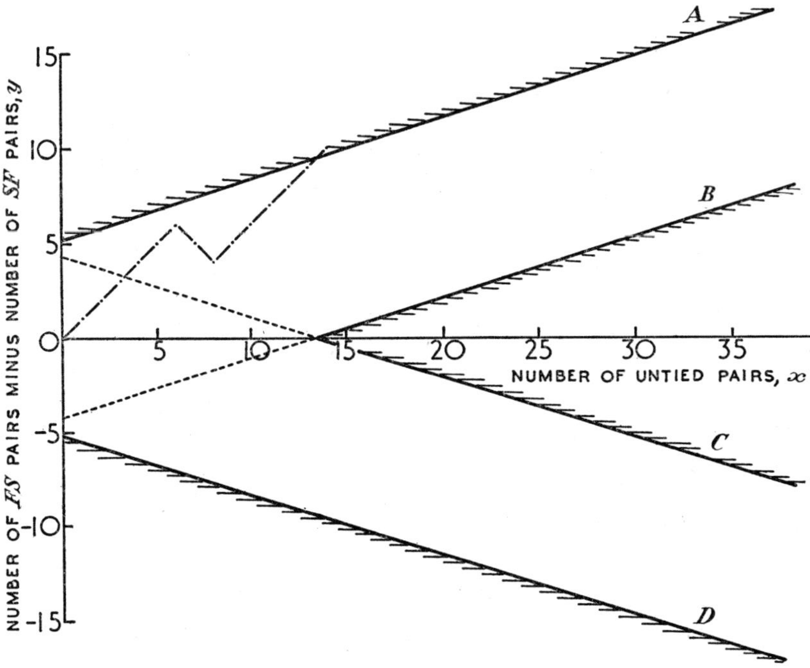

FIG. 3. Boundaries for a sequential test for the difference between two proportions, with a sample path based on the data of Table II.

when the control treatment consists of an inert substance, but becomes a definite possibility when one vaccine is being tested against another.

The sequential scheme may be drawn on a diagram like Fig. 3. Distances (x) along the horizontal axis represent the number of untied pairs; distances (y) along the vertical axis represent the difference between the number of *FS* pairs and the number of *SF* pairs. Another way of expressing this is that at the beginning of the trial the sample line starts at the origin; for each *FS* pair the line continues one step in a 'north-easterly direction', and for each *SF* pair one step in a 'south-easterly direction'. The positions of the four lines A, B, C, and D, which constitute the boundaries in Fig. 3, are determined by the choice of θ_1. The equations of these lines are as follows:

$$A: y = a_1 + bx \qquad C: y = a_2 - bx$$
$$B: y = -a_2 + bx \qquad D: y = -a_1 - bx$$

where the coefficients a_1, a_2, and b depend on θ_1, and may be obtained from Table I. (Alternative methods of graphic representation have previously been suggested. Armitage (1950) and Bross (1952), for instance, plotted the number of *FS* pairs against the number of *SF* pairs. The present method provides a closer analogy with that used in Fig. 1 for the sequential t-test.) As soon as the sample path crosses the upper boundary A, the trial ends and the conclusion is drawn that the new treatment is significantly better than the control. If the lower boundary D is crossed, we conclude that the control treatment is significantly better than the new treatment. If the sample path enters the area

TABLE I

Sequential Test for Difference between Two Proportions

Coefficients in equations for boundaries, a_1, a_2, and b; average sample sizes and equivalent fixed sample size, expressed as numbers of untied pairs.

Critical values of θ, to be detected with a probability of 0·95		Coefficients in equations of boundaries			Approximate average sample size (expressed as number of untied pairs)			Number of untied pairs in equivalent fixed-sample-size test
					when $\theta = \frac{1}{2}$	when $\theta = \theta_1$ or θ_0	at maximum	
θ_1	$\theta_0(= 1-\theta_1)$	b	a_1	a_2	$E_0(x)$	$E_1(x)$	$E_m(x)$	
0·55	0·45	0·0501	36·3	29·6	870	660	1,080	1,294
0·60	0·40	0·1007	17·9	14·7	215	160	270	319
0·65	0·35	0·1524	11·8	9·6	95	70	115	138
0·70	0·30	0·2058	8·6	7·0	51	40	63	75
0·75	0·25	0·2619	6·6	5·4	31	25	38	46
0·80	0·20	0·3219	5·2	4·3	21	17	25	30
0·85	0·15	0·3882	4·2	3·4	15	12	17	20
0·90	0·10	0·4650	3·3	2·7	10	9	11	14
0·95	0·05	0·5640	2·5	2·0	7	7	7	9

between the portions of B and C shown as continuous lines in Fig. 3, the trial ends, no significant difference between the treatments having been established. An extension of this middle boundary is provided by the dotted portions of B and C: if *both* these dotted lines are crossed before any of the other boundaries are reached, the trial ends, again with no significant difference shown.[2]

In addition to the coefficients a_1, a_2, and b, which determine the boundaries, Table I shows the approximate number of untied pairs required, on the average, before a decision is reached: first (in the column headed $E_0(x)$) when the treatments are equally effective, so that $\theta = \frac{1}{2}$; secondly (in that headed $E_1(x)$), when θ is equal to either of the critical values θ_0 and θ_1; and thirdly (in the column headed $E_m(x)$), at its maximum value, which will occur when θ is about mid-way between θ_0 and $\frac{1}{2}$, or mid-way between $\frac{1}{2}$ and θ_1, so that the sample path tends to wander up one of the two side channels in Fig. 3. As an illustration, Fig. 4 shows the approximate average number of untied pairs required for different values of θ, in the scheme whose boundaries are illustrated in Fig. 3. These boundaries were chosen to give $\theta_0 = 0{\cdot}2$ and $\theta_1 = 0{\cdot}8$. Table I and Fig. 4 show that $E_0(x) = 21$, $E_1(x) = 17$, and $E_m(x) = 25$. The last column of Table I shows the number of untied pairs required in the equivalent fixed-sample-size test; it will be observed that this is always greater than the maximum average sample size in the corresponding sequential test. In the test illustrated in Figs. 3 and 4, for instance, the equivalent number of untied pairs in the fixed-sample-size test is 30, whereas $E_m(x) = 25$. Thus, if the sequential scheme shown in

[2] In an earlier paper (Armitage, 1950, p. 142) it was incorrectly stated that the effect of omitting these dotted lines was negligible. The effect may in fact be quite appreciable.

Fig. 3 is used, and if it unfortunately happens that θ is approximately 0·65, so that the sample path tends on the average to wander along the upper channel, the sampling fluctuations will ensure that only rarely does the path continue very far without hitting one of the boundaries, and the average value of x required for a decision will be no more than 25. In an individual trial, of course, the value of x required may be much greater than the average of 25, and

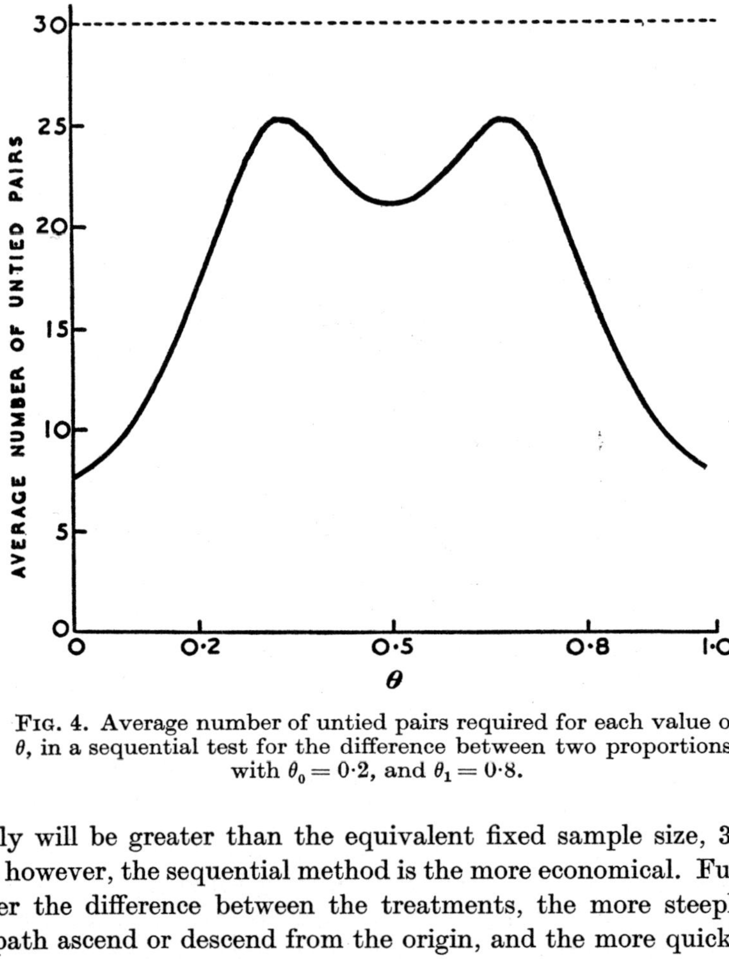

FIG. 4. Average number of untied pairs required for each value of θ, in a sequential test for the difference between two proportions, with $\theta_0 = 0{\cdot}2$, and $\theta_1 = 0{\cdot}8$.

frequently will be greater than the equivalent fixed sample size, 30. On the average, however, the sequential method is the more economical. Furthermore, the larger the difference between the treatments, the more steeply will the sample path ascend or descend from the origin, and the more quickly will one or other of the outer boundaries be reached.

The entries in the last four columns of Table I are all expressed as the number of untied pairs. The average number of pairs in the trial, tied as well as untied, will of course be higher. This average total number has not been tabulated, because it depends not merely on the value of θ, but on the particular values of p_1 and p_2, which cause θ to take that value. For given values of p_1 and p_2, the average number of pairs required altogether in the trial is obtained by multiplying the appropriate entry in Table I by

$$k = \frac{1}{p_1(1-p_2)+p_2(1-p_1)}.$$

Similarly, an approximation to the total number of pairs in the equivalent fixed-sample-size test is obtained by multiplying the entry in the last column of Table I by k.

The boundaries shown in Fig. 3 have been chosen to satisfy the requirements in the imaginary trial of a vaccine described earlier in this section. In that example we chose $\theta_0 = 0{\cdot}2$, $\theta_1 = 0{\cdot}8$. From Table I, the equations of the lines A, B, C, and D are:

$$A: y = 5{\cdot}2+0{\cdot}322x \qquad C: y = 4{\cdot}3-0{\cdot}322x$$
$$B: y = -4{\cdot}3+0{\cdot}322x \qquad D: y = -5{\cdot}2-0{\cdot}322x.$$

In order to illustrate the use of the sequential scheme shown in Fig. 3, let us imagine that a trial of a vaccine has been carried out on randomly selected groups from some population with home-exposure 'escape' rates of $p_1 = 0{\cdot}2$ among uninoculated children, and $p_2 = 0{\cdot}5$ in the inoculated group. As we have seen, these values of p_1 and p_2 give $\theta = 0{\cdot}8$ (which was the value chosen for θ_1), and we should therefore expect the sequential trial almost certainly to yield a significant result. Using a table of random sampling numbers, I obtained, for the first 50 pairs of subjects, the results shown in Table II. Each uninoculated child has a probability of 0·2 of escaping the infection, and 0·8 of being attacked; each inoculated child has a probability of 0·5 of escaping, and 0·5 of being attacked. The children escaping the infection are shown in Table II as successes (S), those who are attacked as failures (F). The sample path corresponding to the results of Table II is shown in Fig. 3. It will be seen that the upper boundary was reached at the 14th untied pair; the number of untied pairs required was rather less than the average of 17 shown in Table I. The average number of pairs of both kinds will be

$$\frac{17}{(0{\cdot}5)(0{\cdot}8)+(0{\cdot}2)(0{\cdot}5)} = 34;$$

the number actually required is seen from Table II to be 45, rather higher than the average. An equivalent fixed-sample-size test, based only on the untied pairs, would require 30 untied pairs. The usual fixed-sample-size test, of course, is not restricted to the untied pairs alone. Such a test would require approximately

$$\frac{30}{(0{\cdot}5)(0{\cdot}8)+(0{\cdot}2)(0{\cdot}5)} = 60 \text{ pairs of observations;}$$

the number of untied pairs, out of these 60, would vary from sample to sample, but on the average would be 30.

In the planning of a sequential trial the choice of θ_0 and θ_1 may present some difficulties. The procedure would usually be to make a preliminary estimate of the 'control' success-rate, p_1, and then consider what value of p_2, greater than p_1, would constitute such an important advance in treatment that the trial should be designed to detect the improvement. These values of p_1 and p_2 would determine a preliminary value of θ_1, and reference to columns 6 to 8 of Table I would indicate how many untied pairs would be required on the average. Multiplication by k provides estimates of the total number of pairs required.

If the organizers of the trial, bearing in mind that these averages may well be exceeded in any particular trial, consider them too high, a revised value of θ_1 must be chosen. Eventually a compromise will be reached between the requirements of sensitivity in detecting small differences (which tend to increase the length of the trial) and those of economy (which tend to decrease the length).

The sequential t-test. We shall consider, as before, trials in which subjects are paired on entry, one member of each pair being allocated to the control group,

TABLE II

Artificial Example to illustrate Sequential Test for Difference between two Proportions

Trial of a vaccine; F indicates failure (attack during home exposure), S indicates success (escape from infection).

Pair number	*Member of pair* *Uninoculated*	*Member of pair* *Inoculated*	*Type of untied pair*	*Pair number*	*Member of pair* *Uninoculated*	*Member of pair* *Inoculated*	*Type of untied pair*
1	*F*	*F*	..	31	*S*	*S*	..
2	*F*	*F*	..	32	*S*	*S*	..
3	*F*	*S*	*FS*	33	*F*	*S*	*FS*
4	*F*	*F*	..	34	*F*	*F*	..
5	*F*	*F*	..	35	*F*	*S*	*FS*
6	*F*	*S*	*FS*	36	*F*	*F*	..
7	*F*	*F*	..	37	*F*	*S*	*FS*
8	*F*	*S*	*FS*	38	*F*	*S*	*FS*
9	*F*	*S*	*FS*	39	*F*	*F*	..
10	*F*	*F*	..	40	*S*	*S*	..
11	*F*	*F*	..	41	*F*	*F*	..
12	*F*	*S*	*FS*	42	*S*	*S*	..
13	*F*	*F*	..	43	*S*	*S*	..
14	*F*	*F*	..	44	*F*	*F*	..
15	*F*	*F*	..	45	*F*	*S*	*FS*
16	*F*	*F*	..	46	*F*	*S*	*FS*
17	*F*	*F*	..	47	*F*	*S*	*FS*
18	*F*	*S*	*FS*	48	*S*	*F*	*SF*
19	*F*	*F*	..	49	*F*	*S*	*FS*
20	*S*	*F*	*SF*	50	*F*	*F*	..
21	*F*	*F*	..				
22	*F*	*F*	..				
23	*S*	*F*	*SF*				
24	*S*	*S*	..				
25	*F*	*S*	*FS*				
26	*F*	*F*	..				
27	*S*	*S*	..				
28	*F*	*F*	..				
29	*F*	*F*	..				
30	*F*	*F*	..				

and the other to the 'new treatment' group. Some measurement is recorded for each subject, and for each pair the difference, d, between the measurement for the subject receiving the new treatment and that for the control subject, is obtained. If the two treatments are equally effective the values of d will, in the long run, fluctuate about a zero mean. If one treatment tends to be better than the other the true mean of the differences, μ_d, will be either greater or less than zero. Suppose the standard deviation of the differences, in the population from which the subjects used in the trial may be regarded as a sample, is σ_d. Then, as a measure of the true difference between the effects of the two treatments, we shall take $\delta = \frac{\mu_d}{\sigma_d}$. It should be noted that δ depends on the population mean and standard deviation, which will in general differ somewhat from the mean and standard deviation of the limited number of values of d obtained in the trial.

In order to determine the rules of procedure in a sequential t-test, we must first decide upon some initial value of δ, representing a 'difference' between the

TABLE III

Sensitivity of the t-Test with Paired Observations

A test on the mean of n differences has a probability of 0·95 of yielding a significant result (at the $P = 0{\cdot}05$ level), when the true mean difference is a multiple δ of the true standard deviation of the differences.

Number of pairs	(n)	10	15	20	30	50	100	200	1000
$\frac{\text{Mean difference}}{\text{s.d. of differences}}$	(δ)	1·29	1·00	0·85	0·68	0·52	0·36	0·26	0·11

effects of the treatments so great that we wish to be fairly certain of detecting it. More precisely, denoting the critical value by δ_1, we are selecting a test having the property that if in fact $\delta = \pm\delta_1$, then the probability is 0·95 that a significant difference will be obtained. If the treatments are equally effective ($\delta = 0$) a significant difference will be erroneously obtained only once in 20 times. In choosing δ_1, it will frequently be possible to make use of preliminary estimates of σ_d obtained in previous investigations. One would then decide what value of the mean difference, μ_d, would represent an important advance in treatment, and obtain δ_1 on dividing this critical value of μ_d by σ_d. Alternatively, if no estimate of σ_d is available, it may be useful to refer to Table III, which shows the critical values of δ which can be detected (with probability 0·95) by using a classical fixed-sample-size t-test on the mean of n differences. It should be borne in mind that since, say, a value of $\delta = 0{\cdot}36$ can be detected fairly certainly by a t-test with a fixed sample size of 100 pairs, the equivalent sequential test would probably require a smaller number of pairs, but that it might require more. The procedure in a sequential t-test can be regarded as one in which the value of Student's t is calculated at each stage and plotted against n, the number of pairs, on a diagram like Fig. 1. The trial continues until the sample path formed by joining the successive values of t crosses one of the three boundaries, indicating either a significant difference in favour of one or the other treatment, or a non-significant difference. In practice the computation is made lighter by the calculation, at each stage, of the quantity

$$z = \frac{(Sd)^2}{Sd^2}$$

instead of the more usual quantity t. Here d represents the difference, for each pair of subjects, between the reading for the control treatment and that for the new treatment. Sd is the sum of these differences for all the pairs so far observed, and Sd^2 is the sum of squares of the differences. Student's t is given by the expression

$$t = \bar{d}\sqrt{\left(\frac{n(n-1)}{S(d-\bar{d})^2}\right)},$$

$\bar{d}$ being the mean difference. The new quantity z is closely related to t by the formula

$$z = \frac{nt^2}{t^2+n-1}.$$

If this formula is used to change all the boundary values of t, in Fig. 1, to the corresponding values of z, the boundaries of Fig. 5 are obtained. There are now only two boundaries, since z depends on t^2 rather than t, and so the outer

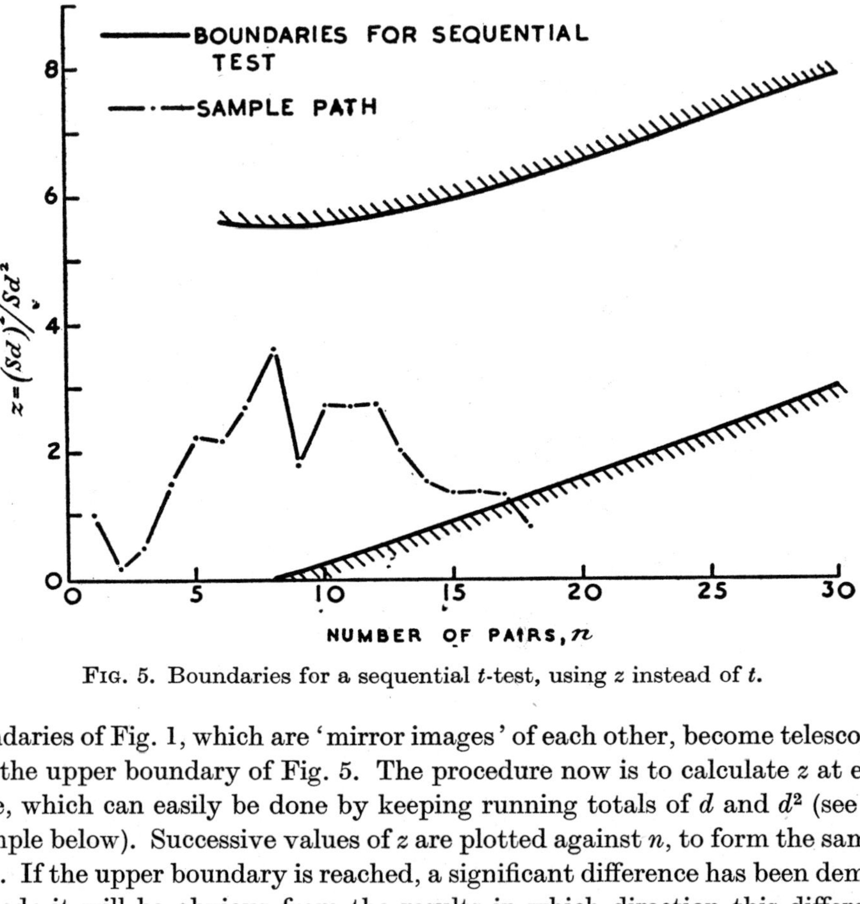

FIG. 5. Boundaries for a sequential t-test, using z instead of t.

boundaries of Fig. 1, which are 'mirror images' of each other, become telescoped into the upper boundary of Fig. 5. The procedure now is to calculate z at each stage, which can easily be done by keeping running totals of d and d^2 (see the example below). Successive values of z are plotted against n, to form the sample path. If the upper boundary is reached, a significant difference has been demonstrated; it will be obvious from the results in which direction this difference lies. If the lower boundary is reached, no significant difference has been found. The sample path shown in Fig. 5 corresponds exactly to that shown in Fig. 1; in the particular set of data from which this path was plotted the trial would have been stopped after 18 pairs, with the conclusion that the treatments did not differ significantly.

In order to calculate the boundaries for a sequential t-test, we must first decide upon the critical value, δ_1 (as explained above). The boundary points for each sample size, n, are given in the National Bureau of Standards (N.B.S.) tables published by the United States Department of Commerce (1951). In these tables the entries in the columns headed '$-\ln 19$' and '$\ln 19$' provide the values of z on the lower and upper boundaries respectively. The test illustrated in Fig. 5, for example, was chosen so as to be 'equivalent' to a fixed-sample-size test with 20 pairs. Table III shows that the critical value, δ_1, is 0·85. Interpolation in the N.B.S. tables, in the columns '—ln 19' and 'ln 19' and half-way between the entries for $\delta = 0{\cdot}8$ and $\delta = 0{\cdot}9$, yields the boundary points for z shown in Table IV (from which the boundaries shown in Fig. 5 have been drawn, and from which the boundaries B, B', and C of Fig. 1 were obtained

TABLE IV

Boundary Points for z in a Sequential t-Test with $\delta_1 = 0{\cdot}85$ (*compare Fig. 5*)

Number of pairs n	*Value of z on* *Lower boundary*	*Upper boundary*
6	..	5·58
7	..	5·51
8	..	5·50
9	0·11	5·51
10	0·23	5·56
11	0·35	5·61
12	0·48	5·69
13	0·61	5·77
14	0·74	5·87
15	0·87	5·97
16	1·00	6·08
17	1·14	6·19
18	1·28	6·31
19	1·42	6·43
20	1·56	6·55
21	1·71	6·68
22	1·85	6·81
23	2·00	6·94
24	2·14	7·07
25	2·29	7·20
26	2·43	7·34
27	2·58	7·47
28	2·73	7·61
29	2·88	7·75
30	3·03	7·89

by transforming back from z to t). The upper boundary starts at $n = 6$; the null hypothesis cannot, therefore, be rejected before the sixth pair of observations. Similarly the null hypothesis cannot be accepted before the ninth pair. The data from which the sample path shown in Fig. 5 has been calculated were obtained in a recent trial of vitamin E in the treatment of intermittent claudication (Hamilton, Wilson, Armitage, and Boyd, 1953).[3] The measurement recorded for each individual is the increase in the average number of circuits walked during the treatment period as compared with the average before treatment. In this trial patients were allotted randomly either to the 'vitamin E' group or to a control group receiving dummy capsules. Within each group the patients have been arranged in serial order, and corresponding members of each group are regarded as forming a pair. The measurements for the first four pairs, and the steps in the calculation of the corresponding values of z, are shown in Table V.

[3] These data were not originally analysed by sequential methods; they are used here only for purposes of illustration.

No method of calculating average sample sizes for sequential t-tests has yet been proposed. Sampling experiments suggest, however, that, for a given value of δ_1, the average sample size required by the sequential test will be lower than the equivalent fixed sample size when in fact $\frac{\mu_d}{\sigma_d} = 0$ (that is on the null hypothesis), and when $\left|\frac{\mu_d}{\sigma_d}\right| \geqslant \delta_1$. When $\frac{\mu_d}{\sigma_d}$ happens to be nearly equal to $\pm\frac{\delta_1}{2}$, the sample paths will tend to wander up the channel in Fig. 5, and the average sample size required for a decision may be slightly greater than the size of the equivalent classical t-test. There is no reason to suppose that this situation would often occur, and, as judged by the number of subjects required in the long run, over a number of trials, the sequential method would almost certainly prove the more efficient.

TABLE V

Example of Calculation for a Sequential t-Test

Data from trial of vitamin E in treatment of intermittent claudication (Hamilton, Wilson, Armitage, and Boyd, 1953); the steps in the calculations are shown for the first four pairs of patients.

Increase in number of circuits for patient in					
Vitamin E group	*Control group*	*Difference, d (Vitamin E minus control)*	*Sd*	*Sd*^{2}	$z = \frac{(Sd)^2}{Sd^2}$
−1·2	2·2	−3·4	−3·4	11·56	1·000
5·8	−0·3	6·1	2·7	48·77	0·150
1·9	−0·7	2·6	5·3	55·53	0·506
14·0	0·8	13·2	18·5	229·77	1·490

Further Remarks about Sequential Trials

Sequential estimation. In addition to a significance test for the difference between the effects of two treatments, it will frequently be informative to estimate the magnitude of that difference and to set confidence limits for the estimated value. In a trial designed to compare the effect of two treatments on temperature, for example, we might wish not merely to assert that one treatment achieves a significantly greater reduction in temperature than the other, but to say further that the mean difference between the treatments is estimated to be 0·5° F., with 95 per cent. confidence limits of 0·3° to 0·7° F. In asserting that the true mean difference lay between 0·3° and 0·7° F., we should have a probability of 0·95 of making a correct statement. The importance of confidence statements in clinical and preventive trials has been emphasized by Hogben and Wrighton (1952). If a trial yields a non-significant difference between the effects of two treatments, a statement of confidence intervals will show whether or not the trial was so insensitive that an appreciable and important difference might have been missed. This approach may well be less important in a sequential trial, where, as we have seen, the statistical procedures can be so arranged before the start of the trial that any difference large enough to be considered important will have a high probability of being detected.

Nevertheless it may be useful to be able to supplement the significance test with a confidence statement about the possible magnitude of the effect. Clearly something in this direction can be achieved merely by considering which boundary has been hit. If the sample path has hit an outer boundary, thus leading to the rejection of the null hypothesis, one can be fairly certain that the true difference is not zero; if the other boundary has been reached, so that the result is non-significant, we can safely assert that the difference (measured in the appropriate scale) is less than the critical value chosen at the beginning of the trial. A narrower interval could be obtained by considering the particular point which was reached on the boundaries. Unfortunately the precise statistical methods for doing this are not yet known. A reasonably good approximation is probably provided by the classical fixed-sample-size methods. Consider, for instance, the example illustrated in Table II. The trial ended at the 45th pair with the statement that the inoculated group had a significantly lower attack rate than the uninoculated group. At that stage the numbers of children attacked (shown as F in Table II) were 26 out of 45 (57·8 per cent.) in the inoculated group, and 36 out of 45 (80·0 per cent.) in the uninoculated group. The observed difference is therefore

$$0{\cdot}800-0{\cdot}578 = 0{\cdot}222,$$

with a standard error of

$$\sqrt{\{(0{\cdot}689)(0{\cdot}311)(1/45+1/45)\}} = 0{\cdot}0976.$$

The 95 per cent. confidence limits for the true difference in attack rates are therefore

$$0{\cdot}222 \pm (1{\cdot}96)(0{\cdot}0976), \text{ that is } 0{\cdot}031 \text{ and } 0{\cdot}413.$$

The true difference, as stated earlier, is 0·3, and is therefore included in the confidence interval. For a survey of the problem of sequential estimation, see Anscombe (1954).

Significance levels. It has been convenient throughout this paper to retain the conventional level of 0·05 both for the significance level (the probability of rejecting, when true, the null hypothesis that the treatments have identical effects), and for what is often called the 'error of the second kind' (the probability of accepting the null hypothesis when the difference between treatments assumes its critical value). But significance levels are arbitrary, and judgements based upon the significance or non-significance of experimental results must be tempered by common sense and by evidence from other sources. It may be that in certain situations workers will require sequential schemes satisfying criteria involving other than the 0·05 level of probability. It seems unlikely, however, that the suggestion of Bross (1952) that a significance level of 0·10 or 0·20 is particularly suitable for clinical trials will find wide acceptance. Once a significant difference has been established in a well-controlled trial, further trials of the same treatments will usually become impossible for ethical reasons. A decision that one treatment is better than another thus becomes virtually irreversible. A risk of 1 in 10 or 1 in 5 of causing the establishment of a quite useless treatment, perhaps more expensive than the equally effective standard treatment which it replaces, appears to be too high.

For simplicity, we have considered only two-sided tests, that is those which are designed to detect differences between treatments in either direction. Furthermore, the tests have been symmetrical, in that (in the test for proportions) the critical values of θ were chosen so that $\theta_0+\theta_1 = 1$, and (in the sequential t-test) the critical values of δ were $\pm\delta_1$. These restrictions can be easily removed if necessary, but details will not be given here.

Closed schemes. The sequential schemes discussed in this paper are of the type known as 'open', in the sense that there is no upper limit to the length of the trial. Although, as we have seen, the schemes may require small average sample sizes, there is a positive, albeit small, chance that a trial will extend beyond any chosen length. This state of affairs is clearly unsatisfactory, and in practice it may be desirable to impose some upper limit on the number of observations required. Unfortunately the extent to which the 'closure' of a scheme affects the probabilities of reaching the various boundaries is not easily calculable. The schemes described by Bross (1952) for testing the difference between two proportions are closed versions of the open schemes described in the present paper, and have been specially constructed to have the required significance levels and 'errors of the second kind'. Only two schemes have so far been constructed (corresponding to two sets of requirements), and unless the requirements for any particular trial happened to coincide with those chosen by Bross, some other method of closure would have to be used. It seems likely that the probabilities of error of the two kinds will not be greatly affected if a sequential scheme is closed at a sample size one and a half to two times as great as that required in the equivalent fixed-sample-size test. For example, the sequential t-test illustrated in Fig. 5 and Table V is equivalent to a fixed-sample-size test with 20 pairs, and could if necessary have been closed at $n = 30$ or 40, the sample path being regarded as having hit whichever boundary it happened to be nearer at the point of closure. The sequential test for a difference in proportions illustrated in Fig. 3 and Table II, being equivalent to a classical test with 30 untied pairs, could have been closed after 45 to 60 untied pairs. If an absolute maximum length of the trial is imposed, and there is no objection to using the allowable maximum period, it will usually be preferable to adopt non-sequential methods. Suppose, for example, that a trial can last two years but no more. If we select a sequential scheme, artificially closed after two years, we have seen that it should be such that the equivalent fixed-sample-size scheme takes not much more than one year. This closed sequential scheme will therefore be less sensitive in detecting differences than the fixed-sample-size scheme with the full two years, and the latter will be the more suitable.

The effect of pairing. In order to simplify the exposition as much as possible, we have considered only tests in which the subjects receiving the control and new treatments are paired in some manner. In discussing the suitability of this device, it is necessary to distinguish between two situations: (A) when members of the same pair tend to be more uniform in response than are members of different pairs, so that their responses tend to be positively correlated; and

(B) when there is no correlation in response between members of the same pair. The third possibility, that of a negative correlation, is unlikely to arise in the present context. In situation (A), any valid test, sequential or otherwise, must take into account the positive correlation between members of the same pair. This situation will arise if the mean value of the response changes throughout the course of the trial. The device of pairing will largely eliminate the trend, and consequently increase the accuracy of the comparison between treatments. In the study of an infectious disease, for instance, the attack rate may change over even a short period of time. In a trial for the treatment of acute or chronic disease the severity of the disease in the patients entering the trial may unavoidably change with time. In situation (B), the device of pairing, although not theoretically necessary, can still be used. The device is, indeed, unavoidable in the sequential test for a difference in proportions, since no simple test is known which does not involve pairing. A sequential t-test can, however, be performed on the unpaired observations (Rushton, 1952), and the existing N.B.S. tables (United States Department of Commerce, 1951) can, with some adaptation, be used in this and more complicated situations. In situation (B) the paired test will be slightly less efficient than the unpaired test; but unless the average sample sizes are small this slight loss of efficiency will not be important, and the paired test will be satisfactory. It should be noted that, in the account of the sequential test for differences in proportions, the formulae given for θ and k, in terms of p_1 and p_2, are valid only in situation (B). In situation (A), for given values of p_1 and p_2 ($p_2 > p_1$), θ and k are both higher than the values given by the formulae, and the average sample sizes required to detect a given difference between p_1 and p_2 are smaller than those obtained from Table I.

If pairing is carried out as the subjects enter the trial, the simplest device would be to ensure that, of each successive pair of subjects, one is allocated (randomly or alternately) to the control group, and the other to the new treatment group. This method, as Hill (1950–1) said, 'may, however, be insufficiently random if the admission or non-admission of a case to the trial turns upon a difficult assessment of the patient and if the clinician involved knows whether the patient, if accepted, will pass to the treatment or control group. By such knowledge he may be biased, consciously or unconsciously, in his acceptance or rejection; or through fear of being biased, his judgement may be influenced.' An alternative method would be to allocate subjects randomly to one or other of the two treatment groups, and then to pair corresponding members of the two groups. By this method the numbers of subjects in the two groups may not be exactly equal at any given stage in the trial, and a few unpaired observations in the larger group may be wasted. This difficulty can be largely overcome by the use of some method of restricted randomization, which ensures that at various stages (say, after every 20 entries) the numbers in the two groups are equal (Hill, 1950–1). Whether or not tests involving pairing are used, it will often be desirable to take into account in the analysis certain subdivisions of the subjects, say by age, sex, or treatment centre. In the pairing method all that needs to be done is to ensure that subjects are paired within each of the sub-groups in which we are interested.

Acknowledgements

I am indebted to a number of colleagues, and other medical research workers, who suggested improvements in the first draft of this paper; to Drs. M. Hamilton and G. M. Wilson for permission to publish, in Table V, some detailed results obtained in their trial of vitamin E in the treatment of intermittent claudication; to Miss I. Allen for computational assistance; and to Mrs. M. G. Young for drawing the figures.

Summary

In a controlled trial to assess the efficacy of prophylactic or therapeutic substances, ethical considerations often require that the results should be subject to continuous analysis as they become available, so that the trial can be stopped as soon as possible. With this sequential type of experimentation the appropriate methods of analysis should be used. In the long run sequential methods are more economical than classical methods, in which the size of the trial is not determined by the results obtained.

A sequential test for the difference between two proportions, and a sequential t-test, are described in detail. For each test the experimenter must decide in advance what difference between the true effects of the treatments he wishes to be fairly certain of detecting, if it exists. The sequential analysis of the results can then be performed by simple graphical methods.

REFERENCES

Anscombe, F. J. (1954) *Biometrics*, **10**, 89.
Armitage, P. (1950) *J. Roy. Statist. Soc.* B, **12**, 137.
Bross, I. (1952) *Biometrics*, **8**, 188.
Hamilton, M., Wilson, G. M., Armitage, P., and Boyd, J. T. (1953) *Lancet*, **1**, 367.
Hill, A. Bradford (1950–1) *Brit. Med. Bull.* **7**, 278.
Hogben, L., and Wrighton, R. (1952) *Brit. J. Soc. Med.* **6**, 89, 205.
Medical Research Council (1950) *Lancet*, **2**, 732.
—— (1951) *Brit. Med. J.* **1**, 1463.
Rushton, S. (1952) *Biometrika*, **39**, 302.
United States Department of Commerce (1951) *Tables to Facilitate Sequential t-Tests* (*Nat. Bur. Standards Appl. Math.* Ser. No. 7), Washington.
Wald, A. (1947) *Sequential Analysis*, New York.

616.832.9–002.5

SPINAL CORD COMPLICATIONS OF TUBERCULOUS MENINGITIS[1]

A Clinical and Pathological Study

By W. D. W. BROOKS, A. P. FLETCHER, and R. R. WILSON
(From the Departments of Medicine and Pathology, St. Mary's Hospital, and the Wright-Fleming Institute, St. Mary's Hospital Medical School, London)

With Plates 19 to 22

Transverse myelitis has been for many years recognized as an infrequent but serious complication of tuberculous meningitis. The earlier literature of the subject, however, is remarkably confused, and is composed mostly of reports of single cases. It was ably reviewed by Wilson (1940). Until the advent of the streptomycin treatment of tuberculous meningitis the study of this complication was difficult, and was largely of academic interest, because the condition usually developed during the terminal phases of an almost invariably fatal illness. Since streptomycin and ancillary therapy has been used, however, many patients have recovered, and a majority have lived far longer with the disease than would otherwise have been the case. Recent papers describing successful treatment of many hundreds of patients with tuberculous meningitis (Choremis, Zervos, Constantinides, and Pantazis, 1948; Medical Research Council, 1948; Rubie and Mohun, 1949; Cairns, 1951; Middleton and Longfield, 1952; Perry, 1952; Somner, 1952; Riley, 1953) have ignored or made only scant reference to spinal cord complications, which have certainly increased in clinical importance and probably also in frequency. Smith and Daniel (1947), however, recorded a case in which tuberculous meningitis was accompanied by a transient episode of subarachnoid haemorrhage and paraplegia. It is also true that the numerous recent reports of the pathology of tuberculous meningitis (Schwarz, 1948; Doniach, 1949; Levinson, Luhan, Mavrelis, and Herzon, 1950; Winter, 1950; Auerbach, 1951) do not directly refer to lesions of the spinal cord. It seemed worth while, therefore, to record our experience of transverse myelitis and associated spinal cord lesions occurring in the course of tuberculous meningitis. The patients so afflicted have been treated under our care during the years 1947 to 1953 at St. Mary's Hospital, London, where a Unit for the investigation and therapy of this disease for the North West Metropolitan Region has been established.

Definition and Incidence

The term 'transverse myelitis' is used here to designate a complete or partial transverse lesion of the spinal cord occurring in the presence of tuberculous

[1] Received October 28, 1953.

meningitis; it does not imply that the neurological lesion was necessarily caused by an inflammatory process in the cord itself. The present communication describes 11 incidents clinically diagnosed as transverse myelitis, occurring in 10 of 80 patients (75 of whom were aged 10 years or more) bacteriologically proved to be suffering from tuberculous meningitis. The crude mortality rate among the 80 patients was 38 per cent.; but neither this rate, nor our recorded incidence of transverse myelitis, is likely to be representative of that occurring in the disease, since it has been the policy of St. Mary's Hospital to accept patients with tuberculous meningitis, however grave their clinical state, who had been treated elsewhere for variable periods of time. Table I shows that transverse myelitis tends to occur late in the disease or after a relapse, so that, by accepting patients often several months after the onset of the disease, the incidence of this complication in the series may have been increased.

A not uncommon complication of tuberculous meningitis with which we have also been concerned is referred to as 'spinal block', by which is meant obstruction within the meninges of the spinal cord to the circulation of the cerebrospinal fluid. It is significant not only because it prevents the effective local action of agents employed in treatment, but also because, as will be shown, it is associated with the development of transverse myelitis. Spinal block has been diagnosed in the present series of cases when a Froin syndrome and a negative Queckenstedt response have both been continuously present for more than three weeks. Where necessary, simultaneous ventricular or cisternal puncture has been combined with lumbar puncture to establish diagnosis, and sometimes the determination of the diffusion rates of antibiotics or dyes has been employed to test the cerebrospinal circulation. Alternatively, when owing to the death of the patient a three-week observation period of the spinal block was impracticable, the combination of a Froin syndrome, a negative Queckenstedt response, and adequate post-mortem confirmation has been accepted as sufficient evidence of the condition. Fifteen of the 80 patients comprising the whole series developed spinal block. All the patients received intrathecal streptomycin by the lumbar route, and in some cases by the ventricular or cisternal route, as well as oral para-aminosalicylic acid or isoniazid with systemic streptomycin.

Illustrative Case Histories of Patients who Recovered

Case 1. A woman aged 25 years was admitted to St. Mary's Hospital in March 1952, two months after the onset of an illness of obscure origin, during which time she had received a short course of streptomycin. The presumptive diagnosis of tuberculous meningitis was confirmed bacteriologically. Her general condition on admission was fair, and treatment produced a steady improvement. During June 1952 she complained of severe aching pain in both legs, the left being the worse. Physical examination revealed signs thought at first to signify a left saphenous vein thrombosis, and heparin treatment appeared to relieve the symptoms. A fortnight later she again experienced severe aching in the legs, and developed a severe flaccid paraplegia involving the legs, glutei, and lower abdominal muscles. Voluntary power in the legs, except for very weak movements of the left foot, was almost absent. The plantar responses were flexor; with the doubtful exception of the left ankle-jerk, the knee- and ankle-reflexes could not be obtained, but she maintained control over both the bladder and the rectum. The next day physical examination revealed diminished sensation to pin-prick over the lower limbs extending up to the T 10 segment; above this level there was a band of hyperaesthesia. During this day the plantar responses became extensor, and the lower abdominal reflexes were found to be absent, as were the knee- and ankle-reflexes. Three weeks later a gradual return of muscle power in the legs became evident. Within six weeks the glutei and trunk muscles were improving, and after two months the knee- and ankle-reflexes returned and the plantar responses became flexor. She commenced to walk with assistance in September 1952, and in October she was discharged to a convalescent home equipped with a physiotherapy department. By January 1953 she was able to walk two miles without difficulty, and by June the strength in her legs was apparently normal, and she stated that she was able to live a normal life without handicap.

Case 6. A woman aged 23 years was admitted to St. Mary's Hospital in January 1949, with a 12-day history of severe headache, vomiting, and malaise. The diagnosis of tuberculous meningitis was confirmed, no other focus of tuberculosis being found. One week after admission a spinal block was detected, and six days later she developed sudden weakness of the legs, together with loss of lower-limb reflexes, and retention of urine and faeces. The plantar responses were flexor. Three weeks later there was some return of muscle power, though at this time she complained of a feeling of numbness in the legs; tests of sensory perception were normal. One month after the onset of weakness it was possible to elicit knee- and ankle-reflexes with difficulty, and she had regained control over the bladder and rectum. The lower limbs were not regarded as clinically normal till four months after the incident. She was discharged in December 1949, walking well and apparently in good health, though the spinal block had not resolved.

She relapsed in January 1950, and one week after admission she complained of inability to move her legs. Examination revealed a severe flaccid paraplegia which again involved the lower-limb muscles, with loss of reflexes and retention of urine and faeces. Some residual power was present in all the affected muscles, but during a period of one week this residual power disappeared, as did the abdominal reflexes, while the plantar responses could not be elicited. A few days later the plantar responses became extensor. By March 1950 she had regained control over the bladder and rectum, the plantar responses were again flexor, and there had been some recovery of voluntary power. Recovery of muscle power was very slow, but it was possible to commence walking exercises in October, and she could walk sufficiently well to be discharged in March 1951. By September 1951 she could walk a mile and do light house-work, while the Queckenstedt response had again become positive after 32 months. By February 1952 the knee- and ankle-reflexes had returned, and she was leading a normal life.

The Clinical Picture of Transverse Myelitis

Tables I and II show the main clinical features and other relevant details of the 10 cases of transverse myelitis. Eight patients rapidly developed a flaccid paraplegia (Cases 1 to 8), while two patients (Cases 9 and 10) showed from the first a spastic paraplegia which progressed to complete interruption of cord function. Only one patient (Case 6) experienced two separate episodes of spinal cord damage.

TABLE I

Details of the 10 Patients who Suffered from Transverse Myelitis

Case number	*Sex*	*Age (years)*	*Tuberculous complications*	*Time after onset of meningitis*	*Time after onset of spinal block*	*Speed of development of lesion*	*Result*
1	F	25	No	5 months	Not present	Hours	Alive and well
2	F	49	Miliary disease	At onset	Not present	Hours	Alive and well
3	F	20	Adult pulmonary	2 months	Not present	Hours	Alive and well
4	M	31	Adult pulmonary	27 months (1 week after a relapse)	1 week	Hours	Died 2 days later
5	M	20	No	8 months (1 week after a relapse)	1 week	Hours	Died 10 days later
*6*a*	F	23	No	1 month	1 week	Hours	Alive and well
6*b*	F	23	No	13 months (2 weeks after a relapse)	10 months	Days	Alive and well
7	F	30	Miliary disease	5 months	3 months	Hours	Alive and well
8	F	18	No	5 months	4 months	Hours	Alive and well
9	F	44	Shoulder and kidneys	5 months	4 months	Weeks	Died 5 months later
10	M	42	Adult pulmonary, and caries of spine	4 months	3 months	Weeks	Died 10 months later

* This was the patient who experienced two episodes of transverse myelitis.

TABLE II

Physical Signs and Course of the Disorder in the 10 Patients with Transverse Myelitis

Case number	*Level of sensory loss determined*	*Ankle- and knee-reflexes*	*Plantar response*	*Abdominal reflexes*	*Bladder or rectum affected*	*Interval to first signs of recovery*	*Able to walk after*
1	T 10	Lost, except left ankle-jerk with reinforcement	Initially flexor, later extensor	Present	No	3 weeks	3 months
2	No	Present	Extensor	Absent	No	3 weeks	6 months
3	T 8	Absent	Not obtained	Present	No	3 weeks	Not yet mobilized
4	T 6	Absent	Not obtained	Absent	Yes	None	Died
5	T 4	Absent	Flexor	Absent	Yes	None	Died
*6*a*	No	Absent	Initially flexor, later extensor	Present	No	3 weeks	4 months
6*b*	No	Absent	Initially flexor, later extensor	Absent	Yes	6 weeks	8 months
7	No	Present on right, absent on left	Extensor	Present	No	1 month	3 months
8	T 6	Present	Extensor	Absent	No	2 weeks	5 months
9	T 10	Initially absent, then + +	Extensor	Absent	Yes	None	Died
10	T 4	+ +	Extensor	Absent	Yes	None	Died

* This was the patient who experienced two episodes of transverse myelitis.

The rapidly developing lesion. The onset of the lesion in Cases 1 to 8 was extremely fast, the full limit of the disability being reached in 12 to 24 hours. The disorder was mainly one of motor function. In those patients in whom a level of sensory loss could be shown, the degree of sensory impairment was definite but relatively slight. One patient (Case 5) showed well-defined sensory loss, but he suffered from a severe spinal lesion, and it is probable that the lesion contributed materially to his early death. Another (Case 4) also experienced a severe lesion with spinal shock, his blood-pressure falling from 130/80 to 90/60. He was stuporose, and the uncertain definition of the level of sensory inpairment was undoubtedly due to that fact. He died two days later. Table II shows that the lower-limb reflexes were usually diminished or absent. The plantar reflexes were frequently absent. Bladder and rectal function was impaired in some patients only; a level of sensory loss could be demonstrated in only half the patients. In Cases 1 to 3 spinal block was not present. In Cases 4 to 8 this complication preceded transverse myelitis by intervals varying from one week to 10 months. Six of these eight patients recovered from their myelitis, and all six began to show some sign of improvement within six weeks. It was, however, months before muscle power had recovered sufficiently to permit walking (slow progress was, of course, partly imposed by the treatment of the meningitis). Five have left hospital and have been followed up for periods of between six months and two years. None of them exhibit any clinical disability due to their previous extensive neurological lesions. Four of the eight patients complained of a poorly localized pain in the legs two to four weeks before the onset of transverse myelitis; in two patients the aching was of such intensity as to require heavy doses of analgesics to permit sleep at nights. Physical examination at this time was entirely negative. It is worthy of emphasis that in our experience the diagnostic significance of pain in the legs is slight, since it frequently occurs in patients being treated for tuberculous meningitis who do not develop evidence of transverse myelitis. It is sometimes of considerable severity, but usually lasts for only two to three weeks. Physical examination has always failed to show any cause, and the symptom usually disappears as suddenly as it comes.

The slowly developing lesion. There were only two patients (Cases 9 and 10) who showed a slowly progressive transverse myelitis, four and three months respectively after developing spinal block. Both were at times irrational and difficult to examine. In these two patients the first signs were those of increasing paraplegia-in-extension, with spasticity in the limbs, increased reflexes, and extensor plantar responses. The development of the lesion was slow and clonus appeared late, but after two and three months respectively paraplegia-in-flexion appeared. Ultimately in both patients there was apparently complete loss of function of the affected segments of the spinal cord. It was not possible to be certain of the level of sensory loss in one patient (Case 9), since her mental state was clouded, but crude tests revealed it to be at about T 10. A myelogram was performed on this patient, and her spinal block was found to have its upper border at T 5–8. The other patient (Case 10) exhibited a level of sensory loss at T 4–6. Both had severe uncontrolled urinary infections, that in the former being tuberculous with superadded pyogenic infection, and that in the latter being associated with the development of decubitus calculi. The presence of these severe urinary infections may have been partly responsible for the change of paraplegia-in-extension to paraplegia-in-flexion. The speed of development, clinical course, and fatal outcome were thus sharply contrasted with the lesions experienced by the majority of the other patients (Cases 1 to 8) with transverse myelitis.

Clinical and Post-Mortem Findings

This section presents the clinical histories and post-mortem findings in nine patients who died with spinal block. Four of them (Cases 4, 5, 9, and 10) had transverse myelitis, and are shown in Tables I and II; the other four patients (Cases 11 to 14) had spinal block without clinical evidence of transverse myelitis. Patient No. 15, who had spinal block, is described separately, since the nature of her neurological lesion could not be determined by clinical examination. The pathological findings are summarized in Table III.

Case 4. A man aged 31 years. Tuberculous meningitis was diagnosed in July 1949, but after a six months' course of treatment he made an apparently complete recovery. Follow-up lumbar punctures had always revealed a cytologically and chemically normal cerebrospinal fluid. In April 1951 he developed miliary tuberculosis, and was treated with a five-month course of chemotherapy. His cerebrospinal fluid remained normal during this treatment, though it was noted that the pressure response to jugular compression was very slow. He was discharged apparently well, but in November 1951 he again developed signs of meningeal irritation, and was transferred to St. Mary's Hospital. On examination he was drowsy and confused, and there were signs of marked meningeal irritation. Lumbar puncture demonstrated a complete spinal block. His condition remained unchanged until, eight days after admission, he suddenly collapsed. Examination revealed a complete flaccid paraplegia with a level of sensory loss at about T 6, though his grave condition precluded accurate localization. He died shortly afterwards.

Post-mortem examination showed widespread tuberculous meningitis, especially marked over the base of the brain and the cord. There was some flattening of the cerebral convolutions, but no hydrocephalus; there were many ependymal tubercles. In the spine, there were obvious tubercles on the inner aspect of the dura in the upper half; in this region the dura and arachnoid were adherent, and in many places the leptomeninges also appeared glued together. These changes were much more pronounced on the posterior aspect of the cord. Microscopically, sections from the cervical and thoracic regions of the cord showed the subarachnoid space to be filled with fibrin and tuberculous tissue. There were endothelioid cell systems of varying size, with some caseation in places; characteristic giant cells and lymphocytic infiltration were also present. Similar lesions beset the inner aspect of the dura. The cord showed superficial oedema; there was also demyelination and histiocyte reaction at some places in the superficial zones and in the posterior columns. Vascular lesions were conspicuous; they affected arteries surrounded by active inflammation, and took the form of fibrinoid degeneration of their coats (Plate 20, Fig. 7). In most vessels the media alone was affected. Where the intima also showed fibrinoid change, it was less extensively affected than the media; and in these vessels the internal elastic lamina was interrupted at one or more points. Polymorphs were scattered among the strands of fibrinoid material. One or two small arteries showed obliterative intimal changes. The anterior spinal arteries were normal in the sections examined. It seemed impossible that these meningeal lesions could have developed in so short a time as eight to ten days.

Case 5. A man aged 20 years. This patient was treated elsewhere from November 1949 to May 1950 for proven tuberculous meningitis, and though clinically well he was discharged from hospital with an abnormal cerebrospinal fluid. In June 1950 he was readmitted to hospital with a relapse of his condition. Three days after admission his lumbar cerebrospinal fluid was found to be evenly blood-stained, and a complete spinal block was present. Next day there was gross weakness of the lower limbs, loss of reflexes, and diminished sensation to pin-prick up to T 4. He was transferred to St. Mary's Hospital, and examination confirmed the above signs, though by this time the weakness of the lower limbs had increased and urinary retention had developed. Death occurred 10 days after the onset of the spinal block.

The brain at post-mortem showed some flattening of the convolutions. There were tubercles on the basal arachnoid, and on that over the superior surface of the cerebellum; there was some exudate in the cisterna chiasmatis. The third ventricle was slightly dilated; ependymal tubercles were scattered throughout the ventricles, mostly in the fourth. The cord was surrounded by thick semi-translucent exudate over all its length except the upper cervical part. There were small haemorrhages in the cord substance at C 7 and C 8, and softening and blurring of pattern at T 1–7. Microscopic examination of the cord showed the subarachnoid space at T 1 to be filled by masses of endothelioid cells, lymphocytes, and giant cells, and some fibrous tissue. The inner aspect of the dura was also affected. The cord itself showed scattered haemorrhages and foci of demyelination. A number of arteries showed marked fibrosis, which not only surrounded the vessels but was seen also in the intima, with sometimes considerable constriction of their lumina. At T 5 meningitic fibrosis was more marked than at T 1; in places there was fibrous fusion of dura and arachnoid. Similar arterial lesions were present here also. At T 8 and T 12 the meningitis appeared considerably older, fibrosis was much more advanced, fusion of dura and arachnoid more extensive, and arterial lesions comparatively few. It was clear that the meningeal lesions were of several months' duration at least.

Case 9. A woman aged 44 years. She became ill during February 1952, and was transferred to St. Mary's Hospital, where in addition to tuberculous meningitis she was also found to suffer from renal tuberculosis. Spinal block developed in March, and persisted till death. She made little response to treatment, and further deteriorated in June, when ventriculography revealed grossly dilated ventricles and suggested the presence in addition of a subtentorial block. Paraplegia-in-extension developed gradually, as well as a chronic urinary infection, during July; by September complete paraplegia-in-flexion was present. A myelogram performed in October showed an almost complete spinal block at T 5 (Plate 22, Fig. 11). She died in January 1953.

At autopsy the cerebral ventricles were moderately dilated. The meninges over the base and around the brain-stem were somewhat fibrotic. From about the first thoracic segment downwards there was a considerable degree of fibrous obliteration of the subarachnoid space; this obliteration was most marked below the mid-thoracic level. Throughout the thoracic levels the central grey substance of the cord showed much softening and cavitation, so that the cord as a whole was irregularly deformed. On microscopic examination, in most of the cord sections there was no active tuberculosis; only one or two foci were found, and they appeared to be in course of fibrous healing. There was great softening and disorganization not only of the grey but also of the white matter of the cord. The meninges were fibrotic; except in the cervical region, the dura and arachnoid were in many places indistinguishably fused into a single dense fibrous membrane, which in the lower thoracic and lumbar regions was extensively attached to the surface of the cord (Plate 19, Figs. 2 and 3). Vascular damage was surprisingly slight; in two lumbar segments there was some reduction of the lumen of the anterior spinal artery by intimal fibrosis, but it was only of moderate degree.

Case 10. A man aged 42 years. Pulmonary tuberculosis was diagnosed in 1940. After a year's sanatorium treatment he remained well till September 1950. A chest X-ray then revealed widespread chronic pulmonary tuberculosis. In May 1951 he complained of pain in the back, and a carious lesion between T 7 and T 8 was detected, together with a large paravertebral abscess. He developed tuberculous meningitis in July 1951, and was transferred to St. Mary's Hospital. On admission his general condition was fair, but after a sharp subarachnoid haemorrhage in August he became desperately ill, and a spinal block developed, which persisted till death. During September 1951 he improved, but during October he developed spasticity of the lower limbs, with increased reflexes and extensor plantar responses. During January 1952 a urinary infection developed and flexor spasms became severe, and by the end of this month complete paraplegia-in-flexion was present. Decubitus calculi formed, and he gradually deteriorated and died in September.

Post-mortem examination showed moderate hydrocephalus, with gelatinous exudate round the base of the brain. In some areas the spinal dura was adherent to the arachnoid. The upper and lower regions of the cord were somewhat soft; the mid-thoracic region was considerably flattened anteroposteriorly, with the meninges closely adherent to its surface. A fibrotic tuberculous change affected the anterior parts of thoracic vertebrae 7 and 8 and the disk between; there was no deformity. There was fibrosis and some caseation of the soft tissues related to these vertebrae, but no epidural abscess. Microscopic examination revealed a quiescent fibrotic lepto- and pachymeningitis. Around the flattened part of the thoracic cord the various membranes were fused together by fibrosis and scarcely distinguishable (Plate 19, Fig. 1); this fusion was seen also in the lumbar region. There was considerable softening of the parenchyma of the cord at all levels; various parts of grey and white matter were affected, but in the flattened region the ventral parts were specially involved and had largely disappeared, so that the remnants of the central canal were found within a millimetre of the meninges. At several levels there was considerable intimal fibrosis of the anterior spinal artery and other arteries in the obliterated subarachnoid space (Plate 20, Fig. 5). Some arteries showed fibrous thickening throughout their walls. Five contiguous blocks were taken from the flattened region. In one, obliterative changes were most marked in arteries in the posterior part; in another the anterior spinal artery was almost completely obliterated, but in most it was almost normal.

The following autopsy reports refer to the patients who died with spinal block but with no clinical finding indicative of cord lesions.

Case 11. This young woman of 19 years died after eight months' illness. Spinal block was present for one month before death. The base of the brain showed extensive thick fibrinous exudate, which filled the basal cisterns. Many tubercles were seen; they extended down the brain-stem to the cord, being sufficiently numerous in the mid-cervical region to obliterate the subarachnoid space. Microscopically, the dura and arachnoid over the cervical cord showed fibrinocaseous tuberculosis filling the subdural and subarachnoid spaces. The cord itself was little affected. Only one or two small arteries showed fibrinoid degeneration of their walls, and in none was there any intimal fibrosis or reduction of lumen. This appearance contrasted sharply with the state of affairs at the brain-stem, where most arteries showed advanced obliterative changes.

Case 12. This woman of 44 years was ill for seven months before death, spinal block being present for the last two months. The brain showed typical tuberculous meningitis, with much thick basal exudate; there was moderate internal hydrocephalus. The cord in its lower thoracic part was surrounded by adhesions, formed of tuberculous material, much thicker posteriorly than anteriorly. Microscopic examination showed that over the lower thoracic cord both dura and arachnoid were affected by fibro-endothelioid tuberculosis, with little caseation and little fibrin. Some vessels in the subarachnoid space showed slight or moderate fibrous thickening of the intima, a few showed acute changes (Plate 20, Fig. 4), but many vessels appeared normal. The cord was normal. A section of cerebral cortex showed a tuberculoma discharging into the subarachnoid space.

Case 13. A woman of 20 years, whose illness lasted two months; throughout the second month there was spinal block. There was slight flattening of the cerebral convolutions. The base of the brain and the brain-stem showed typical tuberculous meningitis, with many tubercles and much subarachnoid exudate. Dense adhesions surrounded the cord in its upper thoracic part, and similar but less extensive adhesions were found in the lower part. Microscopically, the spinal meningeal changes were fairly uniform in type at all levels. The tuberculous process was rather chronic, with little or no caseation but considerable endothelioid-cell accumulations, around which were strands of fibrous tissue, with fine collagen fibres here and there among the endothelioid cells. The dura was affected as well as the arachnoid (Plate 21, Fig. 9); in some places the two membranes were fused. Vascular changes were very irregularly distributed. In some sections it was hard to find a vessel that was not normal, while in others as many as half the arteries, of various sizes, showed fibrous periarteritis and endarteritis; but the reduction of the lumen was seldom serious. No fibrinoid lesions were seen. Sections of the cord appeared to be normal.

Case 14. This girl of 15 years was ill for five months; spinal block was present during the last two months. The subarachnoid space at the base of the brain was filled with fibrinocaseous exudate. The cervical cord appeared almost normal, but over the dorsal and lumbar regions the meninges were matted together, tubercles being clearly visible. Microscopically, the subarachnoid space over the thoracic cord was obliterated by masses of fibrin and caseous material. Caseation was very considerable; there was some endothelioid-cell reaction, but few giant cells. The arachnoid membrane itself was partly destroyed, and the subarachnoid tubercles passed out through the gaps and merged with a vascular and finely fibrotic granulation tissue, which arose from the inner surface of the dura. All these changes were more marked posteriorly than anteriorly. Some of the larger vessels showed moderate intimal thickening. The cord appeared normal.

The following case is reported separately because the available clinical information seemed inadequate to permit its inclusion in the main series.

Case 15. A girl of 17 years was admitted elsewhere to hospital in January 1952, with a 14-day history of headache, vomiting, and abdominal pain. Examination of the nervous system revealed signs of meningeal irritation only, but the findings on lumbar puncture were diagnostic of tuberculous meningitis. A course of intramuscular and intrathecal streptomycin was started, but after 12 days the intrathecal streptomycin was stopped, since a persistent spinal block had developed. The patient's condition deteriorated, and she was transferred to St. Mary's Hospital a month after the start of treatment. Examination showed a comatose, wasted, and incontinent girl. Both fundi showed papilloedema, and there was weakness of the right lateral rectus and left medial rectus muscles. The arm-reflexes were absent, and the left arm was weak. There was weakness of both legs, the knee- and ankle-reflexes were unobtainable, the right plantar response was equivocal, and the left extensor. She died 12 hours after admission.

TABLE III

Post-Mortem Findings in the Cord

All patients had spinal block, and all had dural tuberculosis.

Case number	*Myelitis (clinical)*	*Fibrin*	*Caseation*	*Meningeal fibrosis*	*Lesions of vessels*		*Lesions of cord**
					Frequency	*Type*	
4	Acute	Yes	Moderate	Little	Many	Fibrinoid	Slight†
5	Acute	Little	Little	Yes	Variable	Fibrous endarteritis	Slight†
9	Gradual	No	No	Much	Few	Fibrous endarteritis	Much softening
10	Gradual	No	No	Much	Many	Fibrous endarteritis; medial fibrosis	Much softening
11	No	Yes	Yes	No	Few	Fibrinoid	No
12	No	Little	Little	Some	Few	Fibrous endarteritis	No
13	No	Little	Little	Some	Variable	Fibrous endarteritis and periarteritis	No
14	No	Much	Much	Little	Few	Fibrous endarteritis	No
15	Probable	Much	Much	No	Many	Fibrinoid; thrombosis; fibrous endarteritis	No

* This term excludes simple oedema of the cord, but includes such changes as demyelination and histiocyte reaction.

† See detailed report in text.

There was a slight turbidity under the basal arachnoid, which was studded with minute tubercles. The spinal dura was tense; the subdural and subarachnoid spaces were obliterated by semi-translucent greyish material, so plentiful that in effect the cord and its membranes formed a structure almost solid throughout its length (Plate 21, Fig. 8). On microscopic examination, the inner aspect of the dura was entirely covered with tuberculous tissue at all levels; this tissue was up to 1·0 mm. thick, and was composed largely of systems of endothelioid cells and giant cells. The subarachnoid space was distended by tuberculous tissue with a good deal of caseation, and also by a remarkable amount of fibrin, as much as 2·5 mm. thick in places (Plate 21, Fig. 10). These changes embraced the whole circumference of the cord, but were much more pronounced posteriorly. The vessels were extensively and often seriously damaged. Many small arteries, especially those near the cord, were considerably damaged by fibrinoid change, in some cases with great reduction of the lumen; in one case thrombosis had occurred (Plate 20, Fig. 6). Some of the larger arteries showed oedema and cellular infiltration of the intima. At T 8 the anterior spinal artery showed gross fibrotic endarteritis; at T 12 there was thrombosis of a fair-sized vein in the posterolateral region close to the cord. Microscopically the cord was apparently normal.

The Relationship of Transverse Myelitis to the Presence of Spinal Block

The data in Table I show that spinal block and transverse myelitis are frequently found in the same patient. The problem as to whether this is a real or a coincidental association has been examined by using the data derived from the whole series of 80 patients. The total number of patients developing spinal block was 15. One patient has had to be excluded from statistical analysis, since she developed a terminal neurological lesion which could not during life be accurately localized by clinical examination (Case 15). Fourteen patients with spinal block were observed for a total period of 68 months until death or discharge from the hospital, the average period of observation being 4·8 months (standard deviation 6·3 months, range two weeks to 12 months). Eight incidents of transverse myelitis, involving seven patients, were recorded in this group of 14 patients. These eight incidents of transverse myelitis could be divided into six of acute onset and two of gradual onset. Since 10 patients who later developed spinal block were initially observed among those without spinal block, the group without spinal block numbered 75 patients. These 75 patients were exposed to the risk of developing transverse myelitis in hospital for a total period of 419 months. Three cases of transverse myelitis of the acute type occurred in this group.

Since three patients experienced an episode of transverse myelitis after a relapse of meningitis, it follows that the calculation of any period of exposure to the risk of developing transverse myelitis based on periods of hospital treatment must be unreliable. Furthermore, since patients were followed up for long periods after leaving hospital, the unit of exposure to risk has been taken as the individual case rather than the patient-month. There were 75 exposures to risk in the group without spinal block, resulting in three incidents of acute transverse myelitis, and 14 exposures to risk in the group with spinal block, resulting in seven incidents of transverse myelitis (five of acute onset and two of insidious onset). Using the Fisher 'exact test', we find $P = 0{\cdot}0005$. Similarly, counting only acute incidents, we have three episodes in the 75 patients without spinal block, and five episodes in the 14 patients with spinal block, which gives $P = 0{\cdot}002$. Both these differences are statistically highly significant, and strongly suggest that the association of spinal block and transverse myelitis is real rather than coincidental. The validity of these conclusions is strengthened by three facts: (1) the mean observation period in the patients without spinal block was 5·6 months, while in the spinal-block group it was 4·8 months; (2) ten patients appeared in both groups; (3) only seven episodes of transverse myelitis were counted as having occurred in the spinal-block group, whereas there were really eight episodes (two in one patient). These facts suggest that the difference between the respective attack rates is even more significant than has been shown.

The Relationship of Spinal Block to Mortality

The patients with spinal block had a very heavy mortality rate, 10 of the 15 patients dying, while of the patients with free cerebrospinal circulation 21 died out of 65. These figures give χ^2 (with Yates correction) $= 4{\cdot}711$, P being between 0·02 and 0·05. But the denominators here are individual cases, and the 10 cases with both a preliminary normal phase and later a spinal-block phase have been put into the spinal-block group. This results in the spinal-block group having a longer observation period than the normal group, which might bias the figures so as to give an excessive mortality rate in the spinal-block group. A better construction is to employ again the concept of exposure to risk, using the individual case as the unit of exposure, since by far the greatest mortality of treated tuberculous meningitis occurs in the first two months of treatment. The figures now become 21 deaths among 75 cases in the group without spinal block, and 10 deaths among 15 cases in the group with spinal block; $\chi^2 = 6{\cdot}64$ $(0{\cdot}001 < P < 0{\cdot}01)$. This is again a highly significant statistical difference, and suggests that the development of a spinal block was prejudicial to the patient's chance of survival.

Several factors are believed to influence the mortality rate in tuberculous meningitis, and so the two groups were tested for the following differences: (1) time of survival; (2) clinical condition at onset of the disease (fair or grave); (3) the presence of complicating tuberculosis outside the central nervous system; (4) the actual year of treatment. Statistical testing showed that the differences between the two groups thus examined were in no case significant. It was concluded that the development of a spinal block was prejudicial to the patient's chance of survival.

The Pathological Evidence

Three problems are of particular interest: the relationship of lesions of vessels to spinal cord damage; the mechanism of spinal block; and the possible summation of the effects of spinal block and vascular lesions upon the spinal cord.

The vessels. The lesions of vessels observed in the present series are similar to those reported previously for cerebral vessels (Smith and Daniel, 1947; Doniach, 1949; Winter, 1950; Levinson, Luhan, Mavrelis, and Herzon, 1950; Auerbach, 1951). Three of the papers cited stress the fact that vascular lesions are found only in vessels surrounded by exudate. Our findings bear out this observation. A proportion of our sections were taken from regions of the spinal cord thought at post-mortem examination to be normal. Microscopically, however, every section had some signs of past or present meningeal inflammation, if only a sprinkling of lymphocytes. In sections showing such minimal evidence of inflammation, vascular lesions were always scanty; but every affected vessel had evidence of tuberculous inflammation in intimate relation to it. Affected vessels were not found in the few parts of sections where there were no signs of inflammation. By contrast, in areas where there was widespread inflammation there were usually many affected vessels. The attention of the authors mentioned above has been mainly concerned with cerebral tuberculous meningitis, and with the serious cerebral infarcts which often result from damage to the arteries. Such infarcts were found in the cord in only two (Cases 9 and 10) of the nine patients mentioned in the present report who came to autopsy. None of our other fatal cases showed this feature, though in all cases there was severe spinal meningitis. A possible reason for this apparent sparing of the cord is the nature of its blood-supply; for there is a very free anastomosis between the vessels lying opposite adjacent cord segments, so that even complete obstruction of a number of vessels might not significantly reduce the supply of blood to the cord. In fact it was seldom that as many as half the vessels in any one section were so damaged that they appeared unable to pass any blood; usually the majority showed only moderate stenosis. In view of the anastomosis it is not surprising that, though lesions of vessels are common, cord destruction or damage is uncommon. Those patients who had suffered from transverse myelitis (Cases 4, 5, and 15 probably) showed numerous lesions of vessels at autopsy; whereas those patients (Cases 11 to 14) in whom there was no clinical myelitis showed comparatively few. Case 15 is interesting in that thrombosis was found in a small artery and in a vein. No other case in our series showed vascular thrombosis. Winter (1950) commented that he did not observe arterial thrombosis, and Doniach (1949) did not observe thrombosis in either arteries or veins. Cases 9 and 10 were examples of paraplegia of gradual onset. At autopsy both showed fibrosis and fusion of the dura and arachnoid, with much old softening of the cord. Obliterative vascular lesions were conspicuous in Case 10, as was expected, but they were surprisingly slight in Case 9, from which it appears that arterial stenosis is not essential for producing ischaemia of the cord. It is suggested that fibrous solidification of the meninges might well impede the flow of blood through numerous smaller vessels, especially those in which pressure is lowest. This would be aggravated by the gradual contraction of the fibrous tissue, which might lead also to compression of the cord itself (Plate 19, Fig. 1).

The mechanism of spinal block. Autopsy in Cases 4, 11, 14, and 15 showed considerable amounts of fibrin in the spinal subarachnoid space, which clearly must have played an important part in causing the spinal block. The subarachnoid accumulations of endothelioid cells were in some places bulky enough to fill a high proportion of the space; and dural tuberculosis in some cases was so gross that it must have contributed to the block by restricting the expansion of the arachnoid, if not by actual compression. It seems that, in this respect at least, tuberculosis of the dura is more important in the spine than in the cranium. Oedema of the cord would have little effect by itself, but might well play a part in the presence of the other processes.

The summation of block and vascular lesions. In every case with spinal block the subdural and subarachnoid spaces were partly filled by tuberculous tissue, caseous matter, and fibrin, or by some combination of them. In every such case there were some vascular lesions and consequent impairment of blood-flow. If the meningeal spaces were to be suddenly obliterated by outpourings of fibrin or a rapid increase of tubercles, the vessels would be more or less compressed and the blood-flow further impeded. It seems a natural consequence that spinal block should predispose to cord damage. It is realized that histological examination of the cord may fail to disclose evidence of damage corresponding to clinically observed disturbance of function, especially when, as in Cases 4, 5, and 15, death follows within a few days of the onset of transverse myelitis. Patients (Cases 1, 2, 3) who survived an acute episode of transverse myelitis without spinal block, and those (Cases 4 to 8) in whom spinal block and transverse myelitis both occurred, probably differed only in the degree to which exudates were present. The quantity of exudate was gross enough to produce changes which could be detected by manometric methods in Cases 4 to 8, but insufficient to be detected in Cases 1, 2, and 3.

Discussion

Earlier diagnosis and improved treatment of tuberculous meningitis have resulted in greater attention being paid to complications arising during its treatment. Transverse myelitis must rank as a serious complication causing both death and disability, and clinical and pathological evidence points conclusively to the primary importance of tuberculous exudate in its pathogenesis. The evidence discussed here is considerably strengthened by the work of Doniach (1949) and Winter (1950), who independently noted that arteritis found at post-mortem examination in patients who had died from tuberculous meningitis was virtually confined to those vessels which were buried in exudate. The association between spinal block and the development of transverse myelitis, shown above, would support this contention. Arterial lesions in varying numbers were present in the spinal cords taken from our nine patients who had died with spinal block. Four of the nine showed no signs of spinal cord damage during life, though clinical examination during the terminal stage of this illness is admittedly inexact. This finding suggests that many of these vascular lesions may be clinically silent. Indeed, two of our 80 patients had spinal block for four months and 14 months respectively, and showed no clinical evidence of cord damage. The gradual onset, and slow, relentless progress of the paraplegia in Cases 9 and 10 is in sharp contrast to the lesions experienced by the other patients. Post-mortem examination in Cases 9 and 10 demonstrated that, in addition to lesions of tuberculous arteritis, these patients' cords were surrounded by fibrous tissue derived from old exudate. It seems likely that some of the cord damage found here was caused by fibrosis rather than by tuberculous arteritis. The demonstration that mortality was significantly higher in patients with spinal block emphasizes the dangers of unresolved exudate in this condition. The same danger is apparent when the clinical course and pathology in Cases 4 and 5 are remembered.

A happy feature of the present series has been that six out of 10 patients with myelitis have almost completely recovered from initially severe neurological lesions. Apart from the therapy of meningitis, the only treatment used in the acute stage was passive movement of all joints through the full range of movement twice a day, with splinting to prevent deformity. During the stage of recovery active exercises were insisted upon; two patients derived considerable psychological benefit from a course of galvanic stimulation. The presence of levels of sensory impairment in some patients localized the lesions in the thoracic or lumbar segments of the cord; in the patients who died, arterial lesions were found in these regions. The clinical picture in several patients (especially in those with no level of sensory loss) suggested a cauda equina lesion, but the fact that the bladder and rectum were spared weighed strongly against this diagnosis. The neglect in the literature of transverse myelitis complicating tuberculous meningitis suggests that it may occur mostly in older subjects, who have suffered less frequently than younger persons from the disease. However, it is possible that the complication carries a higher mortality rate and is more difficult to diagnose in younger persons. In any case, experience suggests that tuberculous meningitis is today occurring proportionately more frequently in the older age-groups, a finding which is in line with the later age incidence of primary tuberculous infection in the population.

It might be thought that more effective chemotherapy would reduce the incidence of complications such as transverse myelitis occurring during the treatment of tuberculous meningitis, but this appears unlikely; for, while the mortality of this disease in St. Mary's Hospital has dropped by over two-thirds during the past few years, the incidence of non-fatal complications has risen. The introduction of para-aminosalicyclic acid, and later of isoniazid, has not altered this trend. It is clear, from the histories and pathological findings we have reported, that chemotherapy and antibiotics can have only a restricted effect when the spinal fluid circulation is arrested, as in spinal block. If the therapeutic agents (intrathecal or otherwise) are to have effective access to the tubercle bacilli, then the circulation of cerebrospinal fluid must be as free as possible. Block is caused by the combined effects of accumulations of endothelioid cells, fibrous tissue, and fibrin. Of these, only fibrin can conceivably be rapidly dispersed by natural or artificial means. And if fibrin could be swiftly removed it could carry two advantages: first, the block would be relieved, and secondly the chances of permanent meningeal fibrosis would be reduced. For these reasons we emphatically support the view of Winter (1950) that an 'effective therapeutic agent must . . . rapidly dissipate the fibrin exudate'. It is also clear that early prophylactic use of such an agent would be more effective than its therapeutic use under conditions of established or incipient block.

It is a pleasure to acknowledge our indebtedness to Professors Sir Alexander Fleming and Robert Cruickshank, in whose beds these patients were investigated and treated, and from whom invaluable advice and help were constantly forthcoming: to Drs. D. H. Brinton and H. Edwards, whose help with the difficult neurological problems frequently posed by these patients was unfailing: to Dr. C. C. S. Pike, for help with the morbid anatomy of Case 5; and to Dr. P. Armitage, of the Medical Research Council, Statistical Research Unit.

Summary

1. Investigation and treatment of 80 patients with tuberculous meningitis at St. Mary's Hospital during the years 1947 to 1953 showed that 15 developed spinal block and 10 developed transverse myelitis. In one patient two separate incidents of transverse myelitis occurred.

2. The main clinical features of both these complications of tuberculous meningitis are discussed, and statistical analysis shows that there is a significant correlation between the two.

3. This association receives support from the morbid anatomical findings in the four patients with transverse myelitis who died, and in the five further patients with spinal block who also came to post-mortem examination.

REFERENCES

Auerbach, O. (1951) *Amer. Rev. Tuberc.* **64,** 419.
Cairns, H. (1951) *Arch. Dis. Childh.* **26,** 373.
Choremis, K., Zervos, N., Constantinides, V., and Pantazis, S. (1948) *Lancet,* **2,** 595.
Doniach, I. (1949) *J. Path. Bact.* **61,** 253.
Levinson, A., Luhan, J. A., Mavrelis, W. P., and Herzon, H. (1950) *J. Neuropath. Exp. Neurol.* **9,** 406.
Medical Research Council (1948) *Lancet,* **1,** 582.
Middleton, J. W., and Longfield, A. N. (1952) *Texas Rep. Biol. Med.* **10,** 629.
Perry, T. L. (1952) *J. Pediat.* **40,** 687.
Riley, E. A. (1953) *Amer. Rev. Tuberc.* **67,** 613.
Rubie, J., and Mohun, A. F. (1949) *Brit. Med. J.* **1,** 338.
Schwarz, J. (1948) *Amer. Rev. Tuberc.* **57,** 63.
Smith, H. V., and Daniel, P. (1947) *Tubercle,* **28,** 64.
Somner, A. R. (1952) *Brit. Med. J.* **2,** 356.
Wilson, S. A. K. (1940) *Neurology,* Vol. i, 596. London.
Winter, W. J. (1950) *Amer. Rev. Tuberc.* **61,** 171.

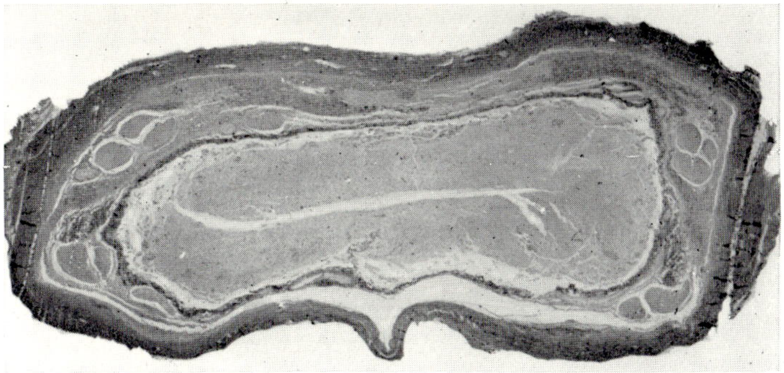

FIG. 1. Case 10. Transverse section of mid-thoracic cord and meninges, showing disorganization and flattening of cord and fibrous fusion of meninges. (Haematoxylin and van Gieson, ×6·5)

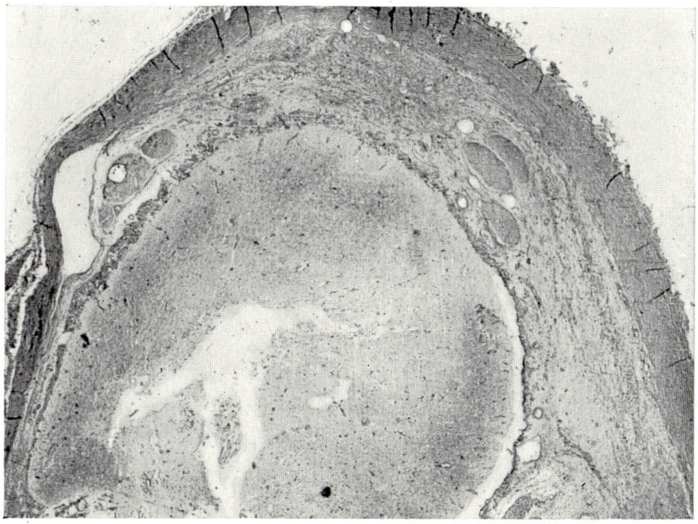

FIG. 2. Case 9. Part of transverse section of lumbar cord and meninges, showing meningeal fibrosis, and softening and cavitation of cord. (Ventral fissure in bottom left corner.) (Haematoxylin and van Gieson, ×9·5)

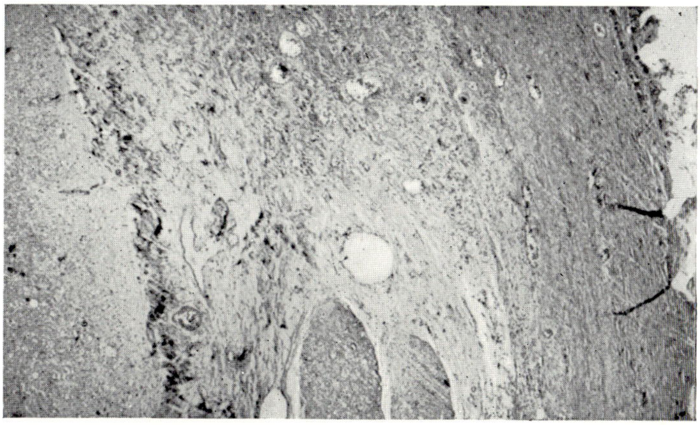

FIG. 3. Case 9. From upper right part of Fig. 2; the cord is on the left, the dura on the right, and parts of two nerve rootlets at the bottom. The virtual solidification of the meninges is apparent. (Haematoxylin and van Gieson, ×30)

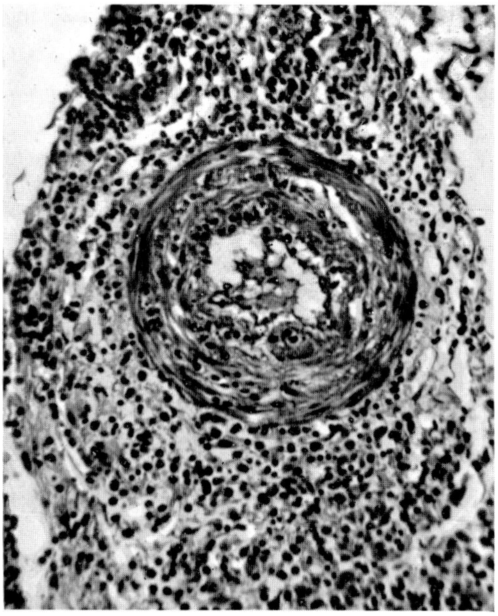

FIG. 4. Case 12. An artery with acute swelling of the intima, and infiltration of the intima and media by polymorphs. Around the vessel are many histiocytes, with some lymphocytes and polymorphs. (Haematoxylin and eosin, ×180)

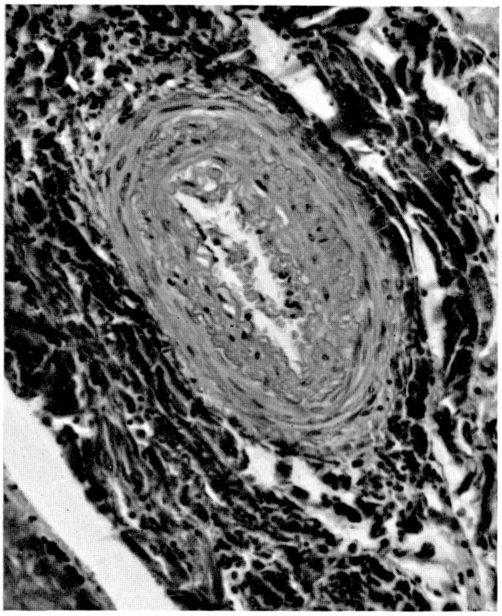

FIG. 5. Case 10. An artery surrounded by dense fibrosis; the intima is thickened by fine fibrosis, which makes it appear slightly darker than the comparatively narrow media. (Haematoxylin and van Gieson, ×180)

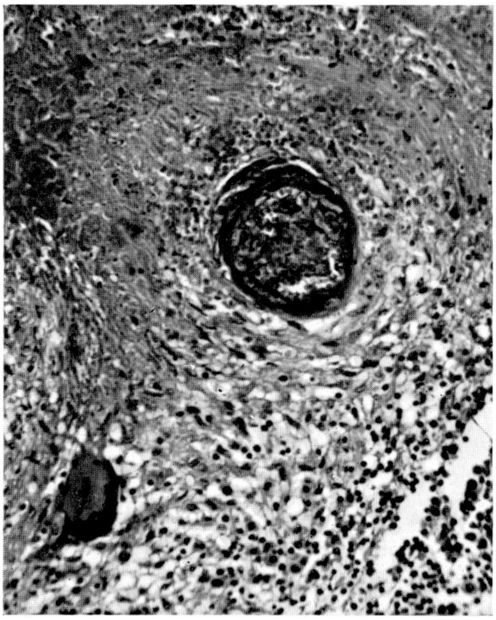

FIG. 6. Case 15. Fibrinoid change and thrombosis of a small artery involved in the tuberculous process. A typical giant cell is seen at the bottom on the left. (Haematoxylin and eosin, ×180)

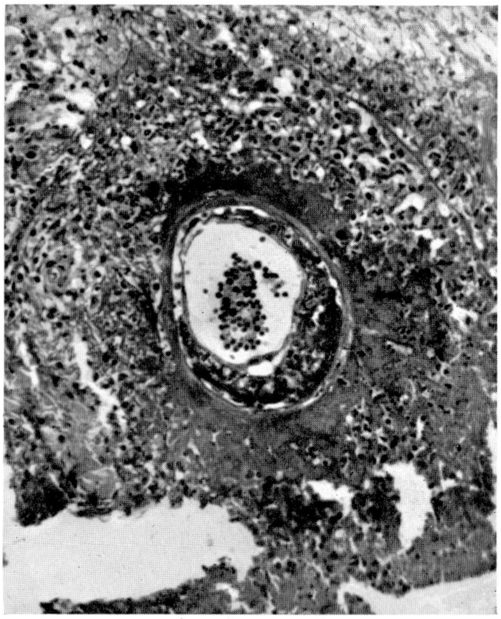

FIG. 7. Case 4. Fibrinoid change in the media and intima of a small artery. The cells scattered round it are mainly polymorphs. (Haematoxylin and eosin, ×180)

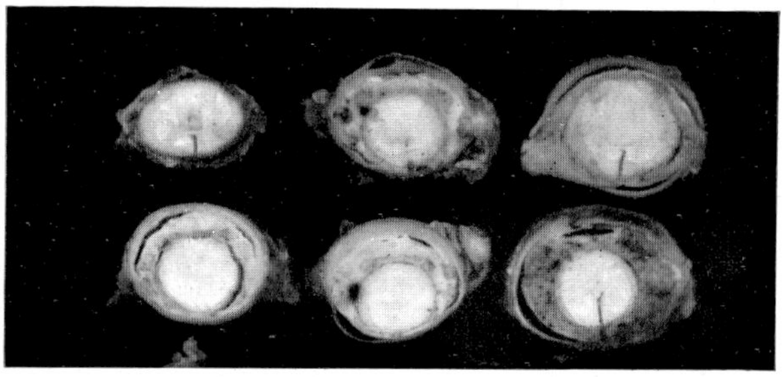

FIG. 8. Case 15. Transverse slices of cord and meninges, showing subdural and subarachnoid spaces obliterated by both dural and subarachnoid inflammation. The cervical, thoracic, and lumbar regions are represented. (Natural size)

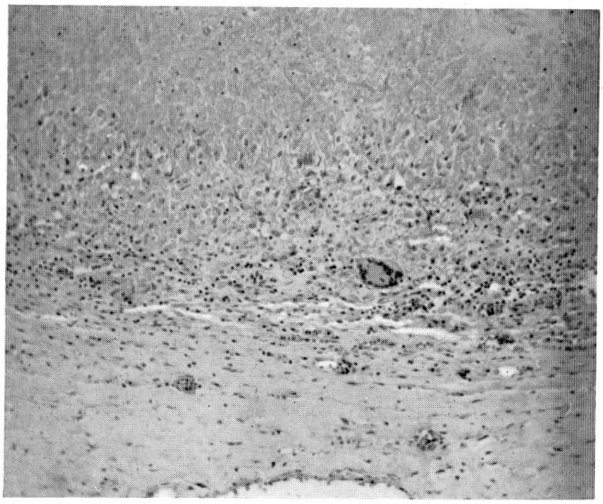

FIG. 9. Case 13. Typical tuberculous inflammation of the inner aspect of the dura. (Haematoxylin and eosin, ×100)

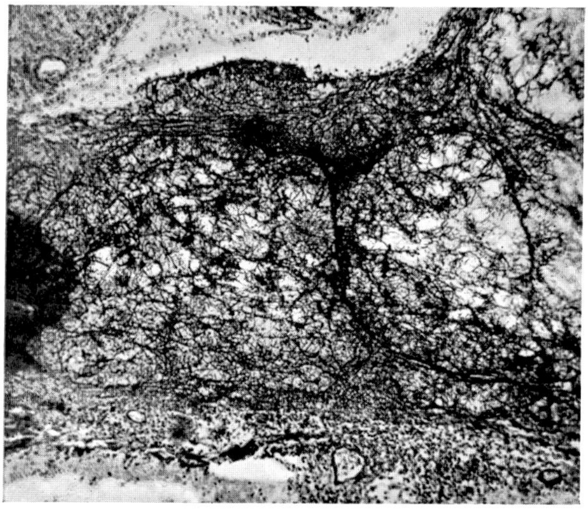

FIG. 10. Case 15. Dense meshwork of fibrin in the subarachnoid space. The cord is at the bottom, part of a root at the top on the left. (Gram, ×74)

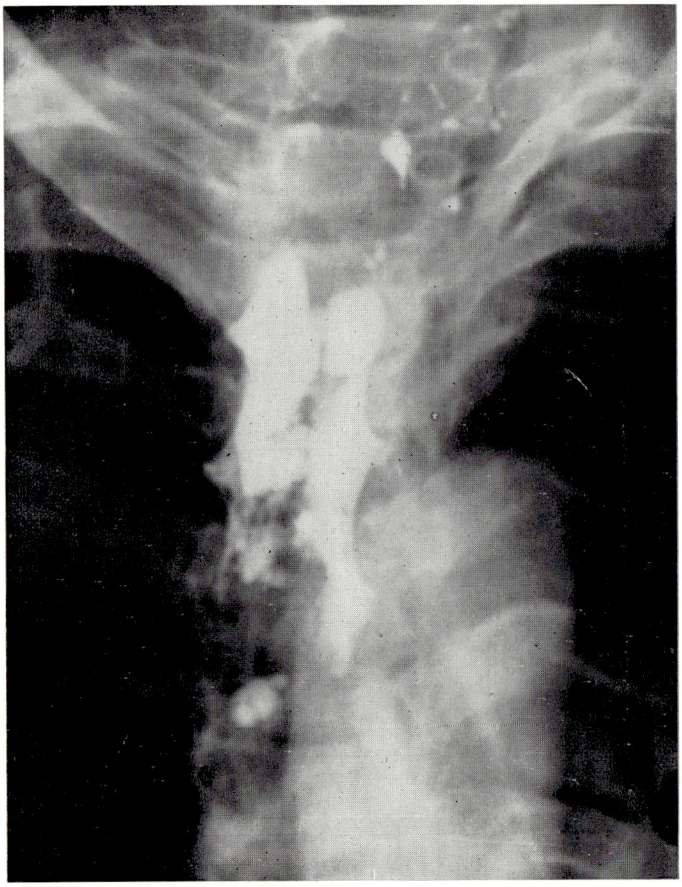

FIG. 11. Case 9. Myelogram showing irregular filling and spinal block at T5 to T8

612.323.21: 606.3-07

STUDIES OF UROPEPSINOGEN EXCRETION IN GASTROINTESTINAL DISORDERS[1]

By W. SIRCUS

(From The Royal Infirmary, Sheffield)

ALMOST a century has passed since the existence of a proteolytic substance in urine was first reported (Brücke, 1861). Fifty years ago the origin of this substance was demonstrated in dogs by Frouin (1904), who showed that its presence in the urine was not due to absorption of proteolytic enzyme by the intestine, but resulted from secretion into the blood-stream at the level of the stomach. By correlating the output of pepsin in the gastric juice with the level of excretion of the urinary enzyme, Gottlieb (1925) found that a close relationship existed between the two substances, and concluded that the urinary product was the inactive proenzyme pepsinogen. No application of these findings to clinical investigation was made until 1946, when Farnsworth, Speer, and Alt, using a technique of assay described by Anson and Mirsky (1932-3) and modified by Bucher, Grossman, and Ivy (1945), reported on the excretion of the enzyme in normal subjects and in cases of anaemia. A close quantitative correlation between the excretion of pepsin in the gastric juice and the excretion of pepsinogen in the urine was shown by Janowitz and Hollander (1950), who demonstrated that the relative rate of release of zymogen into the stomach and into the blood was of the order 99:1 under basal conditions. This correlation justified the use of uropepsinogen assay as a measure of gastric pepsin-formation, and their findings were confirmed by Spiro, Reifenstein, and Gray (1950), who showed an exact quantitative and time relationship between the increases in gastric pepsin secretion and in uropepsinogen excretion under the stimulation of adrenocorticotrophic hormone. The excretion of uropepsinogen has been shown to be fairly consistent in the individual subject, with only small daily fluctuations (Podore, Broh-Kahn, and Mirsky, 1948*a*), and although Bucher (1947) reported a progressive increase in excretion in subjects taking a high-protein diet, ordinary fluctuations in diet produced no significant variation.

Attempts to utilize the assay of uropepsinogen excretion for diagnostic purposes have been made by Podore, Broh-Kahn, and Mirsky (1948*b*), Mirsky, Block, Osher, and Broh-Kahn (1948), and Janowitz, Levy, and Hollander (1950), and, since the present studies were started, by Hirschowitz (1953). All reports have paid insufficient regard to the factor of varying activity in those disorders which are classically remittent, and to possible variations of function during different phases of activity of the disease. All previous studies have utilized various modifications of the Anson-Mirsky technique of assay, with a

[1] Received September 4, 1953.

haemoglobin substrate. In the present investigation it was thought desirable to use a substrate which was generally available and easily prepared, and which gave sufficiently accurate and reproducible results. A modification of the dehydrated-plasma method described by Hunt (1948) for estimating gastric pepsin was found suitable. The purpose of the present studies was to re-examine the possibility of utilizing uropepsinogen estimation for diagnostic purposes, to investigate the excretion of uropepsinogen over a wide field of disorders of the stomach and duodenum, and to pay particular regard to the output of uropepsinogen in relation to the state of activity of cases of duodenal ulcer.

Present Investigation

Two hundred and fifty-six subjects were studied, and the urine excreted during 12 or 24 hours was collected under toluene from each subject on two or more occasions. In the method used for estimation the substrate is prepared from big-pool dehydrated plasma rejected as unfit for transfusion purposes. Two gm. of plasma are dissolved in 100 ml. of distilled water and filtered through Green's 904 paper. The filtrate is then treated with HCl to give a pH of 2·0 as measured by glass electrode at 18° to 22° C. This substrate will remain stable for 72 hours at 6° C. A 1-ml. sample of the timed and measured output of urine from the subject under investigation is mixed with an equal volume of HCl of pH 2·0. A series of pairs of test tubes, one containing 5 ml. of the substrate and the other 10 ml. of trichloracetic acid (4 per cent. w/v), is placed in a thermostatically controlled water bath at 37° C.; 1 ml. of the urine-HCl mixture is added to the tube containing substrate, and mixing obtained by agitating the tubes outside the bath. After two hours' incubation the trichloracetic acid from the other tube is poured into the substrate-urine mixture to stop digestion. Meanwhile the remaining 1 ml. of the urine-HCl mixture has been added to 10 ml. of trichloracetic acid and 5 ml. of substrate, and this mixture serves as a control. The incubated and control mixtures from each pair of tubes are filtered through a Whatman No. 1 paper, and 15 minutes later 2 ml. of the filtrate from each are pipetted into conical flasks containing 20 ml. of 0·25 N NaOH. The flask is rapidly swirled, and immediately 3 ml. of a 1:3 water-diluted Folin and Ciocalteau phenol reagent are run into the flask and mixed by swirling. The flasks are allowed to stand 20 to 30 minutes, and the blue colour which develops is estimated in an absorptiometer using a filter at 600 mμ. The difference between the blank and the incubated specimen is compared on a calibrated curve with the colour produced by a standard solution of tyrosine at a concentration of 0·15 mg. per ml. The period of two hours' incubation was chosen because it was proposed to investigate a number of cases in which peptic activity would be very slight, and short incubation periods might give unreliable results in such cases.

The reproducibility of the substrate and the accuracy of the method were demonstrated by the following experiments. Samples of plasma from five different batches from various supply centres were used to estimate the uropepsinogen in a single urine specimen, and the coefficient of variation of the results was found to be $\pm 4{\cdot}73$ per cent. Five measurements of the peptic activity of each of three specimens of urine were made with substrate taken from a single batch of plasma, and showed an overall mean coefficient of variation of $\pm 3{\cdot}3$ per cent.

The excretion is recorded as the output in uropepsinogen units in 24 hours, where 1 unit = the amount of enzyme releasing the spectrophotometric equivalent of 1 mg. of *l*-tyrosine from 0·1 gm. of plasma-protein substrate in two hours' digestion at 37° C. The symbol $U.U.^{P}$ has been adopted in this report to mean units of uropepsinogen in a plasma-protein assay.

Results

1. *Controls.* There were 41 male and 20 female control subjects, ranging in age from 20 to 79 years. They included healthy students and nurses, and patients, some ambulant and some in bed, who were free from gastro-intestinal and renal disorders. Table I shows that age had no consistent effect on excretion,

TABLE I

Age Distribution and Mean Uropepsinogen Excretion in Controls

		Age in years					
	Sex	*20–29*	*30–39*	*40–49*	*50–59*	*60 and over*	*Total*
Number of persons:	M	18	4	4	9	6	41
	F	5	3	5	4	3	20
Total		23	7	9	13	9	61
							Mean
Mean 24-hour excretion ($U.U.^{P}$):	M	291	309	380	148	238	262
	F	319	257	200	253	286	262
Both sexes . . .		297	287	280	180	254	262

and that the mean excretion was identical in both sexes (in male subjects 262 $U.U.^{P}$ (standard deviation ± 122) in 24 hours; in female subjects 262 $U.U.^{P}$ (s.d. ± 132) in 24 hours). The range in male subjects was 32 to 621 $U.U.^{P}$, and in female subjects 102 to 522 $U.U.^{P}$.

2. *Duodenal ulcer* (70 cases). The mean 24-hour excretion for the whole group, irrespective of age, sex, or the state of activity of the lesion, was 494 $U.U.^{P}$ (range 140 to 1,820 $U.U.^{P}$, s.d. ± 264). This is almost double the normal mean rate of excretion.

Sex factor. There was no significant difference between the sexes, the mean excretion in the 52 male patients being 495 $U.U.^{P}$ (s.d. ± 207), and in the 18 female patients 443 $U.U.^{P}$ (s.d. ± 106); ($t = 1{\cdot}03$; not significant at the 10 per cent. level of P.)

Length of history. No consistent change in the excretion of uropepsinogen was associated with different lengths of history (Table II). In Table II no allowance is made for the state of activity of the lesion at the time of investigation. When the 27 cases of duodenal ulcer in which the disorder was in remission at the time of investigation were alone considered, there was still found to be no change in the excretion of uropepsinogen with different lengths of history (Tables III *a*, III *b*). The criteria adopted for a state of remission were the absence of symptoms of any kind or degree for at least one month, the absence

TABLE II

The Excretion of Uropepsinogen in Duodenal Ulcer according to Sex and Length of History

	History in years	*Number of cases*	*Mean length of history in years*	*Mean age in years*	*Mean excretion (U.U.ᵖ/24 hrs.)*
Male patients:	0–4	20	2·35	39·7	523 (i)
	5–9	7	7·4	41·7	471 (ii)
	10–19	10	13·0	48·3	525 (iii)
	20 and over	15	26·6	56·1	509 (iv)
Female patients:	0–4	2	3·75	45·0	268 (v)
	5–9	6	5·8	50·0	474 (vi)
	10–19	8	11·0	47·1	503 (vii)
	20 and over	2	20·0	50·0	284 (viii)

Significance of differences between the groups:

i and ii: $t = 0{\cdot}514$. Not significant at 10% level of P.
i and iv: $t = 0{\cdot}160$. ,, ,, ,, ,, ,, ,, ,,
ii and iii: $t = 0{\cdot}551$. ,, ,, ,, ,, ,, ,, ,,
ii and iv: $t = 0{\cdot}372$. ,, ,, ,, ,, ,, ,, ,,
iii and iv: $t = 0{\cdot}159$. ,, ,, ,, ,, ,, ,, ,,

TABLE III *a*

Excretion of Uropepsinogen in Cases of Duodenal Ulcer during Remission, related to Length of History

Number of cases	*Length of history*	*Mean excretion (U.U.ᵖ/24 hrs.)*
9	Under 5 years	416 (i)
18	Over 5 years	382 (ii)
27		

Difference between i and ii by t test: $t = 0{\cdot}372$. Not significant at 10% level of P.

TABLE III *b*

Excretion of Uropepsinogen related to Length of History and Duration of Remission

	Duration of remission under 6 months		*Duration of remission over 6 months*	
Length of history in years	*Number of cases*	*Mean excretion (U.U.ᵖ/24 hrs.)*	*Number of cases*	*Mean excretion (U.U.ᵖ/24 hrs.)*
Under 5 . .	8	439	1	231
Over 5 . .	12	377	6	392
	20		7	

of any signs, including epigastric tenderness, and the absence of occult blood from the stools.

State of activity of disorder. A striking difference was observed in the excretion of uropepsinogen between patients in active relapse and those in remission at the time of investigation (Table IV). When considered in relation to sex and to the state of activity of the disorder, there was found to be a considerable fall in the excretion of uropepsinogen during the remission phase in both sexes, the output in female patients returning to normal (Table V). The effect of length of

TABLE IV

State of disorder	*Number of cases*	*Mean excretion (U.U.^{p}/24 hrs.)*	*Standard deviation*
Active . . .	43	559	±278
Remission. . .	27	393	±210

$t = 2{\cdot}74$, which is significant at 1% level of P.

TABLE V

Excretion of Uropepsinogen in relation to Activity of Lesion and to Sex

State of disorder	*Sex*	*Number of patients*	*Mean excretion (U.U.^{p}/24 hrs.)*	*Standard deviation*
Active	M	28	594 (i)	±317
	F	15	485 (ii)	±226
Remission . . .	M	24	413 (iii)	±215
	F	3	232 (iv)	±33

Significance of differences between active and remission phase:
i and iii: $t = 2{\cdot}41$. Significant at 2% level of P.
ii and iv: $t = 2{\cdot}48$. Significant at 5% level of P.

TABLE VI

Comparison of Excretion-rates of Uropepsinogen after 3 Months' Interval and in relation to Activity of Lesion

Patient	*Sex*	*Age (years)*	*Previous state of lesion*	*Previous excretion (U.U.^{p}/24 hrs.)*	*Later state of lesion*	*Later excretion (U.U.^{p}/24 hrs.)*
A. Showing no change in phase of activity:						
D1	F	48	Active	290	Active	340
D2	M	27	Active	809	Active	904
D3	M	40	Remission 3 months	1,184	Remission 8 months	252
B. With change from activity to remission:						
D4	M	33	Active	621	Remission 3 months	270
D5	F	39	Active	576	Remission 3 months	439
D6	M	59	Active	792	Remission 3 months	486
C. With change from remission to activity:						
D7	M	63	Remission 15 months	411	Active 3 weeks	400
D8	M	45	Remission 3 months	242	Active 2 months	720
D9	F	24	Remission 1 month	290	Active 2 months	448

remission on excretion was not fully appreciable, as insufficient patients with a remission of more than six months' duration were investigated:

Number of patients	Duration of remission	Mean 24-hour excretion
18	1 to 6 months	407 U.U.^{p}
7	6 to 12 months	343 ,,
2	1 to 2 years	445 ,,

There is no significant difference between these results by the t test. At the time of writing nine of the patients with duodenal ulcer have been reinvestigated after an interval of three or more months. Change in the state of activity of the lesion, assessed clinically, had occurred in six. The results are compared in Table VI.

3. *Benign gastric ulcer* (35 cases). There were 21 male and 14 female patients in this group. The mean excretion for the whole group was 332 U.U.P in 24 hours (s.d. ±203); but seven of the patients had a concomitant duodenal ulcer. When these were excluded, the results for the remaining 28 patients showed a mean excretion of 279 U.U.P in 24 hours (s.d. ±169). Thus patients with gastric

TABLE VII

Analysis of Studies of Uropepsinogen Excretion in Cases of Gastric Ulcer according to Site of Ulcer and Sex of Patient

Group	*Number of patients*	*Sex*	*Mean excretion (U.U.P/24 hrs.)*	*Standard deviation*
All cases	35	M+F	332 (i)	±203
Gastric ulcer alone	28	M+F	279 (ii)	±169
Gastric and duodenal ulcer	7	M+F	535 (iii)	±202
Gastric ulcer alone: effect of site:				
Ulcer in upper two-thirds	23	M+F	377 (iv)	±192
Ulcer in lower third	5	M+F	301 (v)	±81
Effect of sex:				
A. Gastric ulcer alone:				
Ulcer in upper two-thirds	12	M	311 (vi)	±212
	11	F	240 (vii)	±92
Ulcer in lower third	4	M	338 (viii)	±33
	1	F	150	..
B. Gastric ulcer with and without associated duodenal ulcer:				
Ulcer in upper two-thirds	14	M	387 (ix)	±263
	13	F	291 (x)	±172
Ulcer in lower third	7	M	357	±46
	1	F	150	..

Significance of differences between the groups:

i and ii: $t = 1{\cdot}11$. Not significant at 10% level of P.
ii and iii: $t = 3{\cdot}28$. *Significant at 1% level of P.*
iv and v: $t = 1{\cdot}04$. Not significant at 10% level of P.
vi and vii: $t = 1{\cdot}044$. Not significant at 10% level of P.
vii and viii: $t = 0{\cdot}306$. Not significant at 10% level of P.
ix and x: $t = 1{\cdot}11$. Not significant at 10% level of P.

ulcers uncomplicated by a duodenal ulcer (the incidence of which in the group was 20 per cent.) have an excretion not significantly different from that of the controls, but the presence of a duodenal ulcer results in an elevated excretion of uropepsinogen. Furthermore, the mean excretion in the group of seven patients who had gastric ulcers associated with a duodenal ulcer was 535 U.P.P in 24 hours (s.d. ±202), which is similar to the rate of excretion in active duodenal ulcer alone.

Effect of the site of the ulcer. Of the 28 cases of uncomplicated gastric ulcer, in 23 the ulcers were placed in either the middle or upper third of the stomach, and only five ulcers were at or below the incisura angularis. The mean output of uropepsinogen in the former group was 377 U.U.P in 24 hours (s.d. ±192), and in the latter group 301 U.U.P (s.d. ±81). There were 12 male patients who had a high or mid-stomach ulcer and a mean excretion of 311 U.U.^{P} in 24 hours (s.d. ± 212), and 11 female patients who had a mean excretion of 240 U.U.^{P} in 24 hours (s.d. ± 92). Four of the five low gastric ulcers were in male patients, and the mean excretion was 338 U.U.^{P} (s.d. ± 33).

4. *Partial and total gastrectomy.* During the period of these studies 10 subjects who had had a partial gastrectomy for peptic ulceration, more than one year

TABLE VIII

Uropepsinogen Excretion more than One Year after Partial Gastrectomy

Patient	*Sex*	*Symptom-complex*	*Findings by X-ray and gastroscopy*	*Excretion (U.U.^{P}/24 hrs.)*
G1	M	Recurrent epigastric pain	Stomal ulcer	120
G2	M	Epigastric pain	Probable stomal ulcer	108
G3	M	No dyspepsia; bronchitis	Nil	56
G4	F	Classical dumping syndrome	Nil	60
G5	M	Steatorrhea; malnutrition	Nil	Nil
G6	M	Flatulence and distension	Hiatus hernia of stump	Nil
G7	M	Classical dumping syndrome	Nil	Nil
G8	F	Malnutrition; avitaminosis	Nil	Nil
G9	M	Biliary vomiting	Afferent loop distension	Nil
G10	M	Flatulence and malnutrition	Nil	Nil

TABLE IX

Uropepsinogen Excretion before, and 10 Days after, Partial Gastrectomy

			Excretion (U.U.^{P}/24 hrs.)	
Patient	*Sex*	*Disorder*	*1 day before operation*	*10 days after operation*
G11	M	Chronic duodenal ulcer	2,226	112
G12	M	Chronic gastric ulcer	252	Nil

previously, were seen and investigated. Nine had been admitted for investigation of recurrent gastrointestinal symptoms, and one with an upper respiratory tract infection. Two were found to excrete an amount of uropepsinogen just

TABLE X

Excretion of Uropepsinogen in Haematemesis, according to Aetiology

Lesion	*Number of cases*	*Mean excretion (U.U.^{P}/24 hrs.)*
Chronic duodenal ulcer	10	788
Chronic gastric ulcer	2	363
Haemorrhagic diathesis	2	259
Acute peptic ulcers	3	218
Aspirin gastritis	1	598
Oesophageal varices	1	127

below the normal range; a stomal ulcer was revealed by X-ray in one, and in the other considered probable. Two others excreted small amounts of uropepsinogen (Table VIII). The urine from two other subjects was investigated one day before and 10 days after subtotal gastrectomy for chronic peptic ulceration, and a marked fall in output was revealed in each case (Table IX). The urine from two subjects who had had total gastrectomy performed one year previously was found to contain no uropepsinogen.

5. *Haematemesis and melaena.* Of 23 patients urgently admitted with haematemesis and melaena during the present studies, the diagnosis was unknown in 19 cases at the time of admission. As soon as possible after admission urine was collected for investigation. The results in the 19 cases (Table X) and the details of the subsequent investigation and diagnosis (Table XI) show that, of the

TABLE XI

Details of Investigation of Cases of Haematemesis

Patient	*Sex*	*Symptom-complex*	*Results of investigation*	*Uropepsinogen excretion (U.U.^{P}/24 hrs.)*
H1	M	Repeated symptomless haematemesis during 9 years	All negative except teliangectasia	239
H2	M	1 day dyspepsia with pain; syncope; haematemesis	All negative. Clinically acute peptic ulcer	180
H3	F	6 aspirins daily for 2 weeks for fibrositis	All negative	598
H4	F	10 years' remittent dyspepsia. Attack began 5 days prior to bleeding	Clinically duodenal ulcer. X-ray: doubtful duodenal ulcer	576
H5	F	Repeated haematemesis during 11 years	2 negative gastroscopies. 8 negative barium meals. Generalized capillary abnormality proved by skin microscopy	292
H6	M	10 years' remittent preprandial epigastric pain	X-ray negative 3 weeks after haemorrhage. Clinically chronic duodenal ulcer	953
H7	M	3 years' remittent dyspepsia. 2nd haematemesis	Gastric ulcer in lesser curvature (X-ray and gastroscopy)	123
H8	M	5 years' dyspepsia. Previous melaena	Benign gastric ulcer at operation	604
H9	F	5 years' dyspepsia	Chronic duodenal ulcer (X-ray)	828
H10	M	22 years' remittent dyspepsia	Chronic duodenal ulcer (X-ray)	475
H11	M	14 days' interscapular pain	All negative. Clinically acute peptic ulcer	284
H12	M	8 years' remittent dyspepsia	X-ray: chronic duodenal ulcer	736
H13	F	Sudden haematemesis. No previous dyspepsia	X-ray: persistent irregularity of duodenal cap. Clinically acute peptic ulcer	192
H14	M	3 years' remittent dyspepsia. Pain of 'hunger' type	X-ray: duodenal ulcer	580
H15	M	1 month epigastric pain, 2 hours after food: melaena 1 week before admission	X-ray: pyloric crater. Operation: benign juxtapyloric ulcer	900
H16	F	10 years' flatulent dyspepsia. Haematemesis 6 months previously in U.S.A.	X-ray: oesophageal varices	127
H17	M	2 years' remittent dyspepsia. Epigastric pain 2 hours after food and at night	Gastroscopy: nil. X-ray: chronic duodenal ulcer	828
H18	M	15 years' remittent dyspepsia. Haematemesis 2 years ago	X-ray: chronic duodenal ulcer with deformed cap	1,245
H19	M	12 years' remittent dyspepsia. Epigastric pain 2–3 hours after food	X-ray: chronic duodenal ulcer	762

12 patients whose excretion of uropepsinogen was above normal at the time of the haemorrhage, 10 were subsequently found to have a duodenal ulcer, one a gastric ulcer, and the other a probable aspirin gastritis. Of the seven patients with a normal or low excretion one was shown to have a chronic gastric ulcer, and two haemorrhagic diathesis; three, in whom investigation revealed no cause, were clinically diagnosed as having acute peptic ulcers, and in one

TABLE XII

Excretion of Uropepsinogen in Secondary Dyspepsia

Patient	*Sex*	*Age (years)*	*Clinical details*	*Final diagnosis*	*Excretion (U.U.P/24 hrs.)*
S1	M	50	4 years' vague dyspepsia. Emphysema. Bronchiectasis	Bronchiectasis	342
S2	M	38	14 years' dyspepsia. Mines Safety Officer. Occupational anxiety state	Psychosomatic dyspepsia	161
S3	F	51	3 years' flatulent dyspepsia. X-ray: rolling hiatus hernia	Hiatus hernia	304
S4	F	55	Flatulent dyspepsia, borborygmi, abdominal distension. Emotional factors present	Psychosomatic dyspepsia	221
S5	M	70	Recurrent transient epigastric pain lasting few minutes. Wassermann reaction negative. Thrombosis of inferior vena cava	Vascular syphilis. Autonomic system involved	234
S6	F	72	9 months' indigestion. Chronic bronchitis. Emphysema	Chronic bronchitis	247
S7	M	28	2 years' bizarre dyspepsia. Psychopathic features	Psychosomatic dyspepsia	142
S8	F	59	7 years' history of nausea and abdominal discomfort, associated with headache	Post-menopausal migraine	260
S9	M	43	3 years' flatulent dyspepsia. Severe anxiety state from gunshot-wound disfigurement of face	Chronic anxiety state	610
S10	F	47	10 years' flatulent dyspepsia, menopausal	Migraine and menopause	296

haemorrhage was due to oesophageal varices. The mean excretion in the 10 cases of haematemesis and melaena (788 U.U.P) was significantly higher than the mean excretion in the 43 cases of uncomplicated but active duodenal ulcer, which was 559 U.U.P (Table IV); $t = 2{\cdot}66$, which is significant at the 1 per cent. level of P.

6. *Secondary dyspepsia.* Studies were made of 15 cases of dyspepsia in which full investigation had excluded any inflammatory, ulcerative, or neoplastic lesion of the stomach or duodenum (Table XII). The output of uropepsinogen was found to be normal in all but one, a case of chronic anxiety. The mean excretion for the group was 282 U.U.P in 24 hours (s.d. ± 125), which is very similar to that found in the controls. All the cases were reviewed again after three months, and five patients, in whom a somatic lesion of the nature indicated above was subsequently suggested, have been excluded from the group results.

7. *Anaemia with apparent achlorhydria.* Twelve cases of iron-deficiency

anaemia, confirmed by blood and marrow investigation, were studied. Eight patients showed an excretion of uropepsinogen which was half that of the control series, or less, and four excreted none at all. One patient had a normal uropepsinogen output; eleven had shown complete achlorhydria on ordinary fractional gastric analysis in the ward, with tea and a single injection of 0·5 mg. histamine base as stimuli. In each case the fractional analysis was repeated,

TABLE XIII

Uropepsinogen Excretion in Anaemia compared with Response to Histamine

Patient	*Clinical features*	*Response to ward fractional test meal*	*Maximum response to triple histamine test (mg. HCl per ml. juice)*	*Uropepsinogen output (U.U.P/24 hrs.)*
A1	Iron deficiency (simple)	No free acid	1·97	102
A2	Iron deficiency (simple)	No free acid	1·8	106
A3	Iron deficiency (simple)	No free acid	0·3	147
A4	Iron deficiency (simple)	No free acid	1·1	130
A5	Iron deficiency (simple)	Some free acid	Not tested	279
A6	Iron deficiency (simple)	No free acid	2·9	95
A7	Iron deficiency. Cirrhosis of liver	No free acid	1·46	60
A8	Iron deficiency (simple)	No free acid	Not tested	90
A9	Iron deficiency. Atrophic gastritis	No free acid	Nil	Nil
A10	Iron deficiency (simple)	No free acid	Nil	Nil
A11	Iron deficiency (simple)	No free acid	Nil	Nil
A12	Iron deficiency (simple)	No free acid	Nil	Nil

with three doses of histamine base, 1·0 mg., 0·5 mg., and 0·5 mg., as the sole stimulus, and a production of free acid resulted in six cases. A correlation was observed between the excretion of uropepsinogen and the response to the triple histamine test (Table XIII).

8. *Neoplasms of stomach.* Thirteen subjects with tumours of the stomach were investigated; twelve of the tumours were shown at gastroscopy and laparotomy to be malignant, and one to be a leiomyoma, confirmed by histology. The mean excretion in the patients with malignant tumours was 197 U.U.P in 24 hours (s.d. ± 191). This mean is considerably lower than that found in the controls, but has no value in the diagnosis of carcinoma. The patient with a leiomyoma excreted 579 U.U.P in 24 hours. On clinical and radiological evidence this tumour was thought to be a carcinoma, but the fractional test meal revealed a high output of free acid, and this evidence of an overactive gastric mucosa was confirmed by the uropepsinogen excretion. One subject, in whom a juxtapyloric ulcer was diagnosed on X-ray, was reported at gastroscopy to have a 'Type IV carcinoma of the antrum'. The uropepsinogen output was 900 U.U.P in 24 hours. A laparotomy was performed, and a benign juxtapyloric peptic ulcer was disclosed, and confirmed by histology.

9. *Pernicious anaemia.* Twelve cases of anaemia, proved by marrow studies and response to therapy to be pernicious anaemia, were investigated. The range of uropepsinogen excretion for the group was 0 to 70 U.U.P in 24 hours, and the mean 17 U.U.P in 24 hours (s.d. ± 24). An attempt was made in eight cases to

correlate the uropepsinogen output with the response of the stomach to the triple histamine test. A production of acid, electrometrically recorded, resulted from the histamine injections in only one patient, who was one of the group excreting uropepsinogen. In all the four patients who produced no uropepsinogen, histamine failed to stimulate the release of any acid (Table XIV).

TABLE XIV

Uropepsinogen Excretion in Pernicious Anaemia Compared with Response to Histamine

Patient	*Sex*	*Age (years)*	*Result of fractional test meal*	*Response to triple histamine test*	*Excretion (U.U.ᴾ/24 hrs.)*
P1	F	39	No acid	No acid	70
P2	F	50	No acid	No acid	51
P3	F	47	No acid	Not tested	19
P4	M	46	No acid	No acid	19
P5	M	52	No acid	Fall in pH of 2 units	50
P6	M	60	No acid	No acid	Nil
P7	M	47	No acid	No acid	Nil
P8	M	61	No acid	No acid	Nil
P9	F	60	No acid	Not tested	Nil
P10	F	50	No acid	Not tested	Nil
P11	F	67	No acid	Not tested	Nil
P12	F	65	No acid	No acid	Nil

Discussion

The accepted methods of gastric analysis are unsatisfactory partly because of the artificial nature of the tests, and partly because the uncontrollable effects of the emptying of the stomach make it difficult to acquire quantitative data. The serial test meal described by Hunt and Spurrell (1951) facilitates the quantitative measurement of the parietal-cell secretion, but subjects the patient to repeated tests for several days, and is not therefore practicable for clinical use; and an *in vitro* modification of the test (Hunt, 1953) has confirmed the misleading possibilities of any method of gastric analysis which fails to allow for the emptying factor. The measurement of the excretion of uropepsinogen has the advantage of providing a readily repeatable quantitative estimation of peptic cell function with the minimum of disturbance to the patient, and without the aid of artificial stimuli. The results of such measurements reported above confirm the value of the assay both as an aid to diagnosis and as a tool for physiological research. Previous studies of the excretion of uropepsinogen in disease have not satisfactorily demonstrated the value of the investigation, either because of lack of sufficient subjects for statistical analysis, or because of the limited nature of the field studied. Thus Farnsworth, Speer, and Alt (1946) studied only normal subjects and cases of pernicious anaemia. Podore, Broh-Kahn, and Mirsky (1948*b*) failed to differentiate between gastric and duodenal ulcers, and reported a series of cases of secondary dyspepsia but provided no clinical data. Janowitz, Levy, and Hollander (1950) studied only four cases of gastric ulcer, and their group of duodenal ulcers included anastomotic ulcers.

Hirschowitz (1953) considered only cases of peptic ulcer. All these studies, and one by Eastcott, Fawcett, and Rob (1953), reported since the present work was completed, have failed to allow for the possible coexistence of duodenal and gastric ulcers, which in the present study occurred in 20 per cent. of the gastric ulcer group and 10 per cent. of the duodenal ulcer group; they have also failed to consider the relation of their results in gastroduodenal ulceration to the state of activity of the lesion at the time of investigation, in spite of the known remittent nature of these disorders, and the suggestive demonstrations by Watkinson (1951) and Vanzant, Osterberg, Alvarez, and Rivers (1933) that gastric secretion varies with the state of activity of a gastric or duodenal ulcer.

From the results of the present investigation a number of features emerge which have not previously been described. A highly significant difference was found between the mean rates of excretion of uropepsinogen in active duodenal ulcer and in cases in remission. The 43 patients with active ulcers had a mean excretion of 559 U.U.P in 24 hours, compared with 393 U.U.P in 24 hours in the 27 patients in remission. This fact provides evidence that the differing phases of activity in duodenal ulcer, clinically assessed, are associated with changes in the pattern of gastric secretion; it supports the findings of Watkinson (1951) as regards gastric pH levels in peptic ulcer, and those of Vanzant, Alvarez, Eusterman, Dunn, and Berkson (1932), who reported that the *concentration* of pepsin, in studies of gastric analysis made in cases of duodenal ulcer, altered with the state of activity of the lesion. In their report symptom-free patients had pepsin values within the normal range, but with a higher mean value than the normal average, whereas patients with active ulcers had pepsin values outside the normal range, with a mean value 2·5 times that found in the cases in remission. No significant difference was found between the rates of excretion of uropepsinogen in male and female patients with duodenal ulcer, when the results were considered without relation to the state of activity of the lesion at the time of assay. When this factor was taken into account, a difference between the sexes appeared in the degree to which the uropepsinogen excretion varied during the different phases of ulcer activity. While the excretion in both sexes tended to return towards normal during a clinical remission (the mean 24-hour excretion in male patients was 594 U.U.P in activity and 413 U.U.P in remission, and in female patients 485 U.U.P in activity and 232 U.U.P in remission), the excretion in male patients remained significantly above normal in remission, but in female patients it returned to normal. This finding is in accord with the reports of Vanzant, Alvarez, Eusterman, Dunn, and Berkson (1932), and of Perman (1935), that the mean acidity in response to an Ewald test meal was lower in female than in male ulcer patients, although with active ulcers the response in female patients was still above normal. In an analysis of the relation of output of uropepsinogen to the duration of remission at the time of assay, only seven cases were available in one group, so that no conclusion of significance could be drawn. The figure of 343 U.U.P as the mean 24-hour excretion in patients between the sixth and 12th months of remission, compared with 407 U.U.P in patients with a remission of less than six months, can therefore only remain suggestive. But, in the nine follow-up cases available at the time of writing, a marked change in the rate of excretion of uropepsinogen is seen in five of the six cases in which the phase of activity has altered, and, in one patient who had an extremely high output in early remission, the excretion rate had fallen to normal after the remission had persisted for eight months. There is evidence (Shay, Gershon-Cohen, and Fels, 1942) that the presence of an ulcer in the duodenum interferes with the normal mechanism for inhibiting the production of free acid in an empty stomach, and it has been shown experimentally by Grossman, Greengard, Woolley, and Ivy (1944) that the output of pepsin is inhibited by the presence of fat in the duodenum and by the parenteral administration of enterogastrone. Hence it is possible that the activity of the peptic cells is influenced by the extent of, and state of activity of, an ulcer in the duodenum interfering with the enterogastrone mechanism.

In cases of gastric ulcer the mean rate of excretion of uropepsinogen was found to be normal only when patients with an associated duodenal lesion had been excluded. When they were included, the mean excretion for the whole group rose considerably, because the seven patients with dual lesions had a mean excretion in 24 hours of 535 U.U.P, which is similar to that found in the entire group of duodenal ulcers. This finding implies that the presence of a gastric ulcer does not usually interfere with the function of the peptic cells, whereas the concomitant presence of a duodenal ulcer is associated with a greatly increased peptic activity. The report of Hirschowitz (1953), that ulcers distal to the lesser curvature of the stomach were associated with excretion rates similar to those in duodenal ulcer, was not confirmed.

After partial gastrectomy the results of fractional gastric analysis are unreliable, owing to the rapid emptying of the remnant and the contamination by intestinal contents, but the results reported in the present group of gastrectomy cases appear to offer a simple quantitative test of the glandular function in the stomach remnant, without any of the disadvantages of the methods of fractional analysis. Such a test would be valuable in post-operative assessment of the success of surgery. Of particular diagnostic value is the possibility of excluding anastomotic ulcer as the cause of a post-gastrectomy dyspepsia in which uropepsinogen excretion is found to be absent. Eastcott, Fawcett, and Rob (1953) recently reported that, after partial gastrectomy, all their six patients with duodenal ulcer continued to excrete amounts of uropepsinogen which were greater than the average normal in their control subjects. They also stated that even after total gastrectomy the output of uropepsinogen was only reduced by half. The results obtained in the present study do not confirm their findings. Their findings also conflict with all previous reports of the effects of total gastrectomy on uropepsinogen excretion in man and experimental animals (Frouin, 1904; Bucher and Ivy, 1947; Spiro, Reifenstein, and Gray, 1950; Janowitz, Levy, and Hollander, 1950); these facts suggest that their method of assay should be reconsidered.

The results in the cases of haematemesis and melaena suggest a diagnostic usefulness in providing evidence for the presence of a duodenal ulcer before

X-ray is advisable. The mean output of uropepsinogen in the 10 cases in which haematemesis and melaena proved to be due to a chronic duodenal ulcer was significantly higher than the mean output in 43 cases of uncomplicated but active duodenal ulcer. This fact suggests either that massive bleeding is associated with heightened peptic activity, or that duodenal ulcer patients who excrete an unusually large amount of uropepsinogen are more prone to haemorrhage. This problem could be resolved by serial estimations of uropepsinogen excretion during and after haematemesis, and by a prolonged clinical follow-up of patients with duodenal ulcer who have been found to have an unusually high output of uropepsinogen.

In the cases of iron-deficiency anaemia a correlation was found between the output of uropepsinogen and the response of the parietal cells to a triple dose of histamine, when the normal test meal, with a single injection of histamine (0·5 mg.), had shown achlorhydria. This correlation suggests that the estimation of uropepsinogen may provide a more reliable test of gastric secretory function in the anaemias than the usual fractional analysis. In the group of cases of pernicious anaemia a complete absence of uropepsinogen was associated with complete refractoriness of the parietal cells to histamine in four patients. One of the patients, who excreted a small amount of uropepsinogen, also showed a small but definite response to a triple histamine test when acidity was measured electrometrically, the pH of the juice falling by two units after histamine stimulation. These results suggest that the functions of the peptic and parietal cells usually fail concomitantly in the anaemias associated with degrees of gastric atrophy, but that occasionally either one of the two groups of cells retains its function a little longer, or a small proportion of the endocrine component of the peptic secretion continues after the exocrine component has ceased to appear. The absence in true achlorhydria of the 'washing-out' effect of the hydrochloric acid on pepsin granules (Babkin, 1950) may also, perhaps, result in an apparent total achylia, when some pepsinogen may still be produced and be excreted from the blood-stream in the urine. In pernicious anaemia the acid usually disappears from the gastric juice before the pepsin (Whitby and Britton, 1946).

From the results of the present study it may be concluded that the determination of the excretion of uropepsinogen is of value in the investigation of gastrointestinal disorders, and that further studies may add to the understanding of disordered alimentary function in peptic ulceration and the anaemias.

I wish to thank Professor D. H. Smyth, Professor E. J. Wayne, and Dr. H. Cohen for their criticism of the drafts of this report, and for many helpful suggestions. I am indebted to Dr. H. P. Brody for the facilities of his Unit, from which most of the patients were drawn, to Dr. K. H. Hardy for providing patients and facilities at Wharncliffe Hospital, and to Professor D. H. Smyth for the laboratory facilities at the Department of Physiology of Sheffield University. Dr. E. Blackburn kindly provided the plasma used in these studies. My thanks are also due to the students and nurses who volunteered for control studies, and to Sister Smith and Sister Brent for their care and co-operation in collecting specimens.

The studies were made during the author's tenure of a Clinical Research Fellowship of the United Sheffield Hospitals Endowment Fund.

Summary

With a substrate made from dehydrated human plasma, the excretion of uropepsinogen has been measured in normal subjects and in cases of duodenal ulcer, gastric ulcer, secondary dyspepsia, carcinoma of the stomach, partial and total gastrectomy, haematemesis, iron-deficiency anaemia, and pernicious anaemia.

The mean output of uropepsinogen in duodenal ulcer was almost double that found in normal subjects, and change in the state of the lesion, clinically assessed, was accompanied by a corresponding rise and fall of uropepsinogen excretion, with differences between the sexes in the degree of change.

The mean output in cases of gastric ulcer was within normal limits, when patients with an associated duodenal ulcer were excluded.

No uropepsinogen was excreted by patients who had had total gastrectomy, or by the majority of those who had had partial gastrectomy. Stomal ulcers existed in the two patients who showed a relatively high excretion.

In patients suffering from haematemesis of unknown origin, a high output of uropepsinogen showed a significant correlation with the subsequent disclosure of a duodenal ulcer.

In patients who suffered from dyspepsia not due to disease in the gastro-intestinal tract, with one exception, the excretion rate was normal.

In cases of iron-deficiency anaemia the excretion of uropepsinogen was always less than half the mean output of the controls, and in some cases was absent. A close correlation existed between the uropepsinogen output and the response of the parietal cells to a triple-dose histamine test.

The mean excretion of uropepsinogen in pernicious anaemia was extremely low, and more than half the patients produced no measurable quantity. One of the group excreting uropepsinogen also excreted a small amount of hydrochloric acid in response to a triple-dose histamine test.

Patients who had carcinoma of the stomach excreted less uropepsinogen than normal subjects, but the finding has no diagnostic value.

It is considered that the measurement of uropepsinogen is of value in clinical investigation, and as a research tool for further gastrointestinal studies.

REFERENCES

Anson, M. L., and Mirsky, A. E. (1932–3) *J. Gen. Physiol.* **16**, 59.
Babkin, B. P. (1950) *Secretory Mechanism of the Digestive Glands*, 2nd ed., New York.
Brücke, E. (1861) *Sitz.-Ber. Akad. Wiss. Wien*, **43**, 601.
Bucher, G. R. (1947) *Gastroenterology*, **8**, 627.
—— Grossman, M. I., and Ivy, A. C. (1945) Ibid. **5**, 501.
—— and Ivy, A. C. (1947) *Amer. J. Physiol.* **150**, 415.

Eastcott, H. H. G., Fawcett, J. K., and Rob, C. G. (1953) *Lancet,* **2,** 1068.
Farnsworth, E. B., Speer, E., and Alt, H. (1946) *J. Lab. Clin. Med.* **31,** 1025.
Frouin, A. (1904) *Compt. rend. Soc. biol. med.* **56,** 204.
Gottlieb, E. (1925) *Skand. Arch. Physiol.* **46,** 1.
Grossman, M. I., Greengard, H., Woolley, J. R., and Ivy, A. C. (1944) *Amer. J. Physiol.* **141,** 281.
Hirschowitz, B. I. (1953) *Lancet,* **2,** 66.
Hunt, J. N. (1948) *Biochem. J.* **42,** 104.
—— (1953) *Guy's Hosp. Rep.* **102,** 157.
—— and Spurrell, W. R. (1951) *J. Physiol.* **113,** 157.
Janowitz, H. D., and Hollander, F. (1950) *Federation Proc.* **9,** 67.
—— Levy, M. H., and Hollander, F. (1950) *Amer. J. Med. Sci.* **220,** 679.
Mirsky, I. A., Block, S., Osher, S., and Broh-Kahn, R. H. (1948) *J. Clin. Invest.* **27,** 818.
Perman, E. (1935) *Acta. chir. scand.* Suppl. **77,** 38.
Podore, C. J., Broh-Kahn, R. H. and Mirsky, I. A. (1948*a*) *Federation Proc.* **7,** 95.
—— —— —— (1948*b*) *J. Clin. Invest.* **27,** 834.
Shay, H., Gershon-Cohen, J., and Fels, S. S. (1942) *Amer. J. Digest. Dis.* **9,** 124.
Spiro, H. M., Reifenstein, R. W., and Gray, S. J. (1950) *J. Lab. Clin. Med.* **35,** 899.
Vanzant, F. R., Alvarez, W. C., Eusterman, G. B., Dunn, H. L., and Berkson, J. (1932) *Arch. Int. Med.* **49,** 345.
—— Osterberg, A. E., Alvarez, W. C., and Rivers, A. B. (1933) *J. Clin. Invest.* **12,** 557.
Watkinson, G. (1951) *Gastroenterology,* **18,** 377.
Whitby, L. E. H., and Britton, C. J. C. (1946) *Disorders of the Blood,* 5th ed., London.

616.34–008.337:547.475.2

ASCORBIC ACID REQUIREMENTS AND URINARY EXCRETION OF *p*-HYDROXYPHENYLACETIC ACID IN STEATORRHOEA AND MACROCYTIC ANAEMIA[1]

With a Description of the Paper-Chromatographic Technique for Identification of Hydroxyphenylic Acids

By R. J. BOSCOTT AND W. TREVOR COOKE

(From the Department of Anatomy, Birmingham University, and the Queen Elizabeth Hospital, Birmingham)

DURING an investigation of patients with steatorrhoea, it was found that the administration of ascorbic acid had to be continued for an unusually long time before significant amounts were excreted in the urine. Moreover, the total amounts administered were much greater than those usually considered adequate to saturate patients with long-standing scurvy. It was noticed, too, that none of the usually accepted symptoms or signs of clinical scurvy were present in these patients, an observation similar to those made by Foy and Kondi (1939) and by Alt, Chinn, and Farmer (1939) upon patients with macrocytic anaemia of nutritional origin. A second feature of our patients was the frequency of refractory or poorly responding macrocytic anaemia. Three typical case reports are appended (Cases 1, 2, and 3).

In considering whether these two observations are related, it will be recalled that May and his colleagues have demonstrated a relationship between megaloblastic anaemias and ascorbic-acid deficiency in monkeys (Salmon and May, 1953; May, Nelson, and Salmon, 1949; May, Hamilton, and Stewart, 1952). Nichol and Welch (1950) demonstrated that ascorbic acid is necessary in the transition of folic acid to folinic acid, while another common factor is that patients with either pernicious anaemia in relapse or scurvy excrete abnormal amounts of *p*-hydroxyphenyl compounds in the urine (Dobriner, Lavin, and Rhoads, 1942; Rogers and Gardner, 1949; Swendseid, Burton, and Bethell, 1943). The identification of the latter compounds has hitherto entailed tedious chemical analysis, but the development of a suitable technique by paper chromatography (Boscott, 1952 *a*, *b*, *c*) allowed the investigations of patients with steatorrhoea and macrocytic anaemia to be extended to study in detail the nature of the acidic *p*-hydroxyphenyl compounds present in their urine. The principal abnormal component thus detected in the phenolic acid fraction of acid-hydrolysed urines was *p*-hydroxyphenylacetic acid. The object of the present paper is to report the details of these investigations, and to discuss the

[1] Received October 20, 1953.

clinical and chemical significance of the coexistence of *p*-hydroxyphenylacetic acid and the abnormal requirements of ascorbic acid with the presence of a refractory macrocytic anaemia.

Methods

Twenty-four-hour collections of urine were made from normal subjects and in-patients; glacial acetic acid (5 ml.) and chloroform (5 ml.) were used as a preservative. The urine specimens were thereby maintained at pH 4 to 6, thus preventing oxidation of the polyphenolic compounds present. All drugs, and in particular phenolic and related compounds such as phenolphthalein, aspirin, and synthetic vitamin K (α-methylnaphthoquinone), were withheld from patients for at least 48 hours prior to the urine collection.

Urine hydrolysis and extraction. The specimens were subjected to hydrolysis with hydrochloric acid to liberate phenols and phenolic acids from their glucuronides, ethereal sulphates, and aceturic acids. An aliquot portion of urine, equivalent to a 6- or 12-hour output, was hydrolysed by boiling under a reflux condenser for 30 minutes after the addition of 15 volumes per cent. concentrated HCl (A.R.). Two hundred ml. of benzene were added from the beginning to effect some extraction of the organic compounds, and to minimize destruction of the more acid-labile compounds released during the hydrolysis. One-fiftieth of the 24-hour specimen of urine was adequate if only the strongly acidic fraction was sought, the other reagents being scaled down accordingly. The benzene layer was separated, and the remaining hydrolysed urine was saturated with NaCl and again extracted four times with one-quarter its volume of ether.

The combined benzene and ether extracts were extracted four times with one-quarter their volume of saturated $NaHCO_3$ solution, to which 0·5 per cent. $Na_2S_2O_5$ had been added to prevent oxidation of polyphenolic compounds, for example pyrocatechol. The combined alkaline extracts were extracted with $\frac{1}{20}$ volume of ether, which was rejected, then carefully acidified with concentrated HCl to pH 3 to 4, after saturation with NaCl and the addition of a shallow layer of ether to control the foaming. This procedure also prevented the adherence of the liberated gummy phenolic acids to the glass. The organic acids were extracted three times with one-quarter volume of ether. The combined ether extracts of the separated organic acids were then washed twice with $\frac{1}{20}$ volume of saturated NaCl solution, before the removal of the ether by distillation. The residue (Fraction 1; Boscott, 1952 *a*, *b*, *c*) was dissolved in sufficient 95 per cent. ethanol to make the volume up to 5 ml. Aliquots equivalent to $\frac{1}{2000}$ and $\frac{1}{200}$ part of a 24-hour specimen of urine were analysed by two-way chromatography as previously reported (Boscott, 1952 *a*, *b*, *c*).

Chromatography. The method used is a combination of the partition method for phenolic acids developed by Bray, Thorpe, and White (1950) with the electrolyte-solution method of Boscott (1952 *a*, *b*, *c*) and the capillary-ascent technique of Williams and Kirby (1948). Whatman paper no. 542 has been found the most satisfactory paper for the methods employed. The ethanol solution of organic acids was applied near to the corner of a sheet of paper (16 in. × 10·5 in.) by means of a fine-pointed capillary tube. A stream of air at room temperature was blown on the under side of the paper to aid in the evaporation of the alcohol, so that the diameter of the resultant spot was restricted to 0·4 in. The paper, stapled to form a rigid cylinder, was equilibrated for at least 12 hours with the more aqueous (lower) phase of the solvent system, consisting of benzene two volumes, glacial acetic acid two volumes, and water one volume. Development with the benzene-rich (upper) phase by the capillary-ascent technique took from 10 to 12 hours (10·5 in.). Water-repellent compounds present in the extract have Rf. values approaching 1·0, and therefore do not interfere with development by the aqueous solvent system used subsequently. The paper was dried in a fume-cupboard at room temperature, restapled, and further developed in the direction at right angles to the previous one, with 20 per cent. w/v aqueous KCl solution at 34° C., in a thermostatically controlled water-jacketed oven. The ascent (16 in.) of the electrolyte took from 10 to 12 hours. The paper was dried either at room temperature or in a current of warm air.

Detection of the spots. Tests 1 to 4, when applied consecutively, allowed the detection of most of the components present by the use of only one chromatogram.

Test 1. Fluorescence of the chromatogram at neutral pH in the ultraviolet light (Wood's glass filter). Fluorescent zones were outlined with pencil. The fluorescent acids thus detected have not yet been identified.

Test 2. Micro-droplets of 90 per cent. v/v H_2SO_4 were applied to the chromatogram at intervals of $\frac{3}{4}$ in. by means of a fine-pointed capillary tube. Changes in previous fluorescent zones and the formation of new fluorescence were noted. Indole-acetic acid gave a green fluorescence with this test.

Test 3. The papers were then sprayed with 10 per cent. Na_2CO_3 solution and dried at room temperature. Colour and fluorescent changes were noted. The indole-acetic acid zone gave a magenta colour in the area treated previously with 90 per cent. H_2SO_4. Homogentisic acid, when present, gave a brown colour, due to oxidation at alkaline pH. Several unidentified acidic compounds not detected by Test 1 were then revealed as fluorescent zones. Only some of the compounds detected previously by fluorescence fluoresced differently with the alkali, thereby facilitating the detection of a number of compounds which overlapped partially. The two substances, *m*- and *p*-hydroxybenzoic acid, which were situated close together, were differentiated by Test 3, only the former acid fluorescing violet with the alkali.

Test 4. The papers were finally sprayed with a mixture of nine volumes of 10 per cent. w/v Na_2CO_3 solution and one volume of diazotized 'I.C.I. 5091' (diethylaminoethyl-*p*-aminophenylsulphone), prepared by mixing equal volumes of ice-cold 10 per cent. w/v 'I.C.I. 5091', 10 per cent. v/v concentrated HCl, and 5 per cent. w/v $NaNO_2$. This reagent coupled with all the phenolic acids present to produce coloured azo compounds. If Test 3 were omitted, unidentified compounds giving pink and yellow colours with 10 per cent. w/v Na_2CO_3 alone

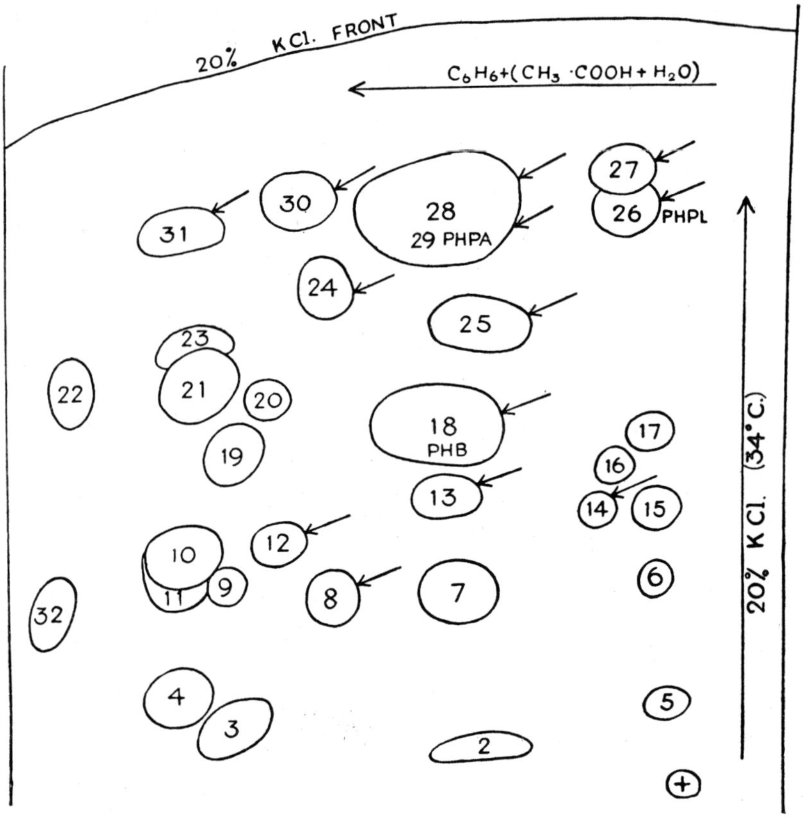

FIG. 1. Two-way chromatogram of the strongly acidic phenolic fraction of urine. Compounds indicated with arrows are found in the urine from a rat receiving a synthetic diet devoid of phenolic compounds other than tyrosine.

TABLE OF CHROMATOGRAM COMPONENTS

Component	*Colour of dye*	*Identity, where known*	*Component*	*Colour of dye*	*Identity, where known*
1	..	Origin	17	Yellow	..
2	Orange	..	18	Orange	*p*-hydroxybenzoic acid
3	Red	..	19	Orange	..
4	Mauve	Ferulic acid	20	Pink	..
5	Yellow	..	21	Red	..
6	Yellow	..	22	Orange	..
7	Orange	..	23	Violet	..
8	Orange-pink	..	24	Orange	..
9	Magenta	Syringic acid	25	Orange-yellow	..
10	Red	Vanillic acid	26	Red	*p*-hydroxyphenyllactic acid
11	Violet	..	27	Orange	*m*-hydroxyphenyllactic acid
12	Pink	..	28	Orange	*m*-hydroxyphenylacetic acid
13	Mauve	..	29	Red	*p*-hydroxyphenylacetic acid
14	Pink	..	30	Orange-pink (weak)	*o*-hydroxyphenylacetic acid
15	Orange-yellow	..	31	Violet	..
16	Orange-yellow	..	32	Red	..

would be indicated erroneously as coloured azo compounds. The absorption spectra of several of the azo compounds from phenolic acids have been described (Boscott, 1950–1). Other diazonium reagents tested did not produce a range of coloured compounds that could be so readily differentiated visually as those obtained with the reagent described, although some were undoubtedly more sensitive. Diazotized sulphanilic acid and *p,p'*-diaminodiphenylsulphone gave a moderately good differentiation, but the detection with these reagents of *p*-hydroxyphenylacetic acid located in the *m*-hydroxyphenylacetic acid zone was then not possible. A typical chromatogram is illustrated diagrammatically in Fig. 1, and a list of the components detected by Test 4 is given in the Table.

Ascorbic-acid estimation in human urine specimens. Urine was collected over metaphosphoric acid, of which the amount varied according to the period over which the urine was collected, either two-hourly for three collections or during 24 hours. The specimens were diluted after collection to ensure a constant concentration of metaphosphoric acid. Ascorbic acid was estimated by a modification of the dichlorophenolindophenol method (Hawk, Oser, and Summerson, 1947).

Results

1. *Ascorbic-acid saturation tests.* Six healthy normal subjects, on a daily dosage of 600 mg. ascorbic acid, excreted one-third of the test dose (600 mg.) in the first six hours after three to seven days' treatment. In six patients with steatorrhoea and megaloblastic anaemia, doses totalling 13·5 to 20 gm. were administered over periods varying from 23 to 40 days before significant amounts were excreted in the urine. The maximum that was excreted in any one patient was 176 mg. in the six hours following the administration of the test dose, after 40 days of therapy. The administration of large amounts of ascorbic acid intramuscularly in Cases 1, 2, and 3 did not result in any more rapid saturation.

2. *Chromatography.* The Table below Fig. 1 gives a description of the ether-soluble phenolic acids which we have encountered in human urine. Dietary experiments on animals (Boscott and Greenberg, 1953) and on human beings (Boscott and Bickel, 1953) suggest that many of these substances are derived from benzenoid compounds other than the phenylalanine, tyrosine, and tryphophane present in food. Of the remaining substances detected, only compounds 18, 26, and 29 are known to be tyrosine metabolites. *m*-hydroxyphenylacetic acid (28) and *o*-hydroxyphenylacetic acid (30) are believed to be derived from phenylalanine (Boscott and Bickel, 1953). Aterman, Boscott, and Cooke (1953) have demonstrated that *p*-hydroxyphenylacetic acid (PHPA) and *p*-hydroxyphenyllactic acid (PHPL) are the usual abnormal components of the strongly acidic phenolic fraction of the urine from scorbutic guinea-pigs, and that they are no longer excreted in the urine of these animals after the administration of ascorbic acid for several days. In the present studies employing chromatography, as opposed to previous experiments on tyrosyluria, test doses of tyrosine were not necessary; but it was found advisable to use acid-hydrolysed rather than non-hydrolysed urine for the preparation of the extracts,

since some of the phenolic acids were present in a conjugated form, and therefore less readily extractable by ether.

Only four of 25 normal subjects examined excreted significant amounts of PHPA in the urine. If three or four daily supplements of 100 mg. of ascorbic acid were administered, PHPA was no longer excreted; the excretion of the other phenolic acids was not altered. PHPA (compound 29) was detected as a

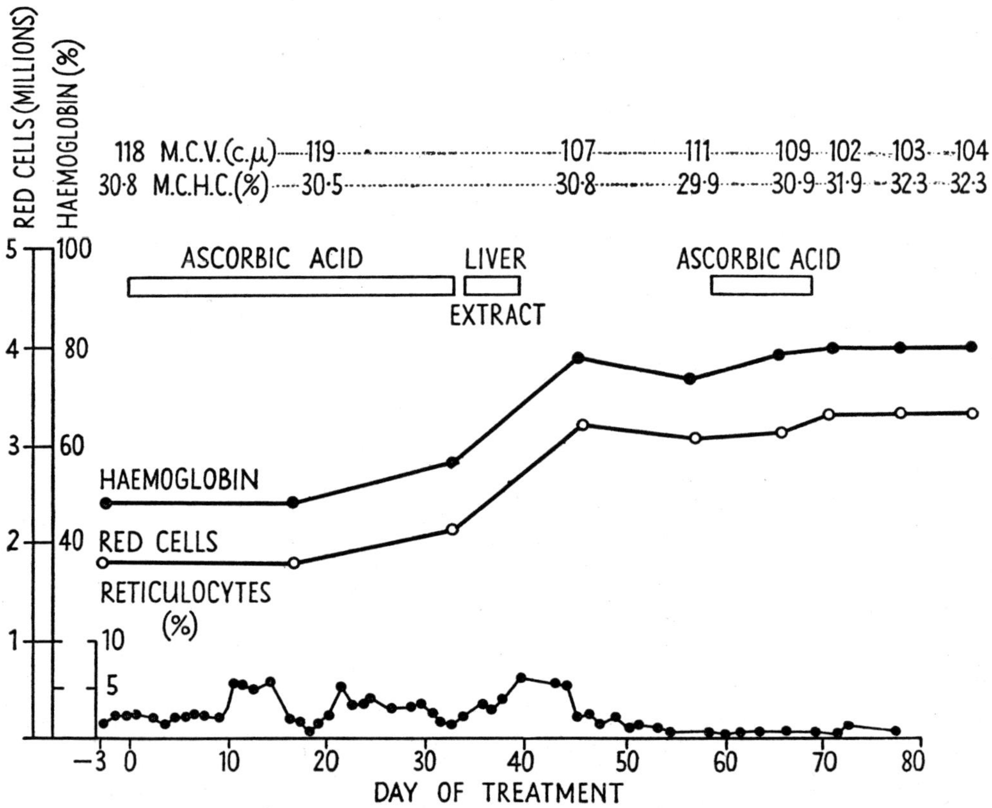

FIG. 2. Case 1. Haematological response to ascorbic acid administration in a 58-year-old man with idiopathic steatorrhoea and megaloblastic anaemia. Crude liver extract was given in error; a response occurred and megaloblasts disappeared from the bone-marrow. No further response was obtained with ascorbic acid subsequently.

M.C.V. = mean corpuscular volume.
M.C.H.C. = mean corpuscular haemoglobin concentration.

red-dye derivative, located in the same position as an orange dye (compound 28) which was found to be formed much more rapidly than the red PHPA dye, when the chromatogram was sprayed with diazotized 'I.C.I. 5091'. The urine specimens from 20 patients with both steatorrhoea and macrocytic anaemia usually contained amounts of PHPA adequate to obliterate completely the orange dye with an intense red one. The response of these patients to ascorbic acid therapy, as judged by the disappearance of this red dye, was very much slower than that seen in the few normal subjects excreting PHPA; thus greatly increased doses of ascorbic acid and longer periods of treatment were required before PHPA excretion was significantly reduced. Five patients with megaloblastic anaemia of pregnancy excreted PHPA in amounts comparable to those found in patients with idiopathic steatorrhoea. On the other hand, in five patients with pernicious anaemia, PHPA was present in small amounts only, and disappeared during specific treatment. In neither of these two groups of patients was the response to ascorbic acid saturation determined. Most of the

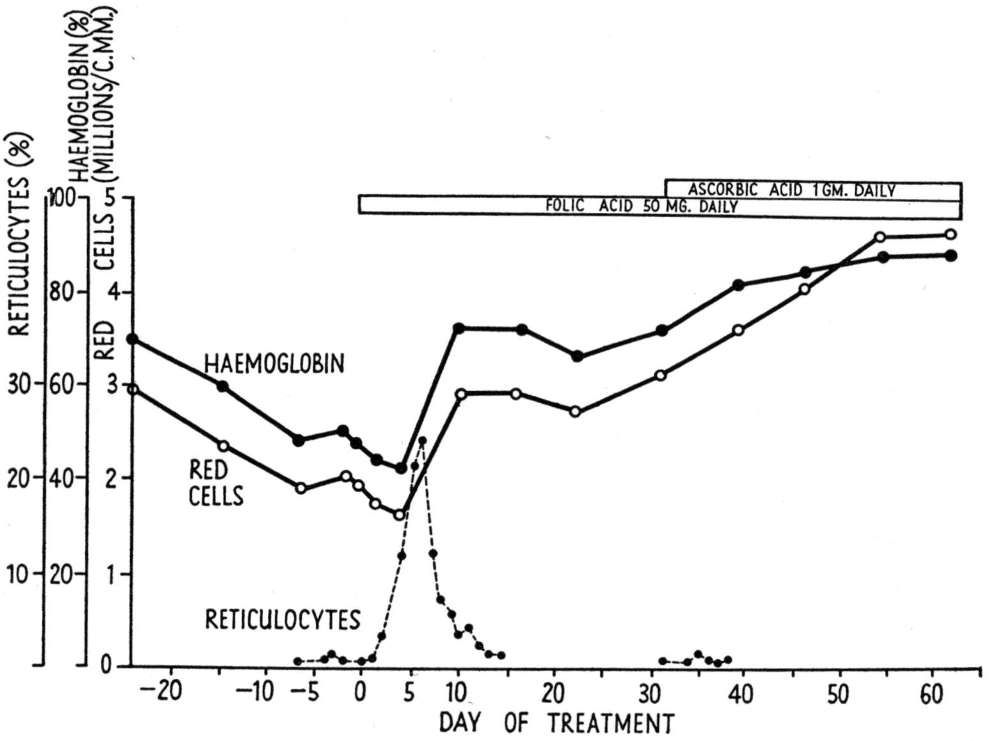

FIG. 3. Case 4. Haematological response to folic acid and ascorbic acid in a 38-year-old woman with idiopathic steatorrhoea and a megaloblastic anaemia. *p*-hydroxyphenylacetic acid was strongly present in the urine prior to the administration of ascorbic acid. Only traces remained 30 days later.

patients with liver disease (16 out of 18), rheumatoid arthritis (five out of six), and thyrotoxicosis (five patients), also excreted PHPA in the urine, but, like the normal subjects, did not do so after the administration of a relatively small amount of ascorbic acid, such as 100 mg. daily for three to four days. In the patients with steatorrhoea PHPA excretion was unaffected by the administration of cortisone, ACTH, vitamin B_{12}, or folic acid. One patient with idiopathic steatorrhoea excreted much less PHPA after the administration of methionine. Only rarely has the presence of PHPL been encountered in our patients, and on these occasions PHPA was present in comparatively large amounts. Among other compounds, indole-acetic acid was detectable by Tests 2 and 3 in the urine of the patients with steatorrhoea. A full report on the 50 components detected in the strongly acidic fraction of acid-hydrolysed urines will be given elsewhere.

3. *The effect of ascorbic-acid administration upon the blood picture.* The observations in Case 1 provided the stimulus for the present investigation. Though this patient appeared initially to be suffering from scurvy, subsequent observations showed that only slight haematological response was obtained with ascorbic acid, and with the continuing purpuric lesions the initial diagnosis could not be sustained. The haematological findings are depicted in Fig. 2. At this

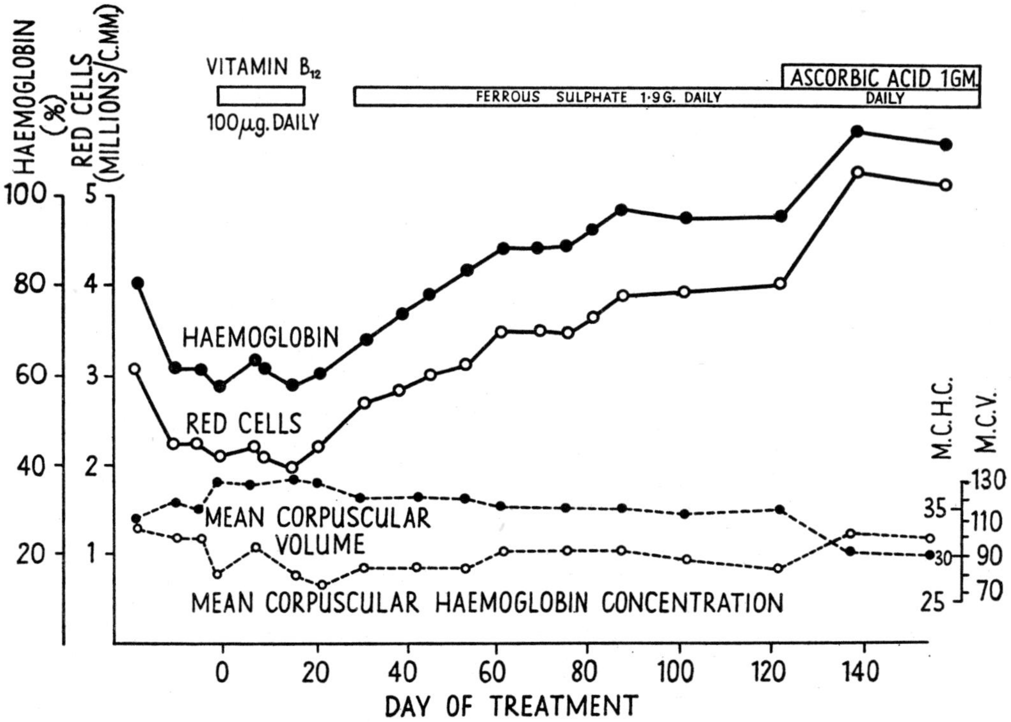

FIG. 4. Case 5. Haematological response to vitamin B_{12}, ferrous sulphate, and ascorbic acid in a 47-year-old woman with jejuno-ileitis and a megaloblastic anaemia. *p*-hydroxyphenylacetic acid was strongly present in the urine until the administration of ascorbic acid. After this it gradually disappeared; at the same time the blood picture showed a significant change.

stage the possibility that ascorbic acid might have to be given in association with folic acid, vitamin B_{12}, or iron, had not been realized. In our later observations this treatment was given, and Figs. 3 and 4 show the haematological details of two such patients (Cases 4 and 5). In both instances PHPA, which was excreted in the urine in large amounts prior to the administration of ascorbic acid, gradually disappeared after a long period of its administration. Case histories of these two patients are given in the Appendix.

Discussion

The finding of *p*-hydroxyphenylacetic acid (PHPA) in certain samples of urine recalled the incidental observations of Dobriner, Lavin, and Rhoads (1942) that this compound was spectroscopically detectable in the urine of patients suffering with pernicious anaemia or refractory macrocytic anaemia.

It has long been known that certain other hydroxyphenyl compounds are found in urine when tyrosine metabolism is disturbed. Thus *p*-hydroxyphenylpyruvic acid (PHPP) and *p*-hydroxyphenyllactic acid occurred in the urine of scorbutic patients, and of guinea-pigs to whom test doses of tyrosine had been administered. Levine, Dann, and Marples (1943) had shown that premature infants who were fed with cow's-milk mixtures free of vitamin C and rich in protein, or to whom a large dose of tyrosine had been given, also excreted *p*-hydroxyphenyllactic acid in the urine. These errors in tyrosine metabolism were rectified by the administration of ascorbic acid. *p*-hydroxyphenylacetic acid has not, however, been previously demonstrated in association with ascorbic-acid unsaturation in man. Its association with ascorbic acid deficiency has been adequately confirmed by its demonstration in the urine of guinea-pigs before they had become fully scorbutic, and by its production from *p*-hydroxyphenylpyruvic acid in the absence of ascorbic acid (Sealock and Goodland, 1951; Le May-Knox and Knox, 1951; Boscott and Aterman, 1953). It seems unlikely that the finding of PHPA in the urine of our patients was an artefact arising from the *in vitro* oxidation of *p*-hydroxypyruvic acid (PHPP), although such a possibility exists, since we were able to demonstrate the presence of PHPA in an old commercial sample of PHPP. The principal reason for this conclusion lay in the similar high ratios of PHPA to *p*-hydroxyphenylbenzoic acid in the hydrolysed and non-hydrolysed urines of scorbutic guinea-pigs. The presence of *p*-hydroxyphenylacetic acid in human urine may therefore be a sensitive indication that more ascorbic acid is required than that being consumed in the diet.

The metabolism of tyrosine has been well reviewed by Lerner (1953) and Berg (1953). Consideration of the possible metabolic pathways for the production of PHPA from tyrosine might indicate points of clinical significance. Two possible metabolic pathways (*A* and *B*) are indicated in Fig. 5. If route *A* is blocked at the transamination stage, a defect in the production or utilization of either pyridoxal phosphate (O'Kane and Gunsalus, 1947) or α-ketoglutarate might be present. Pyridoxic acid, an oxidation product of pyridoxine, is required as an activator of folic acid conjugase (Scott, Hill, and Norris, 1949). This enzyme exists in the blood-stream of various species of animals, including man, and is capable of splitting the conjugates of folic acid to yield free folic acid (Simpson and Schweigert, 1949) and glutamic acid or its peptides. It is of interest, too, that glutamic acid is oxidized to α-ketoglutaric acid. Of the two alternative pathways (*A* and *B*), however, route *B* may be the more probable, since the occurrence of PHPL in these samples of urine would require an additional block in the conversion of PHPP to PHPL. In favour of route *B*, Roka (1952) has demonstrated that kidney tissue, in contrast to liver tissue, converts tyrosine into PHPA, and Ewins and Laidlaw (1910–11) have shown that the administration of tyramine to dogs leads to the excretion of PHPA as the chief recognizable metabolite in the urine.[2]

[2] Boscott (1954, unpublished work) has detected chromatographically *p*-hydroxybenzal-hydantoin, an artefact derived from urinary *p*-hydroxyphenylpyruvic acid and urea by

Even if the biochemical relationship between tyrosine, *p*-hydroxyphenylacetic acid, and ascorbic-acid inadequacy may be demonstrated, it still remains to consider how this deficiency may come about in patients whose diet contains normal quantities of ascorbic acid. Observations that patients with both megaloblastic anaemia and steatorrhoea required large amounts of ascorbic acid before significant amounts of this vitamin were excreted in the urine, were

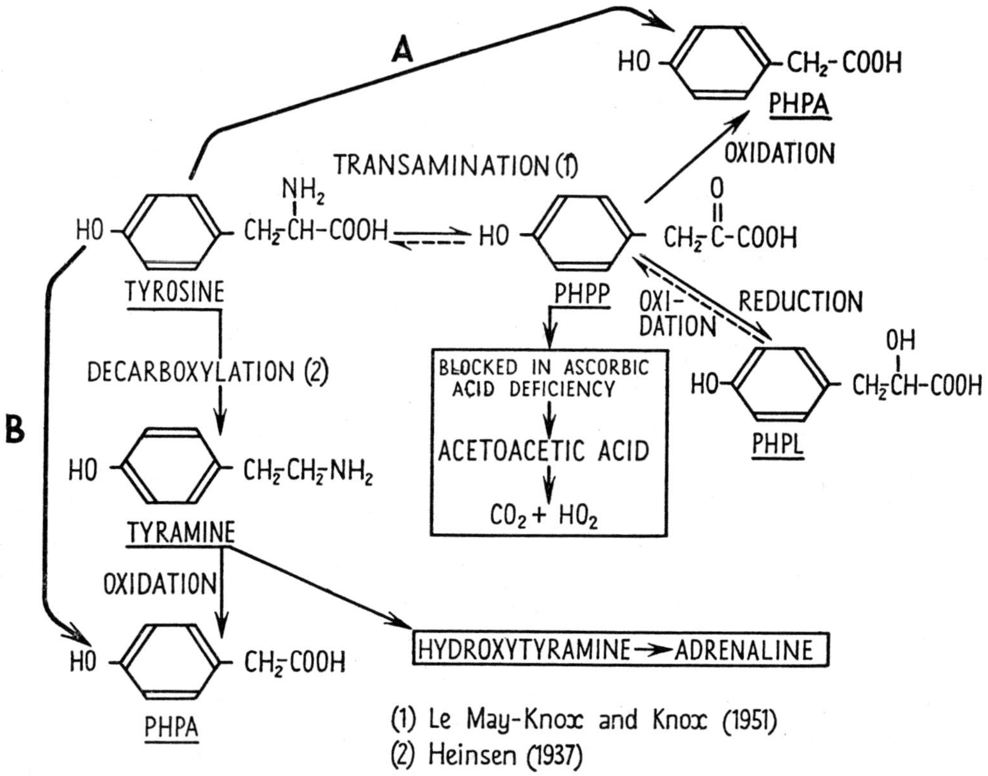

FIG. 5. Schematic representation of two possible metabolic pathways for the conversion of tyrosine to *p*-hydroxyphenylacetic acid.

paralleled by the protracted excretion of PHPA. Both normal subjects and patients with liver disease, rheumatoid arthritis, or thyrotoxicosis who excreted PHPA in their urine promptly responded to ascorbic-acid therapy, and the excretion of *p*-hydroxyphenylacetic acid was rapidly reduced to zero. In the patients who had steatorrhoea the slow reduction of PHPA in the urine after ascorbic-acid therapy may indicate an abnormal utilization or requirement of this vitamin. None of the latter patients showed clinical signs of scurvy, but

a condensation reaction, in acid-hydrolysed urines from subjects depleted of ascorbic acid. This artefact was found to be present in abnormal amounts in the acid-hydrolysed urines from untreated patients with refractory megaloblastic anaemia. Therefore metabolic pathway *A* does take place, at least to some extent, but without significant conversion of *p*-hydroxyphenylpyruvic acid to *p*-hydroxyphenyllactic acid by reduction. The latter observation may possibly be paralleled by an increased oxidation of ascorbic acid by the tissues of patients with refractory megaloblastic anaemia.

those that were studied required 13 to 20 gm. of ascorbic acid to reach saturation, whereas the scorbutic subject is reported to require only 6 gm. (Lowry, 1952). All aspects of vitamin-C metabolism therefore cannot be implicated, and, since the patients did not respond normally to injected ascorbic acid, the results were not likely to be due entirely to impaired absorption of the vitamin, as was suggested by both Borne (1939) and Mohr (1939). These workers also commented upon the difficulty in obtaining evidence of ascorbic-acid saturation in patients with steatorrhoea.

In 1947 Cartwright found it impossible to express any definite opinion as to the need for ascorbic acid in haematopoiesis, but since then the intimate role of ascorbic acid in the prevention of certain experimental megaloblastic anaemias, and in the adequate utilization of folic acid, has been conclusively demonstrated. Thus May, Nelson, and Salmon (1949) were unable to produce megaloblastic anaemia in monkeys who were fed on a diet poor in folic acid, unless a chronic deficiency of ascorbic acid was present. Nichol and Welch (1950) demonstrated that the conversion of folic acid to folinic acid was catalysed by ascorbic acid, even though the intermediate stages were not clear. May, Hamilton, and Stewart (1952) have shown that megaloblastosis in the marrow did not develop in the scorbutic monkey unless the level of free folinic acid in the liver was low. Treatment with either folinic acid or ascorbic acid restored the marrow to normal, and caused the accumulation of folinic acid in the liver. Holly (1951) has claimed that the administration of vitamin B_{12} plus ascorbic acid is effective in the megaloblastic anaemias of pregnancy, which are refractory to vitamin B_{12} alone.

The part played by folic acid in the metabolism of tyrosine is by no means clear. Woodruff and Darby (1948) found that folic acid was able to replace the function of vitamin C in the metabolism of *p*-hydroxyphenyl derivatives in scorbutic guinea-pigs. Rodney, Swendseid, and Swanson (1949) also found that tyrosine metabolism was deranged in the absence of folic acid, and that normal oxidation was restored by folic acid. Extremely large doses of folic acid (90 mg. daily) were required in infants to prevent the hydroxyphenyluria resulting from adding tyrosine to the diet (Morris, Harpur, and Goldbloom, 1950). Against these observations, Govan and Gordon (1949) found little change in the excretion of these derivatives in the urine of premature infants given folic acid. Boscott and Aterman (1953) could not detect any change in the excretion of either PHPA or PHPL in the urine of scorbutic guinea-pigs when treated with folic acid, but did find some diminution of these compounds when the animals were treated with a high dosage of folinic acid administered orally. Our patients with steatorrhoea continued to excrete PHPA when given folic acid 50 mg. daily, while our patients with pernicious anaemia excreted little or none. Girdwood (1953) has reported that the absorption of folic acid is impaired in idiopathic steatorrhoea. It might be argued that the finding of *p*-hydroxyphenylacetic acid in the urine of our patients was due merely to a deficiency of folic acid; but both our experimental findings and the clinical findings in our patients are against such an interpretation. To sum up, there appears to be evidence of a defect in tyrosine metabolism which is less rapidly rectified by ascorbic-acid therapy in patients with steatorrhoea than in other subjects. It does not appear to be due to an absorption defect or to a primary dietary deficiency, but any conclusions further than this must be speculative.

While this paper has been concerned with the presence of *p*-hydroxyphenylacetic acid in the urine, other phenolic acids and polyphenols, such as pyrocatechol, were also encountered in abnormal quantities in the urine. Any of these substances might well have acted as a 'toxic metabolite' needing excess of ascorbic acid for its detoxication, and in this way making less available for synergism with folic and folinic acid in blood formation. While this explanation might account for the relative lack of ascorbic acid, there still remains no explanation for the increased excretion of phenolic acids. It can only be conjectured that this increase in its turn may depend upon the katabolism of unusual compounds absorbed from the deranged intestine of a patient with steatorrhoea. Our own observations on patients with this syndrome suggest that neither folic acid, vitamin B_{12}, nor ascorbic acid, when administered alone, can be guaranteed to restore the blood picture to normal, but that intensive ascorbic-acid therapy appears to synergize the effects of folic acid and vitamin B_{12} in some patients with megaloblastic anaemia as, for example, in the two cases described. For the present we consider that the refractory macrocytic anaemia, the abnormal ascorbic-acid utilization, and the disturbed tyrosine metabolism in these patients are manifestations of a common underlying metabolic error. Further controlled dietary experiments, and subsequent examinations of the urine with the techniques described in this paper, may provide more clues as to the fundamental defects both of the macrocytic anaemias and of the steatorrhoea syndrome.

APPENDIX

Case Reports

Case 1 (Fig. 2). J. D., a bachelor aged 58 years, had been forced to give up work owing to increasing exertional dyspnoea and angina cruris, and for four months prior to admission had been living in a working hostel on unemployment pay, often drinking five to six pints of beer each night and smoking 15 cigarettes daily. He had lost three stone in weight since stopping work, and had developed swelling of the ankles during the previous six weeks. On examination he had mild peripheral glossitis, angular stomatitis, a purpuric rash on the arms and legs, and minimal pitting oedema of the ankles. The peripheral arteries were sclerotic, and the blood-pressure 180/110. Laboratory examinations showed: red blood-cells 1,810,000 per c.mm., haemoglobin 6·6 gm. per 100 ml., white cells 3,850 per c.mm., and a normal differential count; cell volume 21 per cent.; mean corpuscular volume 117·2 c.μ; mean corpuscular haemoglobin concentration 31·4 per cent.; platelets 117,000 per c.mm.; bleeding time $2\frac{1}{2}$ minutes; complete clotting time 12 minutes. Sternal puncture showed the presence of megaloblasts, and the fractional test meal showed the presence of free HCl. Other values were: serum-proteins, albumin 3·9 gm., and globulin 1·7 gm. per 100 ml.; total serum-cholesterol 172 mg. per 100 ml.;

serum-iron 170 mg. per 100 ml. The van den Bergh test was negative. The glucose-tolerance test showed a maximum rise of 25 mg. per 100 ml. A barium meal excluded a gastric neoplasm, but showed a deficiency pattern of the small intestine.

A provisional diagnosis of malnutrition was made, and the possibility of scurvy seriously entertained. His subsequent course and the persistence of purpura eventually excluded the latter diagnosis. The occurrence of an attack of diarrhoea with pale stools for 24 hours led to the examination of the stools. Repeated fat balances revealed absorption varying between 55 and 75 per cent. The administration of ascorbic acid had no significant effect upon the red cells and haemoglobin. Its excretion was estimated after the administration of 600 mg. ascorbic acid by mouth, and after 4·6 gm. had been administered during 10 days. Only 12 mg. were excreted in the first six hours after ingestion of the test dose. After a further 10 days, in which 7·2 gm. were administered, the six-hour excretion was still only 37 mg. Five hundred mg. of ascorbic acid were then administered intramuscularly daily for 12 days. At the end of this time 300 mg. were administered intravenously. In the three hours before injection 9 mg. were excreted, and the same amount was excreted in the three hours after injection. Ascorbic-acid administration was then stopped for 16 days. At the end of this time the plasma ascorbic acid was 0·44 mg. per 100 ml., and the 24-hour output of ascorbic acid was 2·3 mg. Ascorbic acid was again administered, 300 mg. four times a day for 10 days. An excretion test following the administration of 600 mg. orally and 300 mg. intravenously resulted in the excretion of 176 mg. in the first six hours.

Case 2. H. B., a bachelor aged 49 years, was admitted on account of swelling of the ankles and a severe purpuric rash, of 12 months' duration and sufficiently severe to be completely disabling. Ten years previously he had had a similar illness, during which he had lost two stone in weight, and which had lasted two years. Though a single man and living in a hostel, he appeared to have taken an adequate diet. On examination his nutrition was fair, with no evidence of recent loss of weight. There was no glossitis. There was an extensive purpuric rash below the knees and on the left wrist, and oedema of both ankles. No abnormality was found in the heart, lungs, or abdomen. The blood-pressure was 130/85. Laboratory examinations showed: red blood-cells 3,840,000 per c.mm., haemoglobin 12·4 gm. per 100 ml., white cells 8,200 per c.mm., with a normal differential count; mean corpuscular volume 94·5 c.μ.; mean corpuscular haemoglobin concentration 37·1 per cent.; platelets 310,000 per c.mm.; bleeding time 2 minutes; initial clotting 9½ minutes, and complete clotting 19 minutes. Clot retraction was normal, and prothrombin time 85 per cent. of normal. Serum-albumin was 3·6 gm., and globulin 3·7 gm. per 100 ml.; total serum-cholesterol 160 mg. per 100 ml.; plasma-fibrinogen 267 mg. per 100 ml., and plasma ascorbic acid 1·0 mg. per 100 ml. Hess's test was negative. Fat-absorption, on repeated tests, varied between 65 and 75 per cent. X-ray of the small intestine showed a deficiency pattern. Free HCl was shown to be present by the test meal.

An initial ascorbic-acid saturation test, following an oral dose of 600 mg., showed 7 mg. excreted in the first six hours. After daily administration of 600 mg. for 10 days and daily estimation of ascorbic-acid excretion, the amount in the first six hours had slowly risen to 30 mg. This response was not increased by the administration of 300 mg. intramuscularly on alternate days and 300 mg. intravenously on the other days for six days, the amounts remaining at the same level, 28 mg., 27 mg., and 31 mg. A dosage of 600 mg. was continued by mouth, and in one final excretion test, performed 23 days after the onset of therapy, that is after the administration of 13·8 gm. of ascorbic acid, 150 mg. were excreted in the first six hours. His attacks of purpura and gravitational oedema continued.

Case 3. M. W., a married woman aged 46 years, was admitted on account of lack of energy and febrile attacks, associated with a haemorrhagic rash and swelling of the legs, during the previous three years. The attacks consisted of periodic bouts of loss of energy and appetite, lasting about one month every two or three months. For one week during the attack a bright red rash affected the legs, trunk, and arms, together with swelling of the wrist and ankle joints. The attacks were also associated with glossitis and ulcers in the mouth, and with a high temperature, with much sweating. She denied any intestinal upset. She had had four children. Though she stated that she had been anaemic most of her life, she gave no history of any serious illness. On examination there were several fading purpuric spots on the lower abdomen, a mottled red and purple rash on the anterior aspect of the right leg, and considerable pitting oedema extending up to the knee. The left leg showed only fading spots, and no oedema. Examination of the heart, lungs, abdomen, and central nervous system gave normal results. The blood-pressure was 105/70. Laboratory examinations showed: red blood-cells 2,580,000 per c.mm., haemoglobin 8·6 gm. per 100 ml., white cells 3,000 per c.mm., with a normal differential count; mean corpuscular volume 128·3 c.μ.; mean corpuscular haemoglobin concentration 25·9 per cent.; platelets 417,00 per c.mm. Sternal puncture showed occasional megaloblasts, but principally large atypical normoblasts. Bleeding time was 3 minutes; initial clotting time 10 minutes, complete clotting time 16 minutes, and prothrombin time normal. Serum-albumin was 3·1 gm. and globulin 3·7 gm. per 100 ml. Total serum-cholesterol was 283 mg. per 100 ml. The van den Bergh test was negative. Plasma ascorbic acid was 0·57 mg. per 100 ml. Fat-absorption varied between 54 and 73 per cent. Radiology of the small intestine showed a deficiency pattern. Free HCl was shown to be present by the fractional test meal. An ascorbic-acid excretion test showed 15 mg. in the first six hours. After administration of 6 gm. in 10 days this amount had risen to 20 mg. After a further 4 gm. in six days, and a test dose of 600 mg. by mouth and 300 mg. intravenously, only 40 mg. were excreted in six hours. After a further 6 gm. given orally in 10 days, the test result after 600 mg. by mouth and 300 mg. intravenously had risen to 94 gm.

Case 4 (Fig. 3). M. Y., a married woman aged 38 years, the daughter and cousin of patients suffering with idiopathic steatorrhoea, had had episodic diarrhoea and ill health for some years. After a severe attack of influenza six months prior to admission, she had lost weight and become severely anaemic. On admission her blood count showed 1,650,000 red cells per c.mm., and haemoglobin 42 per cent., with mean corpuscular volume 109·0 c.μ., and mean corpuscular haemoglobin concentration 32·2 per cent. Sternal puncture showed megaloblasts, a fractional test meal histamine-fast achlorhydria, and a fat balance 86 per cent. absorption. The response to therapy, which paralleled the improvement in her weight and clinical condition, is shown in Fig. 3. Prior to the administration of ascorbic acid the urine contained large amounts of *p*-hydroxyphenylacetic acid. After the administration of ascorbic acid, 1 gm. daily for 14 days, a saturation test after 600 mg. had been taken by mouth showed that only 37 mg. were excreted in the first six hours. At this stage only a trace of PHPA was present in the urine.

Case 5 (Fig. 4). B. W., a married woman aged 47 years, had been seen two years previously on account of extensive cicatrizing jejuno-ileitis. She was admitted in severe relapse, having lost three stone in weight and become grossly dehydrated and hypokalaemic. After rehydration and restoration of electrolyte equilibrium, her blood count fell to 2,320,000 red cells per c.mm. and 62 per cent. haemoglobin, with mean corpuscular volume 117·4 c.μ. Gross steatorrhoea was present. Sternal puncture revealed large numbers of megaloblasts. She was placed upon a high-protein, low-fat diet for the period of study depicted in Fig. 4. PHPA was present in large amounts until the administration of ascorbic acid, when it gradually disappeared. At the time of her discharge from hospital she was ambulant, and her general condition was relatively satisfactory. Subsequently she has maintained her condition, the most recent blood count, six months after her discharge, showing 4,800,000 red cells per c.mm. and 106 per cent. haemoglobin, with mean corpuscular volume 95·6 c.μ.

Acknowledgements

We are greatly indebted to Miss M. A. Cooke for technical assistance in the chromatographic investigations. We wish also to thank Mr. Garfield Thomas, Biochemist, and Dr. F. Neale, Assistant Biochemist, Queen Elizabeth Hospital, for the ascorbic-acid determinations, and Dr. A. L. P. Peeney, Director of Clinical Pathology, Birmingham United Hospitals, for the haematological investigations.

Summary

1. Chromatographic methods for the study of p-hydroxyphenyl compounds in the urine are described.

2. The occurrence of p-hydroxyphenylacetic acid in specimens of human urine is reported, with particular reference to patients with steatorrhoea.

3. The difficulty in 'saturating' with ascorbic acid patients who have steatorrhoea and macrocytic anaemia is reported. This defect was not due to a primary dietary deficiency or to difficulty in absorption.

4. The presence of p-hydroxyphenylacetic acid in the urine was found to be the result of deranged tyrosine metabolism and ascorbic-acid inadequacy, and should be regarded as a sensitive indication of the need for more ascorbic acid than is present in the diet.

5. Haematological responses to ascorbic-acid administration are reported in three patients, and the relationship of ascorbic acid to haematopoiesis is discussed.

REFERENCES

Alt, H. L., Chinn, H., and Farmer, C. J. (1939) *Amer. J. Med. Sci.* **197,** 229.
Aterman, K., Boscott, R. J., and Cooke, W. T. (1953) *Biochem. J.* **55,** xvii.
Berg, C. P. (1953) *Physiol. Rev.* **33,** 145.
Borne, G. A. (1939) *Nederl. tijd. geneesk.* **9,** 1082.
Boscott, R. J. (1950–1) *J. Endocrinol.* **7,** 154.
—— (1952*a*) 2nd International Biochemical Congress (Paris) Abstracts, p. 349.
—— (1952*b*) *Biochem. J.* **51,** xlv.
—— (1952*c*) *Chem. and Ind.* 472.
—— and Aterman, K. (1953). Unpublished observation.
—— and Bickel, H. (1953) *Biochem. J.* **56,** i.
—— and Greenberg, S. M. (1953) Ibid. **55,** xviii.
Bray, H. G., Thorpe, W. V., and White, K. (1950) Ibid. **46,** 271.
Cartwright, G. E. (1947) *Blood,* **2,** 111.
Dobriner, K., Lavin, G. I., and Rhoads, C. P. (1942) *Cancer Research,* **2,** 79.
Ewins, A. J., and Laidlaw, P. P. (1910–11) *J. Physiol.* **41,** 78.
Foy, H., and Kondi, A. (1939) *Lancet,* **2,** 360.
Girdwood, R. H. (1953) Ibid. **2,** 52.
Govan, C. D., and Gordon, H. H. (1949) *Science,* **109,** 332.
Hawk, P. B., Oser, B. L., and Summerson, W. H. (1947) *Practical Physiological Chemistry,* 12th ed., London.
Heinsen, H. A. (1937) *Zts. physiol. Chem.* **245,** 1.
Holly, R. G. (1951) *Proc. Soc. Exp. Biol. Med.* **78,** 238.
Le May-Knox, M., and Knox, W. E. (1951) *Biochem. J.* **48,** xxii.
Lerner, A. B. (1953) *Advances in Enzymology,* Vol. 14, New York.
Levine, S. Z., Dann, M., and Marples, E. (1943) *J. Clin. Invest.* **22,** 551.
Lowry, O. H. (1952) *Physiol. Rev.* **32,** 431.
May, C. D., Nelson, E. N., and Salmon, R. J. (1949) *J. Lab. Clin. Med.* **34,** 1724.
—— Hamilton, A., and Stewart, C. T. (1952) *Blood,* **7,** 978.
Mohr, W. (1939) *Dtsch. Zts. Verdauungs- u. Stoffwechselkr.* **2,** 142.
Morris, J. E., Harpur, E. R., and Goldbloom, A. (1950) *J. Clin. Invest.* **29,** 325.
Nichol, C. A., and Welch, A. D. (1950) *Proc. Soc. Exp. Biol. Med.* **74,** 52.
O'Kane, D. E., and Gunsalus, I. C. (1947) *J. Biol. Chem.* **170,** 433.
Rodney, G., Swendseid, M. E., and Swanson, A. L. (1949) Ibid. **179,** 19.
Rogers, W. F., and Gardner, F. H. (1949) *J. Lab. Clin. Med.* **34,** 1491.
Roka, L. (1952) 2nd International Biochemical Congress (Paris) Abstracts, p. 302.
Salmon, R. J., and May, C. D. (1953) *J. Lab. Clin. Med.* **41,** 376.
Scott, M. L., Hill, C. H., and Norris, L. C. (1949) *Federation Proc.* **8,** 249.
Sealock, R. R., and Goodland, R. L. (1951) *Science,* **114,** 645.
Simpson, R. E., and Schweigert, B. S. (1949) *Arch. Biochem.* **20,** 32.
Swendseid, M. E., Burton, I. F., and Bethell, F. H. (1943) *Proc. Soc. Exp. Biol. Med.* **52,** 202.
Williams, R. J., and Kirby, H. (1948) *Science,* **107,** 481.
Woodruff, C. W., and Darby, W. J. (1948) *J. Biol. Chem.* **172,** 851.

616.151.5–056.7

FAMILIAL FACTOR V DEFICIENCY: THE PATTERN OF HEREDITY[1]

By C. S. KINGSLEY

(From the Institute for Pathology, Beatrix Street, Pretoria)

Owren (1947*a*) reported extensively on the behaviour and properties of a plasma factor necessary for the normal conversion of prothrombin to thrombin, and described the first case of haemorrhagic diathesis due to deficiency of this factor. He named it 'the fifth coagulation factor' or 'factor V', and the disease resulting from its deficiency 'parahaemophilia' (Owren, 1947*b*). Later he renamed factor V 'proaccelerin' (Owren, 1951). Previously Quick (1943–4) had described the same factor as 'component A of prothrombin', but he later named it 'labile factor' (Quick, 1947). Other workers dealing with what is now acknowledged to be the same substance (Alexander, Flynn, Mann, Owren, and Seegers, 1952) used other names for it; 'accelerator factor' (Fantl and Nance, 1946), 'plasmatic co-factor of thromboplastin' (Honorato, 1947), and 'plasma ac-globulin' (Ware, Guest, and Seegers, 1947). Other less well-known names have recently been introduced by other authors. For the purpose of the present communication Owren's original term 'factor V' will be used. This report considers two families. The first, v. d. W., has already been reported by Brink and Kingsley (1952). At that time, however, factor V assays were not done, and family members were regarded as normal on the basis of normal prothrombin times. The three patients concerned have now been observed for more than three years. The diagnosis has been confirmed repeatedly. No abnormality has been demonstrated in their prothrombin, factor VII, fibrinogen, or platelets. The second family, Mz., has not yet been reported elsewhere.

Note on the Methods Used

Prothrombin time was determined according to the method of Quick (1945). Times for the normal controls were between 11 and 12 seconds throughout. Factor V assays were done by the method of Stefanini (1951). A separate reference curve was constructed for each batch of aged plasma. The reliability of aged plasma as a substrate was confirmed by re-examining some of the cases by the same method, but with the aged plasma replaced by plasma from a known patient. Eight persons, including the whole Mz. family, were examined by the latter method only. Although in most cases the examinations were carried out only once, in some they were repeated up to six months later with substantially the same results.

[1] Received November 28, 1953.

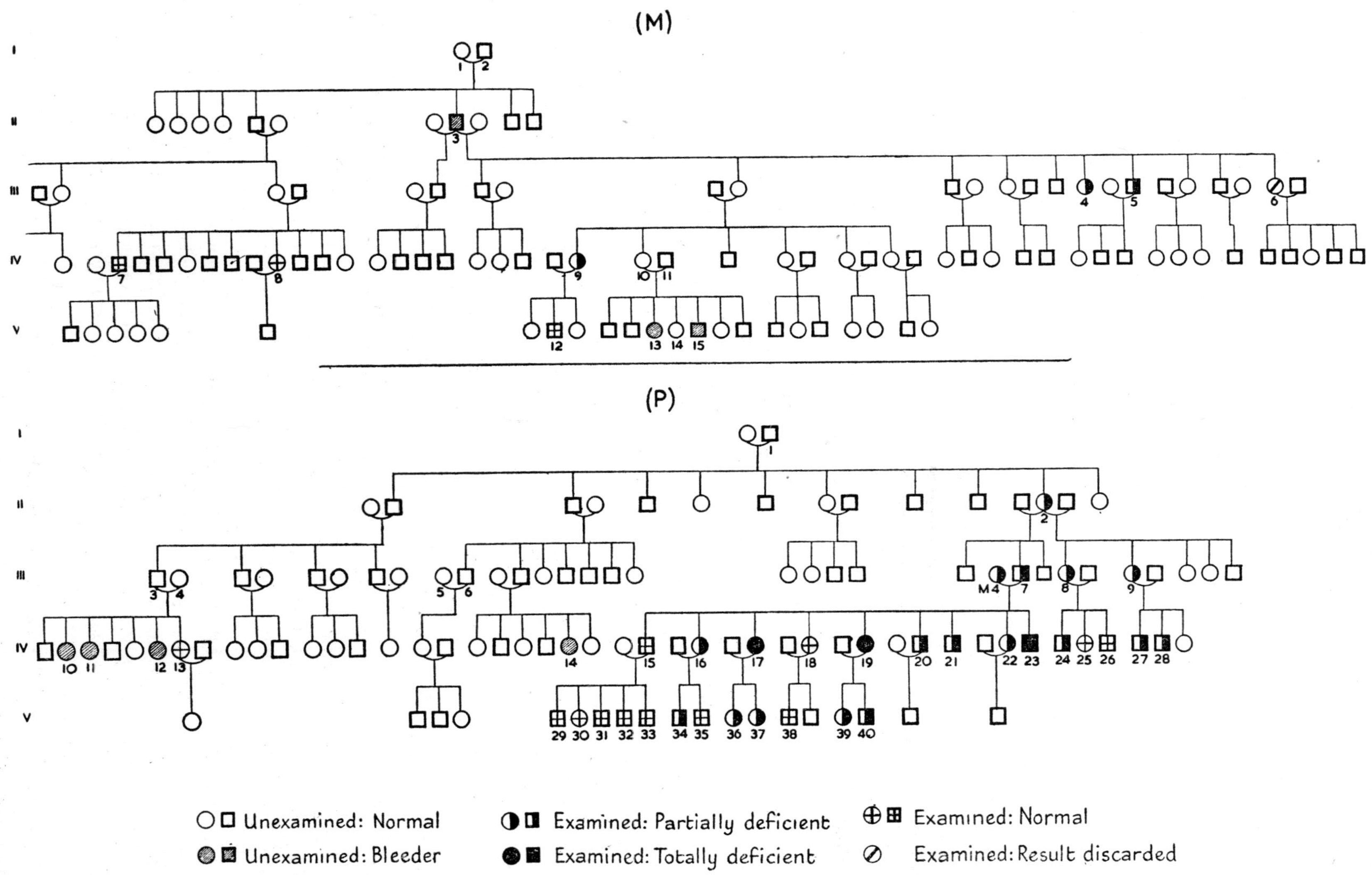

FIG. 1. Factor V deficiency in the v. d. W. family: (M) maternal, (P) paternal pedigree. Circles denote female, squares male members. Infantile deaths from other causes than haemorrhage, and family groups about which no definite history could be obtained, are not shown.

Findings

The results of the factor V assays performed on the v. d. W. family are summarized diagrammatically in Fig. 1. The three patients, shown as P17, P19, and P23, were found to have less than 5 per cent. of normal factor V activity. Since it is known that blood platelets contribute some activity towards restoring the prothrombin time of aged plasma (Mann, Hurn, and Magath, 1947; Ware, Fahey, and Seegers, 1948), and since the plasmas used in these assays were rich in platelets, it is probable that these patients are in fact totally deficient. Members displaying factor V activity above 80 per cent. of normal are shown as 'examined: normal'. All the members shown as partially deficient have no haemorrhagic tendency, but factor V activity ranging between 40 per cent. and 60 per cent. of normal, except in the cases of M5, P8, P21, and P28, in whom values of 68 per cent., 66 per cent., 24 per cent., and 64 per cent. of normal were recorded respectively. Family members who were not examined, and who lack a clear history of haemorrhagic diathesis, are shown as 'unexamined: normal'. 'Unexamined bleeders' are people about whom a definite history of haemorrhagic diathesis exists. Except when influenced by recent transfusion of blood or plasma, the prothrombin time in the three patients has consistently been longer than 36 seconds. In the partially deficient members normal times were usual, but distinct prolongation to between 13 and 14 seconds was encountered in a single examination of M5, and in repeated examinations of P34, P36, P37, and P39. In P21 and P22 the prothrombin time was intermittently prolonged, in the former up to 16 seconds and in the latter up to 13·4 seconds. Doubtfully prolonged times of 12·2 and 12·3 seconds were recorded in single examinations of P2 and P9. In the case of M6 examinations were done, but the results were discarded because at the time the patient was severely ill with cirrhosis of the liver, congestive cardiac failure, and empyema, which caused her death soon afterwards.

From the available information there appears to be little doubt that in this family the partially deficient members are the heterozygous carriers of the disease, while the totally deficient patients are homozygous for the defective gene. Since both maternal and paternal great-grandfathers (shown as M2 and P1 respectively in Fig. 1) bore the same surname, v. d. W., other people of this surname were examined at random in an attempt to find carriers. Of 20 persons so examined, one, A. J. v. d. W., was found to have a prothrombin time varying between normal and 13·4 seconds and factor V activity 40 per cent. of normal. He is not aware of a haemorrhagic diathesis in his family.

It seemed probable that M2, P1, and A. J. v. d. W. derived the faulty gene from a common ancestor. Accordingly, with the aid of the Archives of the Union of South Africa, the ancestry of these people was ascertained. The result is shown in Fig. 2. The first v. d. W. to arrive in South Africa, G, had eight children. The youngest son, N, proved to be the common forefather sought. Thus his second child, A, was the grandfather of M2; his fifth child, J, was the father of P1, and A. J. v. d. W. is descended from his youngest child, H, in the fourth generation. Further, since the defective gene is obviously a rare one, it appeared probable that some of the matings resulting in 'bleeder' children, which are so prominent in this family history, were in fact consanguinous through the same lines. It has so far not been possible to trace the ancestry of M1 or M11 or the maternal pedigree of P14, but P4 was found to be a direct descendant of N through his youngest child, H.

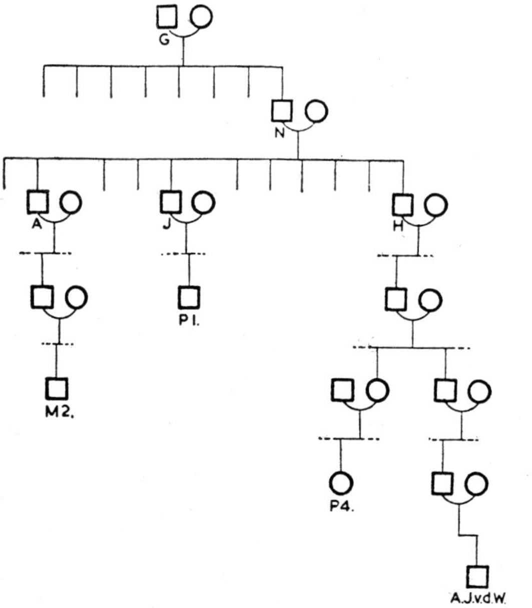

FIG. 2. v. d. W. family. Diagram to show consanguinity of carriers.

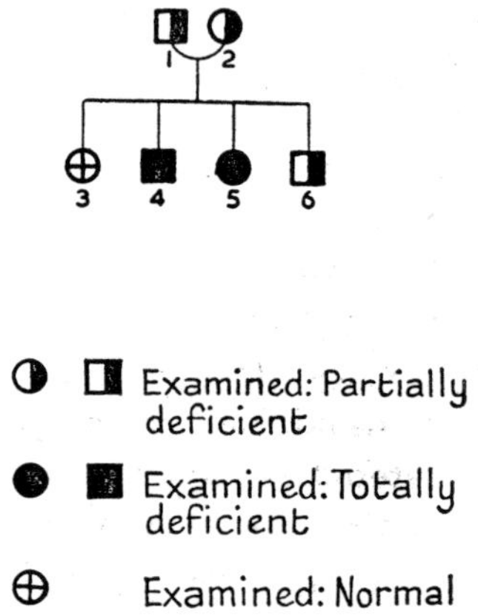

FIG. 3. Factor V deficiency in the Mz. family.

N was born nearly 200 years ago; he was christened in 1757. Since either he or his wife was a carrier of the defect, it is apparent that the faulty gene has now been propagated in South Africa for about 170 years at least. Moreover, the chances of a marriage between two carriers, with the resultant possibility of affected children, is considerably increased by the fact that the country has a comparatively small white population. It is therefore not surprising that a second family showing an identical pattern of heredity was discovered recently. The ancestry of this family is not yet available, but family surnames on the maternal side, and religious affiliation, suggest relationship to the v. d. W. family. The findings for this new family, Mz., are summarized below.

Case histories (refer to Fig. 3)

Mz.4. A boy born in 1946. Apart from two episodes of severe, but not alarming, haemorrhage after tooth-extraction at the ages of four and six years, he has revealed no evidence of haemorrhagic diathesis. The coagulation defect was discovered on routine examination of the family.

Mz.5. A girl born in 1947, the proposita in this family. She was well until the age of three years, when ever-present small subcutaneous bruises were observed, and repeated spontaneous epistaxis began, sometimes lasting up to

12 hours. Since the age of five years, spontaneous bleeding from the mouth has become apparent. At the age of five and a half years tonsillectomy resulted in severe haemorrhage, necessitating blood transfusion, which promptly arrested the bleeding. Shortly afterwards transfusion had again to be resorted to in order to control loss of blood following tooth-extraction, and she was sent for investigation of the haemorrhagic diathesis.

Both parents, and two other siblings, have shown no tendency to abnormal haemorrhage. The findings relating to the coagulation defect are summarized diagrammatically in Fig. 3. The two children Mz.4 and Mz.5 have prothrombin times of 38·4 seconds and 40–41 seconds respectively. Ten-per-cent. additions of their plasmas to that of a known factor-V-deficient patient does not have any shortening effect on the prothrombin time. On the other hand, the prolonged prothrombin time of normal plasma treated with tricalcium phosphate is restored by addition of their plasmas. Both parents are partially deficient in factor V; the father, Mz.1, has a prothrombin time of 12·8 seconds and factor V activity 29 per cent. of normal, and the mother, Mz.2, a prothrombin time of 14 seconds and factor V activity 30 per cent. of normal. The two remaining children have normal prothrombin times, and Mz.3 has a normal factor V activity (103 per cent.), but Mz.6 has a factor V activity 42 per cent. of normal.

Discussion

Though the defective gene behaves clinically as a recessive in these two families, haematologically it is roughly of equal potency to the normal gene, resulting in factor V activity in the region of 50 per cent. of normal in heterozygotes. But the finding of activity as low as 24 per cent. and as high as 68 per cent. of normal in some cases argues a degree of variable expressivity; so that it seems possible that, at the one extreme, cases will be found in which the gene expresses itself sufficiently strongly to assume partial dominance and produce haemorrhagic symptoms in the heterozygous state, while, at the other extreme, it may be so poorly expressed as to render the detection of carriers impossible by the methods employed in the present study. Although unequivocal cases of either of these two possibilities were not found in these families, it is possible that some of the cases reported in the literature may provide examples of both. No evidence of a familial tendency was found in Owren's original case (Owren, 1947*b*), or in the cases reported by Stohlman, Harrington, and Moloney (1951) and Brennan, Monto, and Shafer (1952). In other reports, while the familial nature was obvious, no coagulation defect was demonstrated in the parents of the patients (de Vries, Matoth, and Shamir, 1951; Alexander and Goldstein, 1952). The father of the patient reported by Frank, Bilhan, and Ekren (1950) had haemorrhagic symptoms, but information regarding his mother was not available, while in the case recently reported by Redner, Scalettar, and Weiner (1953) the mother had a suggestively prolonged prothrombin time, but the father was normal. Most authors have not given details about the methods used for examination of the parents of patients, but it is possible that the failure to detect the abnormality in these people may have been due to poor expressivity of the gene.

As has been demonstrated above, the patients who have prothrombin times in the region of 40 seconds or more are either totally deficient in factor V or possess a negligible concentration of the factor. Alexander and Goldstein (1952), using different methods, recorded identical findings in their three cases. It may therefore be reasonably assumed that patients with only moderately prolonged prothrombin times, such as those of de Vries, Matoth, and Shamir (1951) and Stohlman, Harrington, and Moloney (1951), still have considerable factor V activity. It is possible, therefore, that they are heterozygotic, and represent cases in which the expressivity of the gene is so pronounced as to assume partial dominance over the normal. The partial deficiencies of factor V recently described by Owren (1953) in a mother and two sons, one of whom had a mild haemorrhagic diathesis, bear a striking resemblance to the findings recorded above in the heterozygotic carriers of the disease. The finding of normal prothrombin times in patients who nevertheless have considerable factor V deficiency supports the experimental findings of Alexander and de Vries (1949) and Munro and Munro (1947).

Note. The above account represents a summary of which the details are available in the author's doctorate thesis presented at the University of Pretoria, South Africa.

Summary

The hereditary mechanism of familial factor V deficiency in two families is described. It is shown to be transmitted by a gene which, although clinically recessive in these families, nevertheless has a potency roughly equal to its normal counterpart.

In addition it is shown that the gene displays a degree of variable expressivity, and it is suggested that cases may be encountered in which the gene is either completely recessive or partially dominant.

The cases reported in the literature are briefly reviewed in the light of this pattern of heredity.

REFERENCES

Alexander, B., and de Vries, A. (1949) *J. Clin. Invest.* **28**, 24.

—— Flynn, J. E., Mann, F. D., Owren, P. A., and Seegers, W. H. (1952) *Blood Clotting and Allied Problems* (*Appendix*), Trans. 5th Conference, J. Macy Jnr. Found., N.Y., p. 329.

—— and Goldstein, R. (1952) *Amer. J. Med.* **13**, 255.

Brennan, M. J., Monto, R. W., and Shafer, H. C. (1952) *Amer. J. Clin. Path.* **22**, 150.

Brink, A. J., and Kingsley, C. S. (1952) *Quart. J. Med.* N.S. **21**, 19.

Fantl, P., and Nance, M. (1946) *Nature*, **158**, 708.

Frank, E., Bilhan, N., and Ekren, H. (1950) *Acta haematol.* **3**, 70.

Honorato, R. (1947) *Amer. J. Physiol.* **150**, 381.

Mann, F. D., Hurn, M., and Magath, B. (1947) *Proc. Soc. Exp. Biol. Med.* **66**, 33.

Munro, F. L., and Munro, M. P. (1947) *Amer. J. Physiol.* **149**, 95.

Owren, P. A. (1947*a*) *Acta med. scand.* Suppl. **194.**
—— (1947*b*) *Lancet,* **1,** 446.
—— (1951) *Scand. J. Clin. Lab. Invest.* **3,** 168.
—— (1953) *Amer. J. Med.* **14,** 201.
Quick, A. J. (1943–4) *Amer. J. Physiol.* **140,** 212.
—— (1945) *Amer. J. Clin. Path.* **15,** 560.
—— (1947) *Lancet,* **2,** 379.
Redner, B., Scalettar, H., and Weiner, M. (1953) *Pediatrics,* **12,** 5.
Stefanini, M. (1951) *Lancet,* **1,** 606.
Stohlman, F. Jnr., Harrington, W. J., and Moloney, W. C. (1951) *J. Lab. Clin. Med.* **38,** 842.
de Vries, A., Matoth, Y., and Shamir, Z. (1951) *Acta haematol.* **5,** 129.
Ware, A. G., Guest, M. M., and Seegers, W. H. (1947) *J. Biol. Chem.* **169**, 231.
—— Fahey, J. L., and Seegers, W. H. (1948) *Amer. J. Physiol.* **154,** 140.

616.056.52: 616.12–008.331.1

THE EFFECT OF WEIGHT REDUCTION UPON THE BLOOD-PRESSURE OF OBESE HYPERTENSIVE WOMEN[1]

By A. P. FLETCHER

(From The Wright-Fleming Institute of Microbiology and St. Mary's Hospital, London)

EXTENSIVE studies have conclusively demonstrated that obese persons exhibit a greater incidence of hypertension than do persons of normal weight (Hartman and Ghrist, 1929; Short and Johnson, 1939; Robinson, Bruce, and Mass, 1939–40; Levy, White, Stroud, and Hillman, 1946; Boynton and Todd, 1948; Master, Garfield, and Walters, 1952). Furthermore it is clear that the greater the degree of obesity, the greater is the incidence of hypertension at all ages. The 'Minnesota experiment' (Keys, Henschel, and Taylor, 1947) showed that normal men maintained on low-calorie diets for long periods, so as to lose approximately a quarter of their body-weight, experienced a fall of both systolic and diastolic blood-pressure. These falls of blood-pressure were reversed when normal weight was regained. The review of Brozek, Chapman, and Keys (1948) marshals the scattered evidence from Europe demonstrating that during a period of severe and prolonged food shortage the incidence of hypertension and its complications appears to fall in the community. Wood and Cash (1939) published experiments suggesting that the blood-pressure of dogs, whether raised or normal, rises as weight increases and falls as weight decreases. These facts and clinical observations have led to the hypothesis that weight reduction would lower the blood-pressure of obese hypertensive subjects. Many investigations designed to confirm or refute this hypothesis have been published (Rose, 1922; Terry, 1923; Preble, 1923; Bauman, 1928; Master and Oppenheimer, 1929; Adlersberg, Coler, and Laval, 1946; Bram, 1947; Green and Beckman, 1948; Martin, 1952). The majority of these authors believed that weight reduction causes a fall in the blood-pressure of obese patients with hypertension, but the authors have not agreed as to the extent and significance of the fall. The value of these studies is difficult to assess, since some authors disregarded the fact that the initial blood-pressure readings of a series are frequently higher than the later ones; none of them was able to employ a control group of obese hypertensive patients who did not reduce their weight, and in no case did the experimental design allow for the error introduced by the fact that blood-pressure readings taken by the indirect method are influenced by the arm-girth of the subject. Weight reduction, and consequently arm-girth reduction, being an essential part of the investigation, the error due to this factor may have been considerable. The present investigation was designed in the belief that adequate control groups could obviate these uncertainties.

[1] Received December 14, 1953.

Selection of Patients

The number of obese women attending the out-patient department was many times greater than the number of obese men, so that, in order to eliminate the influence of sex from the analysis, the experimental groups included only women. One hundred and fifty-five obese women were seen during the period of the investigation, and all patients who completed at least four months' treatment were included in it. Women were classified as being obese when their body-weight was at least 20 per cent. in excess of their maximum ideal weight. The maximum ideal body-weight was obtained from the Tables of the Metropolitan Life Insurance Company (1942), which provide a range of weight for persons of varying height and body build. A subjective assessment of body-build into three categories had to be made: small-framed, medium-framed, and large-framed. In fact, the distinction between obese and non-obese patients was easily made. The patients were classified as suffering from systolic hypertension if the systolic blood-pressure exceeded 150 mm. Hg on each of the first three blood-pressure readings. Patients were regarded as suffering from diastolic hypertension if the diastolic blood-pressure exceeded 100 mm. Hg under similar circumstances. Patients not classified as suffering from either systolic or diastolic hypertension were entered in the groups showing normal blood-pressure. If a patient had a systolic blood-pressure exceeding 150 mm. Hg and a diastolic blood-pressure exceeding 100 mm. Hg, she was included in both the systolic hypertensive group and the diastolic hypertensive group. Of the obese hypertensive patients who lost weight there were 38, all of whom were entered in the systolic hypertensive group, since in all cases the blood-pressure exceeded 150 mm. Hg. In only 30 of these patients did the diastolic blood-pressure exceed 100 mm. Hg, these 30 constituting the diastolic hypertensive group of patients who lost weight. The other groups were formed on similar criteria (Table I). No patient in the investigation was suffering from 'malignant' hypertension or from nephritis, and all patients who had oedema were excluded from the series.

Technique of blood-pressure estimation. All blood-pressure readings were taken personally, with the technique recommended by the Cardiac Society of Great Britain and Ireland (1939). A standard mercurial sphygmomanometer was used with a 13-cm.-width bag, the length of the bag cover being increased so as to obviate bulging around large arms (Cardiac Society, 1939; Bordley, Connor, Hamilton, Kerr, and Wiggers, 1951). All readings were taken to the nearest 5 mm. Hg, using the right arm. At the initial interview the blood-pressure was taken after a period of 20 minutes' recumbency on a couch; a second reading was taken after another 10 minutes' recumbency. One week later the blood-pressure was again taken after a 15-minute period of recumbency. The lowest figure recorded at the three readings was used to separate the patients into those having normal or raised blood-pressure, and this figure was taken as representing the patient's blood-pressure at the start of the experiment. The patient attended monthly, the blood-pressure again being taken after 15 minutes' rest on a couch. The final blood-pressure reading for each patient was the last recorded in these circumstances, any patient failing to complete four months' treatment being discarded from the series. The duration of treatment is given in Tables II, III, and IV.

Reduction of weight. Each patient, clad only in a dressing-gown, was weighed at every attendance on an accurate pair of jockey scales. The weight of the dressing-gown was subtracted from the gross weight in order to obtain the patient's weight. Patients were requested to void urine prior to the interview. Weight was reduced by prescribing a 600-calorie diet, and trying to persuade the patients to keep to it. A more liberal diet of 1,000 calories was usually allowed towards the end of treatment. Inspection of the weight-loss data suggests that even the successfully treated patients in fact ingested a diet nearer to 1,000 than to 600 calories. Arm-girth measurements were made with a steel tape midway between the acromial process and the medial epicondyle of the humerus.

Experimental Design

It is clear from experiments involving the simultaneous measurements of blood-pressure by the indirect method (sphygmomanometer) and by the direct method (Hamilton manometer), that the indirect estimation gives results of satisfactory accuracy when a 13-cm.-width cuff is employed for adults with a 'normal' arm-girth (Steele, 1942; Kotte, Iglauer, and McGuire, 1944). It is equally clear that if a 13-cm.-width cuff is used on adult arms of greater than 'normal' girth, the blood-pressure recorded will be greater than the true reading (Ragan and Bordley, 1941; Wendkos and Rossman, 1943). Weight reduction will result in a reduction in arm-girth, and, if the indirect method of estimation is used, will give rise to an apparent fall in blood-pressure, even if the true blood-pressure remains constant. Although the reduction of arm-girth for each patient can be measured, the data at present available are insufficient to calculate an accurate correction. Ragan and Bordley (1941) have shown that the discrepancy between the direct and the indirect methods of blood-pressure determination is similar at high and low pressures, and that the discrepancy is related to the arm-circumference. Furthermore it was demonstrated that in adult arms of large girth, where the 13-cm. cuff gave too high a reading, the 20-cm. cuff gave too low a reading. The reason for the false reading given by the indirect measurement in certain circumstances would seem to lie in the differing pressure exerted by the standard cuff on the limb artery of arms of different girth (Thomson and Doupe, 1949).

Repeated direct determinations of blood-pressure were clearly impracticable under out-patient conditions, and this fact rendered it necessary to examine further the contention of Ragan and Bordley (1941) that the discrepancy between the direct and indirect methods of blood-pressure determination is independent of the height of the blood-pressure. Data from all the large series of simultaneous indirect and direct blood-pressure determinations in the literature (Ragan and Bordley, 1941; Steele, 1942; Kotte, Iglauer, and McGuire, 1944; Roberts, Smiley, and Manning, 1953) were combined, excluding only cases in which valvular disease of the heart was present. These combined readings covered a complete range of blood-pressure determinations, from low to high. The correlation coefficient between systolic direct blood-pressure determinations and systolic indirect blood-pressure determinations (174 paired readings) was 0·894, and the regression of direct blood-pressure on indirect blood-pressure ($y = bx+c$) was $y = 0{\cdot}97x+5{\cdot}5$, with a standard deviation of 16·7 mm. For diastolic blood-pressure a plot of the readings showed increasing discrepancies at extremes of diastolic blood-pressure, so that the figures were worked out for the range 60 mm. to 140 mm. diastolic blood-pressure, which amply covered all variations met with in the present investigation. The correlation coefficient (152 paired readings) was 0·69, and the regression of direct on indirect readings was $y = 0{\cdot}92x - 3$, with a standard deviation of 16·3 mm. Since the regression line for complete independence of discrepancy on height of blood-pressure would be $y = x+0$, it can be stated with a high degree of confidence that the discrepancy between direct and indirect blood-pressure readings is independent of the actual height of the blood-pressure.

These findings indicated that a satisfactory estimate of the arm-girth discrepancy could be obtained by reducing the weight of a group of women with normal blood-pressure. Furthermore, this procedure would be likely to give an inflated estimate of the discrepancy, since the blood-pressure in these women, also, might fall because of their loss of weight. The use of this estimate to correct any change of blood-pressure experienced by women of the hypertensive group who lost weight would ensure that reduction of arm-girth due to weight loss was not the cause of the change. Two conditions must be fulfilled prior to the application of this estimate. The first is that the patients in each group must be equally obese (Table I), and the second is that the patients in each group must lose an equal amount of weight (Tables III and IV).

The effect of weight reduction on the successfully treated groups was assessed by comparison with suitable control groups of women who were unsuccessfully treated. For the purposes of the analysis that follows, the systolic and diastolic blood-pressures of each patient are considered separately; within these two groups the patients are divided into four sub-major groups:

Group A: obese patients with hypertension who lost at least 14 lb. in weight.

Group B: obese patients with hypertension who lost less than 14 lb. in weight.

Group C: obese patients with normal blood-pressure who lost at least 14 lb. in weight.

Group D: obese patients with normal blood-pressure who lost less than 14 lb. in weight.

The changes in blood-pressure that occurred during the investigation were calculated in mm. of mercury, and also as a percentage change of the initial blood-pressure. Similarly weight changes were shown both as a gain or loss in pounds, and as a percentage of the initial weight.

Details of the main Groups A, B, and C are shown in Table I; Group D is not shown because, owing to the number of patients who failed to complete treatment, its value in the final analysis was small. In each case in Table I, and also in the following Tables, the average figure for the quantity in question is followed by its standard deviation. All differences between groups were tested by means of the Student '*t*' test, except that the χ^2 test was used to compare the distribution of the parous women in the groups, and also for Table V. It was considered necessary to demonstrate that an approximately equal number of women in each group had borne children, since several authors (Browne and Dodds, 1939; Corwin and Herrick, 1927; Herrick and Tillman, 1935) have suggested that an episode of pregnancy-toxaemia might induce a long-standing or permanent elevation of the blood-pressure. Although this view was challenged by Isenhour, Kuder, and Dill (1942), who compared the blood-pressures of groups of nulliparous and parous women and found them to be similar, it was deemed desirable that the groups should be comparable in this respect as well as in others. Table I shows that the experimental groups were comparable with regard to initial obesity and parity, in that the differences were not significant ($P > 0{\cdot}1$),[2] but that Group C probably differed from Groups A and B with regard to age ($P = 0{\cdot}05$). Since Group C was used to estimate the fall in blood-pressure due to reduced arm-girth, this flaw in sampling is probably unimportant. Table I reveals that the hypertensive patients were elderly, extremely obese, and exhibited a moderate to large increase of blood-pressure.

TABLE I

Details of Groups A, B, and C at the Start of the Experiment

Figures in each line are average figures followed by the standard deviation in parenthesis.

	Systolic blood-pressure group			*Diastolic blood-pressure group*		
	A	*B*	*C*	*A*	*B*	*C*
Number of women in groups	38	21	12	30	19	20
Age in years	54·9 (8·7)	57·3 (8·9)	42·3 (15)	54·4 (9·1)	54·7 (9·2)	46·7 (14·1)
Initial blood-pressure (mm. Hg)	195·8 (31·7)	184·3 (18·8)	134·2 (12·9)	115·7 (13·9)	109·7 (8·2)	87·5 (7·3)
Initial obesity (% of ideal body-weight)	144·5 (13·1)	148 (18)	143·2 (17·3)	146·2 (12·7)	149 (19·6)	146·2 (12·7)
Number of parous women in group	28	13	6	21	11	11

Differences between groups: $P > 0{\cdot}1$, except that Group C differs from Groups A and B with regard to blood-pressure ($P < 0{\cdot}001$; groups were selected on this basis), and possibly with regard to age ($P = 0{\cdot}05$).

Results after Treatment

Patients were regarded as successfully treated if at the end of the observation period they had lost more than 14 lb. in weight, and as unsuccessfully treated, or control cases, if at the end of this time they had lost less than this amount of weight. In practice this division proved satisfactory in producing a clear line of demarcation, since the successfully treated Group A lost an average of 33 lb. in weight, and the control Group B an average of 4 lb. Table II compares the obese hypertensive group, which was successfully treated, with the obese hypertensive group which was unsuccessfully treated. Group A patients lost an

[2] P or probability is expressed on the scale 0 to 1, and is employed in the conventional sense, $P = 0{\cdot}01$ indicating a result likely to occur by chance only once in a hundred trials.

average of 33 lb. in weight, and their systolic blood-pressures fell by an average of 33 mm.; their diastolic pressures fell by an average of 16 mm. They lost 17 per cent. of their initial body-weight, and experienced a fall of 17 per cent. of their initial systolic blood-pressure, while the fall of the initial diastolic blood-

TABLE II

Hypertensive Obese Women who Lost Weight (Group A) and Hypertensive Obese Women (Group B) who Failed to Lose Weight at the End of the Experiment

Figures in each line are average figures followed by the standard deviation in parenthesis.

		Systolic blood-pressure			*Diastolic blood-pressure*		
		Group A	*Group B*	*Difference (P)*	*Group A*	*Group B*	*Difference (P)*
Change of blood-pressure	mm. Hg	−32·8 (17·9)	+0·5 (13·8)	< 0·001	−16·5 (9·4)	+1·3 (6·4)	< 0·001
	% of initial pressure	−17·1 (8·5)	+0·6 (7·9)		−15·3 (3·6)	+1·4 (7·9)	
Change of weight	lb.	−32·4 (14·7)	−4·2 (5·8)	< 0·001	−33·2 (15·5)	−4·2 (4·8)	< 0·001
	% of initial weight	−16·7 (6)	−1·8 (2·6)		−16·9 (6·2)	−1·93 (2·6)	
Period of treatment (months)		6·4 (2·5)	5·2 (1·9)	> 0·1	6·5 (2·6)	5·1 (2)	> 0·1

pressure was 15 per cent. These figures when tested against the control Group B are statistically highly significant ($P < 0{\cdot}001$). The duration of observation did not differ significantly ($P > 0{\cdot}1$). The percentage of excess body-weight

$$\frac{\text{weight lost} \times 100}{\text{initial body-weight} - \text{ideal body-weight}}$$

lost by group A was 59 (s.d. 19·9), demonstrating that substantial progress was made in changing the state of these patients from gross to moderate obesity. At the end of the investigation the patients of Group A were approximately 20 per cent. over-weight. It was concluded that the reduction in weight achieved was associated with a statistically significant fall of both systolic and diastolic blood-pressures, these pressures being measured by the indirect method.

The influence of reduced arm-girth. To assess the influence of reduced arm-girth on the recorded blood-pressure readings, the change of blood-pressure in Group C (obese women with normal blood-pressure who lost weight) was compared with the change in Group D (obese women with normal blood-pressure who did not lose weight). This comparison showed that, although the patients in Group C had experienced a fall of blood-pressure, the difference between the two groups was not statistically significant ($P > 0{\cdot}1$). Unfortunately, during the course of the investigation, Group D was reduced through default to seven patients. Although tests of significance can be applied to these numbers, the establishment of negative findings with such data is not convincing. In order to circumvent this difficulty, Group C was compared with the other control Group B. Table III shows the details of this comparison. It is apparent that, when larger groups are used for comparison, women of Group C, whose weight and arm-girth were reduced, experienced a fall in blood-pressure which was statistically significant when measured against that of a group of women who did not lose weight and whose arm-girths remained the same. These figures

Table III

Obese Women with Normal Blood-Pressure who Lost Weight (Group C) and Hypertensive Obese Women who failed to Lose Weight (Group B) at the End of the Experiment

Figures in each line are average figures followed by the standard deviation in parenthesis.

		Systolic blood-pressure			Diastolic blood-pressure		
		Group C	*Group B*	*Difference (P)*	*Group C*	*Group B*	*Difference (P)*
Change of blood-pressure	mm. Hg.	−10·8 (9·1)	0·5 (13·8)	<0·001	−3·5 (7·9)	+1·3 (6·4)	<0·01
	% of initial pressure	−7·8 (5·8)	+0·6 (7·9)		−4·3 (8·2)	+1·4 (7·9)	
Change of weight	lb.	−30 (15)	−4·2 (5·8)	<0·001	−29·9 (13·4)	−4·2 (4·8)	<0·001
	% of initial weight	−16 (6·7)	−1·8 (2·6)		−16 (6)	−1·9 (2·6)	
Period of treatment (months)		7·8 (4·9)	5·2 (1·9)	>0·1	7·6 (4·8)	5·1 (2)	>0·1

suggest that the reduced arm-girth of the successfully treated group may have exerted an influence on the recorded falls of blood-pressure.

Effect of an estimated arm-girth correction. The reasons for regarding the change of blood-pressure experienced by Group C as an inflated estimate of the arm-girth correction have already been discussed. The blood-pressure of Group C patients fell by an average of 10·8 mm. Hg systolic (s.d. 9·1 mm.), and an average of 3·5 mm. Hg diastolic (s.d. 7·9 mm.). Arm-girth measurements were made on 29 of the 50 patients in Groups A and C who lost weight. These 29 patients lost an average of 34 lb. (s.d. 11·2 lb.), with an average reduction in arm-circumference of 3·6 cm. (s.d. 1·8 cm.). Hamilton, Pickering, Roberts, and Sowry (1954) have suggested that for each centimetre of arm-girth reduction a correction of −1·17 mm. Hg for systolic and of −1·14 mm. Hg for diastolic blood-pressure should be applied to readings taken by the indirect method. On this basis of correction Group C appears to provide an excessive estimate of the correction for systolic fall, and an approximately true estimate for diastolic fall, due to arm-girth reduction. The data of Wendkos and Rossman (1943) also support this contention. It will be appreciated, however, that the accuracy of arm-girth measurements is not high, and the suggested estimates for the correction of indirect blood-pressure readings due to this factor are based upon small series. Since arm-girth measurements confirm the belief that the use of data from Group C does not result in an underestimate of the correction required to compensate for the error produced by arm-girth reduction, Group C is directly compared with Group A in Table IV. Although the loss of weight in each of the two groups was similar ($P > 0{\cdot}1$), the fall of both systolic and diastolic blood-pressures was significantly greater in Group A ($P < 0{\cdot}001$ in each case). This comparison shows that arm-girth reduction alone would not account for the fall of blood-pressure experienced by Group A. Furthermore, if the fall of blood-pressure shown by Group A is adjusted by subtracting the figures for arm-girth correction obtained from Group C, and these adjusted figures for

TABLE IV

Hypertensive Obese Women who Lost Weight (Group A) and Obese Women having Normal Blood-Pressure who Lost Weight (Group C) at the End of the Experiment

Figures in each line are average figures followed by the standard deviation in parenthesis.

		Systolic blood-pressure			*Diastolic blood-pressure*		
		Group A	*Group C*	*Difference (P)*	*Group A*	*Group C*	*Difference (P)*
Change of blood-pressure	mm. Hg.	−32·8 (17·9)	−10·8 (9·1)	<0·001	−16·5 (9·4)	−3·5 (7·9)	<0·001
	% of initial pressure	−17·1 (8·5)	−7·8 (5·8)		−15·3 (3·6)	−4·3 (8·2)	
Change of weight	lb.	−32·4 (14·7)	−30 (15)	>0·1	−33·2 (15·5)	−29·9 (13·4)	>0·1
	% of initial weight	−16·7 (6)	−16 (6·7)		−16·9 (6·2)	−16 (6)	
Period of treatment (months)		6·4 (2·5)	7·8 (4·9)	>0·1	6·5 (2·6)	7·6 (4·8)	>0·1

Group A are compared with those of Group B, the differences of the changes in both systolic and diastolic pressure are still statistically significant ($P < 0{\cdot}001$ in each case). This comparison shows that the combination of errors due to arm-girth reduction and variability during the experiment is insufficient to account for the fall of blood-pressure experienced by the Group A patients. Group A patients experienced a real, rather than an apparent, fall of blood-pressure when compared with the unsuccessfully treated patients of Group B.

Measurement error. The precautions taken to avoid error in the measurement of blood-pressure have already been stated. In order to confirm the fact that these precautions were adequate, the blood-pressure differences between Group A and Group B were tested by employing an average of the second and third blood-pressure readings as the initial reading, and an average of the last two monthly readings as the final reading. This procedure resulted in little change in the figures, and the differences between the two groups for both systolic and diastolic pressures still remained highly significant ($P < 0{\cdot}001$).

The correlation coefficients and regression lines. The correlation coefficient (r) for loss of weight in pounds and fall of systolic blood-pressure in mm. Hg, calculated for the combined Groups A and B, is 0·58 ($P < 0{\cdot}001$); the correlation similarly calculated for diastolic pressure is 0·54 ($P < 0{\cdot}001$). Since Groups A and B comprise the total number of hypertensive women under treatment, these correlation coefficients provide additional evidence that loss of weight was significantly associated with both systolic and diastolic falls of blood-pressure readings. A similar calculation for all the patients with normal blood-pressure (Group C and Group D) gives $r = 0{\cdot}46$ ($P = 0{\cdot}05$) for systolic blood-pressure, and $r = 0{\cdot}44$ ($0{\cdot}05 > P > 0{\cdot}02$) for diastolic blood-pressure. These correlations reach the borderline of statistical significance, and show that in these groups, also, loss of weight was associated with fall of blood-pressure. The regression coefficient for systolic blood-pressure was 0·22, indicating that the patients with normal blood-pressure experienced a fall of 2·2 mm. Hg. for each 10 lb. of weight lost. The regression coefficient for diastolic blood-pressure was 0·16, showing that the patients' diastolic blood-pressure fell 1·6 mm. for each 10 lb. of weight lost. These figures confirm the belief that the correction for reduced arm-diameter was approximately correct; but it should

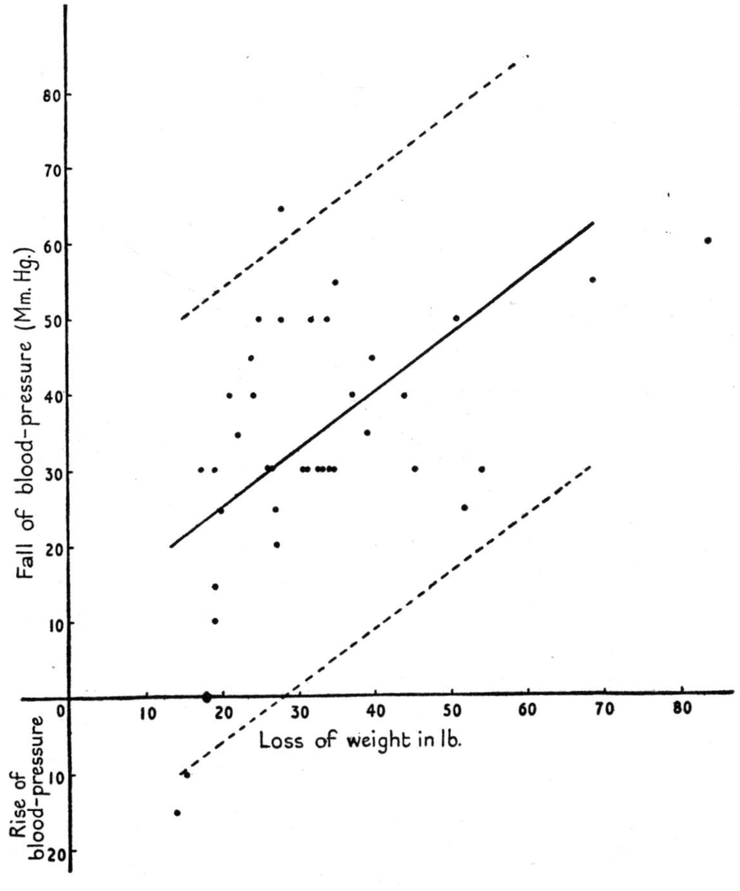

FIG. 1. Relation of fall in systolic blood-pressure to loss of weight in Group A (obese hypertensive women who lost weight).
Correlation coefficient $r = 0{\cdot}61$ ($p < 0{\cdot}001$).
Regression: $y = 0{\cdot}744x + 9{\cdot}7$.
Broken lines above and below the regression line show 95 per cent. confidence limits (= 29·5 mm.).

be noted that the standard deviation from these regression lines is high, being 7·8 mm. in the case of the systolic blood-pressure and 5·7 mm. in the case of diastolic pressure.

The remaining regressions refer only to Group A (obese hypertensive women who lost more than 14 lb. in weight). The correlation coefficient for fall of systolic blood-pressure in mm. Hg and loss of body-weight in lb. is 0·61 ($P <$ 0·001); these data are graphically represented in Fig. 1. The regression coefficient in Fig. 1 implies that patients experienced a fall of 7·4 mm. Hg systolic blood-pressure for each 10 lb. of body-weight lost.[3] The fall of systolic blood-pressure is also well correlated with the percentage loss of initial body-weight ($r = 0{\cdot}53$, $P < 0{\cdot}001$). If the fall of systolic blood-pressure is expressed as a percentage of the initial blood-pressure, this figure correlates well with the percentage loss of initial body-weight ($r = 0{\cdot}5$, $P < 0{\cdot}01$), but correlates less well with the fall of body-weight in lb. ($r = 0{\cdot}31$, $P = 0{\cdot}05$). The correlation

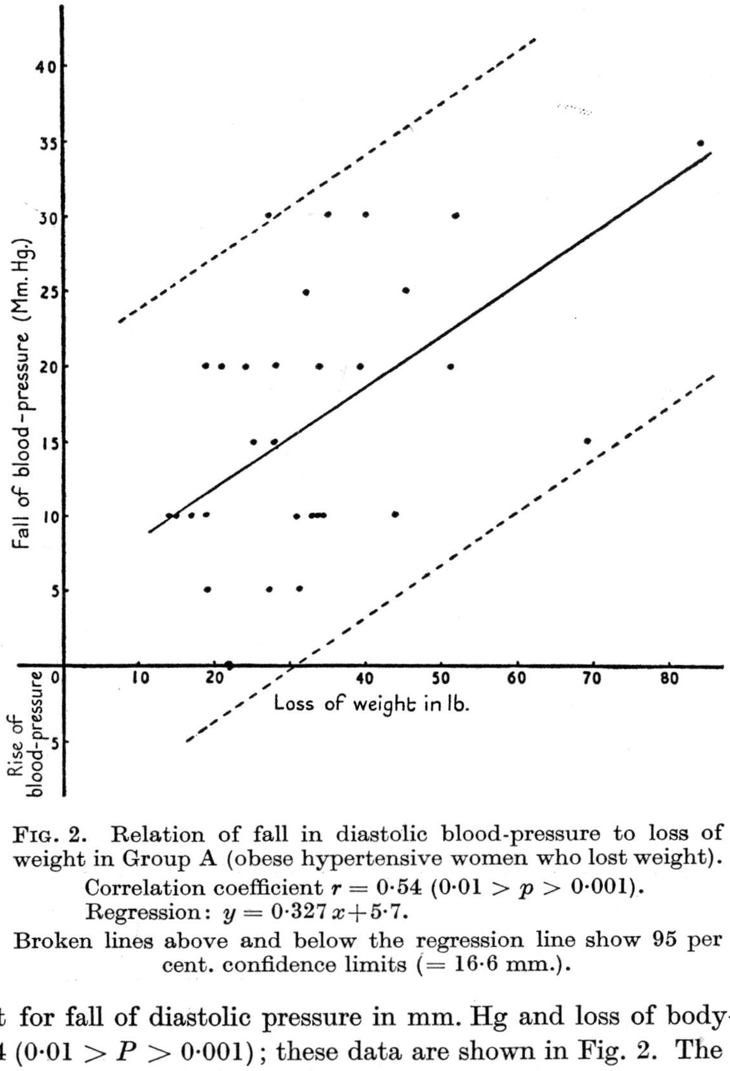

FIG. 2. Relation of fall in diastolic blood-pressure to loss of weight in Group A (obese hypertensive women who lost weight).
Correlation coefficient $r = 0{\cdot}54$ ($0{\cdot}01 > p > 0{\cdot}001$).
Regression: $y = 0{\cdot}327\,x + 5{\cdot}7$.
Broken lines above and below the regression line show 95 per cent. confidence limits (= 16·6 mm.).

coefficient for fall of diastolic pressure in mm. Hg and loss of body-weight in lb. is 0·54 ($0{\cdot}01 > P > 0{\cdot}001$); these data are shown in Fig. 2. The regression coefficient shows that the patients experienced a fall of 3·3 mm. in diastolic blood-pressure for each 10 lb. loss of body-weight. Again the fall of diastolic pressure measured in mm. Hg correlates well with the percentage loss of initial body-weight ($r = 0{\cdot}57$, $P < 0{\cdot}001$), but when this fall of diastolic pressure is expressed as a percentage of the initial pressure its correlation with the loss of

[3] Figs. 1 and 2 show the regression lines and their '95 per cent. confidence limits'. Statistically, 95 per cent. confidence limits are of restricted validity, but in practice they provide a useful measure of the variation about a regression line.

body-weight in pounds, and also with the percentage loss of initial body-weight, is poor, the correlation coefficients not being statistically significant ($P > 0{\cdot}1$).

Follow-up. It was originally hoped that all the patients would be followed up one year after their treatment had ceased, but this proved impossible, and only 19 of the 38 successfully treated Group A patients were seen at this time. Contact with nearly all the control group of 39 patients was lost. Fifteen of the 19 Group A patients had, with the aid of the diet sheets issued, maintained their weights between the limits of 7 lb. above or below their weights at the end of the experiment. The blood-pressures of these 15 patients at the time of follow-up were compared with their blood-pressures at the end of the experiment; the differences between these readings were not statistically different. This incomplete and inadequate follow-up suggests that the fall of blood-pressure obtained at the end of the experiment was sustained.

Discussion

The experimental data, tested for sampling error, variability during the experiment, and error of instrumental measurement, indicate that in this highly selected group of obese hypertensive women a substantial fall of body-weight was accompanied by a true fall of both systolic and diastolic blood-pressure. The demonstration that the results were unaltered when the blood-pressure changes were calculated as percentage changes, rather than stated directly in mm. of mercury, gives confidence that the findings were not biased by the fact that a linear scale for blood-pressure tends to overemphasize the importance of deviations of blood-pressure in the higher ranges (Hamilton, Pickering, Roberts, and Sowry, 1954). It is desirable to stress the fact that these patients were a highly selected and remarkably homogeneous group of elderly, extremely obese, and moderately hypertensive women. Sixty-five per cent. of the patients stated that their obesity had commenced or become severe within the previous 10 years, usually following the menopause. Twenty per cent. of the patients admitted to a recent gain of weight within one year of attending for treatment. Blood-pressure readings prior to attending the out-patient department could be obtained in only a very few cases, so that the date of the onset of the hypertension remained unknown; but the comparatively short history of obesity in a number of the patients may have exerted a significant influence on the results.

It is difficult to compare these results with those of previous studies, since the other investigations differed markedly in design. The most complete and convincing paper is that of Adlersberg, Coler, and Laval (1946), in which the blood-pressure of 54 obese hypertensive patients was followed for an average period of eight months, during which time their weight fell by 9 lb. to 80 lb. These authors found that the blood-pressure was substantially reduced in 39 patients, and was practically unchanged in 15 patients. The falls of blood-pressure corresponding to varying degrees of weight reduction were similar to those found in the present investigation; in fact the similarity was so close that, for fall of systolic blood-pressure, 83 per cent. of their experimental points fell within the

95 per cent. confidence limits shown in Fig. 1, while for diastolic pressure 85 per cent. of their readings fell within the 95 per cent. confidence limits of Fig. 2. The important paper by Lups and Francke (1946–7) describes the blood-pressure response of 520 patients during periods of relative food shortage, severe food shortage, and food abundance, during and after the Second World War, in Holland. Although only one blood-pressure reading could be taken in each phase, because of the difficulties natural to a state of war, this enforced experiment yielded valuable information. It was found that during severe food shortage the regression coefficient for fall of systolic blood-pressure and decrease of weight was 0·268 (statistically highly significant), and during the period of food abundance the regression coefficient for increase of weight and rise of systolic blood-pressure was 0·167 (also highly significant). A similar relationship was found to hold for diastolic blood-pressure. Lups and Francke also found that the blood-pressure of hypertensive patients was altered by the food intake with a significantly greater frequency than that of patients with normal blood-pressure. Brozek, Chapman, and Keys (1948) cited Russian evidence, obtained under similar conditions (siege of Leningrad), leading to similar conclusions.

The mechanism by which obesity may alter the blood-pressure is as yet unknown. Numerous authors have drawn attention to the metabolic burden imposed by obesity, and the subject has been reviewed by Newburgh (1944). It can be calculated that the patients described in the present communication would have shown a basal oxygen consumption from 20 to 60 per cent. in excess of that shown by comparable persons of normal weight. Moreover, their oxygen consumption on exercise would have risen proportionately more than that of normal people, owing to the mechanical handicap of obesity. Taylor, Brozek, and Keys (1952) have shown in an excellent paper that in young, healthy, obese subjects this increase in basal oxygen consumption causes a relatively large increase in arteriovenous oxygen difference, and a relatively small increase of cardiac output. They showed that basal cardiac output was related to body-weight (correlation coefficient (r) = 0·54), to surface area (r = 0·54), to the weight of lean body-mass (r = 0·6), and finally to the weight of fat (r = 0·16). The coefficients of correlation relating basal cardiac work to body-weight, surface area, weight of fat-free tissue, and fat, were found to be 0·50, 0·55, 0·76, and 0·07 respectively. It is likely, as indeed the authors suggested, that the cardiovascular adjustments in the elderly, unfit, obese subject might prove to be much less efficient. The prognosis of hypertension complicated by obesity appears to be better than that of hypertension alone. Bechgaard (1946) followed the fate of 1,000 patients with hypertension, 311 of whom were 20 kg. or more above normal weight, and showed that the mortality was considerably less in the obese groups. The value of Bechgaard's figures is uncertain, since all patients showing a single systolic blood-pressure reading of over 160 mm. Hg were classified as hypertensive. The series of Frant and Groen (1950), although smaller, appears more convincing; they, too, found that the obese hypertensive patient had a better prognosis. These findings, however, are influenced by the exaggeration in readings produced by the fat arm. If indeed obesity contributes to the hypertensive state, this relatively better prognosis might be expected, since the hypertension could be a 'physiological' response to the metabolic burden rather than a response to a definite pathological condition.

It is tempting to speculate on the aetiological importance of the patients' obesity in the genesis of their hypertension. Figs. 1 and 2 show that the blood-pressure response of the individual hypertensive, obese patient is unpredictable, and that estimates of blood-pressure response to weight reduction must be made on a group basis. The regression coefficient, although useful in expressing to a first approximation the relationship between the loss of weight and the fall of blood-pressure, has certain limitations when used for this purpose. It is clear that a linear relationship between these two factors cannot be expected except

TABLE V

Comparison between Group A and Group B in respect of the Number of Patients who Reached 'Normal' Blood-Pressure

Tested at three 'normal' levels for both systolic and diastolic pressure.

	Group A			*Group B*			
Level of 'normal' blood pressure	*Number exceeding 'normal' level at start*	*Number below 'normal' level at end*	*Percentage below 'normal' level at end*	*Number exceeding 'normal' level at start*	*Number below 'normal' level at end*	*Percentage below 'normal' level at end*	χ *and* P
150 systolic	38	15	40	21	0	0	11·2 ($P < 0{\cdot}001$)
160 systolic	35	22	63	19	0	0	17·3 ($P < 0{\cdot}001$)
170 systolic	32	25	78	18	4	22	14·8 ($P < 0{\cdot}001$)
90 diastolic	30	5	17	19	0	0	Expected cell frequency less than 5
100 diastolic	30	11	37	18	0	0	8·56 ($P < 0{\cdot}01$)
110 diastolic	25	24	96	11	8	73	4·18 ($P < 0{\cdot}05$)

over a comparatively narrow range of weight and blood-pressure. These reasons, and general principles, preclude any calculations involving extrapolation beyond the experimental regression point so as to estimate what part of the patients' hypertension was attributable to their obesity.

The fact that the blood-pressure of the group of obese hypertensive patients who lost more than 14 lb. in weight averaged $\frac{196 \text{ (s.d. } 32)}{116 \text{ (s.d. } 14)}$ at the start of the experiment and $\frac{163 \text{ (s.d. } 26)}{99 \text{ (s.d. } 13)}$ at the end, suggests that this group contained many patients whose hypertension was directly or indirectly related to their obese state. Table V shows the number and proportion of women in Groups A and B who attained 'normal' levels of blood-pressure. Owing to the uncertainty as to the correct value for 'normal' blood-pressure, and also in order to avoid a sampling bias in the data, these numbers and proportions have been given with three values for 'normal' systolic blood-pressure, and three values for 'normal' diastolic blood-pressure. The type of comparison shown in Table V is valid only if the frequency distributions for initial blood-pressure in groups A and B are comparable; these frequency distributions were analysed, and shown to be reasonably comparable in that the values for P between the frequency cells exceeded 0·1. Table V shows that, for all levels of 'normal' systolic pressure, a substantial number of Group A patients attained normal levels, and in each case the difference between Group A and Group B was statistically significant. The figures for diastolic pressure are less convincing because of the smaller numbers involved, but here again a substantial number of hypertensive patients reached normal levels of blood-pressure, and the difference between Group A and Group B was significant at the levels of 100 and 110 mm. Hg. These figures suggest that obesity was an aetiological factor of importance in the hypertension of the successfully treated Group A.

Acknowledgements

This investigation was made at Queen Mary's Hospital for the East End, and it is a pleasure to record my indebtedness to the Physicians (Dr. Arnold Osman, Dr. Kenneth Playfair, and Dr. Claude Elman) who allowed me to treat and observe patients under their care. I am most greatful to Professor G. W. Pickering for reading the manuscript and for making several important suggestions, and to Dr. P. Armitage, of the Medical Research Council Statistical Research Unit, whose advice was most valuable.

Summary

1. A group of hypertensive obese women whose weight was reduced experienced a fall of both systolic and diastolic blood-pressure, which was statistically highly significant ($P < 0{\cdot}001$) when compared with a similar group who failed to lose weight.

2. Although blood-pressure was measured by the indirect method, the experiment was designed to give an estimate of the error introduced through the decrease of arm-girth due to loss of weight. This experimental estimate was compared with a second estimate obtained by measurement of the arm-girth before and after weight reduction. These two estimates of error being found to agree, the observed falls of blood-pressure, in the group whose weight was reduced, were corrected to allow for the error of the indirect method of blood-pressure estimation.

3. The corrected fall of blood-pressure in the group of hypertensive obese women whose weight was reduced, when compared with the fall of blood-pressure in the similar group who failed to lose weight, was found to be statistically highly significant ($P < 0{\cdot}001$). It was concluded that weight reduction in this group of obese hypertensive patients had resulted in a true fall of blood-pressure.

4. Calculation of the number of patients who had attained normal levels of blood-pressure at the end of the experiment showed that the difference in favour of the group in which weight was reduced was significant ($P < 0{\cdot}001$) for systolic blood-pressure, and also significant for diastolic blood-pressure ($P < 0{\cdot}01$). It was concluded that obesity had been of aetiological importance in the hypertension of the group of women whose weight was reduced.

REFERENCES

Adlersberg, D., Coler, H. R., and Laval J. (1946) *J. Mt. Sinai Hosp.* **12,** 984.
Bauman, L. (1928) *J. Amer. Med. Ass.* **90,** 22.
Bechgaard, P. (1946) *Acta med. scand.* Suppl. **172.**
Bordley, J., III, Connor, C. A. R., Hamilton, W. F., Kerr, W. J., and Wiggers, C. J. (1951) *Circulation,* **4,** 503.
Boynton, R. E., and Todd, R. L. (1948) *Amer. J. Med. Sci.* **216,** 397.
Bram, I. (1947) *Med. Rec.* **160,** 350.
Browne, F. J., and Dodds, G. H. (1939) *J. Obstet. Gynaec.* **46,** 443.
Brozek, J., Chapman, C. B., and Keys, A. (1948) *J. Amer. Med. Ass.* **137,** 1569.
Cardiac Society of Great Britain and Ireland (1939) *Brit. Med. J.* **2,** 184.
Corwin, J., and Herrick, W. W. (1927) *Amer. J. Obstet. Gynec.* **14,** 783.
Frant, R., and Groen, J. (1950) *Arch. Int. Med.* **85,** 727.
Green, M. B., and Beckman, M. (1948) *New York St. J. Med.* **48,** 1250.
Hamilton, M. F., Pickering, G. W., Roberts, J. A. F., and Sowry, C. S. G. (1954) *Clin. Sci.* **13,** 271.
Hartman, H. R., and Ghrist, D. G. (1929) *Arch. Int. Med.* **44,** 877.
Herrick, W. W., and Tillman, A. J. B. (1935) Ibid. **55,** 643.
Isenhour, C. E., Kuder, K., and Dill, L. V. (1942) *Amer. J. Med. Sci.* **203,** 333.
Keys, A., Henschel, A., and Taylor, H. L. (1947) *Amer. J. Physiol.* **150,** 153.
Kotte, J. H., Iglauer, A., and McGuire, J. (1944) *Amer. Heart J.* **28,** 476.
Levy, R. L., White, P. D., Stroud, W. D., and Hillman, C. C. (1946) *J. Amer. Med. Ass.* **131,** 951.
Lups, S., and Francke, C. (1946–7) *Acta med. scand.* **126,** 449.
Martin, L. (1952) *Lancet,* **2,** 1051.
Master, A. M., Garfield, C. I., and Walters, M. B. (1952) *Normal Blood Pressure and Hypertension,* London.
—— and Oppenheimer, E. T. (1929) *J. Amer. Med. Ass.* **92,** 1652.
Metropolitan Life Insurance Stat. Bull. **23,** 6 (Oct. 1942).
Newburgh, L. H. (1944) *Physiol. Rev.* **24,** 18.
Preble, W. E. (1923) *Boston Med. Surg. J.* **188,** 617.
Ragan, C., and Bordley, J. (1941) *Bull. Johns Hopkins Hosp.* **69,** 504.
Roberts, L. N., Smiley, J. R., and Manning, G. W. (1953) *Circulation,* **8,** 232.
Robinson, S. C., Bruce, R. M., and Mass, J. (1939–40) *J. Lab. Clin. Med.* **25,** 807.
Rose, R. H. (1922) *New York Med. J.* **115,** 752.
Short, J. J., and Johnson, H. J. (1939) *Amer. J. Med. Sci.* **198,** 220.
Steele, J. M. (1942) *J. Mt. Sinai Hosp.* **8,** 1042.
Taylor, H. L., Brozek, J., and Keys, A. (1952) *J. Clin. Invest.* **31,** 976.
Terry, A. H., Jnr. (1923) *J. Amer. Med. Ass.* **81,** 1283.
Thomson, A. E., and Doupe, J. (1949) *Canad. J. Research,* Sect. E, **27,** 72.
Wendkos, M. H., and Rossman, P. L. (1943) *Amer. Heart J.* **26,** 623.
Wood, J. E., Jnr., and Cash, J. R. (1939) *Ann. Int. Med.* **13,** 81.

616.24–002.5–085

A FIVE-YEAR ASSESSMENT OF PATIENTS IN A CONTROLLED TRIAL OF STREPTOMYCIN IN PULMONARY TUBERCULOSIS[1]

Report to the Tuberculosis Chemotherapy Trials Committee of the Medical Research Council

BY WALLACE FOX, IAN SUTHERLAND, AND THE LATE MARC DANIELS

(*From the Tuberculosis and Statistical Research Units of the Medical Research Council*)

IN September 1946 a committee of the Medical Research Council planned the first controlled clinical trial of streptomycin in the treatment of pulmonary tuberculosis. Patients with acute extensive disease were allocated at random to two series: the patients in one series received streptomycin 2 gm. daily for four months in addition to rest in bed; those in the other series received only rest in bed. It will be recalled that at that time the inclusion of the control series was ethically justified by the very limited supplies of streptomycin. Detailed results after the patients had been observed for six months have already been published (Medical Research Council, 1948), and some results at the end of one year were presented in an addendum to that report. Over the period of observation the patients treated with streptomycin fared much better, as a group, than those treated only with rest in bed. The present report gives a comparison of the two series of patients for a period of five years from the start of the trial.

I. *Plan and Conduct of the Trial*

Type of case. The type of case included in the trial was carefully defined as follows: acute, progressive, bilateral pulmonary tuberculosis of presumably recent origin, bacteriologically proved, and unsuitable for collapse therapy; age-group 15 to 30 years. Before acceptance all cases were reviewed by a central panel of clinicians to ensure that they conformed to this definition. Each patient who was accepted for the trial was admitted to one of seven co-operating centres. Treatment was then decided by reference to confidential lists based upon random-sampling numbers. These lists determined whether the patient received streptomycin and rest in bed, or only rest in bed. Full details of this strict procedure will be found in the earlier report (Medical Research Council, 1948). Of 107 patients admitted to the trial, 55 were allocated to the streptomycin (S) series and 52 to the control (C) series. A study of the radiographs taken on entry to the trial has recently been made to determine in each patient the

[1] Received April 8, 1954.

number of zones of the lungs (for definitions see Appendix) showing evidence of disease. This assessment was undertaken by a single independent observer unaware of the treatment allotted to any patient. It demonstrates clearly the extensiveness of the disease in the patients studied, since 52 of the 55 S patients and 51 of the 52 C patients had involvement of six, five, or four zones; the remaining four patients had disease in three zones. All six zones were involved in 38 per cent. of S and 46 per cent. of C patients.

Treatment and observation. All the patients were admitted to the trial between January and September 1947. After a week of preliminary investigation and assessment of clinical condition, each patient entered the trial for a period of six months. Patients in the streptomycin series received streptomycin 2 gm. daily, in four intramuscular injections of 0·5 gm., for a period of four months (a few received rather longer courses); those in the control series received no chemotherapy. Patients in both series remained in bed at the centre for at least the six-month period, and during this time detailed clinical, bacteriological, and radiographic observations were made. From four months onwards the clinician was free to undertake any treatment he wished for patients in either series.

Two-year and five-year assessment. Although some information as to the progress of the patients was obtained one year after the start of treatment, no attempt was made to study their subsequent progress until five years had elapsed since entry to the trial. All the patients were then traced, and assessments of their clinical condition at the end of two and five years were obtained, together with details of the treatment which they had received during the five-year period. Whenever possible a complete series of radiographs for each patient was assembled, and those made on admission to the trial, at four months, at two years, and at five years, were assessed by an independent panel of two radiologists and a chest physician. There are some deficiencies in the radiographic evaluation at two years, because it was the policy in some clinics to destroy the radiographs of patients who died; moreover, in one hospital some of the radiographs of two patients were lost in the flooding of a basement, while in another all the radiographs of one patient were destroyed by fire. Bacteriological analyses were impracticable, since many of the surviving patients, both at two and at five years, no longer had active disease, and examinations for tubercle bacilli had been performed very infrequently.

II. *Comparability of the Two Treatment Series*

Interpretation of long-term comparisons. It was shown in the earlier report (Medical Research Council, 1948) that random allocation had largely equalized the clinical condition of the two series on admission. If anything, there was a greater number of very severe cases in the series treated with streptomycin. Thus during the first four months, when the regimens differed only in the course of streptomycin given to the one series, it was legitimate to ascribe the better progress of these patients to the effects of the streptomycin. After four months, however, the clinicians were free to institute what treatment they felt would most benefit the patient. This fact introduces a complication in the interpretation of the long-term results, which will have been influenced by the varied treatment given after the stipulated four-month period. It should be noted, however, that the initial period of specified treatment came at the acute and frequently critical stage of the disease, when its greatest effect might be expected. Thereafter all the patients in both series presumably received the best treatment available to them, and there is no reason to suppose that one series of patients was more favoured than the other. This point is examined specifically in the following analyses of the additional chemotherapy given to patients in the two series, and of the collapse therapy undertaken, in the five-year period.

Chemotherapy in the first two years. Of the 55 S patients, 14 had a course of streptomycin which was longer than the prescribed four months (one patient was treated for a further two months, two for six weeks, six for one month, and five for two weeks). Apart from these prolongations of the original course of treatment, only four of the 54 S and five of the 42 C patients who survived four months received any chemotherapy between four months and two years after entry to the trial. One S and four C patients had short courses of streptomycin in the next 20 months (a three-month course for one C patient, and five weeks or less for the other four patients); two S patients and one C patient received courses of para-aminosalicylic acid (PAS) (of ten and five months for the S patients, and of three months for the C patient); one S patient had five weeks of streptomycin and subsequently two months of PAS. Quite apart from the cautious attitude of clinicians to the new drugs, streptomycin did not become widely available until the end of 1949, and PAS only began to come into use in the middle of 1948. The value of combining these two drugs was not demonstrated until 1949 (U.S.A. Veterans Administration, 1949; Medical Research Council, 1949, 1950).

Chemotherapy in the next three years. In spite of the greater availability both of streptomycin and of PAS, comparatively little chemotherapy was given to the patients even in the next three years. Twenty-four of the 31 S patients and 10 of the 20 C patients who survived two years received no chemotherapy in the next three years. One C patient had streptomycin alone for three weeks. Four S and two C patients received courses of PAS alone (of nine, six, three months, and one month respectively for the S patients, and of six and five months for the C patients). Two S and two C patients had courses of streptomycin plus PAS (of four and three months respectively for the S patients, and of two months and one month for the C patients). One S patient had 10 months of PAS alone and subsequently three months of streptomycin plus PAS; one C patient had three months of streptomycin alone and subsequently two months of PAS alone; two more C patients each had four months of PAS alone and later two months of streptomycin plus PAS. In addition one C patient received a three-month course of isoniazid alone, and another a nine-month course of thiosemicarbazone. Although a higher proportion of C patients received some chemotherapy, the average duration of the courses was shorter than for the S patients. It may be concluded that, apart from the original course of streptomycin, neither series was more favoured in the chemotherapy administered during the five years after entry to the trial.

Collapse therapy in the first two years. In view of the variety and combinations of collapse measures which were initiated, it is possible to make only broad comparisons between the two series. The recorded incidence of crushes and re-crushes of the phrenic nerve is similar in the two series, but it is certain that some have not been recorded. An artificial pneumothorax or pneumoperitoneum was occasionally abandoned shortly after induction. These reversible forms of collapse therapy have been regarded as established, and included in the analysis, only if they were maintained for at least three months. During the first two years 24 S patients and 18 C patients received one or more forms of collapse therapy. A pneumoperitoneum was established in 14 S patients and 12 C patients. An artificial pneumothorax was established in 13 S patients (bilateral in one case) and in seven C patients (bilateral in four cases). There were two thoracoplasties in the S series, and three thoracoplasties and one extrapleural pneumothorax in the C series. Two S patients had Monaldi drainage.

Collapse therapy in the next three years. In the next three years very little collapse therapy was initiated in either series. A pneumoperitoneum was established in one S and one C patient, and an artificial pneumothorax in two S patients (bilateral in one case) and in one C patient. One S patient had a thoracoplasty. All these patients had already had at least one other collapse measure previously. It should be noted that there were no resections in either series.

Over the five-year period collapse therapy was established for a larger number of S than of C patients; but, as will be shown below, there were more early survivors in the S series, and so more opportunities for surgery. It may be concluded that there are no notable differences in the incidence of established collapse therapy between the two series during the five years.

III. *Results during the Five-year Period*

Mortality in the five-year period. The mortality in the five-year period is analysed in Table I and the Figure.[2] All the deaths were due to pulmonary tuberculosis, except for one S patient who died of monocytic leukaemia after 26 months. The cause of death was confirmed by a post-mortem examination, which also showed 'healing fibrocaseous tuberculosis' (Beven, 1951). Up to the end of the first 18 months there was a considerable difference in the mortality of the two series; by this time 30 (58 per cent.) of the 52 patients in the control series had died, and 19 (35 per cent.) of the 55 patients in the streptomycin series; this difference (like the corresponding differences at six and 12 months) is statistically highly significant. In the next 12 months only three control patients died. The mortality in the streptomycin series, however, continued at the same rate as before, and there were 10 deaths in the corresponding period.

[2] A comprehensive check of the dates of death revealed a minor inaccuracy in the mortality figures at one year which were presented in the addendum to the earlier report (Medical Research Council, 1948).

Thus, after 30 months, 63 per cent. of the control series and 53 per cent. of the streptomycin series were dead, a difference which, although still statistically significant, is much smaller. The streptomycin series maintained a slight

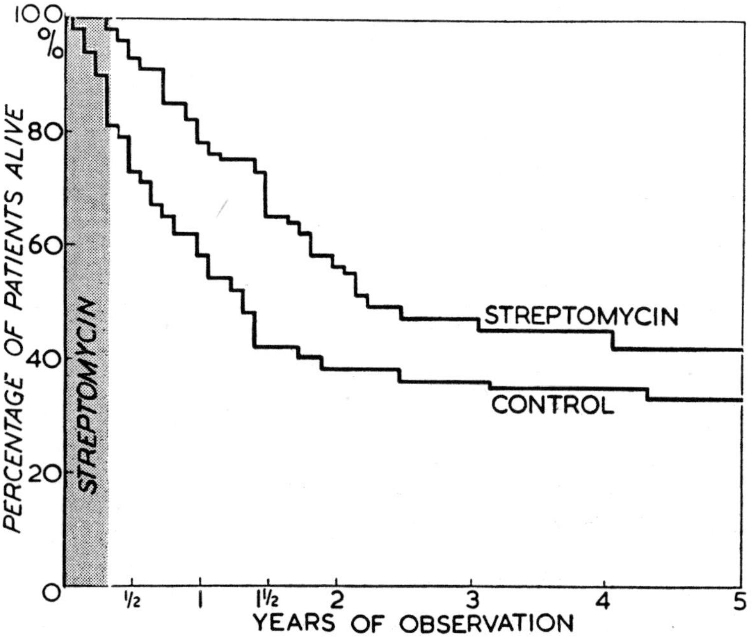

Percentage survival in streptomycin and control series for a five-year period (55 streptomycin and 52 control patients).

TABLE I

Mortality in the Two Treatment Series during the Five-year Period

		Deaths in the first																			
Treatment series	*Number of patients*	*6 months*		*1 year*		*18 months*		*2 years*		*2½ years*		*3 years*		*3½ years*		*4 years*		*4½ years*		*5 years*	
		No.	*%*	*No.*	*%*	*No.*	*%*	*No.*	*%*	*No.*	*%*	*No.*	*%*	*No.*	*%*	*No.*	*%*	*No.*	*%*	*No.*	*%*
Streptomycin	55	4	*7*	12	*22*	19	*35*	24	*44*	29*	*53*	29*	*53*	30*	*55*	30*	*55*	32*	*58*	32*	*58*
Control	52	14	*27*	22	*42*	30	*58*	32	*62*	33	*63*	33	*63*	34	*65*	34	*65*	35	*67*	35	*67*

* Including one non-tuberculous death.

advantage for the remainder of the five-year period, during which time two further control and three further streptomycin patients died.

Clinical assessment at two years. The disease in the survivors at two years was classified by the clinician in charge as quiescent or active (for definitions, see Appendix). The working capacity was recorded as 'full activity', 'modified activity', or 'nil' (for definitions, see Appendix). Patients who were not working were divided into those receiving treatment at home and those who were in a hospital or sanatorium. Table II shows the disease status of the surviving patients in the two series at two years. Of the 31 S patients 61 per cent. had attained quiescence, compared with 30 per cent. of the 20 C patients. Of the 19 S patients who had attained quiescence, 11 had done so in the absence of any collapse therapy or further chemotherapy (apart from prolongations of the original course in four patients). Of the six similar C patients, only one had attained quiescence in the absence of collapse therapy or chemotherapy. Table II also shows that nine of the 31 S patients had returned to full activity, and a further four to modified activity, compared with two and three respectively of the 20 C patients. Over this period the S patients have thus fared better than

TABLE II

Disease Status and Working Capacity of Survivors in the Two Treatment Series at Two Years

Treatment series	Number of patients alive at two years		Disease status: Quiescent		Disease status: Active		Working capacity: Full activity		Working capacity: Modified activity		Working capacity: Nil: At home		Working capacity: Nil: In hospital or sanatorium	
	No.	*%*	*No.*	*%*	*No.*	*%*	*No.*	*%*	*No.*	*%*	*No.*	*%*	*No.*	*%*
Streptomycin	31	*100*	19	*61*	12	*39*	9	*29*	4	*13*	9	*29*	9	*29*
Control	20	*100*	6	*30*	14	*70*	2	*10*	3	*15*	11	*55*	4	*20*

the C patients, not only in respect of mortality but also in the clinical progress of the survivors.

Radiographic changes in the first two years. Radiographic changes in the first two years were assessed by a panel of three members, Dr. L. G. Blair, Dr. A. F. Foster-Carter, and Dr. G. Simon. In making their assessments the members were unaware to which treatment series each patient had been allocated. Four degrees of improvement were allowed—slight, moderate, considerable, and exceptional; and three of deterioration—slight, moderate, and considerable. In evaluating the changes in the first two years, three radiographs were used, namely, those taken on entry to the trial, at four months, and at two years. Intermediate films were studied if these were available and requested. An assessment was first made covering the whole two-year period, and the changes were then apportioned between the first four months (the prescribed treatment period) and the subsequent 20 months. Each panel member interpreted the films at a separate session, and the results were then collated. If there was agreement between two (or all three) of the members on the assessment covering the whole period, and on the apportionment within the period, the agreed readings were accepted as final. Otherwise the films were reviewed and discussed by the members of the panel at a joint session, and a final agreed report was obtained. No comparisons were possible over the first two years for seven S and three C patients; relevant radiographs of five patients had been destroyed or mislaid, those of two were lost in a flood, and of one in a fire; two patients had no radiograph taken at two years (one was too ill to be moved). Of the seven S patients, the disease was quiescent in three and active in four (two of whom died within the next two months). Of the three C patients, the disease was quiescent in one and active in two (one of whom died five months later). The results for the remaining patients are presented in Table III. Of 24 S patients seven showed exceptional improvement and 10 considerable improvement, compared with no exceptional and eight considerable improvements in 17 C patients. When the changes were apportioned, it was found that a higher proportion of S than of C patients improved during the first four months. On the other hand, during the next 20 months the improvements were very similar in the two series.

Changes in cavitation in the first two years. Table IV shows the changes in extent of cavitation during the first two years. The changes were assessed from

TABLE III

Changes in Radiographic Appearances of Survivors in the Two Treatment Series in the First Two Years

Period and treatment series	Total of patients assessed		Improvement: Exceptional		Improvement: Considerable		Improvement: Moderate		Improvement: Slight		No change		Deterioration: Slight		Deterioration: Moderate		Deterioration: Considerable	
	No.	%	No.	%	No.	%	No.	%	No.	%	No.	%	No.	%	No.	%	No.	%
0–2 years:																		
Streptomycin	24*	*100*	7	*29*	10	*42*	2	*8*	1	*4*	1	*4*	3	*13*	0	*0*	0	*0*
Control	17*	*100*	0	*0*	8	*47*	3	*18*	3	*18*	2	*12*	1	*6*	0	*0*	0	*0*
0–4 months:																		
Streptomycin	20†	*100*	0	*0*	2	*10*	6	*30*	10	*50*	1	*5*	1	*5*	0	*0*	0	*0*
Control	15†	*100*	0	*0*	1	*7*	1	*7*	5	*33*	8	*53*	0	*0*	0	*0*	0	*0*
4 months–2 years:																		
Streptomycin	20†	*100*	0	*0*	2	*10*	9	*45*	4	*20*	1	*5*	3	*15*	1	*5*	0	*0*
Control	15†	*100*	0	*0*	2	*13*	5	*33*	4	*27*	3	*20*	1	*7*	0	*0*	0	*0*

* For seven S and three C patients one or the other radiograph was not available.
† For 11 S and five C patients one or the other radiograph was not available.

TABLE IV

Changes in Cavitation on Standard Radiographs in the Two Treatment Series in the First Two Years

Treatment series	Number of patients alive at two years	No initial cavitation	Patients with initial cavitation: Total	Disappearance of cavitation	Cavities smaller or fewer	No change	Cavities larger or more numerous
Streptomycin	24*	5	19	12	4	0	3
Control	17*	0	17	7	3	4	3

* For seven S and three C patients one or the other radiograph was not available.

single postero-anterior radiographs taken on entry to the trial and at two years. No tomograms or radiographs taken in special positions were submitted to the panel. Of the 24 S patients for whom records are available, five had no initial cavitation and did not develop any cavities. In 12 of the remaining 19 S patients, and in seven of the 17 C patients, no cavitation was apparent at two years. Three patients in each series showed more cavitation at two years than on entry to the trial. Thus 37 per cent. of the surviving S patients and 59 per cent. of the surviving C patients still retained cavities visible on a standard radiograph at two years.

Clinical assessment at five years. The disease in patients who survived five years was classified as arrested, quiescent, or active (for definitions, see Appendix). Other aspects of progress were recorded in the same way as at two years. Table V shows the disease status of the patients in the two series at five years. Of the 23 S patients, the disease was arrested in 57 per cent. and quiescent in 26 per cent. The corresponding percentages for the 17 C patients were 29 per

TABLE V

Disease Status and Working Capacity of Survivors in the Two Treatment Series at Five Years

Treatment series	Total of patients alive at five years		Disease status: Arrested		Quiescent		Active		Working capacity: Full activity		Modified activity		Nil: At home		Nil: In hospital or sanatorium	
	No.	%	No.	%	No.	%	No.	%	No.	%	No.	%	No.	%	No.	%
Streptomycin	23	*100*	13	*57*	6	*26*	4	*17*	15	*65*	5	*22*	2	*9*	1	*4*
Control	17	*100*	5	*29*	4	*24*	8	*47*	8	*47*	4	*24*	4	*24*	1	*6*

TABLE VI

Changes in Radiographic Appearances of Survivors in the Two Treatment Series in the Five-year Period

Period and treatment series	Total of patients assessed		Improvement: Exceptional		Considerable		Moderate		Slight		No change		Deterioration: Slight		Moderate		Considerable	
	No.	%	No.	%	No.	%	No.	%	No.	%	No.	%	No.	%	No.	%	No.	%
0–5 years:																		
Streptomycin	22*	*100*	8	*36*	11	*50*	1	*5*	1	*5*	0	*0*	1	*5*	0	*0*	0	*0*
Control	17	*100*	6	*35*	3	*18*	5	*29*	0	*0*	1	*6*	1	*6*	1	*6*	0	*0*
0–2 years: §																		
Streptomycin	20†	*100*	6	*30*	9	*45*	3	*15*	1	*5*	1	*5*	0	*0*	0	*0*	0	*0*
Control	16†	*100*	1	*6*	5	*31*	5	*31*	2	*13*	1	*6*	2	*13*	0	*0*	0	*0*
2–5 years:																		
Streptomycin	19‡	*100*	0	*0*	1	*5*	0	*0*	7	*37*	10	*53*	0	*0*	1	*5*	0	*0*
Control	16‡	*100*	0	*0*	0	*0*	3	*19*	8	*50*	3	*19*	0	*0*	2	*13*	0	*0*

* One S patient was too ill to leave home for a radiograph at five years.
† For three S patients and one C patient one or the other radiograph was not available.
‡ For four S patients and one C patient one or the other radiograph was not available.
§ The assessments for the period 0–2 years in this Table are not necessarily the same as those in Table III, because the five-year assessment utilizes more radiographic information and covers a longer period of time than that made at two years.

cent. and 24 per cent. It is noteworthy that, of the 13 S patients with arrested disease, nine had received neither collapse therapy nor additional chemotherapy (apart from prolongations of the original course in four patients) at any time between four months and five years. Of the five similar C patients, two had received neither collapse therapy nor chemotherapy during the five years. Moreover, all the three C patients whose disease was arrested after collapse therapy underwent a thoracoplasty. Of the four similar S patients, only one had major surgical treatment—also a thoracoplasty. Of the 23 S patients, 15 had returned to full activity and five to modified activity, compared with eight and four respectively of the 17 C patients (Table V). Only one patient in each series was still in a hospital or sanatorium. Over the five-year period the S patients have thus fared better than the C patients, not only in respect of mortality but also in the clinical progress of the survivors.

Radiographic changes in the five-year period. Radiographic changes over the five years were evaluated by the panel in a similar manner to the two-year changes, by using single radiographs taken on entry to the trial, at two years, and at five years, with intermediate films if these were available and requested. The change over the whole period was assessed first, and was then apportioned between the first two and the next three years. The radiographs were read by the panel members at sessions subsequent to those given for the two-year study. Because the five-year assessment utilizes more radiographic information and covers a longer period of time than that made at two years, the category of radiographic change assigned to a patient for the first two years is not necessarily the same in the two assessments. The radiographic information over the five-year period, in contrast to that at two years, is complete except for one S patient, who was too ill to leave home for a radiograph at five years. The results for the remaining patients are presented in Table VI. Nineteen of 22 S patients showed considerable or exceptional improvement, compared with nine of 17 C patients. The numbers with exceptional radiographic improvement were eight S and six C patients. When the changes were apportioned, it was found that a higher proportion of S than of C patients improved during the first two years. On the other hand, during the next three years the changes were similar in the two series; they were also much slighter during this period than in the first two years.

Changes in cavitation in the five-year period. Table VII shows the changes in extent of cavitation during the five-year period. The changes were assessed from single postero-anterior radiographs taken on entry to the trial and at five years. Again no tomograms or radiographs taken in special positions were submitted to the panel. Of the 22 S patients for whom records are available, five had no initial cavitation and did not develop any cavities. In 13 of the remaining 17 S patients, and in 10 of the same number of C patients, no cavitation was apparent at five years. One S patient and three C patients showed more cavitation at five years than on entry to the trial. Thus even after five years 24 per cent. of the surviving S patients, and 41 per cent. of the surviving C patients, retained cavitation visible on a standard radiograph.

Nature of radiographic improvements in the five-year period. The standard radiographs taken on entry to the trial, and at five years, for the 21 S and 14 C patients in whom radiographic improvement had occurred, were submitted to a single independent observer for appraisal of the nature of the improvements which had taken place. The study was made without the observer knowing the treatment of any patient. Improvement was classified under the following headings: resolution, fibrosis, calcification, lobar atelectasis, reduction in cavitation, and disappearance of cavitation (see Appendix). The observer was asked to record only major changes. Resolution was reported in all 35 patients (Table VIII). Disappearance of, or reduction in, cavitation was reported in 15 of the 16 S patients with initial cavitation, and in 11 of the 14 C patients. Calcification occurred in 10 S and five C patients, and fibrosis was recorded in

TABLE VII

Changes in Cavitation on Standard Radiographs in the Two Treatment Series in the Five-year Period

			Patients with initial cavitation				
Treatment series	*Number of patients alive at five years*	*No initial cavitation*	*Total*	*Disappearance of cavitation*	*Cavities smaller or fewer*	*No change*	*Cavities larger or more numerous*
Streptomycin	22*	5	17	13	2	1	1
Control	17	0	17	10	1	3	3

* One S patient was too ill to leave home for a radiograph at five years.

TABLE VIII

Nature of Major Changes in Radiographic Appearances in Patients who showed Radiographic Improvement in the Five-year Period

		Major radiographic change				
Treatment series	*Number of patients with radiographic improvement*	*Resolution*	*Disappearance of cavitation*	*Reduction in cavitation*	*Fibrosis*	*Calcification*
Streptomycin	21	21	13	2	4	10
Control	14	14	10	1	3	5

four S and three C patients. It is thus apparent that, among the survivors who showed radiographic improvement at five years, the major changes consisted in resolution and in disappearance of cavitation. The nature of the improvements was very similar in the two treatment series.

The mortality and course of the disease in the two treatment series have now been described. In the following sections an attempt is made to discover to what extent the mortality in each series depended upon the condition of the patients on admission to the trial and upon their response to the treatment during the first four months.

IV. *Prognostic Factors in Acute Bilateral Pulmonary Tuberculosis in Young Adults*

A study has been made of the extent to which the initial clinical condition and the immediate response to treatment affect the prognosis. The mortality during the five-year period in both the streptomycin and the control series has been related to the condition of the patient on admission to the trial, as judged by extent of cavitation, temperature, erythrocyte sedimentation rate (E.S.R. Westergren), and the number of lung zones involved (on a standard radiograph).

The mortality has also been related to the response to treatment during the first four months as indicated by the radiographic changes, the changes in the E.S.R. and temperature, the sputum positivity, and the emergence of bacterial resistance to streptomycin.

Cavitation. Mortality is associated with the extent of cavitation on admission, as is shown in Table IX. Of the 10 S and 11 C patients with extensive cavitation

TABLE IX

Mortality according to Degree of Cavitation on Admission

	Streptomycin series					Control series				
	Number of patients	Degree of cavitation on admission				Number of patients	Degree of cavitation on admission			
		0	1-plus	2-plus	3-plus		0	1-plus	2-plus	3-plus
Died within 6 mths.	4	1	0	2	1	14	0	2	5	7
„ 6 mths.–1 year	8	0	2	2	4	8	0	4	2	2
„ 1–2 years	12	0	4	5	3	10	2	3	3	2
„ 2–5 years	8	0	2*	4	2	3	1	1	1	0
Alive at 5 years	23	5	5	13	0	17	0	7	10	0
Total	55	6	13	26	10	52	3	17	21	11

* Including one non-tuberculous death.

TABLE X

Mortality According to Temperature on Admission

	Streptomycin series					Control series				
	Number of patients	Average evening temperature during week of preliminary investigation				Number of patients	Average evening temperature during week of preliminary investigation			
		No fever	Under 99° F.	99°–99·9° F.	100° F. or more		No fever	Under 99° F.	99°–99·9° F.	100° F. or more
Died within 6 mths.	4	0	0	0	4	14	0	3	6	5
„ 6 mths.–1 year	8	0	0	3	5	8	0	2	3	3
„ 1–2 years	12	0	2	4	6	10	2	2	5	1
„ 2–5 years	8	0	4	2	2*	3	0	1	1	1
Alive at 5 years	23	3	10	8	2	17	2	8	6	1
Total	55	3	16	17	19	52	4	16	21	11

* Including one non-tuberculous death.

(3-plus) not one survived five years, although those in the streptomycin series did not die so early in the period as the control patients. In contrast, 10 of 19 S patients and seven of 20 C patients with little or no initial cavitation survived for five years.

Temperature. Table X shows the mortality in the two series according to the average evening temperature in the preliminary week of investigation. The same trends appear as for cavitation, the most febrile patients having the worst prognosis. Only two of the 19 S patients and one of the 11 C patients with an average evening temperature of 100° F. or more survived five years, compared with 13 of 19 S and 10 of 20 C patients who had no fever or were in the lowest category of pyrexia.

Other criteria. The differences are slighter, but similar, as regards the sedimentation rate and the number of lung zones involved. Of the 36 S and 29 C patients with an E.S.R. of 51 mm. or more in an hour, 39 per cent. and 24 per cent. respectively survived five years, compared with 47 per cent. of 19 S and

45 per cent. of 22 C patients with a lower E.S.R. At five years 33 per cent. of the 21 S patients and 25 per cent. of the 24 C patients with all six zones involved were still alive, compared with 58 per cent. of the 12 S and 46 per cent. of the 13 C patients with involvement of three or four zones.

TABLE XI

Mortality by Sex and Treatment Series in the Five-year Period

Treatment series	Sex	Number of patients	Deaths in the first: 6 months No.	%	1 year No.	%	18 months No.	%	2 years No.	%	5 years No.	%
Streptomycin	M	22	2	9	7	32	7	32	9	41	13	59
	F	33	2	6	5	15	12	36	15	45	19*	58
Control	M	21	8	38	9	43	12	57	12	57	13	62
	F	31	6	19	13	42	18	58	20	65	22	71

* Including one non-tuberculous death.

TABLE XII

Changes in Radiographic Appearances in the First Four Months related to Mortality in the Five-Year Period*

	Number of patients	Radiographic changes in first four months*: Improvement: Considerable	Improvement: Slight or moderate	No change	Deterioration: Slight or moderate	Deterioration: Considerable
Streptomycin series:						
Died within 4 months	1	..	..	..	..	..
,, 4 months–1 year	11	1	5	1	2	2
,, 1–2 years	12	4	3	2	2	1
,, 2–5 years	8	4†	3	1	0	0
Alive at 5 years	23	16	7	0	0	0
Total alive at 4 months	54	25	18	4	4	3
Control series:						
Died within 4 months	10	..	..	..	..	..
,, 4 months–1 year	12	0	1	1	4	6
,, 1–2 years	10	0	0	3	5	2
,, 2–5 years	3	0	1	0	2	0
Alive at 5 years	17	0	9	5	3	0
Total alive at 4 months	42	0	11	9	14	8

* As assessed in the earlier report (Medical Research Council, 1948).
† Including one non-tuberculous death.

Although the number of patients is comparatively small, further analysis suggests that each of the above criteria is largely independent of the rest as a guide to prognosis. There is no close association between these criteria in the same patient.

Mortality related to sex. The mortality of male and female patients in the two series is set out in Table XI. The five-year mortality was similar for the sexes, but in each treatment series the initial mortality was higher in male patients.

Mortality related to immediate radiographic response. Table XII presents the mortality in relation to radiographic changes during the first four months, as assessed by the original radiological panel (Medical Research Council, 1948). It can be seen that in the streptomycin series 11 patients failed to improve radiographically in the first four months, and all had died within five years. In contrast, of the 43 S patients who showed radiographic improvement, 23 were still alive at the end of the five-year period. In the control series the majority of patients who had deteriorated radiographically in the first four months died subsequently (19 of 22), whereas nine of 11 patients who showed radiographic improvement survived for the five-year period. A corresponding analysis of mortality related to radiographic changes in the first six months yielded similar results, although, as shown in the original report (Medical Research Council, 1948), the tendency of some S patients to deteriorate was evident between four and six months.

Mortality related to immediate clinical response. Similar analyses of changes in the E.S.R. and in the temperature have been made. Ninety per cent. of 21 S patients, and 82 per cent. of 17 C patients, in whom the E.S.R. did not fall in the first four months, died within the five-year period, compared with 34 per cent. of the 32 S and 42 per cent. of the 24 C patients in whom the E.S.R. fell. Of 22 S and 15 C patients in whom the temperature was normal at four months, 32 per cent. and 27 per cent. respectively died within the five years. In contrast, 75 per cent. of the 32 S patients in whom the temperature was elevated, and 77 per cent. of the corresponding 26 C patients, died. Thus changes in the E.S.R. and changes in the temperature are both features of prognostic value.

The figures in Table XII have demonstrated that the prognosis for the 43 S patients who showed radiographic improvement in the first four months was not so favourable as for the corresponding group of 11 C patients. A special study was therefore made of the prognostic value of changes in the E.S.R. and the temperature in the first four months for this group of S patients. At the end of four months the E.S.R. was the same or higher in 14 patients, 12 (86 per cent.) of whom died within the five-year period; in contrast only eight (28 per cent.) died among the 29 patients in whom the E.S.R. fell. Similarly the temperature at four months was elevated in 22 patients, 14 (64 per cent.) of whom died, compared with six (29 per cent.) of 21 patients in whom the temperature at four months was normal. Further analysis suggests that, in this group of S patients who showed early radiographic improvement, the changes in the E.S.R. and the temperature over the same period were each associated independently with the subsequent mortality.

Mortality related to immediate bacteriological response. In Table XIII the mortality in the two series is related to the bacterial content of the sputum at four months. Of nine S patients with specimens negative both on direct examination and on culture, seven were alive at five years, and one of the two deaths was not due to tuberculosis. In contrast only nine of 35 S patients with sputum bacteriologically positive on direct examination at four months survived five years. In the control series, the subsequent experience of patients with specimens positive on direct examination at four months was very similar, only 10 of 30 surviving for five years; three patients were known to have specimens negative even on culture, and all survived five years.

Mortality related to emergence of bacterial resistance to streptomycin. Data concerning the emergence of bacterial resistance in patients in the streptomycin

TABLE XIII

Bacterial Content of Sputum at Four Months related to Mortality in the Five-year Period

	Number of patients with complete results	Results of examinations at four months: Direct examination positive*	Direct examination negative and culture positive	Direct examination and culture negative
Streptomycin series:				
Died 4 months–1 year	10	10	0	0
,, 1–2 years	12	9	2	1
,, 2–5 years	8	7	0	1†
Alive at 5 years	20	9	4	7
Total	50	35	6	9
Control series:				
Died 4 months–1 year	9	9	0	0
,, 1–2 years	10	10	0	0
,, 2–5 years	1	1	0	0
Alive at 5 years	14	10	1	3
Total	34	30	1	3

* Even if culture negative. † One non-tuberculous death.

TABLE XIV

Mortality in the Five Years and Disease Activity in the Survivors, related to Streptomycin Resistance during the First Six Months

	Number of patients	Number with no information available	Patients with information available	Highest streptomycin resistance ratio during first six months: Under 8	8–99	100–999	1,000–7,999	8,000 or more
Died within 1 year	12	2	10	1	1	3	2	3
,, 1–2 years	12	4	8	0	0	3	4	1
,, 2–5 years	8	2	6	0	0	5	1	0
Disease active at 5 years	4	1	3	0	1	2	0	0
,, quiescent at 5 years	6	1	5	1	1	2	1	0
,, arrested at 5 years	13	3	10	3	3	2	2	0
Total	55	13	42	5	6	17	10	4

series during the first six months were incomplete, as no information was obtained from 12 patients, and inadequate information from one patient. Of the remaining 42 patients, 37 (88 per cent.)[3] were known to have harboured resistant bacilli at some time during the six months. In Table XIV the mortality during the five-year period is related to the highest streptomycin resistance ratio obtained during the first six months. Of 31 patients who had organisms with a resistance ratio of 100 or more, 22 (71 per cent.) died in the five years, compared with two (18 per cent.) of 11 patients with less resistant or sensitive

[3] The minor discrepancy between these figures and those in the earlier report (Medical Research Council, 1948) is accounted for by one late result, and by the choice of a resistance ratio of 8 × H37Rv as the lower limit of resistance in place of 10, in accordance with more recent practice.

strains. As in the earlier report (Medical Research Council, 1948), it remains uncertain whether the emergence of high degrees of drug resistance had influenced the subsequent course of the disease, or whether the poor prognosis of this group of patients is no more than a reflection of the emergence of high degrees of resistance in those patients who were most acutely ill on admission. Nevertheless the fact must be stressed that the emergence of high degrees of drug resistance is not always associated with an unfavourable course of the disease. Of the 31 patients known to have had organisms with a resistance ratio of 100 or more, seven had attained quiescence by two years, and the same seven patients had either quiescent or arrested disease at five years.

Discussion

This report presents a long-term follow-up of all the 107 patients in the first controlled clinical trial of streptomycin in the treatment of pulmonary tuberculosis. The patients, all of whom were young adults with acute extensive bilateral disease, were allocated at random to treatment with streptomycin and rest in bed for four months, or to treatment with rest in bed alone. The first report of this investigation (Medical Research Council, 1948), which presented detailed results after the patients had been observed for six months, clearly demonstrated the value of a trial planned in this way. The series of patients treated only by rest in bed permitted a more precise evaluation of the early benefits and limitations of streptomycin therapy, as an addition to rest in bed, than could have been obtained by any other means. It was emphasized in the report, however, that an assessment at six months, even with preliminary results at one year, could be regarded only as a short-term evaluation. The present report gives a comparative assessment of the two series of patients for a period of five years from the start of the trial.

Patients in both series received a variety of treatments after the first four months. Chemotherapy was given subsequently to a limited and similar extent in each series. The incidence of established collapse therapy was also similar in the streptomycin and control series. Thus the only substantial difference between the two treatment series during the five-year period was the short course of streptomycin given to patients in the one series during an acute phase of the disease. In the control series the immediate mortality was very severe, 27 per cent. of the 52 patients being dead within six months of entry to the trial, 42 per cent. within one year, and 58 per cent. within 18 months. Thereafter only five patients died, and at five years 33 per cent. were still alive. In view of the high initial mortality, the number of survivors at the end of five years is unexpectedly large. In the streptomycin series the early mortality was not so great, 7 per cent. of the 55 patients being dead within six months. By 18 months, however, 35 per cent. of the patients were dead, and the mortality continued with comparable intensity for another year, by which time 53 per cent. of the patients had died. Thereafter few deaths occurred, and at the end of the five-year period 42 per cent. of the patients were still alive. Viewed over the whole period, the effect of the course of streptomycin upon the mortality was thus largely one of postponement of deaths, but in addition a small proportion of patients who might otherwise have died were still alive at five years. Mortality figures alone give an incomplete picture of the effects of treatment, and it is important to know the clinical condition of those who survived. At two years the progress of the survivors was considerably better in the streptomycin series, 61 per cent. of the patients having quiescent disease, compared with 30 per cent. of the control patients. A similar difference was apparent at five years, when 57 per cent. of the 23 surviving streptomycin patients had arrested disease, compared with 29 per cent. of the 17 surviving control patients. It is noteworthy that nine of the streptomycin patients attained arrest at five years without later chemotherapy or any collapse therapy, compared with two of the control patients. Thus the course of streptomycin made a decisive contribution to the recovery of some patients. In brief, over the five-year period, the streptomycin series fared better, not only in respect of the number of patients surviving and the clinical condition of the survivors, but also in respect of the numbers who returned to work and the proportions who had considerable or striking radiographic improvement. The benefit to the streptomycin series was, however, less than might have been expected from the findings at six months.

There have been reports on the long-term follow-up of pulmonary tuberculosis treated with streptomycin by Tucker (1949), Canada, Allison, d'Esopo, Dunner, Moyer, Shamaskin, Tempel, and Charter (1950), Moyer and Schwartz (1951), Steinbach, Leiner, Polachek, and Heller (1950), Harden, Payne, McKnight, and Gillem (1951), and McEnery (1953), but none of these studies had a control series. Apart from a follow-up of patients undergoing thoracoplasty with or without streptomycin cover (Murphy and Walkup, 1951), the only controlled trial to report long-term results is that of Long and Ferebee (1950), in which a substantial proportion of the 541 patients has been followed for one year. The plan of this American trial and the dosage of streptomycin were similar to those used in the trial reported here, but the patients were a much less homogeneous group, there being no restriction as to age, duration of disease, or type of lesion. In general the patients had less severe and acute disease than those in the Medical Research Council trial. The American study, like the present report, demonstrated a much higher initial mortality in the control than in the streptomycin series, but there were already signs in the second six months that the effect of streptomycin might be 'a "death delaying" rather than a "life saving" phenomenon' (Long and Ferebee, 1950). The clinical condition of the survivors in the streptomycin series was better than in the control series throughout the year, but the differences between the series decreased as the year proceeded.

A feature of special interest in the present study is that it relates to an acute and very extensive form of pulmonary tuberculosis. It provides valuable information on the prognosis of a grave type of disease, both when unmodified by chemotherapy and when influenced by a course of streptomycin. In the control series the outcome illustrates the extent to which the host, aided by routine medical measures and collapse therapy, can deal with this type of disease (Hart,

1954). The advent of chemotherapy has ensured that no comparable series can ever be studied again.

An analysis of some of the clinical features of the control series on admission to the trial was made to see how these affected the prognosis. The worst prognostic sign was extensive (3-plus) cavitation, for all 11 patients in this category died, nine of them in the first year. An initial pyrexia of over 100° F. was an unfavourable prognostic sign, as were also, although to a less extent, a high initial erythrocyte sedimentation rate and involvement of five or six zones of the lungs (on a standard radiograph). The individual factors usually indicative of acute or extensive disease each carried a relatively bad prognosis. The relationship between mortality and the initial clinical condition was very similar in the streptomycin series, except that, as already stated, the mortality occurred later in the period. Extensive cavitation was again associated with a poor prognosis, for all 10 patients with 3-plus cavitation died, five of them in the first year. A pyrexia of over 100° F., a high initial erythrocyte sedimentation rate, and involvement of five or six zones of the lungs (on a standard radiograph), were likewise bad prognostic signs.

The outcome in the control series was closely linked to the immediate response to treatment, especially the radiographic response. Thus of 22 patients who had radiographic deterioration at the end of four months, only three survived five years. In contrast, of 11 patients who improved initially, nine were alive at five years. These findings suggest that in the control series some patients, owing to a low host resistance, extensive destruction of lung tissue, or overwhelming infection, were incapable of improving, and proceeded steadily downhill. Other patients, with a high host resistance, were able to improve from the outset in spite of severe disease, and had an increased chance of survival. In the streptomycin series the pattern of radiographic response was different. Radiographic improvement occurred in 78 per cent. of patients in the first four months, but nearly half of these patients died within the five years. Initial radiographic improvement was thus not such a good prognostic sign as in the control series. On the other hand all 11 patients who failed to show radiographic improvement died within five years. These findings suggest that the patients who improved initially in the streptomycin series fell into three categories: those with a high host resistance, who would have improved and survived without streptomycin; some patients who might have been expected to die, but who in fact derived decisive and lasting benefit from the streptomycin; and, in addition, a considerable proportion who made only temporary radiographic gains with the drug, and were unable to maintain the initial benefit, presumably because of low host resistance or extensive destruction of lung tissue; these patients subsequently died. This view is supported by the association between the early changes in erythrocyte sedimentation rate and temperature and the subsequent mortality of this group of patients.

An important practical point emerges from the fate of the control series. Acute bilateral disease in young adults is a grave condition, which in the present series, when treated only by rest in bed, carried a mortality of 19 per cent. in the first four months. In addition, 19 of the 22 patients who deteriorated radiographically in the first four months died, 16 of them within the next 14 months. It can therefore be concluded that to delay the start of chemotherapy for a patient with this type of disease may seriously prejudice the chance of survival. The detection of such lesions and their immediate treatment with an effective dosage of combined chemotherapy are a matter of urgency. The start of chemotherapy should not be delayed until the patient is admitted to hospital.

In a previous report on the treatment of the same type of pulmonary tuberculosis (Medical Research Council, 1950) the superiority of streptomycin plus para-aminosalicylic acid over streptomycin alone was demonstrated for a six-month period. A five-year follow-up of the patients in that trial is at present in progress; it should indicate to what extent the superior results in the group receiving combined chemotherapy are maintained over this longer period of time.

Acknowledgements

We regret that it is not possible to name individually the large number of clinicians whose willing co-operation has made this follow-up possible. They provided much clinical data and loaned the radiographs for independent assessment; we wish to thank them for the completeness of the resulting information.

APPENDIX

The following definitions of radiological zones of the lung were used:

Upper zone: the area above a straight line running through the lower borders of the anterior ends of the second ribs.

Middle zone: the area bounded by the above line and one running through the lower borders of the anterior ends of the fourth ribs.

Lower zone: the remainder of the lung below the middle zone.

The definitions of disease activity were taken from the Revision of Section I of the Appendix to the Ministry of Health Memorandum 37/T (Revised), with the one exception that no patient who still had a reversible form of collapse therapy was considered to have 'arrested' disease. The relevant definitions are:

'"*Active cases*". Those not quiescent. All cases discharging tubercle bacilli within the preceding three months should be considered as "active".

'"*Quiescent*". Cases in which the general condition and exercise tolerance are good, having regard to the extent of the lesion; which show no evidence of toxaemia; in which no tubercle bacilli have been found on three consecutive monthly examinations by stained film; and in which changes revealed by other clinical investigations and by serial skiagrams point to retrogression of the tuberculous lesion.

'"*Arrested*". Cases in which the disease has been "quiescent" for a continuous period of at least TWO years.'

The following definitions of working capacity were used:

'*Full activity*'. Patient in full-time employment, or undertaking normal housework.

'*Modified activity*'. Patient in part-time employment, or undertaking limited housework.

'*Nil*'. Patient's activity severely limited, or patient confined to bed.

In the assessment of major radiographic changes the following definitions were adopted:

Resolution: the disappearance or diminution in size of one or more of the lesions.

Fibrosis: (*a*) appearance of linear shadows, *or* (*b*) diminution in size of lesions, associated with sharpening of their outline or increase in their density; often associated with evidence of lung shrinkage, such as tracheal, vessel, or fissure displacement.

Reduction in cavitation: cavities smaller or fewer, or both, on postero-anterior radiographs.

Disappearance of cavitation: disappearance of all cavitation on postero-anterior radiographs.

Summary

All the 107 patients in the first controlled clinical trial of streptomycin in the treatment of pulmonary tuberculosis have now been followed for five years or until death. The patients, who were young adults with acute bilateral progressive pulmonary tuberculosis of recent origin, were allocated at random to treatment with streptomycin 2 gm. daily for four months in bed (55 S patients), or to treatment with rest in bed only (52 C patients).

On entry to the trial the two series had a similar distribution of patients with severe and less severe illness. Neither series was more favoured in the use of chemotherapy, or in the frequency of established collapse measures, after the six months of original treatment and observation in hospital.

Although at the end of six months 7 per cent. of S patients and 27 per cent. of C patients had died, this initial benefit to the S patients was not maintained, and by two and a half years 53 per cent. of the S patients were dead, compared with 63 per cent. of the C patients. There was little further mortality in either series during the remainder of the period.

At two years, 61 per cent. of the 31 surviving S patients had quiescent disease, and 29 per cent. had returned to full activity; the corresponding figures for the 20 surviving C patients were 30 per cent. and 10 per cent. Among the survivors, 71 per cent. of the S patients showed considerable or exceptional radiographic improvement, compared with 47 per cent. of the C series.

At five years, 57 per cent. of the 23 surviving S patients had arrested disease, and 65 per cent. had returned to full activity; the corresponding figures for the 17 surviving C patients were 29 per cent. and 47 per cent. Among the survivors, 86 per cent. of the S patients showed considerable or exceptional radiographic improvement, compared with 53 per cent. of the C series. The major radiographic improvements in each series were resolution of lesions and disappearance of cavitation.

The outcome of the disease in each series was less favourable in patients who had extensive cavitation, high pyrexia, high erythrocyte sedimentation rate, or extensive zonal involvement of the lungs, on admission to the trial. It was also much less favourable in patients who deteriorated radiographically or clinically in the first four months, or who developed organisms highly resistant to streptomycin within the first six months.

The grave prognosis for patients with this type of disease, when treated only with rest in bed, illustrates the importance of starting treatment with a powerful chemotherapeutic combination as soon as the diagnosis has been made.

REFERENCES

Beven, G. (1951) *Brit. Med. J.* **2,** 1442.

Canada, R. O., Allison, S. T., d'Esopo, N. D., Dunner, E., Moyer, R. E., Shamaskin, A., Tempel, C. W., and Charter, W. V. (1950) *Amer. Rev. Tuberc.* **62,** 563.

Harden, K. A., Payne, H. M., McKnight, H. V., and Gillem, N. P. (1951) *Dis. of Chest,* **20,** 392.

Hart, P. D'Arcy (1954) *Brit. Med. J.* In the press.

Long, E. R., and Ferebee, S. H. (1950) *Pub. Health Rep.* **65,** 1421.

McEnery, E. T. (1953) *J. Amer. Med. Ass.* **153,** 627.

Medical Research Council (1948) *Brit. Med. J.* **2,** 769.

—— (1949) Ibid. **2,** 1521.

—— (1950) Ibid. **2,** 1073.

Moyer, R. E., and Schwartz, W. S. (1951) *Amer. Rev. Tuberc.* **64,** 41.

Murphy, J. D., and Walkup, H. E. (1951) *Amer. Surgeon,* **17,** 865.

Steinbach, M. M., Leiner, G. C., Polachek, A. A., and Heller, P. (1950) *Amer. Rev. Tuberc.* **61,** 868.

Tucker, W. B. (1949) Ibid. **60,** 715.

U.S.A. Veterans Administration (1949) *Minutes of the Seventh Streptomycin Conference,* April 1949, pp. 13–15, 25–28.

616.334–007.271: 612.392.6

ELECTROLYTE DEPLETION IN PYLORIC STENOSIS[1]

By D. A. K. BLACK and R. P. JEPSON

(From the Departments of Medicine and Surgery, University of Manchester)

The importance of disordered electrolyte metabolism in pyloric stenosis was perhaps first clearly established by Gamble and Ross (1925); using pyloric ligation in dogs, they demonstrated a loss of sodium as well as of chloride, and suggested that loss of sodium, rather than ill-defined 'toxic factors', was responsible for the circulatory insufficiency and dehydration which patients with pyloric stenosis often show. They noted an increase in plasma-bicarbonate, and ascribed this to an alkalosis induced by loss of chloride in excess of sodium. In the past few years it has become known that to sodium depletion and alkalosis we must add potassium depletion. Hawkins, Hardy, and Sampson (1951) reported potassium depletion in a patient with pyloric stenosis; Lans, Stein, and Meyer (1952) found evidence of potassium depletion in 24 similar patients; and Illingworth (1953) recognized that in patients with pyloric stenosis potassium depletion is common, and should be treated. Although there is good clinical and biochemical evidence of sodium, chloride, and potassium depletion in patients with pyloric stenosis, we have not been able to find adequate information on the relative magnitude of the deficits of these ions; in this paper we present and discuss the results of balance observations in seven patients who had pyloric stenosis, and in four patients who had peptic ulceration without stenosis and were also treated by partial gastrectomy.

Plan of Study and Technical Methods

The general purpose of the investigation was to find out how much sodium, chloride, and potassium patients with pyloric stenosis would retain during preparation for operation and after relief of the obstruction by operation. Retention of electrolytes during repair of deficits has been used to assess the magnitude of the original deficit, for example during recovery from diabetic coma (Nabarro, Spencer, and Stowers, 1952). The results obtained in this way can only be interpreted rather generally, for there is no assurance that complete repair of the electrolyte deficit has been achieved at the end of the observation period, and in the case of potassium it was found that retention during recovery from a deficit was somewhat greater than the original deficit (Black and Milne, 1952). In addition to these general criticisms, we had the special difficulty in the present study that treatment included partial gastrectomy, and surgical procedures in themselves affect the balances of sodium, chloride, and potassium. This 'metabolic response to surgery' has been described in detail by Moore and

[1] Received January 25, 1954.

Ball (1952); we have no new observations to offer on this point, but we determined the magnitude of the response in four patients who had a partial gastrectomy with no preceding stenosis, so that we might know something of the changes attributable to the operative treatment itself on our dietary régime.

All our patients were men in middle or later life. Brief clinical descriptions are given, with the balance results, in the Appendix. Five of the patients presented the clinical picture of vomiting and visible peristalsis, supervening on dyspepsia of varying duration caused by peptic ulcer or gastric neoplasm. Two other patients had not been vomiting, but were found at operation to have a degree of stenosis. Four patients had no stenosis either clinically or at operation. Before operation the patients were having a measured intake of milk, to which sodium or potassium salts were sometimes added, aliquots of the mixed fluid diet being kept for analysis. On the day of operation no fluids were given by mouth, and on the following day only water. Thereafter a milk mixture of increasing strength was given until about a week after operation. Urine was collected in 24-hour specimens; and vomited material, and the results of gastric lavage with water, were collected as available. In some patients part of the electrolyte intake was intravenous. Losses of electrolyte in stools and sweat were not determined; no patient had diarrhoea, or visible sweating except during operation. Blood samples were taken before and at intervals after operation. Serum-sodium, -potassium, -chloride, and -bicarbonate, and the sodium, potassium, and chloride concentration of ingesta and excreta, were determined by standard methods.

Clinical Observations

The dietary régime was well tolerated by all patients until about a week after operation, when they began to be anxious for solid food. Medical and nursing staff with experience of post-gastrectomy convalescence considered that the general condition of the patients compared favourably with that usual in patients after gastrectomy. Nine of the 11 patients made an uncomplicated recovery. One patient of 74 years, with a pyloric cancer, died of pneumonia 12 days after operation. Another patient, in whom a partial stenosis was found at operation, showed no unusual clinical or biochemical features, but his laparotomy wound dehisced on removal of the sutures on the ninth day; the wound was re-sutured, and healed without difficulty. In the five patients who had clinical pyloric stenosis there was considerable variation in respect of the length of history and the extent of clinical dehydration. The two patients who were found at operation to have pyloric neoplasms were more dehydrated, after a shorter history of vomiting, than the three patients with duodenal ulceration. Only three patients were given intravenous fluids, and only two needed considerable amounts of intravenous saline. The absence of clinical dehydration in one patient with duodenal ulcer, who had been vomiting for over a year, was striking; at operation he had a large stomach and a tight stenosis, but he had been taking considerable amounts of alkali before operation. Another patient with duodenal ulcer had the largest stomach, on barium-meal examination, of the series; but he was not clinically dehydrated, although he had had protracted vomiting. It is difficult to assess the amount, as opposed to the duration, of vomiting from the history; and some of the patients may have taken sufficient sodium salts to prevent gross depletion, in spite of their vomiting. Although these five patients were seen consecutively, we cannot of course generalize from them as to the comparative infrequency of severe dehydration in pyloric stenosis; the series was small, and they may have been treated earlier than the average patient with pyloric stenosis. The clinical impression that only two of the five patients were severely dehydrated is supported by the small retention of sodium and chloride during recovery in the other three patients.

Serum-Electrolytes

The results of electrolyte estimations on admission, before treatment, are shown in Table I. One patient (Case 3), who was clinically dehydrated, also had

TABLE I

Serum-Electrolyte Concentrations on Admission
(mEq. per litre)

Case number	*Na*	*K*	*Cl*	*HCO_3*
Patients with clinical pyloric stenosis:				
1	139	4·7	79	44
2	142	4·5	99	31·6
3	129	3·7	84	41·7
4	136	5·0	101	32·9
5	151	6·1	102	30·8
Partial stenosis found at operation:				
6	137	5·4	97	30·8
7	144	4·8	101	26·7
Gastrectomy; stenosis absent:				
8	144	5·9	99	26·6
9	139	5·2	107	28·1
11	138	5·2	105	26·7
Range including 98% of normal subjects (Wootton and King, 1953)	133–152	3·5–5·6	99–108	24–31

a serum-sodium concentration below the normal range (Wootton and King, 1953); in the other patients the serum-sodium fell within the normal range. The serum-potassium concentration was within the lower half of the normal range in three of the five patients with clinical pyloric stenosis, but no single value was abnormally low. There was in fact, in our series, no striking and consistent change in sodium and potassium concentrations in the serum. On the other hand, four of the five patients with pyloric stenosis had an increase in serum-bicarbonate, and the fifth showed a value at the upper limit of normal. Two of the five patients with pyloric stenosis also had a low serum-chloride concentration. An increase in serum-bicarbonate was thus a consistent finding in the patients with pyloric stenosis. During the period of treatment and observation this abnormality was substantially corrected, the average fall in serum-bicarbonate levels being 7·3 mEq. per litre; the final values were 26·3,

29·2, 28·5, 31·7, and 26·5 mEq. per litre, in Cases 1, 2, 3, 4, and 5. Concurrently the serum-chloride concentration increased by an average of 9·6 mEq. per litre, the final concentrations in the same patients being 99, 99, 106, 105, and 104 mEq. per litre. As might be expected in the absence of any notable change in serum-sodium and -potassium concentration, the decrease in bicarbonate and increase in chloride were similar in the individual patient, and in the series these two quantities were significantly correlated ($r = +0{\cdot}928$, $P \simeq 0{\cdot}02$). We have

TABLE II

Cumulative Retention of Electrolytes during Period of Observations (mEq.)

Case number	*Na*	*K*	*Cl*
Patients with clinical pyloric stenosis:			
1	−14	+808	+746
2	+297	+218	+279
3	+1,762	+57	+1,890
4	+602	+255	+770
5	+213	+195	+376
Partial stenosis found at operation:			
6	+42	+1	+108
7	+110	+182	+117
Gastrectomy; stenosis absent:			
8	+82	+32	+137
9	+207	+68	+363
10	+122	+12	+124
11	+43	−71	+50

summarized the results of electrolyte balances in Table II, giving the cumulative balances of sodium, potassium, and chloride after operation. The day-to-day balances of sodium, potassium, and chloride are given in the Appendix.

Sodium Balance (Fig. 1)

The patients without pyloric stenosis had a small positive balance of sodium, averaging 113 mEq., a week after partial gastrectomy. Inspection of the day-to-day balance results shows that sodium retention three days after operation may be somewhat greater, but the general picture is one of moderate sodium retention, variable in duration, as described by various authors (Wilkinson, Billing, Nagy, and Stewart, 1950; Moore and Ball, 1952; Le Quesne and Lewis, 1953; MacPhee, 1953; Ebrill and Naftalin, 1953). The two patients in whom a degree of stenosis was found at operation, without previous clinical effects, were similar in respect of sodium balance to the patients without stenosis. The patients with clinical pyloric stenosis varied considerably in the amount of sodium retention. Two of them retained 213 and 297 mEq. Na, amounts not greatly different from those found in the patients without stenosis. One (Case 4) retained a greater amount of sodium than could readily be accounted for by the operation alone, while another (Case 3) had a very large sodium retention, having received massive saline infusion. The remaining patient (Case 1) retained sodium during preparation for operation, but had no sodium retention after operation; its absence may have been related to the relatively high intake of potassium, maintained on account of his considerable potassium deficit. High potassium intake has been known for many years to promote a negative sodium balance (Bunge, 1873); and we have observed unusually low retention of sodium after operation in two patients, without pyloric stenosis, who were given a high potassium intake. In summary, two of the patients with clinical pyloric stenosis had well-marked sodium depletion, both clinically and as judged by sodium retention during treatment. The other three showed no more sodium retention than is usually found after partial gastrectomy.

Potassium Balance (Fig. 2)

In the patients without pyloric stenosis there was considerable loss of potassium from the body in the first few days after operation, but at the end of a week this had been made up by potassium retention. Transient loss of potassium after partial gastrectomy, like retention of sodium and chloride, is well documented (Wilkinson, Billing, Nagy, and Stewart, 1950; Moore and Ball, 1952; Le Quesne and Lewis, 1953; MacPhee, 1953; Ebrill and Naftalin, 1953). Of the two patients with a partial stenosis found at operation, one was in potassium balance a week after operation, having made up the early loss following operation. The other (Case 7) had a positive balance of 182 mEq. K, which may indicate that he was depleted of potassium when he first came under observation. The patients with clinical pyloric stenosis differed among themselves in respect of potassium. Three of them had a moderate potassium depletion as judged by cumulative retentions, during recovery, of 218, 255, and 195 mEq. K. One patient had a severe potassium depletion, retaining 808 mEq. during recovery; potassium retention of this order has been observed previously in patients with gastrointestinal disease (Martin, Reynolds, Snyder, Berne, Homann, Edmondson, Blatherwick, Fields, Westman, and Westover, 1951). The remaining patient (Case 3) retained only 57 mEq. K; he was the only member of the group who had massive saline infusion, and it is possible that he had not attained potassium balance at the end of the observation period. There is some positive evidence that this was so, in that his serum-potassium fell to 3·2 mEq. per litre, having initially been 3·7 mEq. per litre; and the excretion of potassium in the urine increased during the period of massive saline infusion. To summarize the potassium balance results, four of the five patients with pyloric stenosis had a definite retention of potassium during recovery, moderate in three, considerable in one. The fifth patient did not show a similar retention, but it is probable that at the end of the observation period he was still depleted as a result of saline infusion, his serum-potassium being then only 3·2 mEq. per litre; we have, however, no quantitative assessment of his potassium deficit.

Chloride Balance (Fig. 3)

The patients without pyloric stenosis all retained chloride after operation, the average retention being 168 mEq. The patients with partial stenosis found at operation also retained some chloride. The patients with clinical pyloric stenosis retained large amounts of chloride, and this was most striking in Cases 3 and 4, with severe sodium depletion, and in Case 1, with severe potassium depletion. In Table III we compare the observed retention of chloride, in the five patients with clinical pyloric stenosis, and the change in serum-chloride concentration; we also give the serum-chloride change multiplied by 20, which

TABLE III

Chloride Retention and Change in Serum-Chloride in Patients with Pyloric Stenosis

Case number	*Chloride retention (mEq.)*	*Increase in serum-chloride (ΔCl) (mEq./l.)*	*Estimate of chloride retention which could be accounted for simply by the change in chloride concentration, without increase in extracellular-fluid volume ($\Delta Cl \times 20$)*
1	746	20	400
2	279	1	20
3	1,890	22	440
4	770	4	80
5	376	2	40

Note. In making this calculation we have taken 20 litres as an arbitrary volume exceeding any likely actual extracellular-fluid volume in these patients, and so giving an overestimate of the effect of increase in extracellular-fluid chloride concentration on chloride balance.

is an overestimate of the extracellular-fluid volume (Schwartz, Schachter, and Freinkel, 1949). It is obvious that the change in serum-chloride concentration falls far short of accounting for the positive balance of chloride. Some of this discrepancy could be attributed to expansion of extracellular-fluid volume, each litre of which would represent 100 mEq. Cl. It is difficult to accept this explanation as regards the patients who were not clinically dehydrated, and who retained only comparatively small amounts of sodium; and even in Case 3 the retention of chloride was too great to be related to any likely expansion of extracellular fluid. It seems more likely that some of the retained chloride entered the intracellular fluid, a process which has been suggested as likely on the basis of isotope studies (Deane, Ziff, and Smith, 1952); and we have felt that any attempt to calculate changes in extracellular-fluid volume from changes in chloride balance (Danowski, Greenman, Mateer, Parsons, Weigand, Mermelstein, and Peters, 1951) would not be valid in these patients. We believe, however, that some conclusions of interest emerge from a comparison of the balances of sodium, potassium, and chloride.

Interrelations (Fig. 4)

Two patients (Cases 2 and 5) had a moderate retention of both sodium and potassium. Of the two patients who had severe sodium depletion before treatment, one (Case 4) had a moderate potassium retention during recovery, while the other (Case 3) retained very little potassium in comparison with the other patients with pyloric stenosis. On the other hand the remaining patient (Case 1), with his severe potassium depletion, did not retain sodium during recovery. While moderate depletion of both sodium and potassium existed in two patients, we did not observe in any patient a gross retention of both sodium and potassium; this fact suggests that in pyloric stenosis the factors inducing severe sodium depletion may be different from those producing severe potassium depletion. In order to evaluate the relationship between base retention and retention of chloride, we have subtracted the cumulative balance of chloride from the sum of the balances of sodium and potassium, giving the quantity (Na+K)—Cl. The values for the 11 patients are given in Table IV, together with the corresponding quantity, (Na+K)—Cl, in the dietary intake. In the patients without pyloric stenosis, on the whole more Cl is retained than (Na+K), giving a negative average value for (Na+K)—Cl. In the patients with clinical pyloric stenosis, however, the retention of (Na+K) exceeds that of Cl, except in one patient (Case 3) who was certainly not fully in electrolyte balance at the end of the observation period, and who differed from the others in needing massive saline infusion, and in not taking milk for four days after operation, instead of the usual two days. The average value of (Na+K)—Cl for the four patients without stenosis is —45; for four patients with clinical pyloric stenosis, excluding Case 3, the value is +101; the difference between these means is significant at the level $0{\cdot}05 > P > 0{\cdot}02$ ($t = 2{\cdot}75$). Although in both groups there was in the diet an excess of (Na+K) over Cl, this was on the whole greater in the patients with pyloric stenosis, several of whom were treated with alkaline salts of potassium; and there is in fact some correlation between the dietary (Na+K)—Cl and the observed balance of (Na+K)—Cl ($r = 0{\cdot}68$, $0{\cdot}05 > P > 0{\cdot}02$). The excess of retention of base, however, in these four patients with pyloric stenosis can scarcely be written off as merely a dietary artefact; for it was during this retention of base that they recovered clinically, and their alkali

TABLE IV

Cumulative Retentions of ((Na+K)—Cl) Compared with Dietary ((Na+K)—Cl) (mEq.)

Case number	*Retention of ((Na+K)—Cl)*	*Dietary ((Na+K)—Cl)*
Patients with clinical pyloric stenosis:		
1	+48	+997
2	+246	+730
3	−71	+311
4	+87	+476
5	+32	+847
Partial stenosis found at operation:		
6	−65	+333
7	+175	+825
Gastrectomy; stenosis absent:		
8	−23	+321
9	−88	+232
10	+10	+211
11	−78	+180

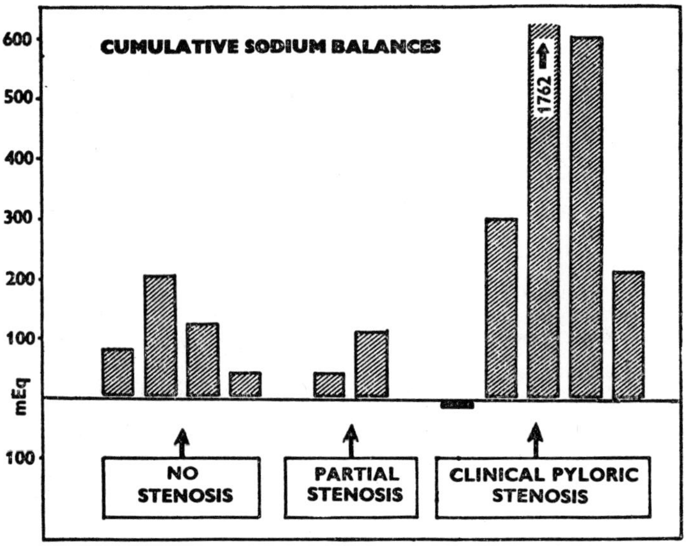

FIG. 1. Cumulative sodium balances. In all the figures each column represents the net retention or loss in a single patient, retention being plotted above the line and loss below it. The order of patients is the same in all the figures: Cases 8, 9, 10, 11 (no stenosis); Cases 6, 7 (partial stenosis); Cases 1, 2, 3, 4, 5 (clinical pyloric stenosis).

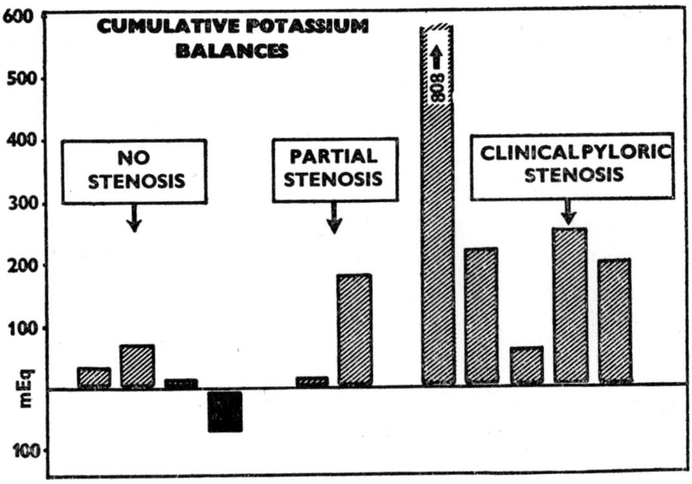

FIG. 2. Cumulative potassium balances.

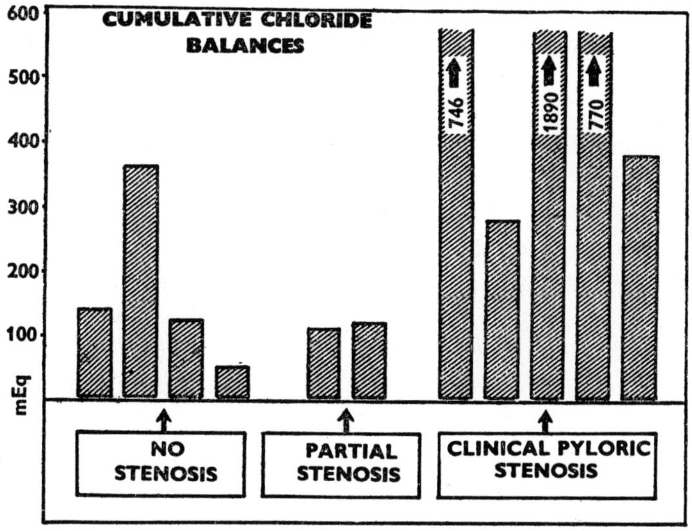

FIG. 3. Cumulative chloride balances.

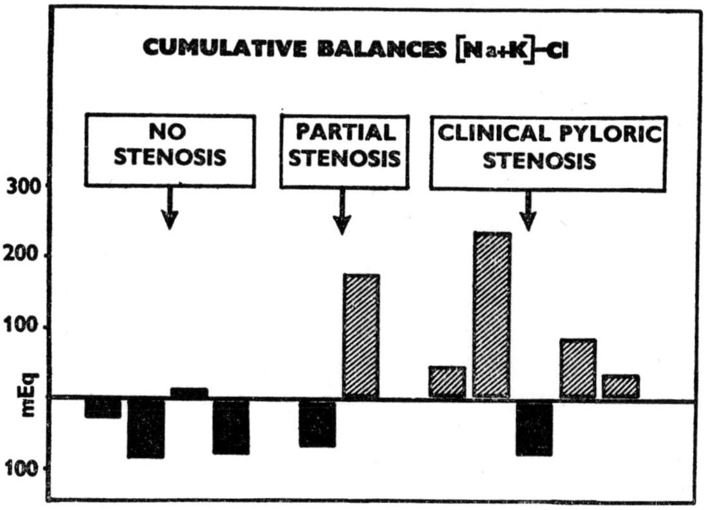

FIG. 4. Cumulative balances of (Na+K)−Cl
(for explanation see text).

reserve fell and the chloride in the serum rose to normal, changes which are the reverse of those to be expected from a dietary excess of base over chloride. We conclude, therefore, that in these four patients retention of (Na+K) in excess of Cl was an integral part of their metabolic recovery; it was favoured by the composition of the diet, and it could not be ascribed to the normal metabolic response to partial gastrectomy.

Discussion

There is no reason to doubt that the raised alkali reserve found in patients with severe pyloric stenosis is related to an alkalosis in the extracellular-fluid compartment. Since we have observed in four patients a return of the alkali reserve to normal in conjunction with a retention of (Na+K) in excess of Cl, we are driven to ask the question 'When is an alkalosis not an alkalosis?' The answer would appear to be 'When it is merely the expression, in those fluids normally accessible to analysis, of a shift of hydrions into the tissue cells.' This statement perhaps needs amplifying. The association of a raised alkali reserve with potassium depletion is well recognized (Darrow and Pratt, 1950). It has recently been suggested (Cooke, Segar, Cheek, Coville, and Darrow, 1952) that this alkalosis in the extracellular fluid may be caused by an exchange of potassium from inside the cells for hydrogen ions derived from the extracellular fluid; in this way the extracellular fluid would become more alkaline, and the cellular fluid more acid. This suggestion was supported by the finding that an extracellular-fluid alkalosis induced by experimental potassium depletion might appear at a time when more (Na+K) than Cl had been lost (Black and Milne, 1952). All four patients with pyloric stenosis who showed (Na+K) retention in excess of Cl during recovery also retained potassium in amounts ranging from 195 to 808 mEq. Concurrently with recovery the alkali reserve fell, and the fall was correlated with the amount of potassium retained over the same period ($r = 0{\cdot}974$, $P \simeq 0{\cdot}02$). We suggest, therefore, that in these four patients the extracellular-fluid alkalosis was related to potassium depletion, and that it was brought about by loss of hydrions from the extracellular fluid in exchange for potassium coming out of the cells. This state of affairs is probably fairly common in patients with pyloric stenosis; we have seen two other patients whose alkali reserve fell when they were given potassium, but we have no information as to their electrolyte balances during recovery.

Our results, obtained during recovery, cannot of course give any direct information as to how this disturbance—potassium depletion associated with extracellular alkalosis—may have arisen. It cannot easily be attributed to loss of gastric secretion *per se*, at least in patients with peptic ulcer, for the analyses of Lans, Stein, and Meyer (1952) show that in the gastric juice of patients with pyloric obstruction from peptic ulcer the chloride concentration always exceeds the sodium, usually by a considerable amount, and the potassium concentration (average 12·6 mEq. per litre) is lower than that of sodium (average 56 mEq. per litre). In patients with obstruction from gastric carcinoma, with no free HCl, the sodium and chloride concentrations were similar (averages of 61 and 58 mEq.

per litre), and the potassium concentration was 10·2 mEq. per litre on an average. Our own analyses of vomit in the two patients with carcinoma show a higher potassium concentration (20 and 26 mEq. per litre), but this is still lower than that of sodium (48 and 105 mEq. per litre) and chloride (68 and 120 mEq. per litre). In spite of the lower concentration of potassium than of sodium in gastric juice, potassium depletion in pyloric stenosis seems to be as common as, if not commoner than, sodium depletion. We would attribute this partly to loss of food, partly to the correction of sodium deficits by alkali treatment, and partly to the greater renal loss of potassium than of sodium in states of depletion.

Some of the potassium lost from the body before treatment in pyloric stenosis can be accounted for by breakdown of cellular tissue; each gramme of nitrogen derived from protein breakdown is associated with about 3 mEq. of potassium (Danowski, Greenman, Mateer, Parsons, Weigand, Mermelstein, and Peters, 1951). Unfortunately we did not estimate the nitrogen balance in our patients, and so cannot definitely say how much of the potassium retention observed by us could be related to protein gain. We are inclined to discount this possibility during the first week after operation, because the operation itself would favour protein breakdown rather than synthesis, and also because uncorrected potassium depletion in itself slows down protein formation (Cannon, Frazier, and Hughes, 1952). It is likely that further potassium will be retained in association with nitrogen as the patients regain their lost weight; but our observations in the first week after operation would not be greatly affected by this process. In patients regaining weight after diabetic coma, Nabarro, Spencer, and Stowers (1952) found little evidence of protein gain before seven to ten days after the beginning of treatment. The main channel of actual potassium loss from the body must be renal, because of the comparatively low concentration of potassium in gastric juice. Berliner, Kennedy, and Orloff (1951) have shown that high rates of potassium excretion are associated with low rates of hydrion excretion, and this effect may well contribute to the acidosis in body-fluids taken as a whole; another factor here is the very low urinary chloride output in some patients at a time when substantial amounts of sodium and potassium are still present in the urine. When an extracellular-fluid alkalosis is once established, the raised CO_2 tension in the plasma will tend to increase bicarbonate reabsorption; and Relman, Etsten, and Schwartz (1953) have suggested that this may be a factor in producing the acid urine sometimes observed in patients with pyloric stenosis. Although this aciduria is usually dubbed 'paradoxical', and indeed is so in relation to the alkalinity of the extracellular fluid, our observations suggest that such a reaction may not be inappropriate to the total acid-base balance, including cells as well as extracellular fluid.

These observations in general support the view of Illingworth (1953) and others, that treatment with potassium has a place in the management of pyloric stenosis. A number of patients (not in our experience a majority) are severely dehydrated, and require intravenous saline, sometimes in large amount; such patients should be given potassium salts by mouth, and we have found an alkaline potassium mixture suitable for this purpose (Black, 1953). Even in pyloric stenosis potassium given in this way is absorbed, at least in part, for we have observed an increase in serum-potassium and a fall in alkali reserve even before operative correction of the obstruction. Patients not clinically dehydrated should not be given intravenous saline, which accentuates potassium loss; but they should be given potassium salts by mouth until they are able to take a normal diet. The dosage of potassium should be of the order of 100 mEq. per day, but larger amounts may be needed in severe potassium depletion. We have not used intravenous potassium in these patients, but would do so in a patient with ileus and a low serum-potassium level. In our view ammonium chloride has no place in the treatment of pyloric stenosis. It may aggravate depletion of extracellular base, even to the point of producing water intoxication (Doxiadis, Goldfinch, and Holt, 1953); and our own observations suggest that, quite apart from this risk, the main deficit to be corrected is not a deficit of chloride, but one of base—sodium or potassium, or both. A good deal of this base, if not all of it, can be given in combination with chloride; but we see no indication for providing chloride without accompanying base, for the sake of achieving a purely biochemical victory over the raised alkali reserve in the plasma.

APPENDIX

BRIEF CLINICAL NOTES AND BALANCE RESULTS

(Intake, output, and balance are expressed in mEq. per day throughout)

1. *Patients with Clinical Pyloric Stenosis*

Case 1

F. K., aged 50. Chronic duodenal ulcer, with pyloric stenosis, and an 80% barium residue at 24 hours. Fair general condition, without obvious dehydration; but he had lost 40 lb. in weight in 8 months, and had massive vomiting for a month before admission. Taking large amounts of alkalies. No complications after operation.

	Intake			*Output*			*Balance*		
Day	*Na*	*K*	*Cl*	*Na*	*K*	*Cl*	*Na*	*K*	*Cl*
1	300	126	350	44	52	62	+256	+74	+288
*2	225	..	225	47	23	1	+178	−23	+225
3	..	126	50	113	75	3	−113	+51	+47
4	19	120	39	67	42	3	−48	+78	+36
5	30	153	59	119	58	6	−89	+95	+53
6	52	260	87	104	46	11	−52	+214	+76
7	54	232	91	93	43	30	−39	+189	+61
8	59	242	100	166	112	140	−107	+130	−40

Case 2

R. B., aged 48. Chronic duodenal ulcer, with vomiting for a year, not causing any clinical dehydration. His abdominal wound burst nine days after operation on removal of the sutures, but healed normally after re-suture.

* Day of operation.

	Intake			*Output*			*Balance*		
Day	*Na*	*K*	*Cl*	*Na*	*K*	*Cl*	*Na*	*K*	*Cl*
1	42	174	48	107	107	112	−65	+67	−64
*2	..	..	..	49	95	54	−49	−95	−54
3	..	..	..	14	50	15	−14	−50	−15
4	92	97	97	3	30	5	+89	+67	+92
5	129	145	145	10	63	25	+119	+82	+120
6	172	192	192	42	76	71	+130	+116	+121
7	188	177	196	101	146	117	+87	+31	+79

Case 3

W. T., aged 60. Carcinoma of pyloric region, with 2 months' massive vomiting. Poor general condition, with dehydration requiring massive saline infusion. No complications after operation.

	Intake			*Output*			*Balance*		
Day	*Na*	*K*	*Cl*	*Na*	*K*	*Cl*	*Na*	*K*	*Cl*
1	775	92	775	31	39	28	+744	+53	+747
2	683	118	765	188	88	170	+495	+30	+595
*3	741	84	805	270	86	324	+471	−2	+481
4	460	34	490	203	96	235	+257	−62	+255
5	..	..	..	28	44	44	−28	−44	−44
6	..	..	..	9	21	15	−9	−21	−15
7	53	89	82	54	49	89	−1	+40	−7
8	44	73	74	124	46	150	−80	+27	−76
9	66	109	119	153	73	165	−87	+36	−46

Case 4

A. G., aged 74. Pyloric carcinoma, with stenosis, and vomiting persistent for 2 months. Fair general condition, but enough dehydration to necessitate considerable saline infusion. In the first few days after operation convalescence was normal, but 12 days after operation he died of pneumonia.

	Intake			*Output*			*Balance*		
Day	*Na*	*K*	*Cl*	*Na*	*K*	*Cl*	*Na*	*K*	*Cl*
1	208	102	242	62	38	53	+146	+64	+189
2	144	96	192	52	51	61	+92	+45	+131
3	63	43	89	134	79	172	−71	−36	−83
*4	200	28	75	29	19	25	+171	+9	+50
5	..	..	..	10	29	8	−10	−29	−8
6	114	58	144	77	24	6	+37	+34	+138
7	91	69	128	42	41	40	+49	+28	+88
8	163	105	207	38	32	35	+125	+73	+172
9	132	102	165	69	35	72	+63	+67	+93

Case 5

S. W., aged 50. Chronic duodenal ulcer, with a very distended stomach on barium examination. Massive projectile vomiting, but no gross dehydration. No complications after operation.

	Intake			*Output*			*Balance*		
Day	*Na*	*K*	*Cl*	*Na*	*K*	*Cl*	*Na*	*K*	*Cl*
1	140	165	181	104	58	71	+36	+107	+110
2	95	105	110	155	100	148	−60	+5	−38
*3	..	..	..	32	78	43	−32	−78	−43
4	..	..	..	29	87	34	−29	−87	−34
5	123	126	155	41	78	56	+82	+48	+99
6	150	169	191	42	88	48	+108	+81	+143
7	169	194	210	61	75	71	+108	+119	+139

* Day of operation.

2. *Patients with Peptic Ulcer who were found at Operation to have Partial Stenosis, but had not had Clinical Pyloric Stenosis*

Case 6

F. B., aged 48. Chronic duodenal ulcer; in good general condition, without dehydration. No complications.

	Intake			*Output*			*Balance*		
Day	*Na*	*K*	*Cl*	*Na*	*K*	*Cl*	*Na*	*K*	*Cl*
1	149	106	200	152	81	166	−3	+25	+34
*2	..	..	..	56	68	85	−56	−68	−85
3	..	..	..	21	65	18	−21	−65	−18
4	56	71	65	14	31	16	+42	+40	+49
5	63	83	77	26	39	19	+37	+44	+58
6	104	111	144	83	95	127	+21	+16	+17
7	104	111	144	82	102	91	+22	+9	+53

Case 7

T. W., aged 63. Chronic duodenal ulcer; in good general condition, without dehydration. No complications.

	Intake			*Output*			*Balance*		
Day	*Na*	*K*	*Cl*	*Na*	*K*	*Cl*	*Na*	*K*	*Cl*
1	219	280	204	217	151	208	+2	+129	−4
2	157	188	177	164	126	170	−7	+62	+7
*3	..	..	..	6	29	15	−6	−29	−15
4	..	96	..	13	140	44	−13	−44	−44
5	90	112	110	3	94	14	+87	+18	+96
6	125	187	138	78	141	61	+47	+46	+77

3. *Patients without Stenosis who had Partial Gastrectomy for Peptic Ulcer*

Case 8

W. B., aged 61. Chronic duodenal ulcer; in good general condition. He had been taking alkalies before operation. No complications.

	Intake			*Output*			*Balance*		
Day	*Na*	*K*	*Cl*	*Na*	*K*	*Cl*	*Na*	*K*	*Cl*
1	25	44	36	139	64	165	−114	−20	−129
*2	..	..	..	18	62	25	−18	−62	−25
3	..	..	..	22	90	23	−22	−90	−23
4	28	50	52	9	44	10	+19	+6	+42
5	35	60	53	12	33	19	+23	+27	+34
6	62	105	99	21	39	42	+41	+66	+57
7	67	116	102	39	57	63	+28	+59	+39
8	70	116	105	59	90	92	+11	+26	+13

Case 9

L. W., aged 35. Chronic duodenal ulcer; partial gastrectomy. Uncomplicated recovery.

	Intake			*Output*			*Balance*		
Day	*Na*	*K*	*Cl*	*Na*	*K*	*Cl*	*Na*	*K*	*Cl*
1	41	63	66	96	71	108	−55	−8	−42
*2	..	..	..	20	93	49	−20	−93	−49
3	..	..	..	8	36	21	−8	−36	−21
4	405	65	448	49	23	18	+356	+42	+430
5	45	70	87	20	34	36	+25	+36	+51
6	82	108	111	51	18	55	+31	+90	+56
7	34	48	51	103	30	106	−69	+18	−55
8	54	77	97	162	66	146	−108	+11	−49

* Day of operation.

Case 10

J. B., aged 44. Long history of gastric ulcer, with some recent loss of weight, but good general condition. No complications after operation.

	Intake			*Output*			*Balance*		
Day	*Na*	*K*	*Cl*	*Na*	*K*	*Cl*	*Na*	*K*	*Cl*
1	132	96	128	177	68	186	−45	+28	−58
*2	..	..	..	45	77	55	−45	−77	−55
3	..	..	..	14	66	17	−14	−66	−17
4	103	62	107	9	39	15	+94	+23	+92
5	65	71	71	6	10	8	+59	+61	+63
6	74	100	86	46	29	45	+28	+71	+41
7	102	104	112	42	24	49	+60	+80	+63
8	108	102	114	141	78	137	−33	+24	−23

Case 11

J. H., aged 55. Chronic gastric ulcer, without stenosis. Good general condition, and no complications after operation.

	Intake			*Output*			*Balance*		
Day	*Na*	*K*	*Cl*	*Na*	*K*	*Cl*	*Na*	*K*	*Cl*
1	134	208	125	95	135	108	+39	+73	+17
*2	..	..	..	26	93	48	−26	−93	−48
3	..	..	..	10	80	14	−10	−80	−14
4	60	48	88	10	54	5	+50	−6	+83
5	40	151	31	11	43	2	+29	+108	+29

* Day of operation.

Summary

The balance of sodium, potassium, and chloride has been determined in the early stages of recovery from pyloric stenosis in five patients treated by partial gastrectomy, and also in another six patients with peptic ulcer, but without symptoms of pyloric stenosis, two of whom were found to have some narrowing of the pylorus at operation. There was considerable quantitative variation among the patients, but in general there was retention of sodium, potassium, and chloride during recovery in the patients who had pyloric stenosis; after operation, in the absence of clinical pyloric stenosis, there was retention of sodium and chloride, but not of potassium. During recovery from pyloric stenosis fixed base (Na+K) was retained in excess of chloride, a finding which could not be accounted for on the basis of gastrectomy *per se*. It is suggested that the extracellular-fluid alkalosis commonly observed in pyloric stenosis is often related to potassium depletion rather than to loss of chloride; in such patients there will be an intracellular acidosis, accounting for the retention of base in excess of chloride during recovery. The therapeutic implications of this hypothesis are discussed.

REFERENCES

Berliner, R. W., Kennedy, T. J., and Orloff, J. (1951) *Amer. J. Med.* **11**, 274.

Black, D. A. K. (1953) *Lancet*, **1**, 353.

—— and Milne, M. D. (1952) *Clin. Sci.* **11**, 397.

Bunge, G. (1873) *Zts. Biol.* **9**, 104.

Cannon, P. R., Frazier, L. E., and Hughes, R. H. (1952) *Metabolism*, **1**, 49.

Cooke, R. E., Segar, W. E., Cheek, D. B., Coville, F. E., and Darrow, D. C. (1952) *J. Clin. Invest.* **31**, 798.

Danowski, T. S., Greenman, L., Mateer, F. M., Parsons, W. B., Weigand, F. A., Mermelstein, H., and Peters, J. H. (1951) Ibid. **30**, 984.

Darrow, D. C., and Pratt, E. L. (1950) *J. Amer. Med. Ass.* **143**, 432.

Deane, N., Ziff, M., and Smith, H. W. (1952) *J. Clin. Invest.* **31**, 200.

Doxiadis, S. A., Goldfinch, M. K., and Holt, K. S. (1953) *Lancet*, **2**, 801.

Ebrill, D., and Naftalin, L. (1953) Ibid. **2**, 411.

Gamble, J. L., and Ross, S. G. (1925) *J. Clin. Invest.* **1**, 403.

Hawkins, C. F., Hardy, T. L., and Sampson, H. H. (1951) *Lancet*, **1**, 318.

Illingworth, C. F. W. (1953) *Peptic Ulcer*, Edinburgh.

Lans, H. S., Stein, I. F., and Meyer, K. A. (1952) *Ann. Surg.* **135**, 441.

Le Quesne, L. P., and Lewis, A. A. G. (1953) *Lancet*, **1**, 153.

MacPhee, I. W. (1953) *Brit. Med. J.* **1**, 1023.

Martin, H. E., Reynolds, T. B., Snyder, E. N., Berne, C. J., Homann, R. E., Jnr., Edmondson, H. A., Blatherwick, N., Fields, I., Wertman, M., and Westover, L. (1951) *J. Amer. Med. Ass.* **147**, 24.

Moore, F. D., and Ball, M. R. (1952) *The Metabolic Response to Surgery*, Springfield, Ill.

Nabarro, J. D. N., Spencer, A. G., and Stowers, J. M. (1952) *Quart. J. Med.* N.S. **21**, 225.

Relman, A. S., Etsten, B., and Schwartz, W. B. (1953) *J. Clin. Invest.* **32**, 972.

Schwartz, I. L., Schachter, D., and Freinkel, N. (1949) Ibid. **28**, 1117.

Wilkinson, A. W., Billing, B. H., Nagy, G., and Stewart, C. P. (1950) *Lancet*, **2**, 135.

Wootton, I. D. P., and King, E. J. (1953) Ibid. **1**, 470.

616.447–008.64

IDIOPATHIC HYPOPARATHYROIDISM[1]

A Study of Three Cases

By P. K. ROBINSON, E. ARNOLD CARMICHAEL, AND J. N. CUMINGS
(From the National Hospital, Queen Square, London)

DURING the past 70 years the syndrome of tetany with diminished serum-calcium and increased serum-phosphorus has gradually become recognized as due to underaction of the parathyroid glands. Accidental removal of, or damage to, the glands during the course of thyroidectomy remains the commonest cause of hypoparathyroidism. The same clinical picture was described by Albright and Ellsworth (1929) in one patient on whom thyroidectomy had not been performed and no cause of the condition could be found. Six such cases were recorded by Drake, Albright, Bauer, and Castleman (1939), and more recently Steinberg and Waldron (1952) reviewed 51 published cases, adding one of their own. Schottstaedt and Gordan (1951) reported a case of idiopathic hypoparathyroidism. Simpson (1952) added two, and Sugar (1953) one, in their reviews of the neurological complications of parathyroid deficiency. In making such a diagnosis it has become necessary to employ the rigid criteria stressed by previous groups of workers, namely (1) a low level of serum-calcium; (2) a high level of serum inorganic phosphorus; (3) chronic tetany; (4) absence of renal insufficiency; (5) normal radiological appearance of the bones, to exclude infantile rickets or adult osteomalacia; (6) absence of chronic defects of intestinal function, such as steatorrhoea or chronic diarrhoea. Albright, Burnett, Smith, and Parson (1942) described three patients who had the above syndrome, but the Ellsworth–Howard test (Ellsworth and Howard, 1934) showed that they failed to respond to intravenous injections of parathormone. The syndrome was called therefore pseudohypoparathyroidism. Cases of spontaneous hypoparathyroidism are rare, and, although the clinical syndromes have been well described in America, there have been few reports in the British literature, and the fundamental nature of the disturbance is as yet poorly understood. Three cases are therefore described, and the results of a metabolic study are given.

Case Histories

Case 1. National Hospital No. 461. This patient was admitted for investigation of epilepsy under the care of Dr. Grainger Stewart in 1934, at the age of 15 years. There was no family history of epilepsy, but the patient had convulsions at the age of seven weeks. They continued for three days, and necessitated admission to Great Ormond Street Children's Hospital. He was given bromide therapy, and the attacks were controlled, except for one which occurred during

[1] Received January 22, 1954.

teething about a year later. He walked and talked at about 18 months, but his first tooth did not appear until 15 months of age. At the age of 14 years he began to suffer from convulsive attacks involving the left arm and leg. In the worst of these he lost consciousness, but never bit his tongue or became incontinent. Examination then revealed him to be 'rather mentally backward'. The left corner of the mouth tended to droop more than the right, but otherwise the cranial nerves were normal. The posture of the outstretched hands was considered abnormal, with wrists semiflexed and fingers extended. There was slight weakness of the left leg, but no sensory loss or ataxia. Pes cavus was recorded, but both plantar responses were flexor. The teeth were 'bad and notched', and all his nails 'had many white flecks on them'. Mr. Williamson Noble considered that the eyes were normal. Cerebrospinal fluid (pressure 140 mm.): 2 cells per c.mm., protein 80 mg. per 100 ml. The Wassermann reaction was negative in blood and cerebrospinal fluid. He was considered to be suffering from idiopathic epilepsy, and was treated with phenobarbitone gr. $\frac{1}{2}$ in the morning and gr. 1 at night. In 1943 he was admitted a second time under the care of Dr. Grainger Stewart for reinvestigation, and he was told at this admission that he was suffering from tetany as well as fits. After his second admission he took phenobarbitone gr. $\frac{1}{2}$ three times a day for four years, and then stopped it.

When admitted for the third time to the National Hospital, under the care of one of us (E.A.C.), in 1950, he complained of 'attacks', loss of breath, 'cramp in the eyes', and tetany. His attacks, which had only occurred four times in seven years, consisted of clenching the teeth, an adversive movement of the head to the right, and forced thinking for about half a minute. There was no loss of consciousness, nor any movement of the limbs. No major convulsions had occurred since the age of 15 years. For seven months prior to admission he had had attacks of laryngeal stridor, and questioning revealed that he had had these 'occasionally' when about nine years old. He had had attacks of carpopedal spasm at the same age, and they had occurred at irregular and long intervals since. During the seven months prior to admission he had had episodes of 'cramp in the eyes' for half a minute at a time, during which his eyes were 'fixed in front of him'. Cramp in the calves, and paraesthesiae in the fingers after holding things for long, had been noticed for some time.

On examination he was a short, round-faced man, who was going bald; height 5 ft. 4 in., span 5 ft. 8 in. His skin was dry, and the nails of the fingers and toes were brittle and cracked. The teeth were carious, hypoplastic, and worn. The lungs, heart, and abdomen were normal. The blood-pressure was 140/90. Chvostek's sign and Trousseau's sign were positive. No weakness or abnormality of tone was found in the limbs, but there was ataxia of the left arm and leg, and the left plantar response was extensor. Small movements of the left toes were poorly appreciated, and vibration sense was depressed at both malleoli. Standing with the eyes shut he swayed to the left. Mr. Williamson Noble reported bilateral lens opacities, situated almost entirely in the lamella, about one-tenth of the thickness of the lens from its surface.

Investigations. The serum-calcium was 4·8 mg. per 100 ml., serum-phosphorus 6·6 mg. per 100 ml., serum alkaline phosphatase 12·2 King–Armstrong units, and serum-protein 6·1 gm. (albumin 4·1 gm.) per 100 ml. The cerebrospinal fluid (pressure 100 mm.) contained no cells, protein 45 mg. per 100 ml., calcium 3·4 mg. per 100 ml., and phosphorus 2·68 mg. per 100 ml. The Wassermann reaction was negative in cerebrospinal fluid and blood. The percentage of faecal fat, estimated on three occasions, was: total, 15, 19, 15; split, 9·1, 12·1, 9·6; unsplit, 5·9, 6·9, 5·4, respectively. X-rays of the skull (Dr. Sutton) showed that calcification in the basal ganglia, recorded six years before, had increased somewhat. It involved the head and body of the caudate nucleus on both sides, and a little calcification was also present in the thalamus on both sides. There was also a suspicion of some deposit in the frontal region. X-rays of the hands (7.1.52) were within normal limits. X-rays of the long bones (Dr. Sutton) were within normal limits; a small osteochondroma was present on the upper medial surface of the right tibia. An intravenous pyelogram (Dr. Bull) showed the dye concentrated by the right kidney only, which was normal apart from slight rotation. Electroencephalography (Dr. Cobb): 'There are no abnormal rhythms of significant amplitude in this symmetrical E.E.G., which contains some fast rhythm and a low-voltage alpha rhythm. Within normal limits.' An electrocardiogram was normal.

Hospital course. The patient had no spontaneous convulsions, but, during investigation with photic stimulation (11 per second) and intravenous injection of leptazol, he had a generalized convulsion beginning in the right arm and spreading rapidly. The arms became abducted at the shoulder, slightly flexed at the elbow, with marked flexion at the wrist and fingers extended. The legs were extended and the feet plantar-flexed, with some extension of the back. The whole appearance was like that of carpopedal spasm. The convulsion was followed after 20 or 30 seconds by a few rapid clonic flexion movements of the arms, and finally by flaccidity. Before treatment it was easy to produce carpopedal spasm with a sphygmomanometer cuff round the arm within one minute of ischaemia. There was very little subjective change during two courses of parathormone, but the Chvostek sign disappeared, and no spasm could be produced in the hand even with 10 minutes of ischaemia. Dihydrotachysterol produced a subjective improvement, and the objective signs of latent tetany disappeared with reversal of the biochemical abnormalities; the patient was discharged free from symptoms, and taking 1 ml. of dihydrotachysterol daily.

Summary. A man of 31 years, who had been subject to generalized and focal fits since childhood. Since the age of nine years he had had intermittent tetany and laryngeal spasm. Examination revealed a man of short stature, with latent tetany, cataracts, dry skin, scanty scalp hair, carious teeth, and calcification of the basal ganglia.

Subsequent progress. The patient remained subjectively well on a maintenance dose of 1 ml. of dihydrotachysterol daily, and because of this he reduced his treatment himself and became careless of his diet. This change resulted in a relapse of the serum-calcium and serum-phosphorus values, and a return of tetany. In spite of this he has had no convulsions during the past three years, and his mental state has not changed markedly. His optic lenses, however, show a little more opacity.

Case 2. National Hospital No. 21653. The patient was admitted to the National Hospital on March 1, 1950, under the care of Dr. M. Kremer. She came from a healthy family, and apart from uncomplicated childhood fevers she had been well until 10 years prior to admission, when she was 18 years old. While walking downstairs her body and legs seemed to stiffen, and she fell headlong. She did not lose consciousness, but every part of her body went stiff. After getting up she had great difficulty in walking, and was unable to hold a knife and fork because her hands had adopted a peculiar attitude; the position described was that of carpal spasm. During the next five or six hours she made a slow recovery. Thereafter she had intermittent attacks of spontaneous carpopedal spasm, lasting a few hours at a time, and occurring once a week. She was irritable and easily tired during this period. Nine years prior to admission she had laryngeal spasm during an attack of generalized stiffness. Such attacks occurred about twice a year until a few weeks before she came into hospital, when they were happening three or four times a week. After questioning, she admitted having occasional left frontal headaches, occasional blurring of vision, and photophobia. She had had fairly frequent attacks of objective vertigo, lasting a few minutes and relieved by lying down. She denied having had any convulsive attack or loss of consciousness.

On examination she was found to be an exceptionally nervous young woman. She reacted in a hysterical manner, and performed poorly on formal intellectual testing. Visual acuity was 6/9 in both eyes, and Mr. Williamson Noble found no evidence of lens opacities. She had a positive Chvostek's sign, but the remaining cranial nerves were normal. There was no weakness, reflex change, sensory loss, or ataxia, of the limbs or trunk, but the slightest exertion produced carpopedal spasms, and Trousseau's sign was positive. General examination gave normal results, and the hair, skin, and nails were healthy. The blood-pressure was 140/90.

Investigations. The serum-calcium was 6·0 mg. per 100 ml., serum-phosphorus 5·28 mg. per 100 ml., serum alkaline phosphatase 7·0 King–Armstrong units, serum-sodium 335 mg. per 100 ml., and serum-potassium 19·2 mg. per 100 ml. The blood-urea was 29 mg. per 100 ml., and the standard urea clearance 76·4 per cent. of normal. The total serum-protein was 6·6 gm. and albumin 3·7 gm. per 100 ml. The percentage of faecal fat, estimated on three occasions, was: total, 27, 20, 24; split, 15·5, 11·0, 12·9; unsplit, 11·5, 9, 11·1, respectively. Otological examination (Dr. Hallpike) showed spontaneous vestibular nystagmus, suggesting an organic lesion of the vestibulo-cerebellar connexions. X-rays of the skull (Dr. Bull) showed a normal size, shape, and bony texture. Symmetrical calcification was present in the caudate nucleus, and in the dentate nucleus of the cerebellum. On X-rays of the long bones (Dr. Moor) the calcium content appeared normal, and no evidence of cysts was detected. X-rays of the kidney areas and the hands (Dr. Davies) showed no calcification in or around the kidneys, and the hands were radiologically normal. On intravenous pyelography (Dr. Sutton) no abnormality was seen. Summary of psychological report (Dr. J. McFie): 'Very poor test scores, with slightly worse performance on "deterioration" tests, may indicate a defective intellectual level (I.Q. 69) with mild impairment, or these results may indicate a severe emotional disturbance (possibly on or masking an organic basis) impairing all performances. I am inclined towards the latter view.'

Hospital course. Clinical assessment of the patient's condition was complicated by hysterical exaggeration, and later by perpetuation of her initial tetanic symptoms. Before treatment, however, Trousseau's phenomenon could be elicited by four minutes' ischaemia, whereas during the course of dihydrotachysterol treatment eight minutes were required to produce a spasm. There was some clinical improvement after dihydrotachysterol, but it did not parallel the biochemical improvement, and the patient remained a therapeutic problem even after discharge, when she had normal serum-calcium and serum-phosphorus levels and was taking 1 ml. of dihydrotachysterol per day.

Summary. A woman of 28 years, who began to have episodes of stiffness of limbs at the age of 18 years. They later became associated with difficulty in breathing. There were no convulsions. Examination revealed a rather short woman exhibiting mild mental impairment and a hysterical personality. There were no cataracts. Chvostek's and Trousseau's signs were easily elicited. There was radiological evidence of calcification of the basal ganglia and dentate nucleus.

Subsequent progress. The patient was cured of her biochemical abnormalities, but there was a hysterical prolongation of her symptoms of tetany, which has necessitated institutional care.

Case 3. National Hospital No. 20278. The patient, aged 59 years, was admitted to the National Hospital under the care of Dr. D. H. Brinton on February 13, 1950. He complained of becoming slower in all his movements, of deterioration of his memory, and of depression. During the five years before admission he had gradually become slower at his work and in his mental processes. His wife had particularly noticed how forgetful he had become. Two years before admission he had had an attack of unconsciousness following one of a course of injections for varicose veins. He had never had any convulsions, but at night his legs gave 'involuntary jumps'. His imitation of these movements showed slight clonic movements of the legs and twitching movement of the ankles. On rare occasions his hands had become locked, but he could not describe their position accurately. When directly questioned he admitted slight deterioration of vision, some clumsiness of the left hand, and a little weakness of both hands. He had complained occasionally to his wife that his head was 'muzzy' and 'dizzy'. His paternal stepbrother was an epileptic. The patient had had 'trigeminal neuralgia' 18 years before, cured by medicine, and a Pott's fracture of the right leg during the First World War.

On examination he was of average build; height 5 ft. 9¼ in., span 5 ft. 11 in. He was going bald, and losing his eyebrows and eyelashes. His expression was mask-like. Psychological testing showed evidence of moderate organic intellectual impairment, with emphasis on the learning defect. He was depressed, and at times tearful. There was depression of the sense of smell, and a moderate degree of high-tone deafness. Visual acuity was 6/12 in both eyes, and the optic fundi looked normal. The slit lamp and corneal microscope (Mr. Williamson Noble) revealed fine cloudy opacities at the level of the outer layer of the adult nucleus and at the junction of the outer and middle thirds of the thickness of the lens. The cranial nerves were normal, and there was no Chovstek's sign. There was slight rigidity of all four limbs, and some tremor of the fingers brought out by movement. There was no weakness, but fine movements were poorly carried out. Trousseau's sign was positive. The deep reflexes were brisk and symmetrical, and the plantar responses flexor. Sensation was normal. The gait was slow and slightly shuffling, 'reminiscent of Parkinsonism'. There were inspiratory and expiratory wheezes over both lung fields. The heart was normal, and the blood-pressure 140/80. The patient was edentulous. Abdominal examination gave a normal result.

Investigations. The serum-calcium was 6·8 mg. per 100 ml., serum inorganic phosphorus 5·1 mg. per 100 ml., serum alkaline phosphatase 6·4 King–Armstrong units, and serum-protein 6·6 gm. (albumin 3·7 gm.) per 100 ml. The blood-urea on 12.2.53 was 41 mg. per 100 ml. The Wassermann reaction in blood and cerebrospinal fluid was negative. The cerebrospinal fluid (pressure 160 mm.) contained 2 cells per c.mm., protein 120 mg., calcium 3·0 mg., and phosphorus 2·5 mg. per 100 ml. The percentage of faecal fat, estimated on three occasions, was: total, 21, 17, 18; split, 13·7, 10·2, 10·9; unsplit, 7·3, 6·8, 7·1, respectively. On X-rays of the skull (Dr. Davies) the vault was normal; there was a considerable amount of stippled calcification throughout the basal ganglia. X-rays of the chest (Dr. Davies) showed some enlargement of the heart outline, chiefly ventricular in type, with a rather wide aortic arch. X-rays of the limbs (Dr. Moor) showed slight osteoporotic changes in the long bones of the right arm, osteoarthritic changes in the right wrist and interphalangeal joints, minimal osteoarthritis in the feet, and in the right leg evidence of an old Pott's fracture. Calcification was seen in the anteroposterior view, lying lateral to the tibia, and might be vascular. In an intravenous pyelogram (Dr. Bull) no abnormality was seen. Electroencephalography (Dr. Cobb): 'For the most part this record is normal, but there are runs of mixed frequency, chiefly about 7 cycles per second, which are bilaterally synchronous. Overbreathing was too poorly performed to have any effect. The degree of abnormality is very slight, and the record is symmetrical.' An electrocardiogram showed left-sided preponderance. Summary of psychological report (Dr. J. McFie): 'A man of previously bright normal intelligence, now showing evidence of moderate organic intellectual impairment, with emphasis on the learning defect and on depressive emotional reaction.'

Hospital course. The patient made very little objective improvement, but he felt better after treatment with dihydrotachysterol, and his 'dizziness' lessened. His wife stated that he became less agitated, anxious, and tense. The ischaemic paraesthesiae observed after putting a cuff round the arm tended to appear later and to be less intense during the course of dihydrotachysterol. There was, however, no change in the dementia, the signs of Parkinsonism, or the lens opacities.

Summary. A man of 59 years, who exhibited signs of mental deterioration during the five years prior to admission. He had had 'attacks' of clonus-like movements in his legs, and at other times his hands might become 'locked'. There was considerable intellectual deterioration, a mask-like facies, and an attitude of flexion. Chvostek's sign was absent; Trousseau's phenomenon was present. There were lens opacities, and X-rays of the skull showed calcification of the basal ganglia.

Subsequent progress. During the past three years the patient has continued treatment with dihydrotachysterol in a maintenance dose of 1 ml. daily. There has been a slight increase in the signs of Parkinsonism, but the optic lenses are unchanged, and his dementia has not noticeably increased. Recent serum analysis has shown the calcium level to be low and the phosphorus level high. Dihydrotachysterol was increased to 2 ml. daily, with improvement in the serum values, and lessening of his retardation.

Clinical Picture

The symptoms of idiopathic hypoparathyroidism are chiefly shown by the nervous system and the ectodermal structures. There may be calcification in the optic lenses, giving rise to cataracts, or in the brain, where it may be dense enough in the region of the basal ganglia and dentate nuclei to show on X-rays of the skull.

Nervous system. The commonest neurological manifestation of this disorder is tetany, which can be most easily demonstrated by Chvostek's and Trousseau's signs, although Kirstein and Kugelberg (1946) found that even the latter sign may be present in 4 per cent. of normal subjects. The carpal spasm in Trousseau's phenomenon might be called the 'positive' motor manifestation of ischaemia in the presence of hypocalcaemia. Kugelberg (1944) noticed the earlier onset of paraesthesiae, and their greater extent and intensity, in patients who had a deficiency of ionized calcium. He found that the paraesthesiae spread centripetally up to or above the elbow, but in 50 normal cases they spread only to a level about the wrist. In Cases 1 and 2 the findings were the same as in Kugelberg's cases. At a stage when the serum-calcium level was low, ischaemic tingling began within a minute, and spread up to the sphygmomanometer cuff above the elbow within three or four minutes. There was a gradual return to normal in both cases as the serum-calcium levels were improved. In Case 1, in which the patient was a more reliable witness, paraesthesiae were absent after 10 days' treatment with dihydrotachysterol. Similar findings were not observed in Case 3, but in view of the paucity of the motor signs produced by ischaemia in this case it is perhaps not surprising that the positive sensory manifestations were few, and the patient's dementia made any accurate observations impossible. In addition to the positive sensory manifestations, it was possible to observe what might be termed negative sensory manifestations in Cases 1 and 2. The centripetal spread of hypaesthesia during compression of the upper arm with a sphygmomanometer cuff, described by Lewis, Pickering, and Rothschild (1931–3) in normal patients, occurred early and spread rapidly in the above patients. When the serum-calcium level was low, such hypaesthesia had extended to the upper part of the dorsum of the hand within four minutes in both cases. A similar degree of sensory impairment took 17 minutes to develop when the serum-calcium had been restored to normal.

The over-excitability of the peripheral nerves may cause spasm or stiffness of a local or generalized nature. Spontaneous pedal spasm may arise suddenly while walking and be of brief duration, so that the foot drags for a second or two, as in Case 2 of Simpson (1952). Drake, Albright, Bauer, and Castleman (1939) recorded, in their Cases 1 and 4, more severe generalized spasm, which caused sudden falling and difficulty in getting up, but without disturbance of consciousness. Wise and Hart (1952) and Simpson (1952) have recorded 'crampy fits', in which carpopedal spasm and involvement of jaw and respiratory muscles led to immobility, dyspnoea, and an inability to talk. More severe spasm of the glottis, as described in Case 3 of Albright, Burnett, Smith, and Parson (1942) and Case 2 of Sutphin, Albright, and McCune (1943), caused a choking sensation, struggling for breath, and cyanosis. In Case 2 of Drake, Albright, Bauer, and Castleman (1939) such attacks were followed by unconsciousness. Thus attacks which begin by a disturbance of a peripheral mechanism may cause profound central effects, and incomplete observation of the episode may lead to a mistaken diagnosis of the primary site of disturbed function. In Cases 1 and 2 of the present series laryngeal spasm had occurred, but it had never been severe enough to cause alarm, nor had consciousness been disturbed by it.

The chief central nervous manifestation of hypoparathyroidism is epilepsy, which Albright and Reifenstein (1948) said may be the only symptom for several years before signs of tetany appear and suggest the true diagnosis. The pattern of such epileptic attacks is diverse. Grand mal has been recorded in many cases, and Albright, Burnett, Smith, and Parson (1942), Sutphin, Albright, and McCune (1943), and Bakwin, Gorman, and Ziegra (1950) recorded cases in which there were episodes consistent with the diagnosis of petit mal. Attacks with twitching of the limbs on one side of the body and turning of the head or eyes to the same side, such as those seen in Case 1 of Simpson (1952) and Case 1 of Sutphin, Albright, and McCune (1943), may suggest a focal lesion in the contralateral hemisphere. Consciousness may not be lost in such unilateral seizures, but it was lost in Case 1 of Wise and Hart (1952). Although description of the attacks in recorded cases is often meagre, it seems from the cases recorded by Sutphin, Albright, and McCune (1943, Case 4), Drake, Albright, Bauer, and Castleman (1939, Case 3), Wise and Hart (1952, Case 1), and Simpson (1952, Case 1) that a true epileptic attack may be accompanied or followed by general or local spasm indistinguishable from that seen in tetany. In Case 1 of the present group there had been generalized convulsions, and apparently focal attacks. It is possible that the clonic movements of the lower limbs described in Case 3 were a manifestation of an over-excitable state in the central nervous system, but the patient had never had a generalized convulsion. Rarely, in hypoparathyroidism, epilepsy may be associated with headache and papill-oedema, so that an expanding intracranial lesion is suspected. The necessity of considering this syndrome, first reported by Albrecht (1923) and recently reviewed by Grant (1953), did not arise in our cases.

It is perhaps surprising that manifestations of disease of the basal ganglia do not occur more often, considering the frequency of punctate calcification in this area. Disease of the extrapyramidal system was noted in the two cases reported by Alexander and Tucker (1949) and Gsell (1950). In Case 3 our patient had a dementia, but on examination he had a well-marked Parkinsonian syndrome, and X-rays showed calcification in the deep grey matter of both cerebral hemispheres. It is evident, however, that intracerebral calcification is not always associated with abnormal neurological signs referable to the affected area, because there were cerebellar signs in Case 1 in the absence of radiological evidence of calcification in the cerebellum, whereas in Case 2 there was calcification in the cerebellum, but no cerebellar signs.

The literature concerning psychosis in tetany was reviewed by Barrett (1919–20), who found no typical psychotic pattern. Various workers have reported cases of psychosis in post-thyroidectomy hypoparathyroidism, and Greene and Swanson (1941) recorded five. They found toxic delirium to be the commonest psychotic disturbance in parathyroid deficiency, although other disorders, including dementia, anxiety, and depression, were seen. Although Mortell (1946) found no improvement in the intellectual function of a patient who had idiopathic hypoparathyroidism, after treatment which had given complete relief of symptoms, Eaton and Haines (1939) noted some improvement of the mental state after adequate treatment. Camp (1947) found that the mental retardation seen in children with parathyroid deficiency improved considerably with treatment. The additional fact that the disorder may be found in the adult with dementia, as seen in Case 3 above, or with a psychotic episode, as described by Steinberg and Waldron (1952), makes early diagnosis and continued therapy all the more important.

Radiological findings. Calcification in the region of the basal ganglia was seen in the X-rays of the skull in all our three cases. It occurred also in the frontal region in Case 1, and in the dentate nucleus in Case 2. Such changes have been noted in idiopathic hypoparathyroidism by Eaton and Haines (1939), in pseudohypoparathyroidism by Medill (1951), and in post-thyroidectomy parathyroid deficiency by Siglin, Eaton, Camp, and Haines (1947). In a review of the pathological basis of such calcification, Camp (1947) stated that there is a colloid deposition in and around the finer cerebral blood-vessels, which subsequently becomes calcified. This colloid deposition was found so frequently in the anterior half of the globus pallidus and dentate nucleus by Ostertag (1929) that its pathological significance might be doubted. Earlier reports by McAlpine (1923) had drawn attention to calcification in these areas in encephalitis lethargica, Huntington's chorea, and paralysis agitans, and, although Lhermitte, Kraus, and McAlpine (1924–5) and Hurst (1926) considered that the histological evidence of calcium was inconclusive, the chemical analyses made by Eaves (1926) showed an abundance of calcium and iron in such deposits. Their presence clearly did not depend upon any specific neurological disease, nor was there evidence of a constant disturbance of calcium metabolism in such cases. The finding of such deposits in hypoparathyroidism is therefore not specific, although in many instances they are conspicuous. Albright and Reifenstein (1948) considered that this ectopic calcification was due to supersaturation of the tissues with calcium phosphate. It is possible that increased serum-phosphorus assists the precipitation of calcium phosphate, but it is certain that, whatever the mechanism, the perivascular colloid has sufficient affinity for calcium to cause its deposition, even in the presence of a low serum concentration.

In discussing the radiological appearance of the long bones, Albright and Reifenstein (1948) considered that one would expect a slightly increased density of bone owing to supersaturation of the tissue-fluids with calcium phosphate. This was the usual finding in their experience, although they had seen osteomalacia with hypoparathyroidism in rare instances. Increased density of the skeleton was seen in one case of Emerson, Walsh, and Howard (1941), although in their second patient, a woman of 56 years, general rarefaction of the bony skeleton was observed. This was attributed to senile osteoporosis, since there was nothing to suggest previous hyperparathyroidism, poor intake of calcium, or deficiency of vitamin D. Peterman and Garvey (1948), and Reynolds, Jacobson, Edmondson, Martin, and Nelson (1952) found evidence of demineralization of the skeleton in their cases, and the latter group of workers considered that the long-standing negative calcium balance was the most likely cause. That a normal radiological appearance of the skeleton may be seen in hypoparathyroidism is shown by the cases reported above.

Electroencephalogram. No specific pattern was found in the electroencephalographic records in hypoparathyroidism made by Odoriz, del Castillo, Manfredi, and de la Balze (1944), and Gotta and Odoriz (1948). Those which were abnormal did not change after administration of intravenous calcium, although there was general clinical improvement. More permanent restoration of the serum-calcium to normal tended to abolish the abnormalities. Varied findings—normal records, slow waves, or continuous generalized dysrhythmia—have been recorded by Kowallis (1941), Sutphin, Albright, and McCune (1943), and Steinberg and Waldron (1952). Some improvement in the records after treatment has been seen in the cases of Taubenhaus and Engle (1945), Mortell (1946), Simpson (1952), and Wise and Hart (1952), although even in these cases overbreathing sometimes revealed a latent abnormality. A different response in the electroencephalogram after treatment was noted by Hansted and Brandt (1953) in two siblings suffering from spontaneous parathyroid deficiency. No abnormality was seen in the record of Case 1 of the present series, although the patient had had clinical epileptic attacks. In Case 3 only was there a very slight abnormality. Such findings are in accord with previous observations that the electroencephalographic pattern in patients suffering from parathyroid deficiency may be normal or abnormal, and if it is abnormal it probably bears a more constant relation to the fundamental electrical activity of the brain than to the serum-calcium level.

Ectodermal structures. Lesions of the ectoderm, such as those described by Cantarow, Stewart, and Morgan (1939) and Emerson, Walsh, and Howard (1941), are met with fairly frequently in hypoparathyroidism. The skin may be dry, coarse, and scaly, the scalp hair thin and patchy, the eyelashes and eyebrows scanty, and axillary and pubic hair absent. The nails may be so deformed and overgrown with skin that the condition resembles a fungus infection. All these changes, however, respond to treatment of the parathyroid deficiency. Sutphin, Albright, and McCune (1943) described five cases of idiopathic hypoparathyroidism (three in siblings) associated with moniliasis, but there was insufficient evidence to assume that the two conditions were causally related, and treatment of the parathyroid deficiency did not alter the nail condition. Enamel deficiency may be seen in the teeth in hypoparathyroidism, with delayed and irregular eruption of the deciduous teeth and retarded development of the permanent teeth. Albright and Strock (1933) found that, when hypoparathyroidism develops before the teeth have entirely formed, aplasia and hypoplasia occur at a point in their development where the deficiency began, and non-calcification can be seen. No such changes were seen in any of our three patients, but the abnormalities observed in the skin and hair in Cases 1 and 3 responded to treatment.

Cataracts. The formation of lens opacities in hypoparathyroidism is very common, although the explanation remains obscure. They occur in other conditions associated with hypocalcaemia, notably in sprue, and do not seem to depend primarily upon the parathyroid deficiency itself. They were observed in two of our cases, being more marked in Case 1, in which the condition had been present since childhood. Treatment seems to have prevented any increase in the opacities, but their density has not lessened. This observation agrees with those of all other workers except Jordan and Kelsall (1951), who reported that the opacities in their patient were less dense and less numerous one year after they had been first noticed and treatment had begun.

Pseudohypoparathyroidism

An outline of the clinical syndrome of parathyroid insufficiency would be incomplete without a reference to pseudohypoparathyroidism. Albright, Burnett, Smith, and Parson (1942) described three patients who showed clinical evidence of spontaneous deficiency of the parathyroid glands, but who had

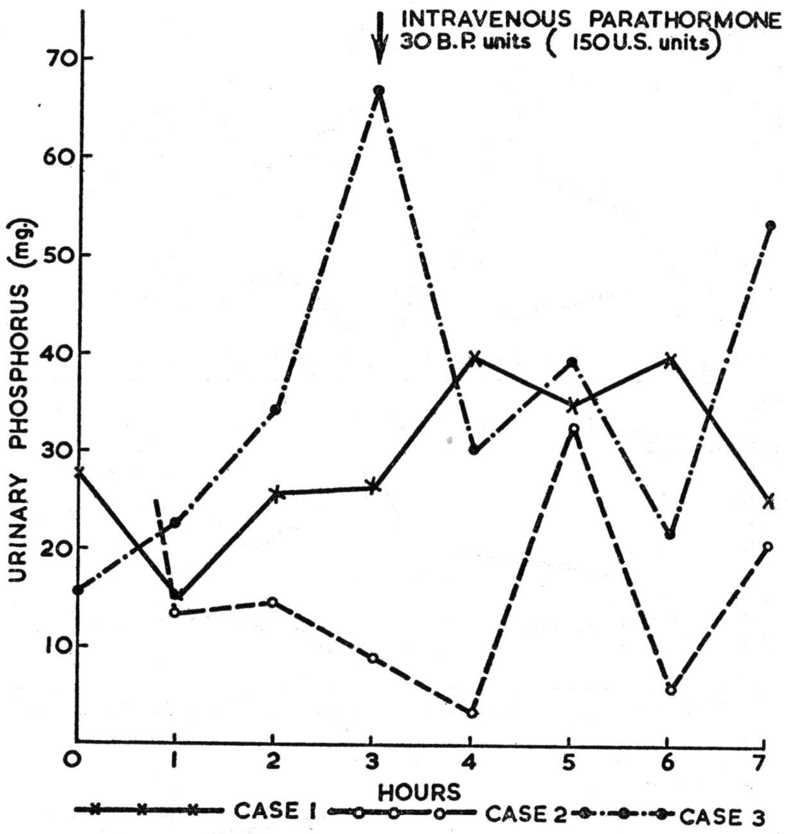

FIG. 1. The effect of intravenous parathormone on the urinary phosphorus.

in addition a resistance to parathormone, a slower response than usual to dihydrotachysterol, a characteristic physical appearance, deformity of the hands, and a tendency to calcification in subcutaneous tissues. An intravenous injection of parathormone failed to produce a 'phosphorus diuresis'. The patients were short and thickset, with unusually round faces, but the most remarkable physical abnormality was brachydactyly. This shortening of the fingers, which is largely due to early closure of the metacarpal epiphyses, leads to a characteristic deformity of the hands, in which the ulnar two fingers are disproportionately short, and the index finger may appear the longest. This feature and the tendency to subcutaneous calcification are discussed by Albright and Reifenstein (1948) and others.

Biochemical Findings

Methods of study. The patients were observed for three months, during which time they had a constant standard diet containing between 750 and 900 mg. of calcium and 800 and 900 mg. of phosphorus per day. This diet proved inadequate to satisfy hunger in Case 1, and the daily intake was increased early

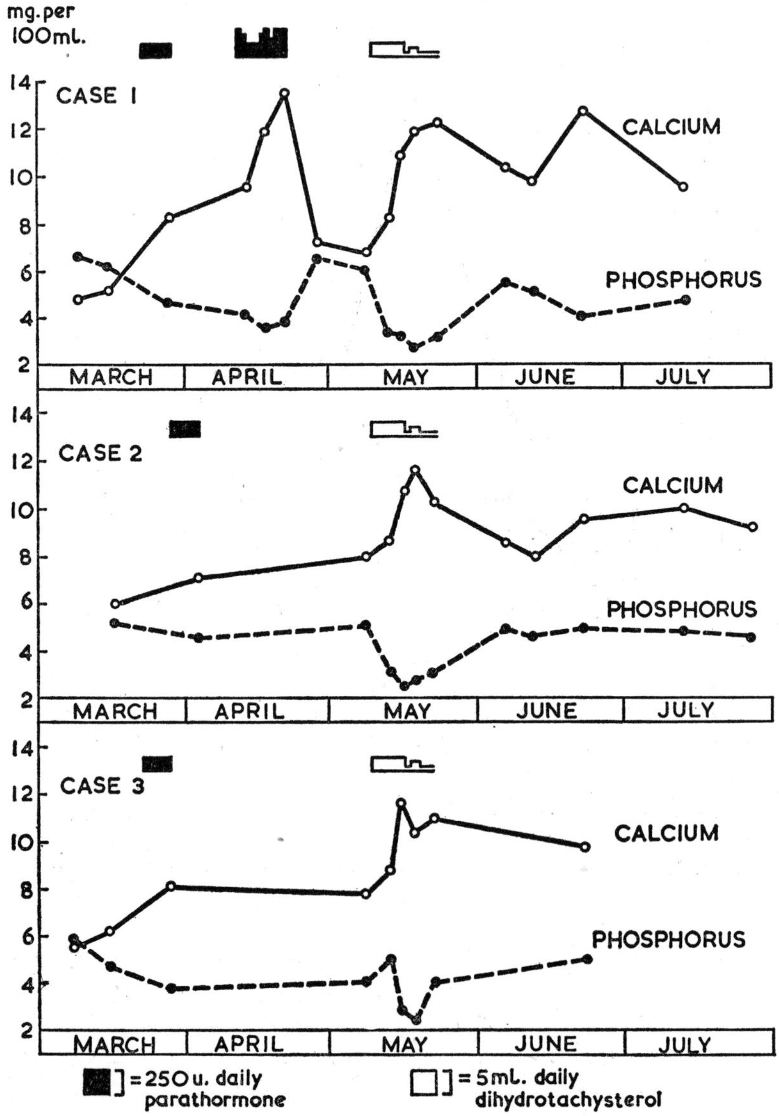

FIG. 2. Serum-calcium and serum-phosphorus values.

in the study to 1·0 gm. of calcium and 1·1 gm. of phosphorus. The fat-content of these diets was 77·2 gm. per day in Case 1 and 75·4 gm. per day in Cases 2 and 3. Twenty-four-hourly specimens of urine, and all stools passed, were collected, and their calcium and phosphorus content estimated by the methods of

Kramer and Tisdall (Harrison, 1947) and Fiske and Subbarow (1925) respectively. Frequent determinations of the serum-calcium and serum-phosphorus were made in specimens of blood taken at the same time of day on each occasion, particularly before, during, and after the three periods in which a study of the calcium and phosphorus balance was carried out. The first period, of four days,

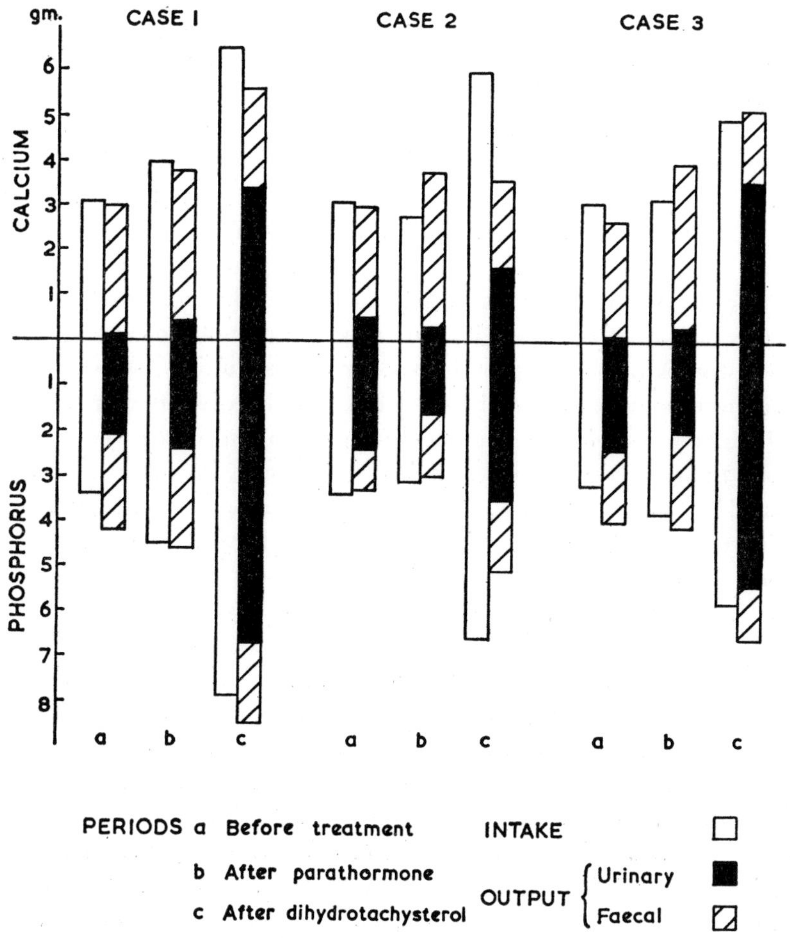

FIG. 3. Calcium and phosphorus balance before and after treatment.

was at the beginning of the patient's stay in hospital, and before any treatment had begun. The second period, also of four days, was after a six-day course of intramuscular parathormone. The third period, of six days, was after 12 days' treatment with dihydrotachysterol. Since the patients were much improved by this treatment, it was continued throughout the third period. Faecal fat estimations (Harrison, 1947), renal investigation, and radiological examination of the long bones excluded alimentary, renal, or general skeletal disease as a cause of the syndrome under investigation. Albright, Burnett, Smith, and Parson (1942) considered that it was possible to distinguish true idiopathic hypoparathyroidism from pseudohypoparathyroidism by using the test described by Ellsworth and Howard (1934), and this test was carried out on our patients. It consists of estimation of the urinary phosphorus in hourly samples taken for three hours before, and three to five hours after, an intravenous dose of 200 U.S. units of parathormone. The normal subject shows an increase of urinary phosphorus, after injection, to 70 mg. per hour; the patient who has idiopathic hypoparathyroidism excretes 100 mg. or more per hour; but the patient who has pseudohypoparathyroidism shows a very slight increase in excretion, which is usually less than 40 mg. per hour.

Results. The Ellsworth–Howard test (using 30 B.P. units of parathormone, equivalent to 150 U.S. units) revealed very small amounts of phosphorus in the urine after intravenous parathormone in all three cases. One isolated value of 53·8 mg. in one hour was the only reading above 40 mg. (Fig. 1). The balance studies showed that all the patients were in positive calcium balance before treatment. Cases 1 and 3 were in negative phosphorus balance, and Case 2 in slightly positive phosphorus balance, before treatment. After parathormone (Fig. 3) there was little change in the excretion of calcium and phosphorus in Case 1, and the balances were unaltered. In Cases 2 and 3 there appeared to be a relative increase in faecal calcium, and the calcium balance became negative. The slight increase in faecal phosphorus in these two cases was insufficient to change the phosphorus balances. It will be noticed, however, that after daily intramuscular doses of 150 B.P. units of parathormone, from the same batch as that which failed to produce a phosphorus diuresis after intravenous injection, there was a slight increase of serum-calcium and a decrease of serum-phosphorus in Cases 1 and 3 (Fig. 2). The changes in Case 2 were not so definite. With larger doses of parathormone, up to 300 B.P. (equal to 1500 U.S.) units daily, in Case 1, the serum values returned to normal. These doses, however, were in excess of the usual therapeutic amounts, and were extremely painful. After dihydrotachysterol there was a marked increase in the urinary calcium and phosphorus (Fig. 4) and a decrease in the faecal calcium and phosphorus. Positive calcium balance was achieved in Case 2, and increased in Case 1, but the changes in Case 3 were only sufficient to reduce the negative balance (Fig. 3). Increased excretion of phosphorus increased the negative phosphorus balance in Cases 1 and 3, but the changes in Case 2 were insufficient to alter the positive balance. In all three cases administration of dihydrotachysterol was followed by a return of the serum values to normal.

Discussion

The clinical syndrome of tetany can be produced by a lowering of the calcium or a raising of the pH of the blood, and Lehmann (1937) and Kugelberg (1944) have shown that these changes are associated with a lowering of the threshold of the peripheral nerves to electrical excitation and a reduced capacity of accommodation. If the disturbance is severe enough, spontaneous activity occurs, giving rise to paraesthesiae and muscle spasm. Lesser degrees of overactivity may be augmented by ischaemia, as in Trousseau's phenomenon, which Lewis (1939–42) showed was due to ischaemia of the nerve-trunk under the occluding

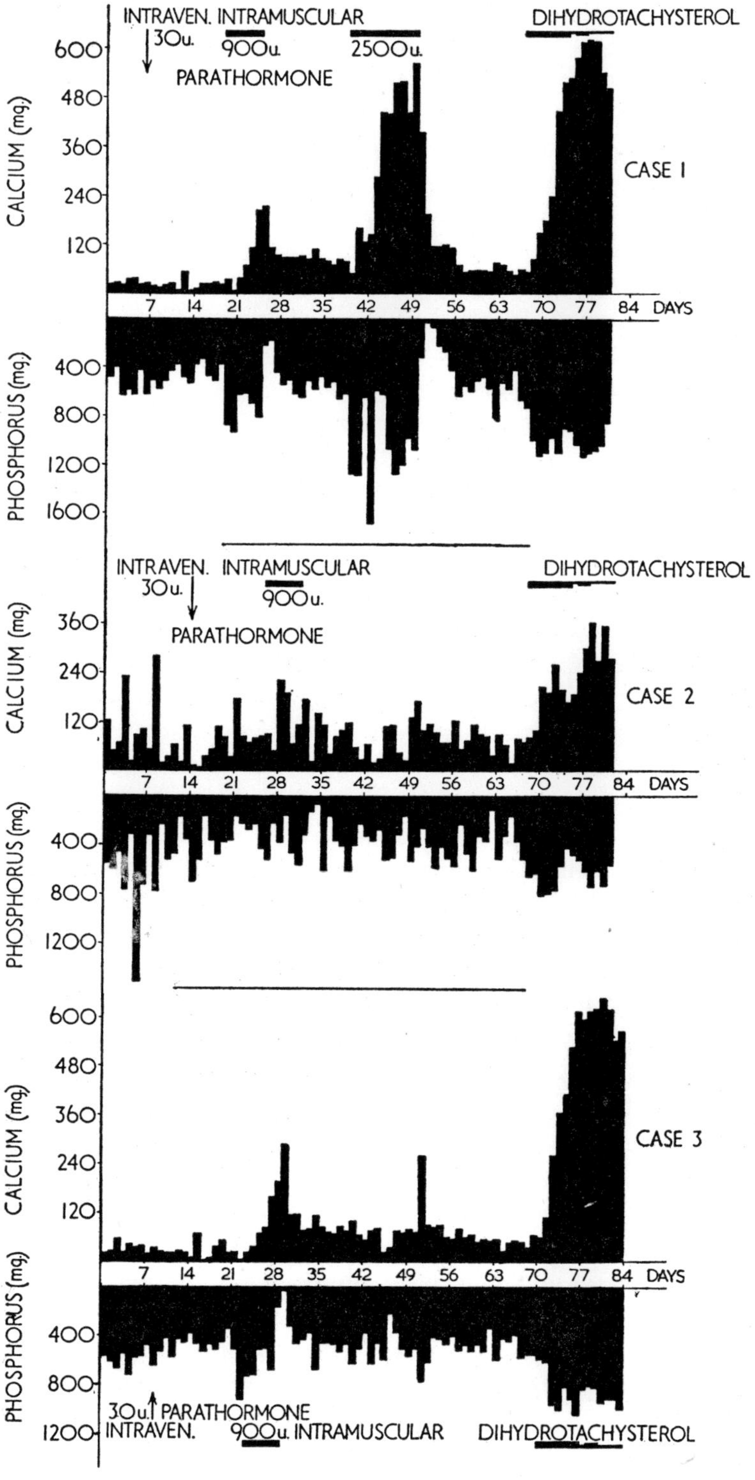

FIG. 4. Charts showing daily urinary excretion of calcium and phosphorus.

cuff. Kugelberg (1944) observed that such overactivity of the sensory and motor nerves, in the hypocalcaemic state, was accompanied by an acceleration of the rate of sensory and motor impairment during ischaemia. Our findings in the above cases confirm this early sensory loss, and show that it is remediable by specific therapy. Since hypocalcaemia appears to induce over-excitability, amounting to spontaneous discharges in the peripheral nerves (Lehmann, 1937), ganglion cells (Bronk, Larrabee, Gaylor, and Brink, 1938), and motor end-plates (Kuffler, 1944), it seems probable that such a state occurs in the central nervous system. Paton, Findlay, and Watson (1916) considered that epilepsy in tetany was due to secondary involvement of the motor cortex, and Sabbatani (1901) showed that the excitability of the cerebral cortex was reduced by the application of isotonic solution of calcium chloride, but was increased by citrate solutions which removed calcium. McQuarrie, Hansen, and Ziegler (1941) considered that with a low mineral intake there was an increase in the tissue-water, with a disturbance of the surface functions of the brain-cell membranes, which permitted the building up of abnormal electrical potentials. A similar increase in water-content of the tissues, resulting in epileptic discharges, occurs in the water pitressin test (Garland, Dick, and Whitty, 1943). In discussing the pathogenesis of papilloedema and fits in hypoparathyroidism, Grant (1953) reviewed the abundant evidence for cerebral oedema in this condition. Such a marked degree of oedema is seen in only a few cases of hypoparathyroidism, but there is evidence that a parathyroid deficiency leads to a disturbance of the water-content of the cell (Ellis, 1928), an electrolyte disequilibrium, and interference with the intracellular metabolism (Imrie and Jenkinson, 1933; McIlwain and Gore, 1951).

The results of biochemical studies of our patients suggested at first that they belonged to the sub-group of patients suffering from pseudohypoparathyroidism, because they failed to excrete phosphorus in the urine after intravenous parathormone. The original description of this sub-group was given by Albright, Burnett, Smith, and Parson (1942), and when Bishop and de Mowbray (1951) demonstrated their case they found that 16 similar cases had been recorded in the literature. Since then isolated cases have been recorded by Bakwin, Gorman, and Ziegra (1950), Reynolds, Jacobson, Edmondson, Martin, and Nelson (1952), Bille (1952), and Wise and Hart (1952). In their analysis of four such cases, Elrick, Albright, Bartter, Forbes, and Reeves (1950) considered that the underlying defect is a genetic one, involving three separate genes concerned with three disorders, namely, a lack of response of the end-organ to parathormone, a dyschondroplasia leading to typical physical habitus and deformity of the hands, and a predisposition to ectopic calcification especially around joints. From a study of the reported cases it is clear that the clinical picture is rarely complete. For example, in the case described by Wise and Hart (1952) the hands and feet were normal, and there was no subcutaneous calcification. In Case 1 of Elrick, Albright, Bartter, Forbes, and Reeves (1950) the points in favour of the diagnosis of pseudohypoparathyroidism were the physical habitus and the poor response to treatment with parathormone, although the Ellsworth–

Howard test gave a result approximating more to the 'normal' than to that usually seen in this group. Reynolds, Jacobson, Edmondson, Martin, and Nelson (1952) have indicated how unreliable the physical habitus may be as a diagnostic sign of pseudohypoparathyroidism, and the implication is that the separation of this sub-group depends primarily on the failure to excrete phosphorus in the urine after intravenous parathormone. It is clear, however, from Cases 1 and 3 of the present series that this failure does not necessarily mean that the patient will not respond to high and repeated doses given intramuscularly, and it has gradually become clear that the biochemical and clinical response to parathormone is uncertain and unpredictable. In discussing the case of pseudohypoparathyroidism described by Bishop and de Mowbray (1951), Prunty spoke of a patient with post-thyroidectomy hypoparathyroidism who made no response to daily injections of 40 B.P. units of parathormone until 200 units had been given intravenously, after which the smaller dose had a very marked effect. It appears, therefore, that the Ellsworth–Howard test may give misleading results, and the experiments of Stewart and Bowen (1952) cast serious doubts on the specificity of this test. For these reasons the present writers consider that too strict a subdivision of a group of cases under the title of pseudohypoparathyroidism is at present misleading, and may prove untenable. They consider further that the cases here described fall into the wider group of idiopathic hypoparathyroidism, although the results of the Ellsworth–Howard test, and the physical habitus in Case 1, suggested at first a narrower definition. It appears indisputable, however, that the resistance of different cases of spontaneous parathyroid deficiency to parathormone varies over a wide range, and some of the most refractory cases respond to dihydrotachysterol, as our patients did. In them the administration of dihydrotachysterol caused an increase in the positive calcium balance with a reduction of faecal calcium; this result suggests an increased absorption, which in turn is followed by an increase in the serum level and a rise in the urinary excretion. In all cases there was an increased urinary excretion of phosphorus, although this was insufficient to change the total phosphorus balance. These findings are in accord with those of Albright, Bloomberg, Drake, and Sulkowitch (1938), who found that dihydrotachysterol appeared to have a greater effect in increasing renal excretion of phosphorus than in increasing the serum-calcium, whereas with vitamin D the reverse was the case. The clinical and biochemical response to dihydrotachysterol suggests that the end-organ is active, and it seems possible that there is a defect in some intermediate stage in the action of parathormone on the kidney, which is circumvented by the use of dihydrotachysterol. Animal experiments reported by Elrick, Albright, Bartter, Forbes, and Reeves (1950) and Wise and Hart (1952) failed to reveal any antihormone activity in the serum of patients who did not respond to parathormone.

Further elucidation of the problem must await the purification and analysis of parathyroid extract, since variation in this substance may account for some of the differing results. At present there is a great deal of evidence of its complex action. Albright and his colleagues consider its main action to be the excretion of phosphorus in the urine, all other findings being secondary to this effect. Milne (1951) and Dent (1953) have both reported experimental evidence for the renal action of parathormone, although the work of others (Collip, 1925; Collip, Clark, and Scott, 1925; Barnicot, 1948; Ingalls, Donaldson, and Albright, 1943) has indicated that it has a direct effect in mobilizing the calcium of the skeleton. The absence of hyperphosphataemia in hyperparathyroidism indicates, however, that this latter action is not the only action of parathormone. The evidence of intracellular migration of phosphate after administration of parathormone (Imrie and Jenkinson, 1933; Tweedy and Campbell, 1944), and the suggestion by Martin and Perkins (1951) that this hormone extract alters the calcium-binding power of serum-albumin, are a further indication that its action is not confined to the kidney or the skeleton. Until these actions are clarified, and until the composition of parathyroid extract is more certainly known, we shall not be able to understand clearly the varied nature of spontaneous parathyroid deficiency.

We wish to thank Dr. D. H. Brinton and Dr. M. Kremer for permission to examine and record details of Cases 3 and 2 respectively. Our thanks are also due to Mr. F. A. Williamson Noble, and to members of the staffs of the Radiological and Applied Electrophysiological Departments, for their help in examining the patients.

Summary

A detailed clinical description of three cases of spontaneous parathyroid deficiency is given. The patients were observed for a period of three months, during which time calcium and phosphorus balance studies were carried out. The daily intake of calcium and phosphorus was known, and the daily excretion in the urine and stools was estimated. Particular attention was paid to the clinical response to treatment with parathormone and with dihydrotachysterol, and the results of studies of the biochemical changes in the blood, urine, and stools, after such therapy, are given. The clinical picture and the biochemical findings are discussed with reference to the work of other authors, and special comment is made on Albright's conception of pseudohypoparathyroidism.

REFERENCES

Albrecht, K. (1923) *Monats. Psychiat. Neurol.* **55,** 55.
Albright, F., Bloomberg, E., Drake, T. G., and Sulkowitch, H. (1938) *J. Clin. Invest.* **17,** 317.
—— Burnett, C. H., Smith, P. H., and Parson, W. (1942) *Endocrinology,* **30,** 922.
—— and Ellsworth, R. (1929) *J. Clin. Invest.* **7,** 183.
—— and Reifenstein, E. C. (1948) *The Parathyroid Glands and Metabolic Bone Disease,* Baltimore.
—— and Strock, M. S. (1933) *J. Clin. Invest.* **12,** 974.
Alexander, S. B., and Tucker, H. St. G. (1949) *J. Clin. Endocrin.* **9,** 862.
Bakwin, H., Gorman, W. F., and Ziegra, S. R. (1950) *J. Pediat.* **36,** 567.
Barnicot, N. A. (1948) *J. Anat.* **82,** 233.
Barrett, A. M. (1919–20) *Amer. J. Insanity,* **76,** 373.
Bille, B. S. V. (1952) *Acta paediat.* **41,** 380.
Bishop, P. M. F., and de Mowbray, R. R. (1951) *Proc. R. Soc. Med.* **44,** 952.
Bronk, D. W., Larrabee, M. G., Gaylor, J. B., and Brink, F. (1938) *Amer. J. Physiol.* **123,** 24.
Camp, J. D. (1947) *Radiology,* **49,** 568.
Cantarow, A., Stewart, H. L., and Morgan, D. R. (1939) *Endocrinology,* **24,** 556.
Collip, J. B. (1925) *J. Biol. Chem.* **63,** 395.
—— Clark, E. P., and Scott, J. W. (1925) Ibid. **63,** 439.
Dent, C. E. (1953) *Proc. R. Soc. Med.* **46,** 291.
Drake, T. G., Albright, F., Bauer, W., and Castleman, B. (1939) *Ann. Int. Med.* **12,** 1751.
Eaton, L. M., and Haines, S. F. (1939) *J. Amer. Med. Ass.,* **113,** 749.
Eaves, E. C. (1926) *Brain,* **49,** 307.
Ellis, M. M. (1928) *Biochem. J.* **22,** 937.
Ellsworth, R., and Howard, J. E. (1934) *Bull. Johns Hopkins Hosp.* **55,** 296.
Elrick, H., Albright, F., Bartter, F. C., Forbes, A. P., and Reeves, J. D. (1950) *Acta endocrinol.* **5,** 199.
Emerson, K., Walsh, F. B., and Howard, J. E. (1941) *Ann. Int. Med.* **14,** 1256.
Fiske, C. H., and Subbarow, Y. (1925) *J. Biol. Chem.* **66,** 375.
Garland, H. G., Dick, A. P., and Whitty, C. W. M. (1943) *Lancet,* **2,** 566.
Gotta, H., and Odoriz, J. B. (1948) *J. Clin. Endocrin.* **8,** 674.
Grant, D. K. (1953) *Quart. J. Med.* N.S. **22,** 243.
Greene, J. A., and Swanson, L. W. (1941) *Ann. Int. Med.* **14,** 1233.
Gsell, O. (1950) *Dtsch. med. Woch.* **75,** 1117.
Hansted, C., and Brandt, S. (1953) *Electroenc. Clin. Neurophysiol.* **5,** 101.
Harrison, G. A. (1947) *Chemical Methods in Clinical Medicine,* London.
Hurst, E. W. (1926) *J. Path. Bact.* **29,** 65.
Imrie, C. G., and Jenkinson, C. N. (1933) *J. Physiol.* **79,** 218.
Ingalls, T. H., Donaldson, G., and Albright, F. (1943) *J. Clin. Invest.* **22,** 603.
Jordan, A., and Kelsall, A. R. (1951) *Arch. Int. Med.* **87,** 242.
Kirstein, L., and Kugelberg, E. (1946) *Acta med. scand.* **124,** 348.
Kowallis, G. F. (1941) *Proc. Staff M. Mayo Clin.* **16,** 129.
Kuffler, S. W. (1944) *J. Neurophysiol.* **7,** 17.
Kugelberg, E. (1944) *Acta physiol. scand.* **8,** Suppl. **24.**
Lehmann, J. E. (1937) *Amer. J. Physiol.* **118,** 600.
Lewis, T. (1939–42) *Clin. Sci.* **4,** 361.
—— Pickering, G. W., and Rothschild, P. (1931–3) *Heart,* **16,** 1.
Lhermitte, J., Kraus, W. M., and McAlpine, D. (1924–5) *J. Neurol. Psychopath.* **5,** 195.
McAlpine, D. (1923) *Brain,* **46,** 255.
McIlwain, H., and Gore, M. B. R. (1951) *Biochem. J.* **49,** xliii.
McQuarrie, I., Hansen, A. E., and Ziegler, M. R. (1941) *J. Clin. Endocrin.* **1,** 789.
Martin, N. H., and Perkins, D. J. (1951) *Lancet,* **2,** 295.

Medill, E. V. (1951) *Brit. J. Radiol.* **24,** 685.
Milne, M. D. (1951) *Clin. Sci.* **10,** 471.
Mortell, E. J. (1946) *J. Clin. Endocrin.* **6,** 266.
Odoriz, J. B., del Castillo, E. B., Manfredi, J. F., and de la Balze, F. A. (1944) Ibid. **4,** 493.
Ostertag, B. (1929) *Virchows Arch.* **275,** 828.
Paton, D. N., Findlay, L., and Watson, A. (1916) *Quart. J. Exp. Physiol.* **10,** 233.
Peterman, M. G., and Garvey, J. L. (1948) *J. Lab. Clin. Med.* **33,** 1620.
Reynolds, T. B., Jacobson, G., Edmondson, H. A., Martin, H. E., and Nelson, C. H. (1952) *J. Clin. Endocrin.* **12,** 560.
Sabbatani, L. (1901) *Arch. ital. biol.* **36,** 416.
Schottstaedt, W., and Gordan, G. S. (1951) *Calif. Med.* **74,** 390.
Siglin, I. S., Eaton, L. M., Camp, J. D., and Haines, S. F. (1947) *J. Clin. Endocrin.* **7,** 433.
Simpson, J. A. (1952) *Brain,* **75,** 76.
Steinberg, H., and Waldron, B. R. (1952) *Medicine,* **31,** 133.
Stewart, G. S., and Bowen, H. F. (1952) *Endocrinology,* **51,** 80.
Sugar, O. (1953) *Arch. Neurol. Psychiat.* **70,** 86.
Sutphin, A., Albright, F., and McCune, D. J. (1943) *J. Clin. Endocrin.* **3,** 625.
Taubenhaus, M., and Engle, H. M. (1945) Ibid. **5,** 147.
Tweedy, W. R., and Campbell, W. W. (1944) *J. Biol. Chem.* **154,** 339.
Wise, B. L., and Hart, J. C. (1952) *Arch. Neurol. Psychiat.* **68,** 78.

616.455–008.64

NON-TUBERCULOUS ADDISON'S DISEASE AND ITS RELATIONSHIP TO 'GIANT-CELL GRANULOMA' AND MULTIPLE GLANDULAR DISEASE[1]

By ANTHONY G. RICKARDS and GEOFFREY M. BARRETT
(From the Departments of Pathology and Medicine, Royal Infirmary, Lancaster)

With Plates 23 and 24

In the original description of the disease which now bears his name, Addison (1855) described one case in which the suprarenal capsules were atrophied. This was the first report of a case of non-tuberculous Addison's disease, and, although it is now known that neoplastic deposits and certain chronic infections may cause cortical destruction, the majority of cases are still attributed to a 'simple atrophy', the cause of which is almost as obscure now as it was 100 years ago. It is maintained by some workers that the non-tuberculous form of the disease is increasing relatively in incidence, and with the improved control of tuberculosis, made possible by modern preventive and therapeutic measures, it is not unlikely that it will soon rival tuberculosis as the most frequent cause of adrenal cortical destruction. In referring to Addison's disease in the present paper we have excluded those cases of acute adrenal failure which sometimes occur in the absence of pre-existing symptoms or signs of Addison's disease. In some of these cases the adrenal glands are destroyed by a sudden haemorrhage or necrosis, but in others autopsy reveals chronic destruction, usually by tuberculosis. In this latter type of case the first symptom or sign of adrenal insufficiency is sudden collapse and death in a person who has previously been in apparent good health, the collapse often being precipitated by some unusual stress, such as a surgical operation. Although the pathological features may be identical with those encountered in the more common form of chronic adrenal destruction, the clinical aspects are so different that we have not referred to them in our discussion of Addison's disease. Three cases of non-tuberculous Addison's disease, all occurring in women, will be described. In addition to the adrenal destruction all the patients showed varying degrees of 'lymphoid thyroiditis' and atrophy, which was severe enough to produce clinical evidence of myxoedema coexisting with Addison's disease in Cases 1 and 2. In the first case the adrenal destruction was part of a giant-cell granulomatous disease, which also affected the anterior lobe of the pituitary gland. Our second patient was a woman who had been under treatment for Addison's disease for several years. At autopsy the adrenal glands were replaced by dense scar tissue, but after careful search multiple nodular granulomata were found in the spleen.

[1] Received February 3, 1954.

The presence of these nodules suggested that at one time the adrenal glands may have been similarly affected, the dense scar tissue representing the end-result of the granulomatous process. The third case we describe is an example of 'simple atrophy' or 'post-necrotic scarring' of the adrenal glands, and showed no evidence of any granulomatous disease.

Three other cases have been reported hitherto in which autopsy study has revealed replacement of the adrenal and pituitary glands by non-caseating giant-cell granulomata, and various theories have been advanced to account for the glandular destruction, the most usual explanation being that the adrenal lesion was secondary to the pituitary destruction, and that the pituitary disease was caused by some unspecified 'anomaly of internal secretion', which somehow gave rise to a giant-cell granuloma of foreign-body type. Simmonds (1917) first suggested this theory, when he originally described four cases of giant-cell destruction of the pituitary gland for which there was no apparent cause. The cases he described occurred in middle-aged or elderly women, who had shown no sign of defective pituitary function during life, and formed part of a study of 2,000 pituitary glands removed as a routine at autopsy. Since his description evidence has been accumulating that some cases of giant-cell involvement of the pituitary gland represent a hitherto unrecognized disease, in which not only the pituitary but the adrenal glands and certain non-endocrine tissue may be affected. The first case we describe is the third example in the literature to show both adrenal and pituitary lesions, and it is the first case in which the patient has come under observation with Addison's disease. From a study of this case, and other cases previously reported and ascribed to various causes, it is apparent that this disease, which will be referred to as 'giant-cell granuloma', is a distinct disease entity with characteristic clinical and pathological features. In the present paper the relationship between giant-cell granuloma and Addison's disease will be discussed, and in a further publication we hope to contrast the various clinical and pathological features of granulomatous destruction of the pituitary gland caused by giant-cell granuloma, syphilis, sarcoidosis, and tuberculosis. After briefly reviewing the literature dealing with the incidence and aetiology of non-tuberculous Addison's disease, we shall discuss its relationship to the various multiple glandular syndromes which were frequently described by early continental workers under the titles of *insuffisance pluriglandulaire* or *multiple Blutdrüsensklerose*, in some of which the pathogenesis was said to be an infective condition which involved several endocrine glands either simultaneously or successively.

Case 1. Giant-cell granuloma affecting adrenal and pituitary glands.

Mrs. A. L., aged 56 years at death, was referred to the out-patient department of the Royal Lancaster Infirmary in March 1951, with a suggested diagnosis of Addison's disease. Four years previously she had commenced to gain weight and to feel vaguely unwell, and she stated that she had 'cracked up completely' after a dental clearance in 1949. The main symptoms had been morning nausea and vomiting, weakness and tiredness, and intolerance of cold. The patient's doctor had recorded a very low blood-pressure and commented on dusky pigmentation present over the hands, neck, and lower abdomen. Examination confirmed the presence of excessive skin pigmentation, and showed dry sparse hair, pretibial myxoedematous pads, and very marked erythema ab igne. The pulse-rate was 58 per minute, and the blood-pressure 145/90; no buccal pigmentation was present, and the diagnosis of Addison's disease was rejected in favour of one of myxoedema, support for which was obtained by the finding of a serum-cholesterol level of 530 mg. per 100 ml. Treatment was commenced with thyroid B.P. gr. $\frac{1}{2}$ three times daily, and was continued at that dosage, as larger amounts of thyroid appeared to increase the patient's nausea. When next seen on July 6, 1951, the patient had lost 14 pounds in weight, but otherwise her condition appeared unchanged; the blood-pressure was recorded as 140/75. Six days later she was admitted to hospital, nausea and vomiting having suddenly become more severe and weakness more profound. The blood-pressure was then only 95/65, and there was slight buccal pigmentation; the serum-sodium was 290 mg. per 100 ml. (123 mEq. per litre), but potassium, chloride, and urea levels were within the normal range; the serum-cholesterol was 375 mg. per 100 ml. A water excretion test performed two days later strongly suggested Addison's disease. Treatment with intravenous saline, deoxycorticosterone acetate 30 mg. subcutaneously, and cortical extract 25 ml. subcutaneously, was commenced. The following day (July 19) the blood-pressure had fallen to 60 mm. systolic, and despite the continuation of intravenous fluid therapy and the administration of larger quantities of cortical extract the patient died on July 20.

Autopsy was commenced half an hour after death. Significant naked-eye lesions were confined to the endocrine system. Both adrenal glands presented an unusual picture of an irregular type of atrophy; the glands were markedly thinned and devoid of lipoid, and showed patchy areas of firm grey tissue within their substance; these areas gave the gland an irregular knobbly appearance. The thyroid gland showed severe fibrotic atrophy, and weighed 7 gm. The pituitary gland and stalk showed no macroscopic abnormality. Microscopic examination showed the following features. *Pituitary.* The gland contained small foci of non-caseating giant-cell granulomata; these were formed by epithelioid and giant cells interspersed with dense lymphoid aggregations; the granulomata were nodular in type, and showed no inclusion matter; examination of the nodules for micro-organisms was negative. The infiltrations were confined to a small area of the anterior lobe adjacent to the pars intermedia (Plate 23, Fig. 1); at least seven-eighths of the anterior lobe was free from disease. The pars nervosa and pituitary stalk were not affected. Both *adrenal glands* showed a constant pattern of apparent total destruction of cortex and medulla by a chronic inflammatory reaction composed of epithelioid cells, lymphocytes, and giant cells, arranged in nodular formation (Plate 23, Fig. 2). No inclusion matter was found within the cells, and stains for micro-organisms were negative. Caseation of the granulomata was not present. The right adrenal contained a small artery showing an extensive panarteritis with inflammation of all its coats (Plate 23, Fig. 3); no other arteries were found to be affected. *Thyroid.* The gland showed marked fibrosis, with heavy lymphocytic infiltrations throughout all areas; plasma cells were plentiful (Plate 23, Fig. 4). The *liver* showed a marked round-cell infiltration into portal tracts. Histological examination of the kidneys, heart, and spleen showed no significant lesions.

Case 2. Fibrotic scarring of adrenal glands with splenic granulomata.

Mrs. D. L., a housewife, aged 51 years at death, was first admitted to the Royal Lancaster Infirmary in 1946, giving a three months' history of increasing lassitude and attacks of abdominal discomfort, nausea, and vomiting. There was a past history of lumbago and sciatic pain. Examination showed a well-nourished woman, with general pallor and with pigmentation of the skin and mucous membranes; the blood-pressure was 82/40, and plasma-electrolyte studies confirmed the diagnosis of Addison's disease. The Mantoux reaction was negative at 1/100, and radiographs showed no calcification in the region of the adrenal glands. Treatment with added dietary salt, eucortone injections, and later with deoxycorticosterone implants, produced normal blood-electrolyte, urea, and glucose levels, but some degree of hypotension persisted, as did the abnormal pigmentation. The necessity for insertion of subsequent DOCA implants could not be judged on the basis of blood changes, since sodium, potassium, and chloride levels remained within the normal range at all times after the initial treatment. The deciding factor was usually the patient's symptoms; at no time after the disease was diagnosed did she feel really well, but tiredness and general malaise usually became more pronounced about six months after each DOCA implant, and further treatment was then considered necessary. In April 1951 it was noticed that the patient's hair was becoming dry and sparse; she admitted to intolerance of cold, and the serum-cholesterol was found to be 309 mg. per 100 ml. Dry extract of thyroid, gr. 1 three times a day, was prescribed, but was discontinued after two weeks owing to increasing nausea. In June 1952 the patient received injections of eucortone 5 mg. daily for one week, and what proved to be her last implant of DOCA was then inserted. Two days later the patient was seen at her home complaining of a feeling of fullness in the head, of dizziness, and of central abdominal pain; examination showed slight oedema of the ankles, and the blood-pressure at 120/80 was the highest ever recorded. Symptoms subsided rapidly after the temporary withdrawal of all dietary salt. In July 1952 the patient appeared definitely myxoedematous, serum-cholesterol estimation gave a value of 365 mg. per 100 ml., and treatment with thyroid extract was recommenced at a dosage of gr. $\frac{1}{2}$ three times a day, increasing to gr. 1 three times a day after two weeks. In September 1952, while engaged in shopping, the patient had severe central abdominal pain and vomited; later in the day she appeared cyanotic and pale, and continued to complain of abdominal pain; her blood-pressure was 115/75, and an electrocardiograph tracing showed no evidence of myocardial infarction. She was admitted to hospital, but died the same night; blood investigations subsequently reported showed normal electrolyte levels, serum-cholesterol 252 mg. per 100 ml., negative Wassermann and Kahn reactions, and no agglutinins against brucella organisms.

Autopsy was performed 12 hours after death. The body was that of a well-built woman, with generalized brown pigmentation especially prominent around the scar tissue overlying the DOCA implants. Pubic hair was scanty, and axillary hair was absent. Other significant autopsy finding included the following. Both adrenal glands were found after some difficulty; they showed a marked degree of atrophy, weighing together 2·5 gm. The thyroid, weighing 31·5 gm., showed superficial scarring, and on the cut surface the general texture of the gland was firmer and paler than normal, and did not show any of the usual colloid appearance. The only other significant findings were a slight generalized lymphadenopathy and an enlarged spleen, weighing 300 gm., which otherwise showed no unusual features on macroscopic examination. Cultures were made of the blood, liver, and spleen for the presence of bacteria, and especially for the brucella group, but no growth was obtained. Microscopic examination showed the following features. *Pituitary.* No significant abnormality was noted. *Adrenals.* Both glands showed similar features: normal cortical tissue was completely destroyed, and was represented by a thick band of fibrous tissue showing no present inflammatory reaction. Within the central part of the dense connective tissue were small areas of residual cells, which were so atypical in morphology and staining reactions that it was difficult to identify them with any certainty as representing medullary or cortical components (Plate 24, Fig. 5). The *thyroid* showed massive lymphoid infiltration into the stroma, with gross atrophy of the vesicles, which appeared as small duct-like structures of non-secretory type. In some areas lymphoid aggregations with germinal centres were present. The *liver* showed marked cellular infiltration into portal tracts; the predominant cell was lymphocytic, but a few eosinophils and plasma cells were present. In view of the splenomegaly and our experience in the first case, in which the adrenal destruction was part of a disseminated granulomatous process, a systematic attempt was made to determine the presence of granulomata. Twenty-five blocks of splenic tissue were prepared; in 22 of these blocks no significant histological abnormality was noted, but in three our search was rewarded by the finding of multiple nodular granulomata of epithelioid type (Plate 24, Fig. 6). These granulomata were surrounded by a rim of lymphocytes, and showed no evidence of caseation. The cells were almost exclusively of epithelioid type, but an occasional poorly formed giant cell was present. About 40 granulomata were encountered in one cubic centimetre of tissue; the nodules varied in size from 44μ to 350μ in diameter. Other pathological features were confined to the gall-bladder, which showed much fibrosis and contained numerous small stones. Histological examination of the following organs showed no special features: heart, ovary, brain, thymus, pancreas, kidney, lungs, and bone-marrow. The skin around the implants showed fibrosis of the dermis and marked pigmentation of the basal layer of the squamous epithelium, as usually seen in Addison's disease.

Case 3. Simple atrophy of the adrenal glands.

Mrs. J. T., aged 28 years at death, had been diagnosed as suffering from Addison's disease by Dr. M. Anderson of South Shields in April 1951. At that time a history was given of extreme weakness and anorexia following an acute upper respiratory tract infection; examination revealed buccal pigmentation and a blood-pressure of only 80/60. Response to eucortone injections was good, and was maintained following DOCA implants. On May 23, 1952, the patient told Dr. Anderson that she had never felt better. On June 7, 1952, she was married and travelled to Windermere for her honeymoon; she arrived in a somewhat exhausted condition, and awoke the following morning with severe bronchial asthma, a condition from which she had never previously suffered. A local practitioner was called and informed of the history of Addison's disease; he found the patient to be in moderately severe status asthmaticus, but with no undue tachycardia, and with a blood-pressure of 110/80. An injection of adrenaline was given with some benefit, and arrangements made for the patient's transfer to hospital, but she died in the ambulance before arrival.

Autopsy (Dr. G. W. Storey) was performed 12 hours after death. The body was that of a frail woman, and showed generalized pigmentation of Addisonian type. Significant morbid anatomical changes were confined to the following organs. Both adrenal glands were very atrophic; the left adrenal was smaller than the right; cortical lipoid was not visible in either gland, and both organs presented as thin greyish structures of irregular outline. The thyroid, weighing 40 gm., was unusually pale and firm, and did not present the usual colloid appearance. The pituitary gland showed no significant change. The lungs showed emphysema of moderate degree; the bronchioles were plugged with mucous casts. The heart was atrophic, weighing 175 gm., and showed fine petechiae over the posterior surface of the epicardium. There were several sub-endocardial haemorrhages within the left ventricle. Microscopic examination of the *adrenal glands* showed complete destruction of cortical tissue, which was densely infiltrated with lymphocytes (Plate 24, Fig. 7); fibrosis was plentiful, and stains for reticulum fibres showed a dense and irregular network throughout both glands. The right adrenal gland showed scanty deposits of haemosiderin. The *thyroid* showed a uniform picture of intense infiltration with lymphocytes, interspersed with small thyroid acini of atrophic type. Numerous giant cells were observed, but as a rule were lying scattered within the gland in haphazard manner, no true nodular formations being seen (Plate 24, Fig. 8). No inclusion bodies were found. The *thymus* showed moderate hypertrophy, and the *liver* showed a moderate lymphocytic infiltration into portal tracts. Histological study of the pituitary, kidneys, ovary, brain, spleen, lungs, uterus, and pancreas showed no noteworthy features.

Incidence of Non-Tuberculous Addison's Disease

Various estimates of incidence have been reported. Wells (1930) stated that the condition accounted for 10 per cent. of all cases of Addison's disease, while Guttman (1930), analysing 566 cases, found a non-tuberculous cause in 20 per cent. of the female and 7 per cent. of the male patients. Guttman showed that the disorder was commoner in women than in men in the proportion of 1·6:1, although Brenner (1928–9), reviewing 47 cases of simple atrophy, had found the sexes to be equally affected. In a series of 7,000 adult necropsies from the Toronto General Hospital, Duffin (1943) encountered 17 cases of Addison's disease, of which 10 were due to tuberculosis and seven were of atrophic type. More recently O'Donnell (1950) has found a relative increase in the incidence of non-tuberculous Addison's disease, while Emerson (1951) has estimated that 50 per cent. of all cases are due to primary idiopathic atrophy.

Aetiology of Non-Tuberculous Addison's Disease

Amyloidosis. The view that generalized amyloidosis affecting the suprarenal glands could cause Addison's disease was first advanced by Bittorf (1910); Riesman (1898) had previously described a case occurring in a man of 60 years of age, but the only sign or symptom of Addison's disease was weakness before death. The illness described by Bittorf occurred in a man of 32 years, who showed gross albuminuria and complained of fatigue and weakness. A curious type of pigmentation which 'suggested that it may have been produced by dyeing his moustache' was the only tangible evidence produced in support of the diagnosis; moreover, autopsy was limited to the examination of only one kidney and suprarenal, and although the gland showed amyloid infiltration there was apparently plenty of easily recognizable cortex. Further instances of the association have been described by Schultz (1912), Schlesinger (1917), Bauer (1922), McCutcheon (1923), Hunter and Rush (1926), Philpott (1928), Bronfin and Guttman (1935), Colton (1935), Mendel and Saibil (1938), Levenson, Tagnon, Goodpastor, Green, Taylor, and Lund (1947), O'Donnell (1950), Heller and Camarata (1950), and Cope and Woodrow (1953). Schultz's patient, a man of

25 years, was found to have amyloidosis of the adrenals complicating recurrent ascites due to 'gummata of the liver'. There was no clinical evidence at all suggestive of adrenal insufficiency, except slight pigmentation. Schlesinger's patient was a man of 47 years, who was found to have amyloidosis due to chronic nephritis. There were signs of cardiac failure, and intense pigmentation of the skin but not of the mucous membranes. In Bauer's case the patient had a systolic blood-pressure of 150, and no pigmentation. In the case described by McCutcheon amyloidosis of the adrenals was associated with a carcinoma of the kidney in a woman of 53 years; the only indication of Addison's disease was diffuse bronzing of the skin, which was most marked over the breasts and back, where the pigmentation was nearly black; this may well have been an example of acanthosis nigricans. Philpott (1928) recorded the case of a man of 45 years with generalized amyloidosis of syphilitic origin; the blood-pressure some days before death was 80/50, and very slight pigmentation developed, shortly before death, over the face and cheek; no electrolyte studies were made. In the report by Hunter and Rush (1926) the diagnosis of Addison's disease in a man of 29 years was made on the finding of hypotension, and of a slight yellow mottling of the gums and thighs which appeared three days before death; at autopsy plenty of recognizable cortical tissue was present. Of the 14 cases described by Bronfin and Guttman (1935), five were classified as clear cases of Addison's disease, five were regarded by the authors as doubtful, and in four the amyloidosis was said to have produced no symptoms. All their cases occurred in patients who had chronic pulmonary tuberculosis. Even in the five cases with 'characteristic signs of Addison's disease' the evidence for the diagnosis is inadequate; in two there was no pigmentation, and in no case was the pigmentation typical. In two of the patients who showed signs of gastrointestinal disturbances during life, tuberculous enteritis was found at autopsy, and in no case were electrolyte studies undertaken. The two cases described by Colton (1935) also occurred in patients who had chronic pulmonary tuberculosis; in the first case there is no record of the blood-pressure, and in the second case bronzing of the skin of the forehead, face, and neck, and a 'marked drop in blood-pressure', were the only indications of Addison's disease. The case described by Mendel and Saibil (1938) occurred in a man with long-standing pulmonary tuberculosis. The blood-pressure was recorded as 88/58, and some irregular brownish pigmentation was noticed about the shoulders and upper part of the back; later he developed some buccal pigmentation. The associated gastrointestinal symptoms may have been due to tuberculous ulceration of the caecum, which was discovered at autopsy; no electrolyte studies were made. Addison's disease was described by Levenson and his colleagues (1947) in a woman who developed amyloidosis after extensive flame burns involving 15 per cent. of the body area; after 12 months in hospital she suddenly collapsed, the blood-pressure was recorded as 85/40, and she revived temporarily after hormone-replacement therapy. Apart from the drop in blood-pressure there were no other indications of Addison's disease. O'Donnell (1950) recorded 29 cases of adrenal amyloidosis, in three of which Addison's disease is said to have developed.

In his first case a woman with pulmonary tuberculosis complained of progressive weakness and anorexia; there was no other evidence of Addison's disease apart from some increased pigmentation of the nipples. In his second case a young woman with chronic pulmonary tuberculosis showed areas of brown pigmentation, which recently had become more prominent, over the face and arms. The blood-pressure was recorded as 90/65, and gastrointestinal symptoms were present, but could have been accounted for by the tuberculous enteritis found at autopsy. O'Donnell's third patient was a young man whose main complaints were weakness, fatigue, and dyspnoea; 'during several months numerous pin-head to pea size macules of varying depths of brownness and with irregular borders had appeared on the upper part of the back, arms and face.' The blood-pressure was recorded as 70/50, and biopsy of skin showed a patchy melanoderma. At autopsy generalized amyloidosis was found, for which there was no apparent cause; gastrointestinal symptoms were not encountered, and electrolyte studies were not made. In the case described by Heller and Camarata (1950) a woman with chronic pulmonary tuberculosis developed generalized pigmentation 'typical of Addison's disease', anorexia, asthenia, and gastro-intestinal disturbances; the blood-pressure was recorded as 80/50. At autopsy the adrenal glands appeared normal, but on microscopy were found to be largely replaced by amyloid deposits; no electrolyte studies were made. Recently Cope and Woodrow (1953) described a further case of adrenal amyloidosis causing Addison's disease in an elderly man in whom a nephrotic syndrome followed chronic bronchitis and emphysema. The blood-pressure fell from 110/70 to 95/60, and generalized pigmentation developed. No gastrointestinal symptoms were encountered, and in the authors' words the 'diagnosis was based on the weakness, pigmentation, and low blood-pressure. The chemical tests, though at a superficial glance confirmatory, are unreliable in the presence of a renal lesion. The destruction of the adrenals in our case may be regarded as confirmatory evidence.' From an analysis of these 27 cases reported in the literature it is apparent that in the majority the evidence for the diagnosis is inadequate; in a few the diagnosis may be correct, but in no case has it been established beyond doubt.

Secondary carcinomatosis. Among his first 11 cases Addison described four in which the disease was attributed to neoplastic destruction of the adrenal glands; in no case, however, was there any adequate evidence for this diagnosis. Further cases have been reported by Poynton, Wright, and Laurent (1933), Fleiner (1889), Aguilar and Bancalari (1940), Madeheim (1941), Strang (1942), Ball (1858), Cayley (1865), Bannwart (1922), Warthin, Crane, and Jackson (1924), Hall and Hemken (1936), and Butterly, Fishman, Seckler, and Steinberg (1952). Study of these reports shows that very few can be accepted as clear cases of Addison's disease. The first of the cases reported by Butterly, Fishman, Seckler, and Steinberg appears to be well substantiated, but in their other cases the diagnosis seems doubtful. In Strang's patient the diagnosis is probably correct, but in none of the other cases can it be established beyond doubt. The view that secondary carcinomatous destruction of the adrenal glands frequently produces symptoms and signs of cortical failure is not supported by critical analysis of published cases, nor by the conclusions of Rowntree and Snell (1931), who could demonstrate no evidence of Addison's disease in 70 cases in which the adrenal glands were invaded by secondary neoplasms.

Specific inflammatory lesions. Certain specific inflammatory lesions of the adrenal cortex have been shown to cause Addison's disease. Butt and Hoffman (1945), in a discussion of pulmonary coccidioidomycosis, reported a case of 'typical Addison's disease with coccidioidal involvement of the adrenals', but gave no further details. Hall and Hemken (1936) described a case of adrenal destruction of coccidioidal origin, but there was no clinical evidence of Addison's disease. Maloney (1952), however, reported two cases of Addison's disease due to chronic disseminated coccidioidomycosis, although in the second of these the organism was not definitely identified. Cases of extensive adrenal involvement in histoplasmosis have been reported by Parsons and Zarafonetis (1945), Manchester (1941), Palmer, Amolsch, and Shaffer (1942), Van Pernis, Benson, and Holinger (1943), Henderson (1940), Thomas and Morehead (1943), Martin and Silber (1944), Ziegler (1946), and Rawson, Collins, and Grant (1948). In one case, described by Van Pernis, Benson, and Holinger, the patient presented a 'generally light-brown appearance', but the blood-chlorides were normal and the blood-pressure was not lowered. This was the only case in which pigmentation was present. In only three cases was hypotension noted, and in these there was no pigmentation. In none of the other patients was there any evidence of chronic adrenal insufficiency during life, and it has yet to be shown that histoplasmosis of the adrenal glands can cause classical Addison's disease. Rawson, Collins, and Grant (1948) reported the first case of adrenal insufficiency due to torulosis. The only indication of adrenal failure was sudden death in a stuporose patient with cryptococcal lesions, and, while the adrenal involvement may have been responsible for the suddenness of death, the authors did not suggest that torulosis is a cause of Addison's disease. Moniliasis associated with Addison's disease has twice been reported (Talbot, Butler, and MacLachlan, 1943; Sutphin, Albright, and McCune, 1943); but in the one case in which necropsy was done the glands showed simple atrophy. Syphilis has been incriminated by several authors. Gordon (1870) originally described a case of Addison's disease which he thought was of syphilitic origin, but autopsy disclosed normal adrenal glands. Hallopeau (1905) reported a further case without pathological confirmation. Gaucher and Gougerot (1911) described two further cases of the association, maintaining that the disease may manifest itself either as a gummatous or as a sclerotic process; in neither case, however, do the criteria exist for the acceptance of the diagnosis. Jacquet and Sézary (1906) and Sézary (1914) described a case of Addison's disease in which enlarged adrenal glands were found in a man, 66 years of age, who had previously suffered from pulmonary tuberculosis and syphilis. Sézary claimed to have demonstrated spirochaetes in the fibrotic glands. This case appears very doubtful, as not only were many of the spirochaetes of 'abnormal shape', but the patient also died of a cerebral haemorrhage, an unusual exitus during the course of Addison's disease. Schaffner and Howard (1916) described a further case in a man of 38 years, but the disease was not confirmed pathologically. Huebschmann (1921) recorded another case in which he suggested that the fibrotic atrophy probably followed a syphilitic infection, but there is very little evidence for this supposition. Fahr and Reiche (1919) recorded five cases of Addison's disease, in two of which they suggested a syphilitic origin; there is, however, no pathological evidence to support this view, and in the only case in which the Wassermann test was done it was negative. Simmonds (1914*a*) recorded involvement of the adrenal glands in congenital syphilis, and suggested that this involvement may produce adrenal insufficiency in later life; but it is clear from analysis of the above reports that it is unlikely that acquired syphilis ever produces Addison's disease. Finally, Hüber (1868) recorded a case of Addison's disease due to destruction of one adrenal gland by hydatid disease; the other adrenal gland was said to be normal, and even the history did not suggest the diagnosis.

Vascular occlusion. Ischaemic atrophy following vascular occlusion was originally suggested as a cause of Addison's disease by Huebschmann (1921); and Rogoff (1944) has shown that partial ligation of the adrenal vessels in animals is followed by selective atrophy of the cortical areas closely resembling the appearances met with in Addison's disease. A comparable case in man has been reported by Silberman, Rowntree, and Orenstein (1950), who have described a remarkable instance of recurrent acute Addisonian crises occurring in a young man, with diffuse vascular disease, in whom thrombosis of the adrenal vessels was responsible.

Idiopathic atrophy. Though we admit that Addison's disease may on very rare occasions be caused by secondary neoplasms, coccidioidomycosis, and vascular occlusion, it is apparent that some other cause or causes must be sought for the large majority of non-tuberculous cases. Many theories have been advanced to account for this group of cases, an early suggestion being that of congenital hypoplasia, put forward by Neusser and Wiesel (1910) and later by Bloch (1920). Authentic cases of congenital aplasia have been recorded by Šikl (1948), Deamer and Silver (1950), and Geppert, Spencer, and Richmond (1950); but it is apparent that such abnormal infants could not be expected to live into the fourth decade, at which age non-tuberculous Addison's disease reaches its maximum incidence. The atrophic process was regarded by Held (1926) as being the result of an inborn constitutional error, and by Bittorf (1908), Schmidt (1926), Huebschmann (1921), and Guttman (1930) as being a simple degenerative process. More recent workers have considered the lesion to be the result of preceding necrosis of the adrenal cortex due to chemical or bacterial toxins (Kovács, 1928; Wells, 1930); and many others have likened the change to the portal fibrosis that follows liver necrosis. That chemical agents can produce selective cortical lesions in experimental animals has been shown by the work of Nelson and Woodard (1948, 1949) with the chlorethane insecticide compound D.D.D., but when administered to a woman with Cushing's syndrome the drug gave no clinical or histological evidence of a similar action in human beings (Sheehan, Summers, and Nichols, 1953). Other experimental work, not known to be applicable to man, is the demonstration by Supplee, Bender, and Kahlenberg (1942) of suprarenal haemorrhages and necrosis in rats fed on a diet deficient in pantothenic acid. Crawford (1951) has described adrenal necrosis or haemorrhage in 14 women who died during pregnancy or the puerperium; massive infection and the toxaemias of late pregnancy, with severe malnutrition, were said to be possible aetiological factors, and she suggested that patients who survive may later develop fibrotic atrophy or 'post-necrotic scarring'. In support of this view she cited the higher incidence of non-tuberculous Addison's disease in women of the fourth decade. Other cases of adrenal haemorrhage or necrosis associated with pregnancy have been described by Hall and Hemken (1936), Dodds (1945), Hurter (1945–6), Way (1947), Burnett (1948), and Arnold, Richer, and Lepore (1949). Haemosiderin deposits within the destroyed cortical tissue are occasionally seen in the chronic non-tuberculous form of the disease, and occurred in the third case we describe. This finding suggests that a similar process may occur in cases not associated with pregnancy; but, while this theory of adrenal cortical necrosis progressing to fibrotic atrophy appears to be the most probable explanation of some cases of non-tuberculous Addison's disease, and has its pathological counterpart in the post-partum pituitary necrosis of Sheehan, there is as yet no conclusive evidence that the adrenal glands behave in the same manner.

Giant-cell granuloma. The first case we describe is an example of giant-cell granuloma affecting both adrenal and pituitary glands, and is of importance because, although previous cases have been described in which the adrenal glands were involved, it is the first case in which the patient came under observation with signs and symptoms of Addison's disease, and incidentally the first case to show signs of myxoedema. Moreover, the anatomical distribution of lesions serves to show that previous theories of the aetiology of giant-cell granuloma are open to question. Symptoms and signs, when present, in other reported cases have usually been those of hypopituitarism, although simultaneous involvement of other endocrine glands has been previously recorded. Some years before Simmonds's (1917) description of his four cases of giant-cell granulomatous involvement of the pituitary of obscure aetiology, Brissaud, Gougerot, and Gy (1908) and Gougerot and Gy (1911) had reported a similar case under the title of *insuffisance pluriglandulaire interne thyro-testiculo-surrénale.* In 1935 Boller and Goedel reported three further cases, in one of which (Case 4) the pituitary, adrenal, and thyroid glands were all involved. The authors regarded this case as an example of multiple glandular disease due to non-caseating tuberculosis, but study of their case leaves little doubt that it represents a further example of giant-cell granuloma. In recording two further cases of giant-cell lesions of the pituitary, Sheehan and Summers (1949) were the first workers to suggest that some of these cases represented a distinct disease entity and were not due to tuberculosis, syphilis, or sarcoidosis, as had been previously suggested. More recently Oelbaum and Wainwright (1950) described a further case occurring in a young man, in whom giant-cell nodules were found in the pituitary and adrenal glands, and one small focus was found in the testis. Doniach and Wright (1951) described two further cases, in one of which the adrenal glands were affected. These authors described a typical destruction of the adrenal glands by giant-cell granulomata indistinguishable from those in the pituitary, and attributed the adrenal atrophy to pituitary failure. They regarded the pituitary granulomata as of post-necrotic origin 'rather than a destructive infiltration by an infective granuloma', but 'were held back from full confidence in this interpretation by the finding of granulomatous lesions, admittedly differing in detailed morphology, in other parts of the body'. Systemic granulomata were also described in these two cases; in one of them an epithelioid granuloma was found in the spleen, and the authors commented on this finding in the following terms: 'the interpretation of the finding of a possible miliary tubercle in the spleen is difficult, it may be simply evidence that the patient was debilitated and had suffered a recent lighting up of an old tuberculous infection'. In the second case described by these authors the occurrence of giant-cell granulomata in the liver was noted. The occurrence of granulomata in non-endocrine tissue appears to be too frequent to be coincidental, and suggests that the endocrine and non-endocrine lesions have a common aetiology. The view that the widespread lesions are part of a disseminated sarcoid type of reaction would also explain the occurrence of the adrenal lesions in our patient (Case 1). In this case the pituitary granulomata were far too small to interfere seriously with glandular function, and the adrenal and pituitary lesions were clearly independent. In previously reported cases of pituitary and adrenal destruction by this type of lesion, the pituitary gland has been completely destroyed by the process. This has led to the theory that the adrenal atrophy was a result of the hypopituitarism, although the appearance of sarcoid-like granulomata in the adrenals could hardly be explained on this basis. The view that the pituitary granulomata appeared as a post-necrotic reaction is not borne out by our knowledge of the subsequent course of the pituitary gland which has undergone necrosis, for in cases of hypopituitarism caused by post-partum necrosis the gland shows varying degrees of atrophy and fibrosis, and is not characterized by a giant-cell granulomatous reaction. The alternative theory originally proposed by Simmonds (1917) also fails to explain the various lesions. In support of Simmonds's view, Roussy and Mosinger (1946) stated that they had occasionally seen giant-cell foci within the pituitaries of old people, both men and women. Sometimes these foci were isolated cells, either lining the walls of the colloid vesicles of the pars intermedia or in the adjacent glandular tissue, and they were sometimes surrounded by lymphocytes, or even epithelioid cells. The authors regarded these lesions as foreign-body reactions, and likened them to the pseudo-tuberculous nodules sometimes found in the thyroid gland. Apart from the fact that there is no evidence that the cells of the pituitary may excrete substances which could excite a foreign-body reaction, the theory entirely fails to explain the occurrence of the extra-hypophyseal granulomata. From the evidence at present available it appears not improbable that the pituitary, adrenal, splenic, hepatic, testicular, and vascular lesions which have been described in this disease are all a manifestation of a generalized sarcoid reaction of unknown aetiology; and, from our knowledge of comparable reactions in the human body arising from infective agents, it seems not unlikely that giant-cell granuloma may also have an infective basis. Other cases of giant-cell granuloma localized to the pituitary have been reported by von Gierke (1914), Guirguis (1944), Herlant (1946), Bastenie, Gepts, and Tagnon (1950), and Bleisch and Robbins (1952).

In our second case symptoms of Addison's disease had been present for six years, but the clinical history had suggested a continuing infective process, there being recurrent episodes of anorexia, lassitude, and fatigue, not explained by deterioration in the plasma-electrolyte pattern, and not accompanied by any increase in hypotension. Moreover, during the patient's numerous admissions to hospital she was frequently found to have a low-grade pyrexia. At autopsy the adrenal glands showed no evidence of an active granulomatous process, being represented by a thick layer of scar tissue. In the spleen, however, were found multiple non-caseating granulomata. Examination for tubercle bacilli and other organisms gave negative results, and at the time of autopsy culture of various tissues, including the spleen, produced no pathogenic organisms. The Wassermann and Kahn reactions during life were negative, and no evidence of generalized Boeck's sarcoidosis was found. The occurrence of these granulomata, of similar type to those found in the adrenal glands of Case 1, suggests the possibility in both cases of a common aetiological process which may still show signs of activity several years after the onset of symptoms of Addison's disease.

Multiple glandular disease. The three cases here described can be considered as examples of multiple glandular disease; for, apart from the adrenal destruction, all three patients showed 'lymphoid thyroiditis', which was severe enough in the first two to produce clinical signs and symptoms of myxoedema. Towards the end of the last century Continental authors frequently described cases of a polyglandular dystrophy which was thought to be due to disease of one endocrine gland, usually the thyroid, destruction of which led to depressed function of other ductless glands (Rumpel, 1896; Ponfick, 1899; Poncin, 1900; Dalché, 1902; Moutard-Martin and Malloizel, 1903; Achard and Demanche, 1906; Gandy, 1906, 1911; Brissaud and Bauer, 1907; Claude and Gougerot, 1907, 1908*a*, *b*; Brissaud, Gougerot and Gy, 1908; Gougerot and Gy, 1911; Sainton and Rathery, 1908; Austrege-Silo, 1908; Rénon, Delille, and Monnier-Vinard, 1908, 1909; Maranon, 1909; Etienne, 1910; Marie and Foix, 1910; Josserand, 1911; Cordier and Françillon, 1911; Murri, 1911; Burnier, 1911; Faure Beaulieu, Villaret, and Sourdel, 1911; Collard-Huard, 1911; Gouillod and Poncin, 1912; Falta, 1923). By 1912 Sourdel was able to review 53 cases from the literature, and added a further 11 of his own. Following the example of Claude and Gougerot (1908*a*) and Laignel-Lavastine (1908), he divided the syndrome into various clinical types, although the difference between these groups is not always clear. In some cases the cause of the defect of pituitary function was obscure, but in others tumours were found, and some were examples of post-partum necrosis; Gouillod and Poncin, for example, gave a good description of the syndrome of hypopituitarism following a severe post-partum haemorrhage at an interval of some years. Claude and Gougerot (1907, 1908*a*), realizing that a number of features, such as loss of secondary sex characteristics, were the result of some undetermined endocrine deficiency, developed the theory of an *insuffisance pluriglandulaire*, suggesting that several endocrine glands might be simultaneously or progressively affected by a destructive process of inflammatory origin. Brissaud, Gougerot, and Gy (1908) and Gougerot and Gy (1911) described a further case of polyglandular disease which they considered to be of infective origin. This case, previously referred to, is an example of giant-cell granuloma, although it was thought by the authors to have a tuberculous origin. The case is of unusual interest, for not only is it the first recognizable description of giant-cell granuloma, but their theory of a simultaneous or progressive destruction of endocrine glands by an inflammatory lesion may possibly be the correct interpretation of the pathogenesis of this disease. In addition to stressing the theory of a single infective agent, these authors also maintained that the clinical picture varied according to the degree of affection of the individual glands. This theory of polyglandular insufficiency eventually fell into disrepute, partly owing to the inclusion of such conditions as acromegaly and Fröhlich's syndrome, which were attributed by Poncet and Leriche (1911) to 'hypophyseal degeneration of tuberculous origin'. The description of hypopituitarism by Simmonds (1914*b*), although inaccurate in some respects, served to reveal the true nature of most of the earlier reported cases of polyglandular disease, and appeared finally to disprove the pluriglandular theory of Gougerot and his collaborators; but to these workers must be credited the recognition that atrophic change, such as loss of axillary and pubic hair, was a consequence of defective endocrine function—a notable advance on the theory of an *infantilisme reversif* advocated by some adherents of the monoglandular school (Gandy, 1906, 1911; Brissaud and Bauer, 1907).

All the cases we describe showed gross disease of the thyroid gland, with intense lymphocytic infiltration and varying degrees of fibrosis and atrophy. Case 1 showed the most severe degree of fibrotic atrophy, and in this patient the symptoms of myxoedema were the most severe (Plate 23, Fig. 4). Case 2 also showed clinical signs and symptoms of myxoedema and, although the thyroid weighed 31 gm. at autopsy, microscopic examination showed very marked lymphoid infiltration and extreme atrophy of vesicles. Case 3 also showed a uniform picture of intense lymphocytic infiltration, with plentiful giant-cells but not arranged in nodular formation; there was marked atrophy of thyroid acini (Plate 24, Fig. 8). In Cases 1 and 2 the glands showed well-formed lymph-nodules with germinal centres. Dubois (1919) described six cases of Addison's disease showing marked lymphoid infiltration into the thyroid, and was the first observer adequately to describe the association, although Sternberg (1914) had previously reported a case. Donath and Lampl (1920) recorded an additional case, and in 1926 Schmidt fully described a further two cases, the association of Addison's disease and lymphoid thyroiditis later becoming known as the Schmidt syndrome. Several other cases were later reported (Hewer, 1923; Shaw and Smith, 1925–6; Kreibig, 1928; Brenner, 1928–9; Susman, 1930;

Wells, 1930; Köhler, 1931; Gowen, 1932; Klingner, 1933; Duff and Bernstein, 1933; Crooke and Russell, 1935; Johnson, 1936; Anderson and Lyall, 1937; Bastenie, 1937; Müller, 1938; Masshoff, 1937–8; Rushton, Cragg, and Stalker, 1940; Heim, 1940; Matisseck, 1941–2; Duffin, 1943; Leonard, 1946; Demol and Herlant, 1947; Moehlig, 1947; Laqueur and Bernstein, 1948; Sorkin, 1949; Silberman, Rowntree, and Orenstein, 1950; Simpson, 1953). In the majority of these reported cases the thyroid infiltration was discovered as an incidental post-mortem finding, but in the cases described by Johnson (1936), Demol and Herlant (1947), Sorkin (1949), and Gowen (1932) both myxoedema and Addison's disease were recognized during life.

Various theories have been advanced to account for the thyroid changes. Brenner (1928–9) was of opinion that the diffuse lymphocytic infiltration was due to the same inflammatory reaction which caused the adrenal destruction, but the evidence for this theory receives little support from the result of more modern study of the relationship between adrenal cortex and lymphoid tissue. Star (1895) was the first observer to note persistence of the thymus gland in Addison's disease, and several authors have shown that generalized lymphoid hyperplasia and thymic hypertrophy constantly follow experimental adrenalectomy (Jaffe, 1924, 1927; Marine, Manley, and Baumann, 1924; Simpson, Dennison, and Korenchevsky, 1934; Reinhardt and Holmes, 1940; Murphy and Sturm, 1947). Conversely it has repeatedly been found that administration of adrenocorticotrophic hormone or adrenal cortical hormone to normal animals is followed by atrophy of lymphatic tissue (Moon, 1937–8; Ingle and Mason, 1938; Ingle, Higgins, and Kendall, 1938; Evans, Moon, Simpson, and Lyons, 1938; Wells and Kendall, 1940; Ingle, 1940; Crede and Moon, 1940; Noble and Collip, 1941; Dougherty and White, 1943; Simpson, Li, Reinhardt, and Evans, 1943). This experimental evidence is supported by the clinical observations in cases of Addison's disease, in which lymphoid and thymic hyperplasia are frequently found (Addison, 1855; Wiesel, 1904; Hedinger, 1907; Bittorf, 1908; Rössle, 1914; Fahr and Reiche, 1919; Wakefield and Smith, 1927; Medlar, 1927; Wells, 1930; Guttman, 1930). Not only is there a close relationship between 'lymphoid thyroiditis' and adrenal cortical destruction, but there is also evidence that the thyroid failure in some instances is preceded by overactivity of the gland. Bastenie (1937) found histological evidence of thyroid overactivity in 13 patients who died from Addison's disease of varying aetiology, but also found marked lymphocytic infiltration and evidence of degenerative changes in other parts of the gland. He was of opinion that adrenal cortical destruction always stimulates thyroid activity in the early stages, but that later degenerative changes supervene with a consequent lymphocytic infiltration. Although Bastenie's patients showed no evidence of Graves' disease during life, other authors have recorded cases of Addison's disease associated with thyrotoxicosis (Courmont, Lesieur, and Thévenot, 1905; Gitman, Ant, and Jacobi, 1943; Etienne, 1910; Elsner, 1923; Chauffard and Girot, 1925; Rössle, 1914; Löffler, 1921; Etienne and Richard, 1926; Brenner, 1928–9; Guttman, 1930; Anderson and Lyall, 1937; Forsham, Thorn, Prunty, and Hills, 1948). Although in some of these cases the diagnosis is questionable, in others it appears to be well substantiated. Recently Sloper (1953) has described the appearance of the thyroid gland in 21 cases of Addison's disease. In nine cases he found conspicuous involutional change, associated in five instances with foci of hyperplasia. He considered that the involutional change was probably due to a diminution in pituitary thyrotrophin output, and described the severe lymphoid infiltration as probably representing an active cellular reaction to the parenchymal involution, or alternatively to diminution in the production of adrenal cortical hormone. Whatever the precise mechanism may be, it is clear that thyroid atrophy and lymphoid infiltration frequently follow adrenal destruction of any type, although they appear to be more commonly encountered in the post-necrotic-scarring group than in the cases due to tuberculosis, possibly because of the tendency to complete destruction of the adrenal glands in the former group.

From the preceding evidence it is apparent that myxoedema rarely develops in cases of Addison's disease which show 'lymphoid thyroiditis', though in some cases the clinical signs and symptoms of adrenal failure may mask the onset of a low-grade hypothyroidism. When hypothyroidism is present, there is evidence that administration of thyroid extract is not without danger. Harrop, Weinstein, and Marlow (1932), and Harrop, Weinstein, Soffer, and Trescher (1933), had noticed that several of their cases of Addison's disease had a lower basal metabolic rate, which responded satisfactorily to thyroid administration, but in spite of this elevation of metabolism their patients showed an exacerbation of their symptoms of adrenal insufficiency; in three cases a typical Addisonian crisis ensued. Other authors have recorded similar cases (Johnson, 1936; Means, Hertz, and Lerman, 1940; Talbott, 1940). A similar danger is said to exist in adrenal atrophy secondary to hypopituitarism (Lerman and Stebbins, 1942). Study of these cases suggests that administration of large doses of thyroid extract in cases of Addison's disease may provoke adrenal failure, but the risk involved would hardly justify withholding the drug altogether.

Conclusion

Study of the present three cases, and of similar cases previously published, suggests that the disease 'giant-cell granuloma' is a specific clinico-pathological entity, which often manifests itself by signs and symptoms of hypopituitarism. It is also apparent that the lesions may not be confined to the hypophysis; they have been described in vascular tissue, spleen, liver, testes, and adrenal glands. Should adrenal destruction occur when the pituitary gland is unaffected or only slightly involved, the patient will come under observation with Addison's disease. It is not possible to know how frequently giant-cell granuloma is responsible for this condition, as the probable result, gross scarring of the adrenal glands, is common to other causes of non-tuberculous cortical destruction. From the clinical viewpoint giant-cell granuloma should be suspected when hypopituitarism occurs in women who have not previously suffered from conditions which may have caused a necrosis of the pars anterior of the pituitary gland, and in both men and women in whom tumour, tuberculosis, and syphilis can be excluded. From the pathological point of view the disease might be more frequently recognized if careful post-mortem search was made for evidence of granulomata in non-endocrine organs in cases of non-tuberculous Addison's disease and hypopituitarism.

We are indebted to Mr. F. Taylor, chief technician, for the photomicrography, and to Mr. G. Radcliffe for technical help. We thank Mrs. Joyce Garnett, Miss Margaret Bird, and Miss Gwynne Alexander for their clerical help. Our thanks are also due to Dr. M. Anderson, of South Shields, for clinical details of Case 1, and to Dr. J. McKeon, of Newcastle-upon-Tyne, for the earlier case records of Case 2. We are much indebted to Mrs. J. L. Neuberg for her help in translating German publications.

Summary

1. Three cases of non-tuberculous destruction of the adrenal glands are described. In two cases Addison's disease coexisted with myxoedema, and in all three cases the thyroid gland showed evidence of 'lymphoid thyroiditis'.

2. Case 1 is an example of a disease which we have referred to as giant-cell granuloma. It occurs predominantly in middle-aged or elderly women, although men may also be affected. Pathologically it is characterized by the presence of non-caseating granulomata, which may be found in various tissues of the body, and sometimes the pituitary and adrenal glands may be affected. The disease usually manifests itself by the insidious onset of hypopituitarism, due to destruction of the anterior lobe of the hypophysis by the granulomatous process, but in the case we describe it was the adrenal glands which were chiefly affected, and although similar lesions were present in the pituitary they were not severe enough to cause any disturbance in glandular function. In a succeeding paper the clinical and pathological features of granulomatous destruction of the pituitary of all types will be contrasted.

3. Our second case was that of a woman who had suffered from Addison's disease for many years. At autopsy the adrenal cortex was replaced by old, dense scar tissue. The spleen was moderately enlarged, and on microscopic study revealed many nodular granulomata which closely resembled the basic lesion in giant-cell granuloma. This finding, in association with certain aspects of the clinical history, suggests that at one time the adrenal glands may have been similarly affected by the granulomatous process, which had since healed, leaving only dense scar tissue.

4. Our third case of Addison's disease occurred in a young woman, in whom the disease followed an acute febrile illness 14 months before her death. This case was one of simple atrophy, or of the 'post-necrotic scarring' type. The various theories of the causation of this group of cases are reviewed.

5. The literature dealing with some aspects of multiple glandular disease is reviewed, and the association of 'lymphoid thyroiditis' and adrenal cortical destruction (Schmidt's syndrome) is discussed.

REFERENCES

Achard, C., and Demanche, R. (1906) *Bull. mém. Soc. méd. hôp. Paris,* **23,** 1305.

Addison, T. (1855) In *A Collection of the Published Writings of Thomas Addison,* London (1868), p. 211.

Aguilar, O. P., and Bancalari, C. A. (1940) *Arch. argent. tisiol.* **16,** 321.

Anderson, I. A., and Lyall, A. (1937) *Lancet,* **1,** 1039.

Arnold, G., Richer, A. G., and Lepore, J. J. (1949) *New Engl. J. Med.* **240,** 1040.

Austrege-Silo, A. (1908). Abstract in *Rev. neurol.* **17,** 1491.

Ball (1858) *Bull. Soc. anat. Paris,* 2nd Ser. **3,** 423.

Bannwart, A. (1922) *Frankfurt. Zts. Path.* **26,** 307.

Bastenie, P. (1937) *Arch. internat. méd. exp.* **12,** 1.

Bastenie, P. A., Gepts, W., and Tagnon, R. (1950) *Sem. hôp. Paris,* **26,** 3157.

Bauer, J. (1922) *Klin. Woch.* **1,** 1595.

Bittorf, A. (1908) *Die Pathologie der Nebennieren und der Morbus Addisonii,* Jena.

—— (1910) *Dtsch. Arch. klin. Med.* **100,** 116.

Bleisch, V. R., and Robbins, S. L. (1952) *Arch. Int. Med.* **89,** 877.

Bloch, R. (1920) *Beitr. path. Anat.* **67,** 71.

Boller, R., and Goedel, A. (1935) *Wien. Arch. inn. Med.* **27,** 41.

Brenner, O. (1928–9) *Quart. J. Med.* **22,** 121.

Brissaud and Bauer (1907) *Bull. mém. Soc. méd. hôp. Paris,* **24,** 39.

Brissaud, Gougerot, and Gy (1908) *Rev. neurol.* **16,** 1354.

Bronfin, I. D., and Guttman, P. H. (1935) *Amer. Rev. Tuberc.* **31,** 1.

Burnett, C. W. F. (1948) *Lancet,* **1,** 249.

Burnier, R. (1911) *Ann. d'ocul.* **145,** 277.

Butt, E. M., and Hoffman, A. M. (1945) *Amer. J. Path.* **21,** 485.

Butterly, J. M., Fishman, L., Seckler, J., and Steinberg, H. (1952) *Ann. Int. Med.* **37,** 930.

Cayley (1865) *Trans. Path. Soc. London,* **16,** 250.

Chauffard, A., and Girot, L. (1925) *Rev. fr. d'endocrin.* **3,** 145.

Claude, H., and Gougerot, H. (1907) *Mém. Soc. biol.* **2,** 785.

—— —— (1908*a*) *Rev. de méd.* **28,** 861, 950.

—— —— (1908*b*) *J. physiol. path. gén.* **10,** 469 and 505.

Collard-Huard (1911). Cited by Sourdel (1912).

Colton, W. A. (1935) *Med. Bull. Vet. Admin.* **12,** 27.

Cope, S., and Woodrow, J. C. (1953) *Post-Grad. Med. J.* **29,** 558.

Cordier, V., and Françillon, G. (1911) *Lyon méd.* **116,** 26.

Courmont, J., Lesieur, C., and Thévenot, L. (1905) Ibid. **104,** 939.

Crawford, M. D. (1951) *J. Path. Bact.* **63,** 365.

Crede, R. H., and Moon, H. D. (1940) *Proc. Soc. Exp. Biol. Med.* **43,** 44.

Crooke, A. C., and Russell, D. S. (1935) *J. Path. Bact.* **40,** 255.

Dalché, P. (1902) *Bull. mém. Soc. méd. hôp. Paris,* **19,** 478.

Deamer, W. C., and Silver, H. K. (1950) *J. Pediat.* **37,** 490.

Demol, O., and Herlant, M. (1947) *Acta clin. belg.* **2,** 343.

Dodds, G. H. (1945) *Brit. Med. J.* **1,** 769.

Donath, J., and Lampl, H. (1920) *Wien. klin. Woch.* **33,** 962.

Doniach, I., and Wright, E. A. (1951) *J. Path. Bact.* **63,** 69.

Dougherty, T. F., and White, A. (1943) *Proc. Soc. Exp. Biol. Med.* **53,** 132.

Dubois, M. (1919) *Berl. klin. Woch.* **56,** 1178.

Duff, G. L., and Bernstein, C. (1933) *Bull. Johns Hopkins Hosp.* **52,** 67.

Duffin, J. D. (1943) *Arch. Path.* **35,** 649.

Elsner, H. L. (1923) *The Prognosis of Internal Diseases,* New York.

Emerson, K. (1951) *Med. Clin. N. America,* **35,** 1283.

Etienne, G. (1910) *Bull. mém. Soc. méd. hôp. Paris,* **29,** 824.

—— and Richard, G. (1926) *Rev. fr. d'endocrin.* **4,** 1.

Evans, H. M., Moon, H. D., Simpson, M. E., and Lyons, W. R. (1938) *Proc. Soc. Exp. Biol. Med.* **38,** 419.

Fahr, T., and Reiche, F. (1919) *Frankfurt. Zts. Path.* **22,** 231.
Falta, W. (1923) *Endocrine Diseases*, London, 3rd ed., p. 453.
Faure Beaulieu, Villaret, and Sourdel (1911) *Presse méd.* **19,** 691.
Fleiner, W. (1889) *Berl. klin. Woch.* 26, 1101.
Forsham, P. H., Thorn, G. W., Prunty, F. T. G., and Hills, A. G. (1948) *J. Clin. Endocrin.* **8,** 15.
Gandy, C. (1906) *Bull. mém. Soc. méd. hôp. Paris,* **23,** 1226.
—— (1911) Ibid. **31,** 837.
Gaucher and Gougerot (1911) *Ann. des mal. vén.* **6,** 321.
Geppert, L. J., Spencer, W. A., and Richmond, A. M. (1950) *J. Pediat.* **37,** 1.
Gierke, E. von (1914) *Verhandl. dtsch. pathol. Ges.* **17,** 200.
Gitman, L., Ant, M., and Jacobi, M. (1943) *Ann. Int. Med.* **19,** 507.
Gordon, C. A. (1870) *Med. Times and Gaz.* **1,** 281.
Gougerot, H., and Gy, A. (1911) *Nouv. iconog. de la Salpêtrière,* **24,** 449.
Gouillod and Poncin (1912). Cited by Sourdel (1912).
Gowen, W. M. (1932) *New Engl. J. Med.* **207,** 577.
Guirguis, Z.-A. (1944) *Thèse de Genève.*
Guttman, P. H. (1930) *Arch. Path.* **10,** 742.
Hall, E. M., and Hemken, L. (1936) *Arch. Int. Med.* **58,** 448.
Hallopeau, H. (1905) *Ann. dermat. syph.* **6,** 638.
Harrop, G. A., Weinstein, A., and Marlow, A. (1932) *J. Amer. Med. Ass.* **98,** 1525.
—— —— Soffer, L. J., and Trescher, J. H. (1933) Ibid. **100,** 1850.
Hedinger, E. (1907) *Frankfurt. Zts. Path.* **1,** 527.
Heim, W. (1940) Ibid. **54,** 250.
Held (1926) *Virchows Arch.* **261,** 600.
Heller, E. L., and Camarata, S. J. (1950) *Arch. Path.* **49,** 601.
Henderson (1940). Cited by Parsons and Zarafonetis (1945).
Herlant, M. (1946) *Acta clin. belg.* **1,** 197.
Hewer, E. E. (1923) *Brit. Med. J.* **1,** 235.
Hüber (1868) *Dtsch. Arch. klin. Med.* **4,** 613.
Huebschmann (1921) *Beitr. path. Anat.* **69,** 352.
Hunter, W. C., and Rush, H. P. (1926) *Ann. Clin. Med.* **5,** 404.
Hurter, L. E. (1945–6) *Proc. R. Soc. Med.* **39,** 581.
Ingle, D. J. (1940) *Proc. Soc. Exp. Biol. Med.* **44,** 174.
—— Higgins, G. M., and Kendall, E. C. (1938) *Anat. Rec.* **71,** 363.
—— and Mason, H. L. (1938) *Proc. Soc. Exp. Biol. Med.* **39,** 154.
Jacquet, L., and Sézary (1906) *Bull. mém. Soc. méd. hôp. Paris,* **23,** 314.
Jaffe, H. L. (1924) *J. Exp. Med.* **40,** 325.
—— (1927) *Arch. Path. Lab. Med.* **3,** 414.
Johnson, R. M. (1936) *J. Amer. Med. Ass.* **107,** 278.
Josserand (1911) *Lyon méd.* **116,** 75.
Klingner, R. (1933) *Zts. klin. Med.* **123,** 242.
Köhler, R. (1931) *Virchows Arch.* **281,** 466.
Kovács, W. (1928) *Beitr. path. Anat.* **79,** 213.
Kreibig, W. (1928) *Frankfurt. Zts. Path.* **36,** 668.
Laignel-Lavastine (1908) *Gaz. hôp. Paris,* **81,** 1563.
Laqueur, G. L., and Bernstein, D. E. (1948) *Stanford Med. Bull.* **6,** 199.
Leonard, M. F. (1946) *J. Clin. Endocrin.* **6,** 493.
Lerman, J., and Stebbins, H. D. (1942) *J. Amer. Med. Ass.* **119,** 391.
Levenson, S. M., Tagnon, H. J., Goodpastor, W. L., Green, R. W., Taylor, F. H. L., and Lund, C. C. (1947) *New Engl. J. Med.* **237,** 152.
Löffler, W. (1921) *Zts. klin. Med.* **90,** 265.
McCutcheon, M. (1923) *Amer. J. Med. Sci.* **166,** 197.
Madeheim, H. (1941) *Frankfurt. Zts. Path.* **55,** 447.
Maloney, P. J. (1952) *Arch. Int. Med.* **90,** 869.
Manchester (1941). Cited by Parsons and Zarafonetis (1945).

Maranon (1909). Cited by Sourdel (1912).
Marie and Foix (1910) Ibid.
Marine, D., Manley, O. T., and Baumann, E. J. (1924) *J. Exp. Med.* **40,** 429.
Martin, W. P., and Silber, B. (1944) *Amer. J. Clin. Path.* **14,** 119.
Masshoff, W. (1937–8) *Beitr. path. Anat.* **100,** 413.
Matisseck, H. (1941–2) *Virchows Arch.* **308,** 700.
Means, J. H., Hertz, S., and Lerman, J. (1940) *Trans. Ass. Amer. Phys.* **55,** 32.
Medlar, E. M. (1927) *Amer. J. Path.* **3,** 135.
Mendel, D. L., and Saibil, M. (1938) *Canad. Med. Ass. J.* **39,** 457.
Moehlig, R. C. (1947) *J. Clin. Endocrin.* **7,** 134.
Moon, H. D. (1937–8) *Proc. Soc. Exp. Biol. Med.* **37,** 34.
Moutard-Martin and Malloizel (1903) *Bull. mém. Soc. méd. hôp. Paris,* **20,** 1428.
Müller, E. (1938) *Ztrbl. allg. Path. path. Anat.* **70,** 289.
Murphy, J. B., and Sturm, E. (1947) *Proc. Soc. Exp. Biol. Med.* **66,** 303.
Murri, A. (1911) *Riforma med.* **28,** 85.
Nelson, A. A., and Woodard, G. (1948) *Federation Proc.* **7,** 277.
—— —— (1949) *Arch. Path.* **48,** 387.
Neusser, E., and Wiesel, J. (1910) *Die Erkrankungen der Nebennieren,* Ed. 2, Leipzig.
Noble, R. L., and Collip, J. B. (1941) *Endocrinology,* **29,** 934.
O'Donnell, W. M. (1950) *Arch. Int. Med.* **86,** 266.
Oelbaum, M. H., and Wainwright, J. (1950) *J. Clin. Path.* **3,** 122.
Palmer, A. E., Amolsch, A. L., and Shaffer, L. W. (1942) *Arch. Dermat. Syph.* **45,** 912.
Parsons, R. J., and Zarafonetis, C. J. D. (1945) *Arch. Int. Med.* **75,** 1.
Philpott, N. W. (1928) Ibid. **1,** 613.
Poncet, A., and Leriche, R. (1911) *Bull. Acad. méd.* **65,** 711.
Poncin (1900) *Lyon méd.* **94,** 127.
Ponfick, E. (1899) *Zts. klin. Med.* **38,** 1.
Poynton, F. J., Wright, G. P., and Laurent, L. P. E. (1933) *Lancet,* **1,** 740.
Rawson, A. J., Collins, L. H., and Grant, J. L. (1948) *Amer. J. Med. Sci.* **215,** 363.
Reinhardt, W. O., and Holmes, R. O. (1940) *Proc. Soc. Exp. Biol. Med.* **45,** 267.
Rénon, L., Delille, A., and Monier-Vinard, R. (1908) *Bull. mém. Soc. méd. hôp. Paris,* **25,** 704.
—— —— —— (1909) Ibid. **26,** 204.
Riesman, D. (1898) *Trans. Path. Soc. Philad.* **18,** 428.
Rogoff, J. M. (1944) *Arch. Path.* **38,** 392.
Rössle (1914) *Verhandl. dtsch. pathol. Ges.* **17,** 220.
Roussy, G., and Mosinger, M. (1946) *Traité de neuro-endocrinologie,* Paris, p. 432.
Rowntree, L. G., and Snell, A. M. (1931) *A Clinical Study of Addison's Disease,* Mayo Clin. Mon., p. 56.
Rumpel (1896) *Neurol. Ctrbl.* **15,** 428.
Rushton, J. G., Cragg, R. W., and Stalker, L. K. (1940) *Arch. Int. Med.* **66,** 531.
Sainton, P., and Rathery, F. (1908) *Bull. mém. Soc. méd. hôp. Paris,* **25,** 647.
Schaffner, P. M., and Howard, T. (1916) *New York Med. J.* **103,** 1026.
Schlesinger, H. (1917) *Wien. klin. Woch.* **30,** 99.
Schmidt, M. B. (1926) *Verhandl. dtsch. pathol. Ges.* **21,** 212.
Schultz, O. T. (1912) *Cleveland Med. J.* **11,** 40.
Sézary, A. (1914) *Gaz. hôp. Paris,* **87,** 1317.
Shaw, A. F. B., and Smith, R. P. (1925–6) *Brit. J. Surg.* **13,** 93.
Sheehan, H. L., and Summers, V. K. (1949) *Quart. J. Med.* N.S. **18,** 319.
—— —— and Nichols, J. (1953) *Lancet,* **1,** 312.
Šikl, H. (1948) *J. Path. Bact.* **60,** 323.
Silberman, D. E., Rowntree, L. G., and Orenstein, H. B. (1950) *Ann. Int. Med.* **32,** 760.
Simmonds, M. (1914*a*) *Virchows Arch.* **218,** 152.
—— (1914*b*) *Dtsch. med. Woch.* **40,** 322.
—— (1917) *Virchows Arch.* **223,** 281.

Simpson, M. E., Li, C. H., Reinhardt, W. O., and Evans, H. M. (1943) *Proc. Soc. Exp. Biol. Med.* **54,** 135.
Simpson, S. L. (1953) *Proc. R. Soc. Med.* **46,** 566.
—— Dennison, M., and Korenchevsky, V. (1934) *J. Path. Bact.* **39,** 569.
Sloper, J. C. (1953) Ibid. **66,** 53.
Sorkin, S. Z. (1949) *Medicine,* **28,** 371.
Sourdel, M. (1912) *Contribution a l'étude anatomo-clinique des syndromes pluriglandulaires,* Paris.
Star, P. (1895) *Lancet,* **1,** 284.
Sternberg (1914) *Verhandl. dtsch. pathol. Ges.* **17,** 233.
Strang, C. (1942) *Newcastle Med. J.* **21,** 126.
Supplee, G. C., Bender, R. C., and Kahlenberg, O. J. (1942) *Endocrinology,* **30,** 355.
Susman, W. (1930) *J. Path. Bact.* **33,** 749.
Sutphin, A., Albright, F., and McCune, D. J. (1943) *J. Clin. Endocrin.* **3,** 625.
Talbot, N. B., Butler, A. M., and MacLachlan, E. A. (1943) *J. Clin. Invest.* **22,** 583.
Talbott, J. H. Cited by Means, Hertz, and Lerman (1940).
Thomas, W. C., and Morehead, R. P. (1943) *N. Carolina Med. J.* **4,** 378.
Van Pernis, P. A., Benson, M. E., and Holinger, P. H. (1943) *Ann. Int. Med.* **18,** 384.
Wakefield, E. G., and Smith, E. E. (1927) *Amer. J. Med. Sci.* **174,** 343.
Warthin, A. S., Crane, A. W., and Jackson, J. B. (1924) *Arch. Dermat. Syph.* **10,** 139.
Way, G. T. C. (1947) *Amer. J. Obstet. Gyn.* **54,** 928.
Wells, B. B., and Kendall, E. C. (1940) *Proc. Staff M. Mayo Clin.* **15,** 133.
Wells, H. G. (1930) *Arch. Path.* **10,** 499.
Wiesel, J. (1904) *Virchows Arch.* **176,** 103.
Ziegler, E. E. (1946) *Ann. Int. Med.* **24,** 1073.

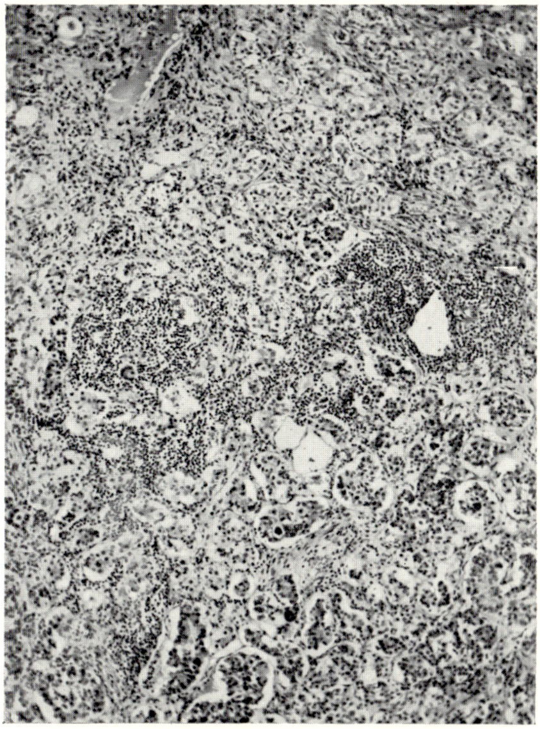

FIG. 1. Giant-cell nodule in pituitary (Case 1) (haematoxylin and eosin, × 72)

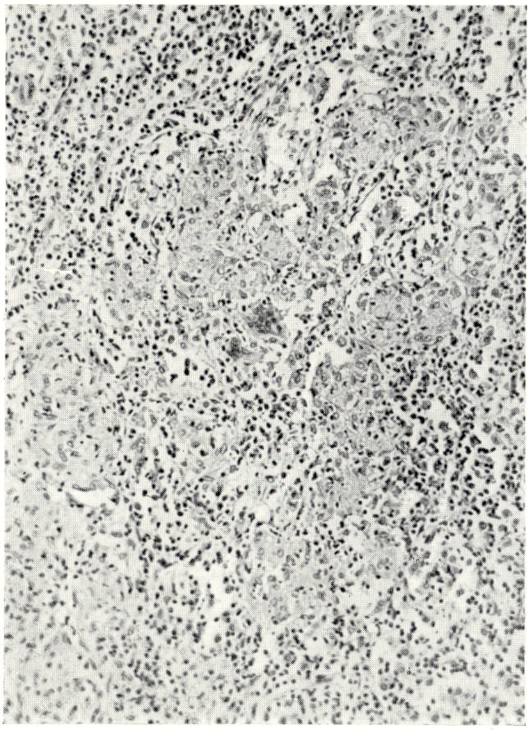

FIG. 2. Giant-cell nodule in adrenal (Case 1) (haematoxylin and eosin, × 134)

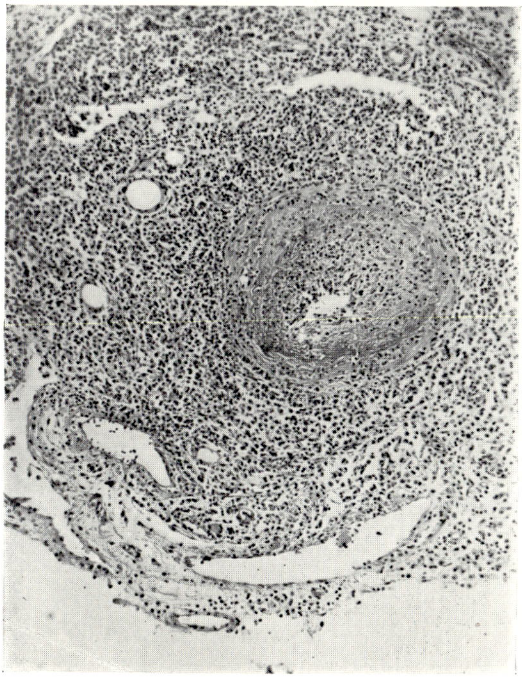

FIG. 3. Arteritis of adrenal vessel (Case 1) (haematoxylin and eosin, × 80)

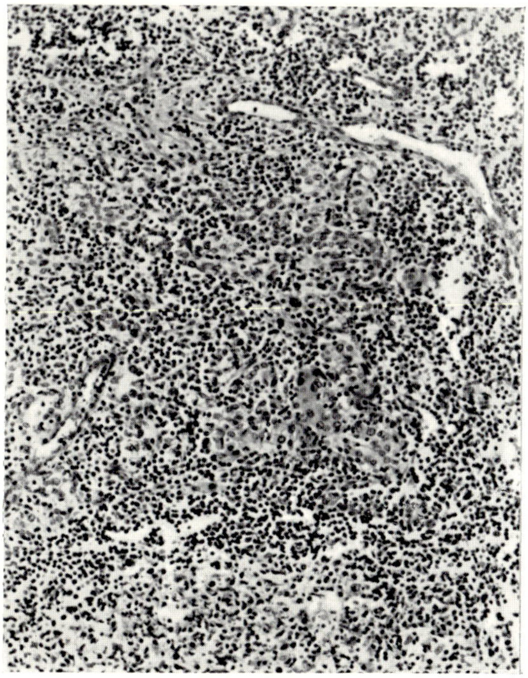

FIG. 4. Lymphoid thyroiditis (Case 1) (haematoxylin and eosin, × 134)

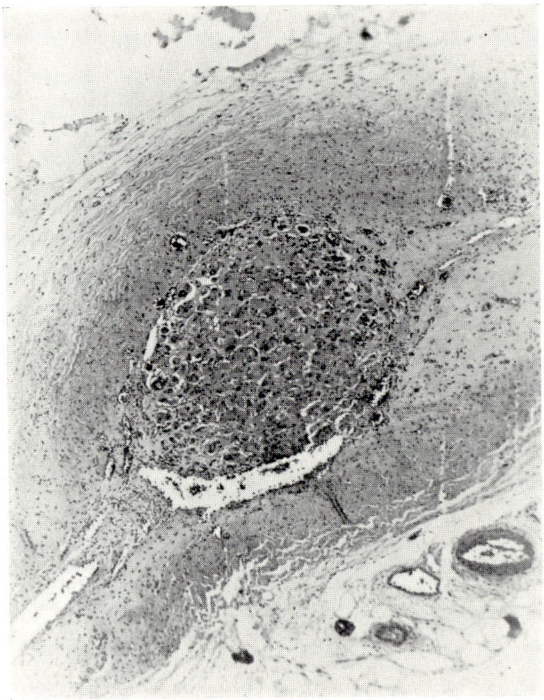

FIG. 5. Fibrotic atrophy of adrenal (Case 2) (haematoxylin and eosin, × 45)

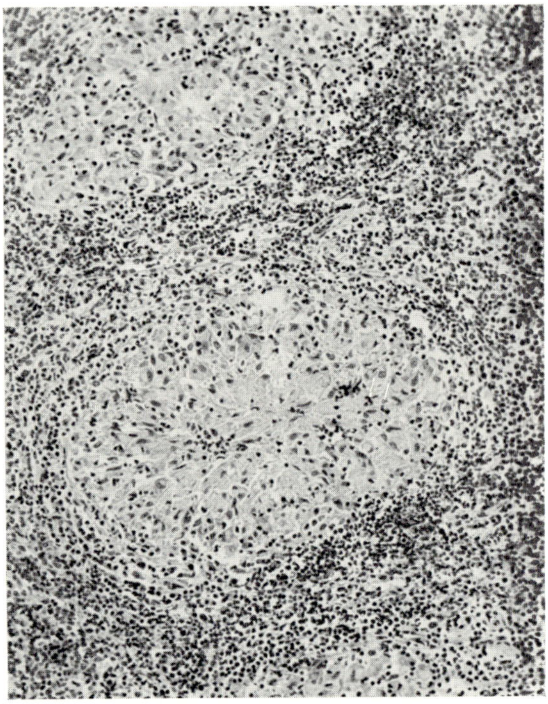

FIG. 6. Splenic granulomata (Case 2) (haematoxylin and eosin, × 134)

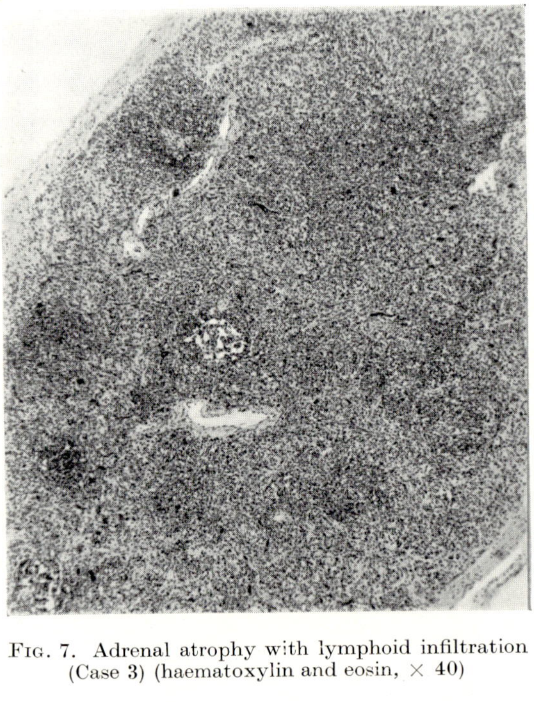

FIG. 7. Adrenal atrophy with lymphoid infiltration (Case 3) (haematoxylin and eosin, × 40)

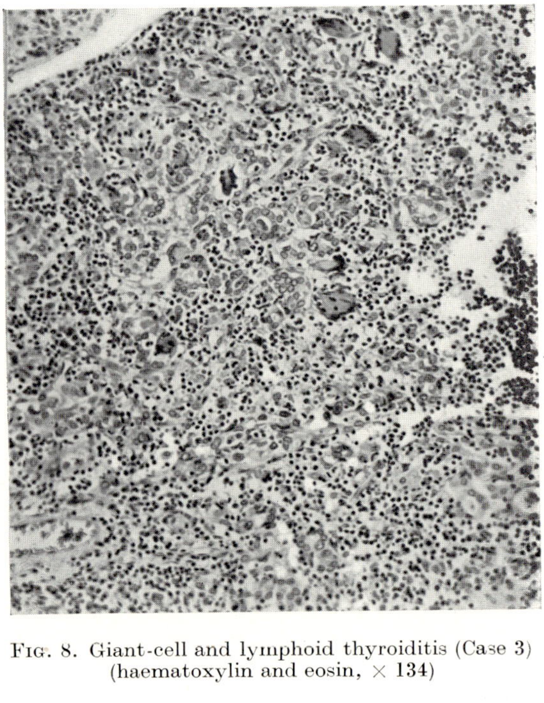

FIG. 8. Giant-cell and lymphoid thyroiditis (Case 3) (haematoxylin and eosin, × 134)

616.831.43-002.7

'GIANT-CELL GRANULOMA' AND THE OTHER PITUITARY GRANULOMATA[1]

By ANTHONY G. RICKARDS and PETER W. HARVEY

(From the Departments of Pathology, Royal Infirmary, Lancaster, and Crumpsall Hospital, Manchester)

With Plates 25 and 26

In another communication dealing with non-tuberculous Addison's disease (Rickards and Barrett, 1954) one case was described in which the adrenal glands were replaced by non-caseating giant-cell granulomatous tissue. This case also showed small foci of giant-cell lesions in the anterior lobe of the pituitary gland. Reasons were advanced which had led us to believe that this disease, which we referred to as giant-cell granuloma, was a distinct clinico-pathological entity. It is the purpose of the present paper to report two further examples of the condition, and to deal particularly with the pituitary manifestations.

Case 1. Giant-cell granuloma affecting the pituitary gland.

Miss M. D., aged 31 years at death, was admitted to Hope Hospital, Salford, in May 1951, complaining of intermittent diarrhoea for the preceding eight years. Her family doctor reported that since the age of 23 years she had been subject to repeated attacks of mucopurulent colitis, which had not appreciably affected her general health until shortly before admission to hospital, when it was evident that she was becoming anaemic and suffering considerable pain. The attacks generally lasted about a month, and were followed by remissions lasting a week or two, but the present attack had persisted for five weeks, and was for the first time associated with nausea and vomiting. She was nulliparous, and her menstrual cycle had always been normal. Physical examination revealed an obviously ill woman, with marked tenderness in the left iliac fossa. Sigmoidoscopy showed the typical features of ulcerative colitis, and she was referred to the medical unit for corticotrophin therapy. Two days after the sigmoidoscopy she suddenly collapsed, with marked pallor and imperceptible pulse; intravenous plasma infusion was commenced, but the patient died the same evening. Her sudden deterioration was unexpected, as immediately beforehand she had appeared to be relatively well.

Autopsy (Dr. J. T. A. Lloyd) was performed on the following day. Significant macroscopic lesions were confined to the following organs: the colon showed extensive ulcerative colitis; the spleen was enlarged to approximately twice its normal size; the pancreas was very firm in consistency, presented none of the normal lobular pattern, and was unusually pale in colour, the whole of the gland being affected; the pituitary gland was markedly enlarged, and bulged out of the fossa; the thyroid gland was of normal size. After death the urinary chlorides were estimated as 3 gm. per litre, and the blood-urea was found to be 200 mg.

[1] Received May 3, 1954.

per 100 ml. Other organs showed no abnormal features. Microscopic examination showed the following features. *Pituitary gland*: the anterior lobe was no longer recognizable; in place of the normal glandular pattern there was a diffuse infiltration with giant cells and epithelioid cells (Plate 25, Figs. 1 and 2), which in a few places were arranged in small nodules; plasma cells and lymphocytes were densely scattered throughout the entire lobe; remnants of anterior lobe tissue could be identified as small cellular clusters embedded within the inflammatory tissue; no foreign bodies were detected, and neither the pituitary stalk nor the posterior lobe showed any abnormal features. The *thyroid gland* showed coarse and irregular fibrous trabeculation throughout its substance, with a moderate lymphocytic infiltration; judged from the histological appearances there was ample active thyroid tissue. The *pancreas* (Plate 25, Fig. 3) showed a uniform and massive fibrosis of its substance, which had almost completely replaced the acinar tissue but had not involved the islets; in some areas there were focal collections of lymphocytes and plasma cells; the pancreatic ducts were denuded of their epithelium, which was replaced by an irregular flat endothelial lining; their walls showed fibrosis and chronic inflammatory cell infiltration; no giant cells or epithelioid cells could be seen. The *colon* showed mucosal ulceration, and the submucosa was densely infiltrated with inflammatory cells. Sections of liver were not available for histological study.

Case 2. Giant-cell granuloma involving the pituitary, hypothalamus, and liver.

Mrs. M. T., aged 54 years at death, was referred by her family doctor to the Manchester Northern Hospital in March 1950. She gave a history of progressive weakness and fatigue during the preceding two years, and shortly before admission she had developed visual disturbances; her family doctor had previously noted albuminuria and hypertension. On examination she was found to have a paralysis of the left abducent nerve; the blood-pressure was recorded as 205/115, although the optic fundi showed no abnormal features, and radiological examination of the chest showed no evidence of pulmonary or cardiac disease. Clinical study suggested a diagnosis of myxoedema, although the origin of the sixth-nerve palsy was not determined; her general condition improved on thyroid treatment, and she was sent home to be kept under observation as an out-patient. She was readmitted 15 months later, having 'suddenly' lost the sight in both her eyes; she also complained of painful 'spasms' in the legs, and suffered from periodic sweating attacks. On admission her blood-pressure was found to be 100/60, and she was almost completely blind, although there were now no signs of the internal strabismus; examination of the nervous system showed her to have absent abdominal reflexes and positive Babinski responses on both sides; radiographs of the skull showed enlargement of the pituitary fossa and erosion of the posterior clinoid processes; examination of the fundi showed bilateral optic atrophy. Serum-calcium and -cholesterol estimations gave results of 9·7 mg. and 280 mg. per 100 ml. Clinically it was considered that the patient was suffering from hypopituitarism due to a pituitary tumour which was involving the optic chiasma. In view of these findings it was decided to confirm the diagnosis of hypopituitarism by an insulin-tolerance test. One unit only of soluble insulin (0·016 unit per kg. body-weight) was administered intramuscularly. Fasting blood-sugar was estimated at 68 mg. per 100 ml. Within one hour the level had dropped to 12 mg. per 100 ml., and hypoglycaemic coma developed; the patient was revived with intravenous glucose, and within two hours her blood-sugar had risen to 64 mg. per 100 ml. The results of this test were so remarkable that it was decided to repeat the investigation, and on the following day a further unit was administered. On this occasion the dose was carefully checked, as it was considered that the first result was probably due to a mistake in the amount of insulin injected; blood-sugar readings were not taken, and the patient showed no untoward reaction throughout the period following injection. Two hours later she suddenly collapsed in hypoglycaemic coma, with a blood-sugar reading of less than 10 mg. per 100 ml. She remained in coma in spite of remedial measures, and died four days later.

Autopsy was performed five and a half hours after death. The body was that of a normally nourished woman 64 inches (162·5 cm.) tall, and weighed 139 lb. (63 kg.). Pubic and axillary hair were virtually absent. Significant macroscopic lesions were confined to the following organs: both lungs showed hypostatic bronchopneumonia; the thyroid and adrenal glands showed severe simple atrophy; the heart weighed 200 gm., and showed dilatation of the left ventricle. The brain (weight 1,220 gm.) showed a tumour involving the tuber cinereum, optic chiasma, and both optic nerves (Plate 25, Fig. 4). The optic nerves were expanded to approximately three times their normal size; median sagittal section (Plate 26, Fig. 5) showed that the tumour was localized to the anterior half of the tuber cinereum; the pituitary stalk could not be identified, as it was embedded in the tumour tissue, and the pituitary gland was replaced by dense scar tissue. Microscopically the *hypothalamus* was extensively replaced by giant-cell granulomata (Plate 26, Fig. 6); the giant cells were large, and in places seemed to lie relatively free within the remains of the nervous tissue, although in other areas there were dense aggregations of lymphocytes and large mononuclear cells. Within the immediately surrounding nervous tissue were found perivascular collections of the same type of cells. In some areas giant cells and epithelioid cells were arranged in the form of non-caseating nodular granulomata. The *pituitary gland* showed almost complete destruction of its substance, which was replaced by dense fibrous tissue containing a few small clusters of residual pituitary cells. Within the fibrous tissue were occasional giant cells, some of which contained uncoloured optically active material (Plate 26, Fig. 7). Adjacent to the fibrotic pituitary gland were many foci of giant-cell granulomata, one area of which showed central calcification. The posterior lobe could not be identified. The *adrenal glands* showed typical atrophy of hypopituitary type, but in some areas the medulla showed patches of diffuse interstitial fibrosis reminiscent of the pituitary scarring. Several blocks of *liver* tissue were prepared in an attempt to identify giant-cell granulomata. In several histological preparations the characteristic nodular foci of epithelioid cells were demonstrated (Plate 26, Fig. 8), and in some lesions typical giant cells were also found; the nodules occurred anywhere within the liver lobule, and were not related to portal tracts. Caseation was not present, and optically active particles were not encountered; stains for micro-organisms were negative. The *pancreas* showed moderate hyperplasia of islet tissue. Histological study of the *lung* showed a terminal bronchopneumonia of about 24 hours' duration. The *thyroid gland* showed gross fibrosis, with a few remaining areas of atrophic glandular tissue; there was an occasional lymphoid germinal follicle. The lymph-nodes, spleen, and kidneys showed no significant lesions apart from atrophic and senile changes.

Comment

These cases are of particular interest in that they show different stages in the development of the disease. In the first patient the lesion is seen to be an active granulomatous process, with little evidence of replacement fibrosis of the pituitary gland and no clinical evidence of hypopituitarism, although the unexpected death of this woman may have been connected with the pituitary destruction. In the second case the lesion has advanced to the stage of almost complete replacement of the pituitary gland by fibrous tissue, although still active in the surrounding brain tissue; in this case overt hypopituitarism was evident. The final stage in the natural history of the disease is seen in the cases described by Sheehan and Summers (1949) under the title of 'healed granuloma': in these two cases the anterior lobe had completely disappeared, leaving an empty sella lined with a tough fibrous-tissue capsule in which occasional foci of giant-cell granulomata were still discernible. In a previous communication (Rickards and Barrett, 1954) attention was called to the various theories regarding aetiology of giant-cell granuloma, and it was pointed out that, in several cases reported under various titles by other workers, nodular granulomata had been found in other organs; the occurrence of these extrahypophyseal lesions appeared to be too frequent to be a coincidental finding, and it appeared likely that cases of giant-cell granuloma affecting the pituitary gland were part of a disseminated granulomatous disease which was probably of infective origin. This view has been further strengthened by the finding of typical nodular granulomata in the liver in our present Case 2. Moreover, in Case W. L. recorded by Sheehan and Summers (1949), a giant-cell lesion was subsequently found in the liver by Sheehan. We have had the opportunity of studying this specimen; it corresponds exactly to those we have described, and it appears not unlikely that extrahypophyseal foci of granulomata will be found in most cases of giant-cell granuloma affecting the pituitary, if careful search is made for such lesions. In Case 1 the pancreas showed extensive fibrosis of its substance which only affected exocrine tissue; as we were unable to demonstrate any granulomatous foci within the gland, it seems likely that the condition was unrelated to the granulomatous disease, and was probably due to an undetected lesion within the main pancreatic duct.

Granulomata of the Pituitary Gland

In view of the close similarity in tissue reactions provoked by sarcoidosis, syphilis, tuberculosis, and giant-cell granuloma, it may be argued that the cases we have designated giant-cell granuloma may be an atypical form of one of these diseases. It was decided, therefore, to review all cases of pituitary granulomata of different types previously reported, and to compare the outstanding clinical and pathological features with those of giant-cell granuloma. This study has revealed marked and characteristic differences between the four groups of cases, and has provided additional evidence that giant-cell granuloma is a disease *sui generis* and unrelated to the other conditions known to be responsible for granulomatous destruction of the hypophysis. In many of the reported cases of syphilis and tuberculosis of the pituitary gland the evidence for the diagnosis is considered inadequate, and several of them may in fact be further examples of giant-cell granuloma; but where any doubt seems to exist we have omitted them, because their inclusion would invalidate any attempt to compare the clinical and pathological features of granulomatous involvement of the pituitary of known aetiology. Tables I to IV show the reported cases of pituitary involvement by giant-cell granuloma, sarcoidosis, syphilis, and tuberculosis. The criteria we have adopted in accepting the diagnosis are summarized at the beginning of each Table, and a list of cases which have failed to satisfy these

TABLE I

Giant-cell Granuloma of the Pituitary Gland

The criteria for the diagnosis of giant-cell granuloma include the histological examination of the gland, which shows non-caseating granulomata, in the absence of signs of syphilis, sarcoidosis, or tuberculosis.

	Patient			Distribution of granulomata		
Author	*Sex*	*Age (years)*	*Signs of pituitary disease*	*Anterior lobe*	*Posterior lobe*	*Stalk*
1. Bastenie, Gepts, and Tagnon (1950).	F	66	Hypopituitarism	yes	n.s.	n.s.
2. ,, ,, ,, ,, .	F	71	Hypopituitarism	yes	n.s.	n.s.
3. Bleisch and Robbins (1952) . .	M	61	Hypopituitarism	yes	no	no
4. Boller and Goedel (1935) . .	F	51	Hypopituitarism	yes	n.s.	n.s.
5. ,, ,, ,, . .	F	69	Hypopituitarism	yes	n.s.	n.s.
6. ,, ,, ,, . .	F	41	Hypopituitarism	yes	n.s.	n.s.
7. Brissaud, Gougerot, and Gy (1908) and Gougerot and Gy (1911) .	M	52	Hypopituitarism; diabetes insipidus	yes	n.s.	n.s.
8. Doniach and Wright (1951) . .	F	43	Hypopituitarism	yes	yes	n.s.
9. ,, ,, ,, . .	M	60	None	yes	no	yes
10. von Gierke (1914) . . .	M	23	Diabetes insipidus	yes	no	yes
11. Guirguis (1944)	F	67	Hypopituitarism	yes	yes	n.s.
12. Herlant (1946)	F	36	Hypopituitarism	yes	yes	yes
13. ,, ,, ...	F	66	Hypopituitarism	yes	n.s.	n.s.
14. Oelbaum and Wainwright (1950) .	M	29	Hypopituitarism	yes	no	n.s.
15. Rickards and Barrett (1954) . .	F	56	None	yes	no	no
16. Rickards and Harvey, present case .	F	31	None	yes	no	no
17. ,, ,, ,, .	F	54	Hypopituitarism; chiasma involved	yes	yes	yes
18. Sheehan and Summers (1949) . .	F	69	Hypopituitarism	yes	no	n.s.
19. ,, ,, ,, . .	F	62	Hypopituitarism	yes	no	no
20. Simmonds (1917)	F	63	None	yes	no	n.s.
21. ,, ,, ...	F	73	None	yes	no	n.s.
22. ,, ,, ...	F	61	None	yes	no	n.s.
23. ,, ,, ...	F	50	None	yes	no	n.s.

n.s. = not stated.

criteria are appended at the foot. In many of these unclassified cases the diagnosis is probably correct, but we have thought it best to exclude all cases of tuberculosis or syphilis in which the diagnosis has not been firmly established by histological examination of the pituitary gland.

1. *Giant-cell granuloma*

As will be seen from Table I, 21 previously reported cases of giant-cell granuloma affecting the pituitary gland have been found. In all cases full post-mortem study has failed to reveal any evidence of syphilis, sarcoidosis, or tuberculosis.

Clinical features. Age. The ages of the patients varied from 23 to 73 years. Only four patients were under the age of 40, and 17 of the 23 cases occurred in patients over the age of 50. The average age of the group was 54 years. This is in marked contrast to the ages of the sarcoidosis, syphilis, and tuberculosis groups. *Sex.* Of the 23 cases, 18 occurred in women. This is again unlike the sex distribution in the sarcoidosis and tuberculosis groups. *Signs and symptoms.* In the 16 cases in which signs of pituitary disease had been present, they were usually those of hypopituitarism, and in only two instances had diabetes insipidus been noted. In seven there was no clinical evidence of pituitary disease. In only one case was there evidence of chiasmal involvement.

Table II

Sarcoidosis of the Pituitary Gland

The criteria for the diagnosis of sarcoidosis include clear clinical or pathological evidence of extrahypophyseal sarcoid lesions, and clear evidence of defective pituitary function for which there is no other apparent cause.

	Patient			*Distribution of granulomata*		
Author	*Sex*	*Age (years)*	*Signs of pituitary disease*	*Anterior lobe*	*Posterior lobe*	*Stalk*
1. Appelmans and van Horenbeeck (1941)	F	16	Diabetes insipidus		No necropsy	
2. Arbuse and Madonick (1938)	F	22	Diabetes insipidus		No necropsy	
3. Barber (1945–6)	M	28	Diabetes insipidus; hypopituitarism		No necropsy	
4. Bleisch and Robbins (1952)	F	33	Diabetes insipidus and hypopituitarism	yes	yes	no
5. ,, ,, ,,	F	72	None	n.s.	n.s.	n.s.
6. ,, ,, ,,	F	77	None	n.s.	n.s.	n.s.
7. ,, ,, ,,	F	64	None	n.s.	n.s.	n.s.
8. Cameron and Dawson (1942)	F	25	Diabetes insipidus		No necropsy	
9. Cowdell (1954)	F	29	None	yes	no	n.s.
10. Elshout (1942)	M	10	Diabetes insipidus		No necropsy	
11. Ernsting and Sillevis-Smitt (1944)	F	31	Diabetes insipidus		No necropsy	
12. Falta and Spitzenberger (1937)	F	43	Diabetes insipidus	yes	yes	n.s.
13. Flandin, Parat, and Poumeau-Delille (1936)	F	56	Diabetes insipidus		No necropsy	
14. Folger (1936)	F	34	Diabetes insipidus		No necropsy	
15. Franceschetti and de Morsier (1941)	M	15	Diabetes insipidus		No necropsy	
16. Gjessing (1916)	F	27	Diabetes insipidus		No necropsy	
17. Glass and Davis (1944)	M	54	Hypopituitarism	yes	yes	n.s.
18. Harrell (1940)	M	26	Diabetes insipidus		No necropsy	
19. Heerfordt (1909)	M	27	Diabetes insipidus		No necropsy	
20. Jersild (1939)	M	15	Diabetes insipidus		No necropsy	
21. Kraus (1942–3)	F	41	Diabetes insipidus	yes	yes	yes
22. Leitner (1949)	M	24	Diabetes insipidus		No necropsy	
23. Lemming (1940)	F	34	Diabetes insipidus		No necropsy	
24. Lesné, Launay, and Sée (1935)	M	10	Diabetes insipidus		No necropsy	
25. Levin (1935)	M	28	Diabetes insipidus		No necropsy	
26. Longcope (1941)	n.s.	n.s.	Diabetes insipidus	yes	yes	yes
27. Longcope and Freiman (1952)	M	31	Diabetes insipidus; hypopituitarism; chiasma involved	yes	yes	yes
28. Merrill and Oaks (1931)	F	43	Diabetes insipidus		No necropsy	
29. Pennell (1951)	M	19	Diabetes insipidus		No necropsy	
30. Posner (1942)	F	2	Diabetes insipidus	yes	n.s.	n.s.
31. Reis and Rothfeld (1931)	F	17	Chiasma involved	no	no	yes
32. Rey, Canepa, and Vivoli (1947)	M	20	Diabetes insipidus		No necropsy	
33. Ricker and Clark (1949)	M	25	None	n.s.	n.s.	n.s.
34. Schüpbach (1936)	M	35	Diabetes insipidus		No necropsy	
35. Snapper and Pompen (1938)	F	16	Diabetes insipidus		No necropsy	
36. Spillane (1952)	M	35	Diabetes insipidus		No necropsy	
37. Teilum (1951)	F	49	None	n.s.	n.s.	n.s.
38. Terpestra (1944)	F	41	Diabetes insipidus; chiasma involved		No necropsy	
39. Tillgren (1935)	M	42	Diabetes insipidus	yes	n.s.	n.s.
40. Wahlgren (1936)	M	42	Diabetes insipidus	yes	yes	n.s.
41. Walsh (1939)	F	34	Diabetes insipidus		No necropsy	

n.s. = not stated.

Four cases with insufficient evidence for the diagnosis of sarcoidosis of the pituitary gland:
Doub and Menagh (1929) M 30; Toulant and Morard (1936) M 17; Gernez-Rieux, Breton, Bonte, and Delwaulle (1948) F 23; Pearson (1954) F 52.

Pathological features. In all cases the pituitary gland was found to be partially or wholly replaced by non-caseating giant-cell granulomata. In all cases the anterior lobe was invaded, and in four (Cases 8, 11, 12, and 17) granulomata were present in the pars nervosa. In several cases doubly refractile particles were found within the giant cells. In four cases (9, 10, 12, and 17) the pituitary stalk was involved; in the remaining cases either it was free from disease or no reference was made to its condition. This anatomical distribution of lesions accords closely with the clinical signs of hypopituitarism.

2. *Sarcoidosis*

Table II summarizes the recorded cases of pituitary involvement in generalized sarcoidosis.

Clinical features. Age. The ages of the patients varied from two years to 77 years, but over 80 per cent. were under the age of 50 years. No age was exempt from the lesion. The average age of the group was 32 years. *Sex.* In this group the sexes were evenly divided. *Clinical findings and symptoms.* Of the patients who had signs of pituitary involvement, more than 90 per cent. presented symptoms of diabetes insipidus. In four cases symptoms of hypopituitarism were encountered, and in another two the association was doubtful. In only one case was hypopituitarism found without being preceded by polyuria and polydipsia.

Pathological features. In 16 cases the pituitary gland was subjected to histological examination, and in all of them typical non-caseating giant-cell foci were found. In those cases in which full details of the histological findings were given, it is apparent that the lesions did not tend to be confined to the anterior lobe, but frequently involved the posterior lobe and infundibulum. It is probably for this reason that diabetes insipidus occurs so much more commonly; there is a greater probability of the hypothalamo-hypophyseal tract, or the supraoptic nuclei, being involved by sarcoidosis before destruction of the anterior lobe is complete, than in the case of the more restricted lesion of giant-cell granuloma. The generalized nature of the lesions of sarcoidosis in lymph-nodes, eyes, parotid glands, bones, lungs, and skin had usually been clinically evident before the onset of pituitary disturbances, and it was the rule for the patient who showed the recognized picture of sarcoidosis to develop suddenly the striking symptoms of diabetes insipidus. This train of events is in marked contrast to the giant-cell-granuloma group of cases, in which there is either the silent development of a pituitary lesion only detected at autopsy, or the slow appearance of hypopituitarism of unknown cause.

3. *Syphilis*

Table III summarizes the reported cases of pituitary involvement in congenital and acquired syphilis; cases of neonatal syphilis have been excluded.

Clinical features. Age. The ages of the patients varied from nine to 78 years, and 65 per cent. of the cases occurred before the age of 50 years. No age was exempt from the lesion, and the average age of the group was 42 years. *Sex.* Women predominated over men in a ratio of approximately two to one. *Clinical findings and symptoms.* In the majority of cases in which signs of pituitary involvement had been present, these were of hypopituitary type, and in four cases death was due to unexplained coma, which may well have been due

TABLE III

Syphilis of the Pituitary Gland (excluding neonatal syphilis)

The criteria for the diagnosis of syphilis of the pituitary gland include positive serological evidence of syphilis, or clear pathological evidence of the disease in extrahypophyseal structures, together with histological examination of the gland.

	Patient			Distribution of granulomata		
Author	*Sex*	*Age (years)*	*Signs of pituitary disease*	*Anterior lobe*	*Posterior lobe*	*Stalk*
1. Barbacci (1892)	n.s.	n.s.	Chiasma involved	n.s.	n.s.	n.s.
2. Beadles (1896 and 1897)	F	41	None	yes	no	no
3. Berblinger (1932)	F	57	None	yes	n.s.	n.s.
4. Chiari (1913)	F	9	Unexplained coma	yes	yes	yes
5. Cohn (1923)	F	43	Hypopituitarism	yes	n.s.	yes
6. Esser (1927)	F	66	None	yes	n.s.	n.s.
7. Farquharson and Graham (1931)	M	50	Hypopituitarism	yes	n.s.	n.s.
8. Fink (1933)	F	34	Chiasma involved	yes	n.s.	yes
9. Fry (1914–15)	M	43	None	yes	n.s.	n.s.
10. Graubner (1925)	F	52	Hypopituitarism	yes	no	no
11. Hektoen (1896)	F	45	n.s.	yes	n.s.	yes
12. Hirsch (1922)	M	55	Hypopituitarism	yes	n.s.	n.s.
13. Hunter (1898)	F	47	n.s.	n.s.	n.s.	n.s.
14. Jaffé (1922)	M	33	None	no	no	yes
15. Jedlicka (1923)	M	Old	n.s.	yes	n.s.	n.s.
16. Josephy (1920)	F	53	None	yes	n.s.	n.s.
17. Kennedy and Fisher (1934)	F	58	Unexplained coma	yes	no	n.s.
18. Kufs (1905)	F	47	None	yes	yes	n.s.
19. Lanza (1949)	M	51	Chiasma involved	yes	yes	no
20. Lindemann (1923)	F	34	Hypopituitarism	yes	n.s.	no
21. Mencarelli (1930)	M	31	None	yes	no	n.s.
22. Nonne (1922)	M	38	Diabetes insipidus	yes	yes	n.s.
23. Pappenheim (1934)	F	33	Diabetes insipidus; hypopituitarism	yes	n.s.	n.s.
24. Pennetti (1928)	M	28	Hypopituitarism	yes	n.s.	n.s.
25. Rössle (1934)	F	52	Hypopituitarism	yes	n.s.	n.s.
26. Schaefer (1919)	F	22	None	no	yes	yes
27. Scholtz (1924)	F	32	None	yes	no	yes
28. Simmonds (1914*a*)	M	78	None	yes	no	no
29. Sokoloff (1896)	F	44	None	yes	yes	n.s.
30. Starck (1908–9)	F	37	None	yes	n.s.	n.s.
31. Stroebe (1905)	F	52	Unexplained coma	yes	yes	yes
32. Troisier (1874)	F	25–30	Unexplained coma	yes	yes	n.s.
33. Virchow (1858)	F	29	Diabetes insipidus; chiasma involved	yes	n.s.	n.s.
34. Weigert (1875)	F	64	n.s.	yes	yes	n.s.
35. Williams (1940)	F	27	Chiasma involved	yes	n.s.	n.s.
36. Woolley (1915)	M	52	n.s.	yes	yes	n.s.

n.s. = not stated.

One hundred and two cases reported as syphilis or probable syphilis of the pituitary gland which do not fulfil the above criteria:

Bauer (1923) F 41; Benda (1914) 3 cases, no details; Berblinger (1927) 1 case, no details; Berblinger (1934) M 50; Bergé and Schulmann (1918) F, age n.s.; Bianchi (1913) F 38; Birch-Hirschfeld (1885), no details; Broussilovski (1925) F 56; Brühl (1931) F, age n.s.; Buday (1923) 2 cases, no details; Camauer (1939) M 40; Camauer and Sacon (1930) M 40; Curschmann (1922) M 1; Cushing (1912) F 57 and M 32; Darley, Gordon, and Neubuerger (1944) M 49; Dolin (1929) M 42, M 46, M 24, and M 19; Drouet and Hamel (1931) M 18; Fahr (1918) F 50; Falta (1923*a*) F, age n.s.; Faure Beaulieu and George (1922) M 44; Feit (1920) M 53; Fink (1926) M 50; von Frankl-Hochwart (1909) 3 cases, no details; Frisch (1921) F 39; Futcher (1902) M 32, M 36, and M 35; Goldzieher (1913) M 32 and M 34; Hemptenmacher, cited by Falta (1923*b*) F 42; Herlant (1946) F 36; Hernandez (1924) M 41; Hirsch and Berberich (1924) F 57; Hutinel and Stévenin (1920) M 13, F 15, F 14, F 11, and F 15; Hval (1937) M 43; Jaffé (1922) M 54; Lancereaux (1868), no details; Lancereaux (1879–81) F 39; Lerman and Means (1945) M 48; Leudet (1860) F 32; Magnus-Alsleben (1926) 1 case, no details; Mann (1922) F 44; Marburg (1922) 2 cases, no details; Marx (1928) M 33; Mathieu (1931) and Mathieu and Grandpierre (1931) F 30; Meyer (1861) F 44; Mingazzini (1920) F 27; Nonne (1916) M 52, M 15, and M 16; Nonne (1922) M 51, M 52, F 17, M 17, M 17, M 18, M 19, M 16, M 17, M 5, F, age n.s., F 18, and M 16; Oelbaum (1952) M 45 and M 46; Oelbaum and Wainwright (1950) M 29; Payenneville and Cailliau (1931) F 28; Plaut (1922) F 50 and M 54; Reiche (1927) F 67; Reuter and Lamprecht (1937) M 26; Reye (1920) F 50; Riecker and Curtis (1932) M 47 and F 41; Schmorl (1914), no details; Skubiszewski (1924) F 37; Turner (1910) F 33; Uthy (1912), no details; Werner (1931) M 50; Westphal (1863) M 48; Winkler (1934) F 38; Wittgenstein and Kroner (1921) F 50; Wood (1909) M 37; Zondek and Koehler (1928) F 32, F 33, and F 34.

to hypopituitarism. In only three cases had symptoms of diabetes insipidus been present. Clinical involvement of the optic chiasma was present in five cases.

Pathological features. The pituitary gland was subjected to histological examination in all cases, and in those in which a full description of the lesions was given it is evident that the disease was not confined to the anterior lobe. In 10 cases the posterior lobe was definitely involved and, judging from the extent of the lesions, it was probably diseased in several other cases in which no specific mention of the posterior lobe was made. In eight cases the infundibulum was said to have been diseased; in 23 cases no reference was made to it, and in five it was described as being normal. In the great majority of cases the lesions were typical gummata with extensive central necrosis, but in three cases they were composed of non-caseating foci of epithelioid and giant cells; in one of these cases (Case 17) multiple non-caseating epithelioid granulomata were found in the liver. This case occurred in a Negress with a strongly positive Wassermann reaction, but the atypical histological appearance raises a doubt as to whether the lesion was an example of giant-cell granuloma complicated by concurrent syphilis. From the pathological point of view the most distinguishing feature between syphilis and giant-cell granuloma of the pituitary gland is the presence or absence of tissue necrosis within the lesions. Moreover, optically active particles are not infrequently present in the lesions of giant-cell granuloma, but have not been reported in gummata of the pituitary gland.

TABLE IV

Tuberculosis of the Pituitary Gland

The criteria for the diagnosis of tuberculosis include histological examination of the gland and the presence of extrahypophyseal tuberculosis.

	Patient			Distribution of granulomata		
Author	*Sex*	*Age (years)*	*Signs of pituitary disease*	*Anterior lobe*	*Posterior lobe*	*Stalk*
1. Berblinger (1939)	F	52	Hypopituitary coma	yes	yes	yes
2. Bock (1924)	M	24	Hypopituitarism	yes	no	yes
3. Fodor, Emerich, and Jankovich (1921)	M	32	Diabetes insipidus; chiasma involved	yes	n.s.	n.s.
4. Froboese (1918)	F	32	Unexplained coma	yes	yes	n.s.
5. von Hann (1918)	F	32	Diabetes insipidus	no	yes	yes
6. Heidkamp (1912)	M	13	Chiasma involved	yes	yes	n.s.
7. Knoll (1922)	M	23	Chiasma involved	yes	yes	n.s.
8. Kraus (1924)	F	23	None	yes	yes	yes
9. Kurzak (1921)	M	20	Chiasma involved	n.s.	n.s.	yes
10. Lancereaux (1889)	F	27	None	n.s.	n.s.	n.s.
11. Lucien and Parisot (1909)	F	65	Polyuria; glycosuria	yes	no	n.s.
12. Oliver (1952)	M	52	Hypopituitary coma	yes	yes	n.s.
13. Raab (1923–4)	F	23	Chiasma involved	yes	yes	yes
14. Schlagenhaufer (1916)	F	27	None	yes	n.s.	yes
15. Wagner (1862)	F	13	None	yes	n.s.	n.s.

n.s. = not stated.

Twenty-three cases reported as tuberculosis or probable tuberculosis of the pituitary which do not fulfil the above criteria:

Beck (1835) M 17; Berblinger (1932), no details; Cerise (1912) F 45; Coleman and Meredith (1940) F 57; von Frankl-Hochwart (1909) 7 cases, no details; Glinski (1913) F 10; Haushalter and Lucien (1908) F 6; Kirshbaum and Levy (1941) F 37 and M 44; Kraus (1924) F 61; Kraus and Reisinger (1924) F 56; Letchworth (1924) M 16; von Meyenburg (1916) F 36; Parsons and Zarafonetis (1945) M 63; Schmidt (1898), no details; Schmorl (1914), no details; Simmonds (1914*b*), no details; Simmonds (1914*c*) F 71; Sommer (1909) F 48; Thaon (1907) M 40; Versé (1914) M 45; Wilder (1946) F 62; Zenoni (1913) F 46.

4. *Tuberculosis*

Table IV summarizes the reported cases of pituitary involvement in tuberculosis. Cases of miliary tuberculosis with pituitary involvement have been excluded.

Clinical features. Age. The ages of the patients varied from 13 to 65 years, but approximately 90 per cent. of the cases occurred before the age of 50 years. Over 80 per cent. occurred in the first four decades. The average age of the group was 28 years. *Sex.* The sexes were fairly evenly divided in this group. *Clinical findings and symptoms.* Hypopituitarism had been a feature of only three cases in this series, and in a further case probably accounted for an unexplained coma. Obesity was described in three cases, in one case associated

TABLE V

Summary of Clinical Features

	Sex		*Age (years)*						
	F	*M*	*< 50*	*> 50*	*Average*	*Diabetes insipidus*	*Hypo-pituitarism*	*Chiasma involved*	*Total*
Giant-cell granuloma	18	5	6	17	54	2	15	1	23
Sarcoidosis	22	18	35	5	32	33	4	1	41
Syphilis	24	11	22	14	42	3	8	5	36
Tuberculosis	9	6	12	3	28	2	3	5	15

with diabetes insipidus and in another with signs of chiasmal involvement. The optic chiasma was clinically affected in five cases, and in three cases polyuria and polydipsia were encountered; in one of these latter cases, however, glycosuria was also present. The outstanding feature of this series is the diversity of symptoms and signs following tuberculous involvement of the pituitary.

Pathological features. The pituitary gland was subjected to histological examination in all cases, and in those in which full details are given it is apparent that the lesions may develop in any part of the pituitary gland. The posterior lobe was involved in eight cases, and in 12 cases the lesion was found in the anterior lobe. The stalk was involved in seven cases, and in the remaining cases it is not described. In all cases evidence of extra-cerebral tuberculosis was present. In only one case could tubercle bacilli be identified in the pituitary granulomata.

Discussion

Table V shows a comparison of the main clinical features of the four different groups of granulomatous disease of the pituitary gland. This analysis of the four groups of cases supports the view that giant-cell granuloma is a distinct disease entity, which conforms neither to the clinical nor to the pathological patterns of sarcoidosis, syphilis, or tuberculosis. The disease is shown to occur predominantly in middle-aged or elderly women, and symptoms when present have been usually those of hypopituitarism. When the granulomatous lesions affect the adrenal glands the patient may come under observation with Addison's disease; this is particularly likely if the pituitary gland is either free from lesions or only very slightly involved. Sarcoidosis of the pituitary gland is shown to be a disease of early adult life, to be evenly distributed between the sexes, and to present almost invariably the symptoms of polyuria and polydipsia. Accepted cases of syphilis have occurred more frequently in women than in men, and the majority of patients have been under 50 years of age. Symptoms, when present, were usually attributable to hypopituitarism, although diabetes insipidus and involvement of the optic chiasma were not infrequent. Tuberculosis of the gland is shown to be predominantly a disease of adolescent or early adult life; no difference has been shown between the sexes; symptoms, when present, were usually those of polyuria and polydipsia, or of involvement of the optic chiasma; signs of hypopituitarism have occurred in only three cases.

We are greatly indebted to the following colleagues for advice and permission to publish these cases: Drs. G. J. Crawford and W. Mackay, of Hope Hospital, Salford; Dr. J. T. A. Lloyd, of the Royal Alexandra Hospital, Rhyl; Dr. R. Sykes, of the Manchester Northern Hospital; Drs. J. Davson and R. A. Bailey, of Crumpsall Hospital, Manchester; and Dr. G. M. Barrett, of the Royal Infirmary, Lancaster. We would also thank Mr. F. Taylor, chief technician, for the photomicrography, and Miss J. Perry for Fig. 4. Our thanks are due to Mrs. J. Garnett and Miss M. Bird for clerical aid, and to Mrs. J. L. Neuberg for her help in translating German publications.

Summary

1. Two cases of giant-cell granuloma affecting the pituitary gland are described. Study of these cases strengthens the belief that giant-cell granuloma affecting the pituitary gland is part of a widespread granulomatous disease. Usually it has manifested itself by symptoms and signs of hypopituitarism, although not infrequently it has been found incidentally at autopsy. One patient previously reported came under observation with Addison's disease.

2. Clinical and pathological comparison of previously reported cases of granulomatous destruction of the pituitary gland suggests that giant-cell granuloma is a clinico-pathological entity distinct from tuberculosis, syphilis, and sarcoidosis.

3. It appears likely that the disease has an infective basis.

REFERENCES

Appelmans, M., and van Horenbeeck, A. (1941) *Ophthalmologica*, **102**, 65.
Arbuse, D., and Madonick, M. (1938) *Amer. J. Med. Sci.* **196**, 222.
Barbacci, O. (1892) Abstract in *Ctrbl. allg. Path. path. Anat.* **3**, 301.
Barber, H. W. (1945–6) *Proc. R. Soc. Med.* **39**, 92.
Bastenie, P. A., Gepts, W., and Tagnon, R. (1950) *Sem. hôp. Paris*, **26**, 3157.
Bauer, J. (1923) *Verhandl. dtsch. Ges. inn. Med.* **35**, 219.
Beadles, C. (1896) *Brit. Med. J.* **2**, 1775.
Beadles, C. F. (1897) *Trans. Path. Soc. London*, **48**, 1.
Beck (1835). Cited by Heidkamp (1912).
Benda (1914). *Verhandl. dtsch. pathol. Ges.* **17**, 233.
Berblinger (1927). Ibid. **22**, 191.
—— W. (1932) *Pathologie und pathologische Morphologie der Hypophyse des Menschen*, Leipzig.
—— (1934) *Endokrinologie*, **14**, 369.
—— (1939) *Schweiz. med. Woch.* **69**, 1217.
Bergé, A., and Schulmann, E. (1918) *Presse méd.* **26**, 618.
Bianchi, G. (1913) Cited by Cohn (1923).
Birch-Hirschfeld (1885). Ibid.
Bleisch, V. R., and Robbins, S. L. (1952) *Arch. Int. Med.* **89**, 877.
Bock, E. (1924) *Virchows Arch.* **252**, 98.
Boller, R., and Goedel, A. (1935) *Wien. Arch. inn. Med.* **27**, 41.
Brissaud, Gougerot, and Gy (1908) *Rev. neurol.* **16**, 1354.
Broussilovski, L. (1925) *Encéphale*, **20**, 734.
Brühl, R. (1931) *Monats. Geburtsh. Gynäkol.* **89**, 330.
Buday, K. (1923) *Klin. Woch.* **2**, 902.
Camauer, A. F. (1939) *Prensa méd. argent.* **26**, 2327.
—— and Sacon, J. I. (1930) *Rev. Asoc. méd. argent.* **43**, 423.
Cameron, C., and Dawson, E. K. (1942) *Edin. Med. J.* **49**, 737.
Cerise (1912) *Rev. neurol.* **23**, 227.
Chiari (1913) *Dtsch. med. Woch.* **39**, 1662.
Cohn, E. (1923) *Virchows Arch.* **240**, 452.
Coleman, C. C., and Meredith, J. M. (1940) *Arch. Neurol. Psychiat.* **44**, 1076.
Cowdell, R. H. (1954) *Quart. J. Med.* N.S. **23**, 29.
Curschmann (1922) *Dtsch. Zts. Nervenheilk.* **74**, 188.
Cushing, H. W. (1912) *The Pituitary Body and its Disorders*, Philad., p. 266.
Darley, W., Gordon, R. W., and Neubuerger, K. T. (1944) *Ann. Int. Med.* **21**, 890.
Dolin, A. O. (1929) *Dtsch. Zts. Nervenheilk.* **110**, 166.
Doniach, I., and Wright, E. A. (1951) *J. Path. Bact.* **63**, 69.
Doub, H. P., and Menagh, F. R. (1929) *Amer. J. Roentgenol.* **21**, 149.
Drouet and Hamel (1931) *Rev. méd. de l'est*, **59**, 661.
Elshout, C. (1942) *Nederl. tijd. geneesk.* **86**, 1473.
Ernsting, W., and Sillevis-Smitt, W. G. (1944) Cited by Leitner (1949).
Esser, A. (1927) *Ctrbl. allg. Path. path. Anat.* **39**, 97.
Fahr, T. (1918) *Dtsch. med. Woch.* **44**, 206.
Falta, W. (1923*a*) *Verhandl. dtsch. Ges. inn. Med.* **35**, 117.
—— (1923*b*) *Endocrine Diseases*, London, 3rd ed. p. 568.
—— and Spitzenberger, O. (1937) *Strahlentherapie*, **60**, 385.
Farquharson, R. F., and Graham, D. (1931) *Trans. Ass. Amer. Phys.* **46**, 150.
Faure Beaulieu, M., and George, P. (1922) *Rev. neurol.* **38**, 694.
Feit, H. (1920) *Med. Klin.* **16**, 421.
Fink, E. B. (1926) *Endocrinology*, **10**, 317.
—— (1933) *Arch. Path.* **15**, 631.
Flandin, C., Parat, M., and Poumeau-Delille, G. (1936) *Bull. mém. Soc. méd. hôp. Paris*, **52**, 1423.

Fodor, Emerich, and Jankovich (1921) Abstract in *Ctrbl. ges. Tuberk-forsch.* **15**, 407.
Folger, H. P. (1936) *Arch. Ophthal.* **15**, 1098.
Franceschetti, A., and de Morsier, G. (1941) *Rev. méd. suisse rom.* **61**, 129.
Frankl-Hochwart, L. von (1909) *Wien. med. Woch.* **59**, 2326.
Frisch, A. (1921) *Med. Klin.* **17**, 1021.
Froboese, C. (1918) *Ctrbl. allg. Path. path. Anat.* **29**, 145.
Fry, H. J. B. (1914–15) *Quart. J. Med.* **8**, 277.
Futcher, T. B. (1902) *Johns Hopkins Hosp. Rep.* **10**, 197.
Gernez-Rieux, C., Breton, A., Bonte, G., and Delwaulle (1948) *J. fr. méd. chir. thorac.* **2**, 376.
Gierke, E. von (1914) *Verhandl. dtsch. pathol. Ges.* **17**, 200.
Gjessing, H. G. A. (1916) *Klin. Monatsbl. Augenh.* **21**, 258.
Glass, S. J., and Davis, S. (1944) *J. Clin. Endocrin.* **4**, 489.
Glinski, L. K. (1913) *Dtsch. med. Woch.* **39**, 473.
Goldzieher, M. (1913) *Ctrbl. allg. Path. path. Anat.* **24**, 281.
Gougerot, H., and Gy, A. (1911) *Nouv. iconog. de la Salpêtrière,* **24**, 449.
Graubner, W. (1925) *Zts. klin. Med.* **101**, 249.
Guirguis, Z.-A. (1944) *Thèse de Genève.*
Hann, F. von (1918) *Frankfurt. Zts. Path.* **21**, 337.
Harrell, G. T. (1940) *Arch. Int. Med.* **65**, 1003.
Haushalter, P., and Lucien, M. (1908) *Rev. neurol.* **16**, 1.
Heerfordt, C. F. (1909) *v. Graefes Arch. Ophthal.* **70**, 254.
Heidkamp, H. (1912) *Virchows Arch.* **210**, 445.
Hektoen, L. (1896) *J. Amer. Med. Ass.* **26**, 1115.
Hemptenmacher. Cited by Falta (1923*b*).
Herlant, M. (1946) *Acta clin. belg.* **1**, 197.
Hernandez, R. A. (1924) *Amer. J. Syph.* **8**, 321.
Hirsch, S. (1922) *Dtsch. Arch. klin. Med.* **140**, 323.
—— and Berberich, J. (1924) *Klin. Woch.* **3**, 483.
Hunter, W. (1898) *Trans. Path. Soc. London,* **49**, 249.
Hutinel, V., and Stévenin, H. (1920) *Arch. de méd. des enf.* **23**, 5.
Hval, E. (1937) *Acta derm.-venereol.* **18**, 64.
Jaffé, R. (1922) *Frankfurt. Zts. Path.* **27**, 324.
Jedlicka, V. (1923) Abstract in *J. Amer. Med. Ass.* **81**, 2072.
Jersild, M. (1939) *Ann. dermat. syph.* **10**, 641.
Josephy, H. (1920) *Zts. ges. Neurol. Psychiat.* **58**, 56.
Kennedy, F. S., and Fisher, J. H. (1934) *Amer. J. Syph.* **18**, 12.
Kirshbaum, J. D., and Levy, H. A. (1941) *Arch. Int. Med.* **68**, 1095.
Knoll, W. (1922) *Wien. Arch. inn. Med.* **4**, 555.
Kraus, E. J. (1924) *Med. Klin.* **20**, 1290.
—— (1942–3) *J. Lab. Clin. Med.* **28**, 140.
—— and Reisinger, A. (1924) *Frankfurt. Zts. Path.* **30**, 68.
Kufs (1905) *Arch. Psychiat. Nervenkr.* **39**, 134.
Kurzak, H. (1921) *Zts. Tuberk.* **34**, 433.
Lancereaux, E. (1868) *Treatise on Syphilis,* New Sydenham Soc., London, **1**, 376.
—— (1879–81) *Traité d'Anatomie Pathologique,* Paris, **2**, 550.
—— (1889) Ibid. **3**, 732.
Lanza, G. (1949) *Arch. de Vecchi anat. pat.* **13**, 585.
Leitner, S. J. (1949) *Der Morbus Besnier-Boeck-Schaumann,* Basel, 2nd ed. p. 76.
Lemming, R. (1940) *Acta med. scand.* **103**, 400.
Lerman, J., and Means, J. H. (1945) *J. Clin. Endocrin.* **5**, 119.
Lesné, E., Launay, C., and Sée, G. (1935) *Bull. mém. Soc. méd. hôp. Paris,* **51**, 1137.
Letchworth, T. W. (1924) *Brit. Med. J.* **1**, 1127.
Leudet (1860). Cited by Falta (1923*b*).
Levin, P. M. (1935) *J. Nerv. Ment. Dis.* **81**, 176.
Lindemann, E. (1923) *Virchows Arch.* **240**, 11.

Longcope, W. T. (1941) *J. Amer. Med. Ass.* **117,** 1321.
—— and Freiman, D. G. (1952) *Medicine,* **31,** 1.
Lucien, M., and Parisot, J. (1909) *Rev. neurol.* **17,** 970.
Magnus-Alsleben (1926) *Münch. med. Woch.* **73,** 510.
Mann, L. (1922) *Dtsch. Zts. Nervenheilk.* **74,** 188.
Marburg (1922) Ibid. **74,** 188.
Marx, H. (1928) *Dtsch. Arch. klin. Med.* **158,** 149.
Mathieu, L. (1931) *Rev. méd. de l'est,* **59,** 246.
—— and Grandpierre, G. (1931) Ibid. **59,** 638.
Mencarelli, L. (1930) *Pathologica,* **22,** 465.
Merrill, H. G., and Oaks, L. W. (1931) *Amer. J. Ophthal.* **14,** 15.
Meyenburg, H. von (1916) *Beitr. path. Anat.* **61,** 550.
Meyer, L. (1861) *Zts. Psychiat.* **18,** 287.
Mingazzini, G. (1920) *Dtsch. Zts. Nervenheilk.* **66,** 336.
Nonne, M. (1916) Ibid. **55,** 29.
—— (1922) Ibid. **74,** 168.
Oelbaum, M. H. (1952) *Quart. J. Med.* N.S. **21,** 249.
—— and Wainwright, J. (1950) *J. Clin. Path.* **3,** 122.
Oliver, L. C. (1952) *Lancet,* **1,** 698.
Pappenheim, M. (1934) *Wien. klin. Woch.* **47,** 148.
Parsons, R. J., and Zarafonetis, C. J. D. (1945) *Arch. Int. Med.* **75,** 1.
Payenneville and Cailliau, F. (1931) *Rev. méd. de l'est,* **59,** 663.
Pearson, J. E. G. (1954) *Brit. Med. J.* **1,** 704.
Pennell, W. H. (1951) *Arch. Neurol. Psychiat.* **66,** 728.
Pennetti, G. (1928) *Riforma med.* **44,** 9.
Plaut, R. (1922) *Dtsch. Arch. klin. Med.* **139,** 285.
Posner, I. (1942) *J. Pediat.* **20,** 486.
Raab, W. (1923–4) *Wien. Arch. inn. Med.* **7,** 443.
Reiche, F. (1927) *Med. Klin.* **23,** 1569.
Reis, W., and Rothfeld, J. (1931) *v. Graefes Arch. Ophthal.* **126,** 357.
Reuter, A., and Lamprecht, I. (1937) *Dtsch. med. Woch.* **63,** 1033.
Rey, J. C., Canepa, E., and Vivoli, D. (1947) *Medicina,* **7,** 451.
Reye (1920) *Med. Klin.* **16,** 1313.
Rickards, A. G., and Barrett, G. M. (1954) *Quart. J. Med.* N.S. **23,** 403.
Ricker, W., and Clark, M. (1949) *Amer. J. Clin. Path.* **19,** 725.
Riecker, H. H., and Curtis, A. C. (1932) *J. Amer. Med. Ass.* **99,** 110.
Rössle, R. (1934) *Verhandl. dtsch. pathol. Ges.* **27,** 152.
Schaefer, H. (1919) *Ctrbl. allg. Path. path. anat.* **30,** 520.
Schlagenhaufer (1916) *Virchows Arch.* **222,** 249.
Schmidt, M. B. (1898) *Ergebn. allg. Path.* **5,** 895.
Schmorl (1914) *Verhandl. dtsch. pathol. Ges.* **17,** 231.
Scholtz, L. (1924) *Arch. f. Dermat. u. Syph.* **147,** 509.
Schüpbach, A. (1936) *Schweiz. med. Woch.* **66,** 1182.
Sheehan, H. L., and Summers, V. K. (1949) *Quart. J. Med.* N.S. **18,** 319.
Simmonds, M. (1914*a*) *Dermat. Woch.* Erganz. **58,** 104.
—— (1914*b*) *Verhandl. dtsch. pathol. Ges.* **17,** 208.
—— (1914*c*) *Ctrbl. allg. Path. path. Anat.* **25,** 194.
—— (1917) *Virchows Arch.* **223,** 281.
Skubiszewski, F. (1924) *Rev. neurol.* **2,** 327.
Snapper, I., and Pompen, A. W. M. (1938) *Pseudo-tuberculosis in Man,* Haarlem, p. 23.
Sokoloff, A. (1896) *Virchows Arch.* **143,** 333.
Sommer, H. (1909) *Zts. Laryng. Rhinol.* **2,** 355.
Spillane, J. D. (1952) *Thorax,* **7,** 134.
Starck, H. (1908–9) *Dtsch. Zts. Nervenheilk.* **36,** 126.
Stroebe, H. (1905) *Beitr. path. Anat.* **37,** 455.
Teilum, G. (1951) *Acta path. microbiol. scand.* **28,** 294.

Terpestra, J. J. (1944) *Nederl. tijd. geneesk.* **88,** 476.
Thaon, P. (1907) *Thèse de Paris* No. 122.
Tillgren, J. (1935) *Brit. J. Dermat. Syph.* **47,** 223.
Toulant and Morard (1936) *Arch. d'ophtalmol.* **53,** 321.
Troisier (1874). *Bull. Soc. anat. Paris,* 3rd Ser. **9,** 25.
Turner, J. (1910) *Rev. Neurol. Psychiat.* **8,** 344.
Uthy (1912). Cited by Jaffé (1922).
Versé (1914) *Verhandl. dtsch. pathol. Ges.* **17,** 236.
Virchow, R. (1858) *Virchows Arch.* **15,** 217.
Wagner, E. (1862) *Arch. Heilk.* **3,** 381.
Wahlgren, F. (1936) *Acta path. scand.* **26,** 168 (Suppl.).
Walsh, F. B. (1939) *Arch. Ophthal.* **21,** 421.
Weigert, C. (1875) *Virchows Arch.* **65,** 212.
Werner, A. A. (1931) *South. Med. J.* **24,** 953.
Westphal, C. (1863) *Zts. Psychiat.* **20,** 481.
Wilder, J. (1946) *Confinia neurol.* **7,** 96.
Williams, J. E. (1940) *Texas St. J. Med.* **35,** 672.
Winkler, F. (1934) *Med. Klin.* **30,** 967.
Wittgenstein, A., and Kroner, K. (1921) *Berl. klin. Woch.* **58,** 1185.
Wood, C. E. (1909) *J. Amer. Med. Ass.* **52,** 700.
Woolley, P. G. (1915) *J. Lab. Clin. Med.* **1,** 155.
Zenoni, C. (1913) *Sperimentale,* **67,** 249 (Suppl.).
Zondek, H., and Koehler, G. (1928) *Dtsch. med. Woch.* **54,** 1955.

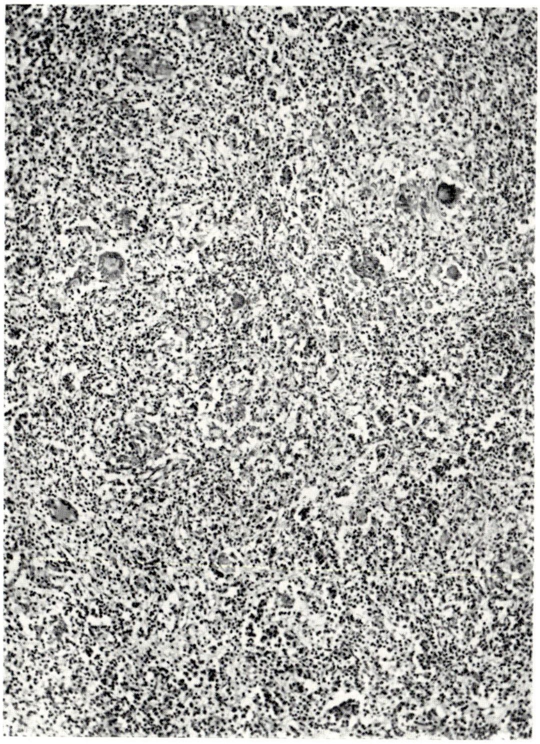

FIG. 1. Diffuse infiltration of anterior lobe with giant cells, epithelioid cells, and lymphocytes (Case 1) (haematoxylin and eosin, $\times 85$)

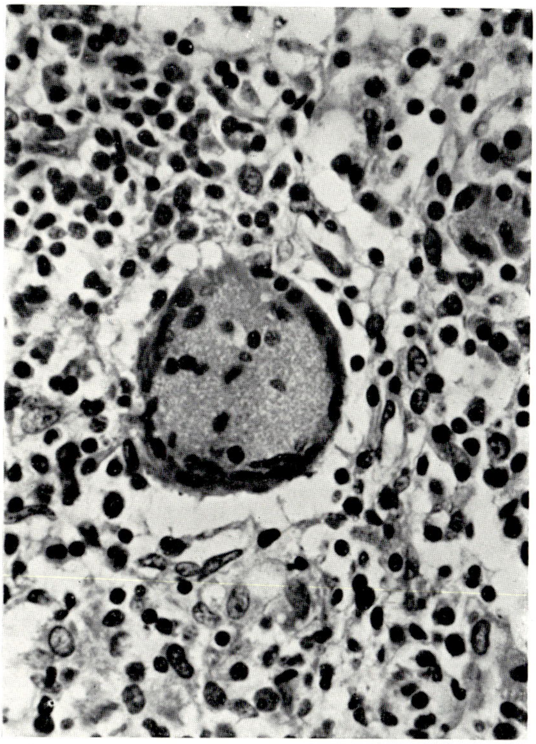

FIG. 2. Giant-cell lesion in anterior lobe (Case 1) (haematoxylin and eosin, $\times 500$)

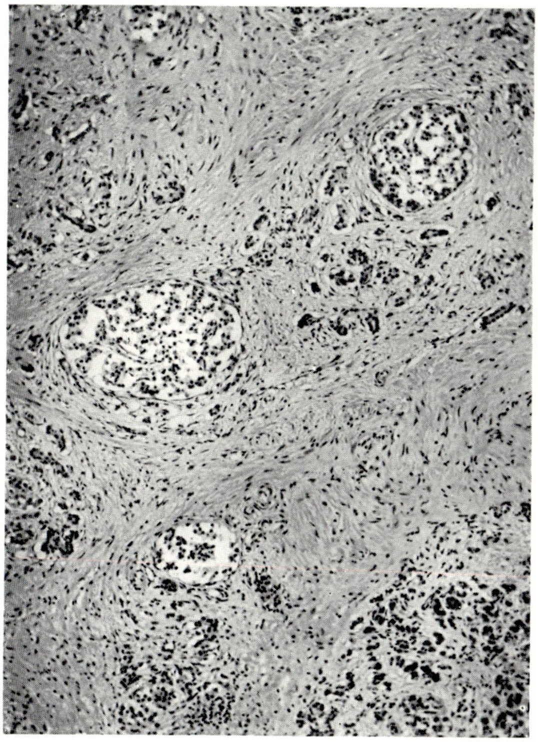

FIG. 3. Fibrosis of pancreas with surviving islet tissue (Case 1) (haematoxylin and eosin, $\times 85$)

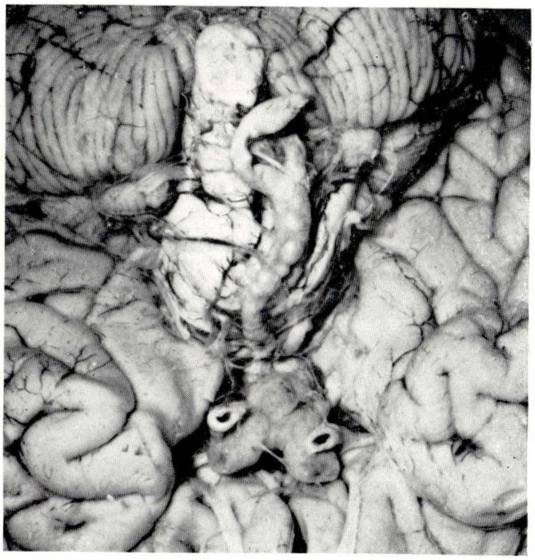

FIG. 4. Giant-cell granuloma affecting optic chiasma (Case 2)

5

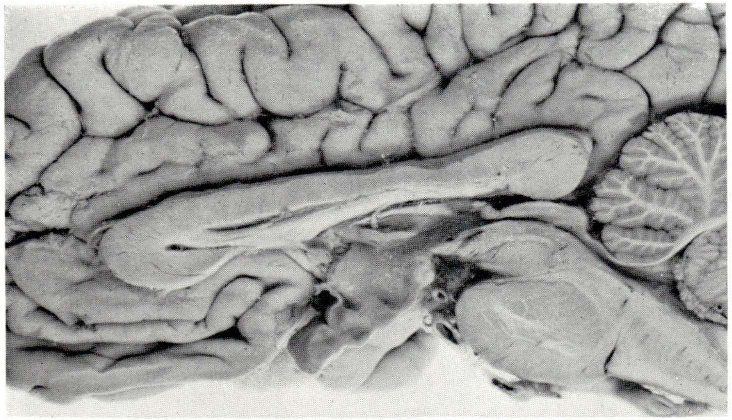

6

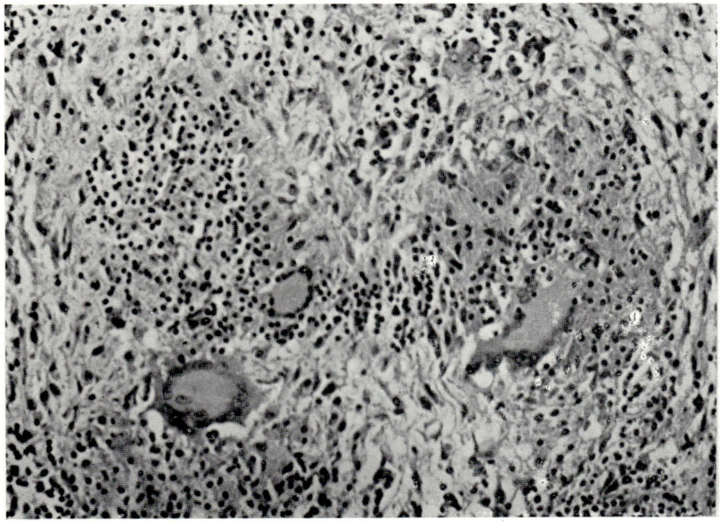

7

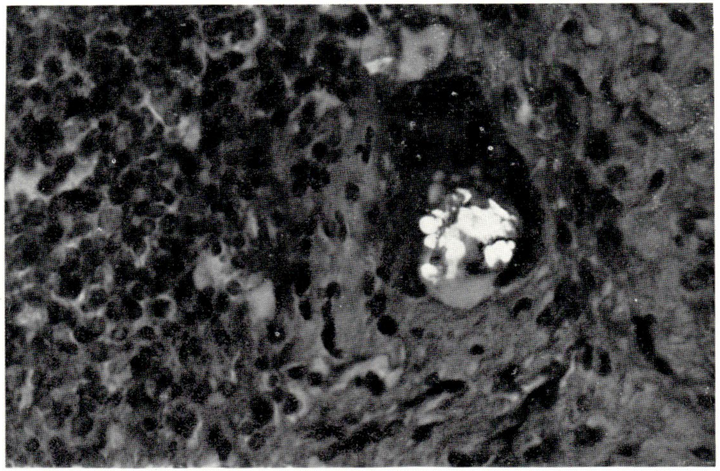

8

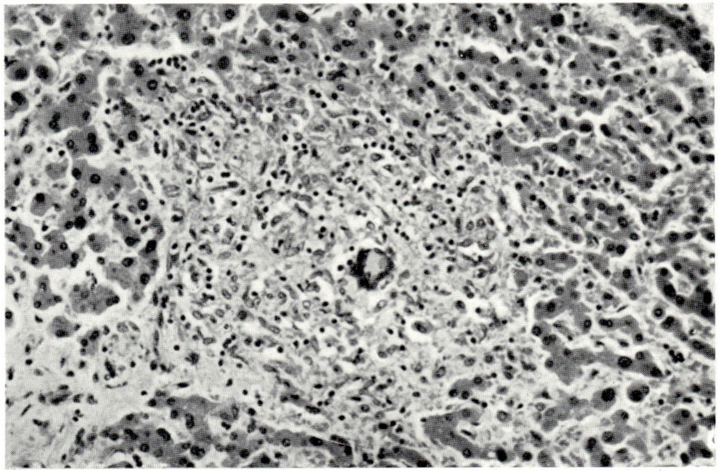

FIG. 5. Localization of giant-cell granuloma to anterior half of tuber cinereum (Case 2)

FIG. 6. Giant-cell granuloma affecting hypothalamus (Case 2) (haematoxylin and eosin, ×170)

FIG. 7. Optically active material in a pituitary giant cell (Case 2) (haematoxylin and eosin under polarized light, ×560)

FIG. 8. A giant-cell granuloma of liver (Case 2) (haematoxylin and eosin, ×170)

617.735:616.12–008.331.1

HYPERTENSIVE RETINOPATHY AND ITS MEDICAL TREATMENT[1]

By ROBERT PLATT

(From the Department of Medicine, Manchester University)

With Plates 27 to 34

THE heart, the brain, the kidney, and the retina are the four organs in which the effects of hypertensive disease most often become apparent either to the patient or to his physician. Heart failure and cerebral haemorrhage or thrombosis are only indirectly related to the height of the blood-pressure, and perhaps depend as much upon the duration of the hypertension and the degree of accompanying arterial disease. The development of hypertensive neuroretinopathy, however, and of renal insufficiency (in a patient whose kidneys were not primarily affected), are signs of the malignant phase of hypertension, and probably depend upon the occurrence of arteriolar necrosis, which is probably closely related to the height of the intra-arterial pressure (Wilson and Byrom, 1941; Byrom and Dodson, 1948). It is a clinical finding with few exceptions that the malignant phase does not occur unless the diastolic pressure is 140 mm. Hg. or more, and in the few apparent exceptions there is often evidence that the diastolic pressure has been at such levels in the recent past. The converse is not true; patients are sometimes seen in whom the diastolic pressure may be 160, or even more, without evidence of a change to the malignant phase.

We have recently treated a series of sufferers from hypertensive retinopathy by medical means, on the assumption that if the diastolic pressure can be kept significantly below 140 by hypotensive drugs the retinopathy should regress. The study of these patients has given us the opportunity also of observing by fundus photography the healing phases of hypertensive retinopathy, and of making some general observations on the retinal disorders of hypertension. Undoubtedly the most efficient drugs in use at the present time for the control of high blood-pressure are those which produce a medical sympathectomy by blocking nervous transmission at autonomic ganglia. Medical sympathectomy is more complete than surgical sympathectomy because the variable distribution of sympathetic nervous pathways, the impossibility of destroying them wholesale, and the tendency to regeneration combine to defeat the surgeon in his attempt to carry out an operation which is both successful and lasting in its effects. The disadvantages of medical treatment with drugs at present in use are the variability of response from case to case, the short duration of action of most of the drugs, the variability in absorption when they are given by mouth

[1] Received May 22, 1954.

(Milne and Oleesky, 1951), and, above all, the fact that they paralyse parasympathetic as well as sympathetic transmission, thus producing undesirable atropine-like side-effects such as dryness of the mouth, paralysis of accommodation, and diminution in peristaltic action, which are irksome and distressing to many patients. The time is therefore not ripe for the planning of a controlled trial of long duration in a large unselected series of hypertensive disease of all degrees of severity, and, owing to the very variable and unpredictable course of human hypertension, nothing less than a full-scale investigation of this type will provide an assessment of the drugs in terms of their value in prolonging life. At present most physicians use hypotensive drugs only in cases of very severe hypertension, especially those already in, or entering, the malignant phase, and even in this group they are reluctant to use these remedies in the presence of severe arteriosclerosis, angina pectoris, or renal failure.

Retinal changes in hypertension may be considered under five headings.

1. *Visible vascular changes.* These have been described by many authors, and consist of narrowing of arterioles, irregularity of their calibre, and changes in their light reflex. Venous compression at arteriovenous crossings is often observed. These changes are probably more closely related to the age of the patient and the duration of hypertension than to the severity of the process or the height of the intra-arterial pressure. Venous compression is well seen in Plate 27, Figs. 1, 2, and 3, showing the retina of a man who was 46 years of age when the first photograph was taken, and in Plate 31, Fig. 12, showing that of a man of 58. It is much easier for the physician to make dogmatic statements about the presence of minor arterial changes when the patient's blood-pressure is already known to him. Such findings are not of much value in prognosis.

2. *Vascular accidents.* These consist of arterial and venous thromboses, central or peripheral. Either may occur in patients with normal blood-pressure, and their occurrence is as impossible to predict, as are the similar accidents of cerebral or coronary thrombosis. It is difficult for the clinician who sees a selected group of patients to state whether any close relationship exists between retinal venous thrombosis and hypertension. The impression is that it does. The fact that the thrombosis can sometimes be seen to start at an arteriovenous crossing (Friedenwald, 1935) perhaps supplies a reason. Plate 28, Fig. 4, shows a central venous thrombosis in a hypertensive subject aged 59. Figs. 5 and 6 (Plate 28) show the two eyes of a patient aged 52 with severe benign hypertension. The left fundus shows only vascular changes, while the right shows thrombosis in the superior temporal branches of both artery and vein, with haemorrhages and the opening out of new vascular channels. The thrombosis occurred when he had been having treatment with subcutaneous hexamethonium bromide for two years. At the time his blood-pressure, which had been 260/160, was frequently in the region of 135/100 when measured with the patient standing within two hours of the injection. The photograph was taken four months after he had noticed a sudden defect of vision in the right eye. He had had a similar attack in the same eye seven years previously. These vascular accidents

may cause a serious and permanent visual defect, which may amount to complete blindness in the affected eye when the central artery or vein is involved, but they have little or no bearing on the ultimate prognosis of hypertensive disease.

3. *Hypertensive neuroretinopathy.* This is the specific retinopathy of the malignant phase of hypertension. It may occur in any case of hypertensive disease if sufficiently severe, irrespective of aetiology. Attempts have been made to distinguish between retinopathy of malignant essential hypertension and that of chronic glomerulonephritis (Keith, Wagener, and Kernohan, 1928), but I agree with Friedenwald (1935) that such distinctions, if they can be made at all, are probably based on differences in the age of the patient, the rapidity with which the hypertension has developed, and the presence or absence of anaemia. Malignant essential hypertension is rarely seen before the age of 40 (Platt, 1948), whereas nephritic or pyelonephritic hypertension and pregnancy toxaemia occur in young persons. It has already been observed that some patients may sustain very high diastolic pressures without this retinopathy developing. These are mostly older subjects with a slowly progressing essential hypertension accompanied by considerable arteriosclerosis. If it be true that hypertensive retinopathy depends on arteriolar sclerosis, often with necrosis of the arteriolar wall (Friedenwald, 1935), and if the observations of Byrom and Dodson (1948) on the production of arteriolar necrosis by a rapid and extreme rise of intra-arterial pressure can be applied to the human subject, it seems possible that in elderly subjects the presence of narrow or inelastic arteries may protect the arterioles from the worst effects of intra-arterial tension. It is certainly rare to see the malignant phase of hypertension develop from any cause in any subject over the age of 55 years.

Hypertensive neuroretinopathy may be the first manifestation of hypertensive disease to cause symptoms. Its ophthalmoscopic appearances have been described by many authors (for example, Fishberg and Oppenheimer, 1930), and are well shown in Plate 29, Fig. 7, Plate 30, Fig. 9, and Plate 33, Fig. 15. In severe, that is acute, cases, where the changes have developed rapidly, the full picture is one of retinal oedema with 'soft' or 'cotton-wool' exudates and haemorrhages. Papilloedema, which is always present, may be obscured by the general retinal and peripapillary oedema (Plate 30, Fig. 9). 'Hard', clearly defined, scintillating exudates, often arranged as a 'fan' or 'star' in the macular region, seem to occur more in cases which are somewhat slower in their development, and are often seen during recovery when 'soft' exudates or retinal oedema are beginning to resolve (Plate 34, Figs. 18, 19, 20), but these distinctions are not to be made dogmatically, for the two eyes of the same patient may show 'soft' exudates as the predominant lesion on one side with a macular star on the other (Plate 30, Fig. 9; Plate 29, Fig. 7). I believe that the development of hypertensive retinopathy is an absolute indication for the urgent use of measures to reduce blood-pressure, unless such measures are otherwise contra-indicated.

4. *Arteriosclerotic retinopathy.* Some authors (Moore, 1917; Fishberg and Oppenheimer, 1930; Pickering, 1934) have distinguished between arteriosclerotic

retinopathy and the foregoing 'neuroretinopathy'.[2] It is certain that in some subjects, mostly in older and more arteriosclerotic patients, the full picture of neuroretinopathy does not develop, and they do not run the rapidly downhill clinical course of malignant hypertension. Nevertheless the retina may show 'hard' exudates and haemorrhages, but without papilloedema or general retinal oedema. The distinction between this condition and neuroretinopathy is probably valuable from the prognostic point of view, but it must be recognized that the two conditions overlap, and that the development of one or the other type of retinopathy probably depends upon factors such as the age of the patient and the degree of arteriosclerosis already existing, and their separation is not to be regarded as absolute. Figs. 11 and 12 (Plate 31) are interesting in this respect, since they show the right and left retinae of a patient of 58 years, photographed on the same day. His complaint was of failing vision in the right eye only. The left eye shows changes which most authors would characterize as arteriosclerotic retinopathy. In the right eye there is papilloedema and a macular star, and although 'soft' exudates are not present neuroretinopathy must presumably be diagnosed. This patient's diastolic pressure was usually about 140.

5. *Papilloedema* may sometimes occur in hypertension without, or before the development of, the other changes of hypertensive neuroretinopathy. This is shown in Plate 27, Fig. 2. Such cases are difficult to distinguish from cerebral tumour. If the diastolic pressure is much below 140, cerebral tumour should be strongly suspected. The relation of papilloedema to raised intracranial pressure has been discussed by Shelburne, Blain, and O'Hare (1932), and by Pickering (1934).

Medical Treatment of Hypertensive Retinopathy

It is of course well established that measures which reduce blood-pressure, such as surgical sympathectomy, and the rice diet (Kempner, 1948), may in successful cases cure the retinal lesions of hypertension. In the series here described we have sought to treat all cases of hypertensive retinopathy with hypotensive drugs of the methonium series administered subcutaneously. In retrospect it is clear that the cases varied considerably in severity; a few, like the one illustrated in Plate 32, Fig. 13, did not show the grosser changes of the acute retinal disorder, and might be considered to be on the borderline between neuroretinopathy and the arteriosclerotic type. Nevertheless some degree of papilloedema, and usually peripapillary oedema, was present in nearly every case (see Table I).

It is not proposed to go into full details of the management of hypertension with the methonium drugs. Since the original paper of Arnold and Rosenheim (1949) this has been well described by several authors (for example, Smirk, 1954). Our earlier patients were given two or three subcutaneous injections of hexamethonium bromide every day, but more recently we have used 'ansolysen',

[2] The terminology used by the authors quoted varies, but the distinction which they make between the two types of retinal disorder is the same.

or 'ansolysen retard'. This is pentapyrrolidinium bitartrate, the 'retard' solution containing in addition polyvidone solution with 0·5 per cent. ephedrine hydrochloride to delay absorption.[3] At present it seems essential to admit all patients to hospital in the first instance, so that resting blood-pressures may be determined and dosage decided. At the same time renal tests and other relevant investigations are carried out, and the patient is taught to give his own injections before discharge. Our present practice is to start with 2·5 mg. of 'ansolysen retard' twice daily and increase the dose gradually until significant falls of blood-pressure are achieved. At this stage the effect often wears off in a few days, and the dosage may have to be increased several times. The whole process often takes about three weeks. Most patients require from 10 to 20 mg. twice daily as their maintenance dose, and it is our experience that when this level is reached further increases are not necessary. Many patients still have a profound fall in blood-pressure after each injection, although they have had a constant dosage for many months. Most of them state that they still feel light-headed within an hour or so of the injection if they stand upright and still, and this is a good guide to dosage in out-patients. The postural fall of pressure on standing is usually still evident several hours after 'ansolysen retard'. Occasional patients are extremely sensitive. One woman was quite unable to stand up after the injection of 0·5 mg. of 'ansolysen', which brought her blood-pressure down from 240/145 to 80/50. In patients with severe renal insufficiency a very cautious dosage must be used, as the drug is slowly excreted. Nevertheless we have treated some patients in whom the blood-urea was as high as 100 mg. per 100 ml., without causing any apparent deterioration of renal function, and in a few cases rapid failure of vision has been arrested and reversed, even though the patient inevitably died of renal failure in due course.

Table I gives some clinical features of the patients treated, and Table II summarizes the results. If one excludes the patients who were not treated or who are too recent to assess, those who discontinued treatment, and those who died too soon for any significant improvement to be observed, it will be seen that all the remaining patients showed retinal improvement, which in the majority of cases was striking, vision being restored to normal although the retinopathy had been severe. In some patients who improved, especially earlier ones, we feel that our control of the blood-pressure was not good enough, and in some it was difficult to obtain good control without side-effects which seriously interfered with the patient's domestic life or occupation. In these respects we feel that 'ansolysen' and 'ansolysen retard' are an advance on hexamethonium, since their effects are longer maintained, making it unnecessary to produce such precipitous falls of pressure as are required with hexamethonium if an effect is to be maintained for some hours. The effect on visual accommodation, which greatly worries some patients, can readily be corrected by the prescription of suitable reading-glasses (usually +2 or +3 D. spherical). These results seem to us to be very encouraging, the restoration of vision bringing happiness and hope

[3] We are indebted to Messrs. May and Baker for supplying us with these solutions before they were marketed.

Table I

Thirty-nine Cases of Hypertensive Retinopathy

Case number	*Sex*	*Age (years)*	*Diagnosis*	*Initial blood-pressure*	*Retinopathy*	*Remarks*
1. *Patients not treated with hypotensive drugs (4 cases):*						
1	F	22	Chronic nephritis	235/135	Gross	Advanced uraemia
2	M	42	Chronic nephritis	240/155	Gross	Died (uraemia)
3	F	54	Essential hypertension	300/170	Macular star. No papilloedema	Arteriosclerotic heart failure
4	F	55	Essential hypertension	250/160	H and E. Early P	Vision not badly affected
2. *Treatment discontinued, or patient died after treatment (18 cases):*						
5	M	32	Chronic nephritis	235/170	Gross	Hexamethonium 6 months. Vision strikingly improved. Died (uraemia)
6	F	52	Essential hypertension	275/135	Early P. Macular H	Deaf, difficult, and stupid. Treatment given up
7	M	28	Chronic nephritis	290/175	Gross	Treated 2 weeks. No better. Died (uraemia)
8	M	41	Essential hypertension	230/160	Gross	Sympathectomy 3 years before. Treated 2 weeks. Died (heart failure)
9	M	49	Essential hypertension	240/125	Gross	Blood-urea 114 mg./100 ml. Treatment stopped
10	M	52	Essential hypertension	260/170	H and E. Slight P	Treated 2 months. Died (cerebral thrombosis)
11	M	45	Essential hypertension	230/175	Gross	Very ill. Heart failure. Hex. abandoned
12	M	48	Essential hypertension	250/160	P only	Treated few weeks. Hemiplegia. Treatment stopped
13	M	32	Essential hypertension	210/140	E right and left. No or early P	Exudates cleared. Left district
14	M	52	Essential hypertension	230/145	Gross	Great improvement in 7 months. Died (cardiac infarction)
15	M	41	Diabetic glomerulosclerosis	260/140	Gross	No improvement. Died (uraemia)
16	M	44	Essential hypertension	240/150	Early P. Exudates	Died (cerebral haemorrhage) at 4 months
17	F	47	Essential hypertension	260/150	Early P. Macular fan	Treatment abandoned. Vision not badly affected
18	M	36	Essential hypertension	280/170	Early P. H and E	Died suddenly (1 month)
19	M	36	Chronic nephritis	230/170	Gross	No improvement. Died (uraemia)
20	M	49	Essential hypertension	225/150	Gross	Great improvement. Died (cerebral thrombosis) at 4 months
21	M	45	Essential hypertension	210/150	Exudates. Little P	Angina. Treatment stopped
22	M	54	Essential hypertension	220/140	Papilloedema++	Coronary occlusion. Treatment stopped
3. *Treatment continues (17 cases):*						
23	F	50	Essential hypertension	280/160	Papilloedema slight. Hard exudates	Hex. 33 months. Improved. Not a good patient
24	M	42	Essential hypertension	230/145	Papilloedema slight. (See Plate 32, Figs. 13, 14)	Hex. 23 months. Retinae clear
25	M	46	Essential hypertension	220/145	P only (Plate 27, Figs. 1, 2, 3)	Hex. 36 months. Retinae clear
26	M	13	Unknown	220/170	Gross (Plates 29 and 30, Figs. 7, 8, 9, 10)	Hex. 15 months. Retinae clear. Then sympathectomy
27	F	50	Essential hypertension	250/180	Gross	Hex. 15 months. Few hard exudates remain
28	F	39	Pyelonephritis	260/170	Gross	Hex. 12 months. Clear
29	F	43	Essential hypertension; pregnancy toxaemia	220/145	Gross	'Ansolysen' 10 months. Clear
30	M	51	Essential hypertension	220/145	Early P. H and E	'Ansolysen' 9 months. Clear
31	M	44	Essential hypertension	260/160	Gross	Hex. 6 months. Few E remain
32	F	53	Essential hypertension	270/145	Gross	'Ansolysen' 4 months. Improved
33	M	38	Tuberculous kidney	270/160	Gross (Plates 33 and 34, Figs. 15 to 20)	'Ansolysen' 4 months. Great improvement
34	M	36	Bilateral hydronephrosis; uraemia	240/155	Gross	Hex. 4 months. Vision much better, but uraemia advancing
35	M	22	Chronic nephritis	260/160	Gross	'Ansolysen' 3 months. Much improved
36	F	39	Essential hypertension (?)	260/150	Macular H. No P	'Ansolysen' 3 months. Improved
37	M	58	Essential hypertension	220/140	Macular star R. (Plate 31, Figs. 11, 12)	'Ansolysen' 2 weeks
38	F	51	Essential hypertension	260/160	Gross	'Ansolysen' 3 weeks. Improving
39	M	49	Essential hypertension	235/140	Gross	'Ansolysen' 2 weeks

Notes. Column 6: 'Gross' means extensive retinopathy with papilloedema (P), exudates (E), and haemorrhage (H).
Column 7: Hex. = Hexamethonium.

to both patient and doctor. Nevertheless Table II also shows only too clearly how bad the prognosis for life remains in an unselected series of patients with hypertensive neuroretinopathy. Obviously the best group of cases for treatment is that in which retinal changes have occurred before renal or cardiac disease is far advanced. These are not necessarily cases of essential hypertension. Some patients with pyelonephritis, for instance, may retain good renal function and run an almost purely hypertensive course.

It is not proposed to give full details of all the patients treated beyond what is contained in Table I, but further notes on some of those whose retinae are

TABLE II

Summary of Results

	Number of patients
Not treated	4
Discontinued treatment	8
Died after treatment (3 showed great visual improvement)	10
Continuing treatment:	
Retina clear or greatly improved	12
Retina improved	2
Too recent	3
Total	39

illustrated may be added. Plate 27, Fig. 1, is from a patient, aged 46 years in 1948, with moderately severe benign essential hypertension (diastolic pressure 110 to 120). In 1951 he noticed blurring of vision, and it was found that he had developed bilateral papilloedema with some small 'hard' exudates (Plate 27, Fig. 2). His blood-pressure was then 220/145. The papilloedema slowly subsided when he was given hexamethonium bromide subcutaneously (Plate 27, Fig. 3). Plates 29 and 30 (Figs. 7, 8, 9, 10) are from a boy, aged 13 years on admission, who had been suffering from headaches for about six months. He then complained of failing vision, and was sent into hospital urgently on account of generalized convulsions. The blood-pressure on admission was 220/170, and he was given injections of hexamethonium bromide subcutaneously every three hours for the first few days. He was maintained on this treatment for 15 months, and the retinopathy completely cleared, with restoration of normal vision, although a scar could still be seen at the left macula. It was then thought advisable for him to have a bilateral lumbodorsal sympathectomy. All investigations, and inspection of the kidneys and suprarenals, have failed to show any cause for his hypertension. He has albuminuria, but renal function remains good. Plate 32 (Figs. 13 and 14) is from a man aged 42 years who had severe essential hypertension. The blood-pressure was variable, being 230/145 when he was seen in the out-patient department, but only about 210/120 on admission. He was satisfactorily treated with hexamethonium bromide subcutaneously, and the retinopathy (which was never severe) has completely subsided. Plates 33 and 34 (Figs. 15 to 20) are from a man aged 38 years who complained of blurring of vision. He had a previous history of pulmonary tuberculosis and of a right nephrectomy for renal tuberculosis. The blood-pressure on admission was 270/160. An intravenous pyelogram showed an apparently normal left kidney, with a satisfactory renal function. The figures show successive changes in the fundus after treatment with 'ansolysen retard' (20 mg. twice daily). It is interesting to note that the macular star became evident as his vision was improving and the retinopathy subsiding.

Smirk (1954), commenting on the regression of the retinal changes in his patients, said: 'Papilloedema cleared in 21 out of 23 patients who were on effective treatment for five months or more; . . . In most instances disappearance of papilloedema takes three to four months, sometimes six months, of intensive treatment; and a reduction of blood-pressure to normal or near normal levels at the trough of the fall is necessary. . . . A clear reduction in the amount of papilloedema should be evident in three to four weeks, with reappearance of a physiological cup or a part of the disk edge. . . . Within the first month of effective treatment soft exudates should have disappeared, there should be no fresh haemorrhages, and as a rule old haemorrhages have been dispersed. . . . Substantial dispersal of hard exudate is unlikely under six months, and some may remain after 12 months, but it will be absorbed in most patients who have been under effective treatment for 12 to 18 months.' With these conclusions I agree. It is to be noted that Smirk excluded cases of nephritis from his series of hypertensive disease in the malignant phase.

Acknowledgements

I have to thank Dr. F. Wemyss Smith and his pupil Raymond Lawton for the retinal photographs, and the Department of Medical Illustration for preparing them for reproduction. I am grateful to all members of my staff who have co-operated in the treatment of the patients.

Summary

The retinal lesions of hypertension are discussed, and illustrated by fundus photography.

The medical treatment of hypertensive retinopathy is described. In most cases, if the patients are not advanced in renal or cardiac failure before treatment is attempted, great improvement in the retinopathy can be achieved, with restoration of vision.

REFERENCES

Arnold, P., and Rosenheim, M. L. (1949) *Lancet*, **2**, 321.
Byrom, F. B., and Dodson, L. F. (1948) *J. Path. Bact.* **60**, 357.
Fishberg, A. M., and Oppenheimer, B. S. (1930) *Arch. Int. Med.* **46**, 901.
Friedenwald, J. S. (1935) In *The Kidney in Health and Disease*, Edd. H. Berglund and G. Medes, Philad.
Keith, N. M., Wagener, H. P., and Kernohan, J. W. (1928) *Arch. Int. Med.* **41**, 141.
Kempner, W. (1948) *Amer. J. Med.* **4**, 545.
Milne, G. E., and Oleesky, S. (1951) *Lancet*, **1**, 889.
Moore, R. F. (1917) *Quart. J. Med.* **10**, 29.
Pickering, G. W. (1934) *Clin. Sci.* **1**, 397.
Platt, R. (1948) *Quart. J. Med.* N.S. **17**, 83.
Shelburne, S. A., Blain, D., and O'Hare, J. P. (1932) *J. Clin. Invest.* **11**, 489.
Smirk, F. H. (1954) *Brit. Med. J.* **1**, 717.
Wilson, C., and Byrom, F. B. (1941) *Quart. J. Med.* N.S. **10**, 65.

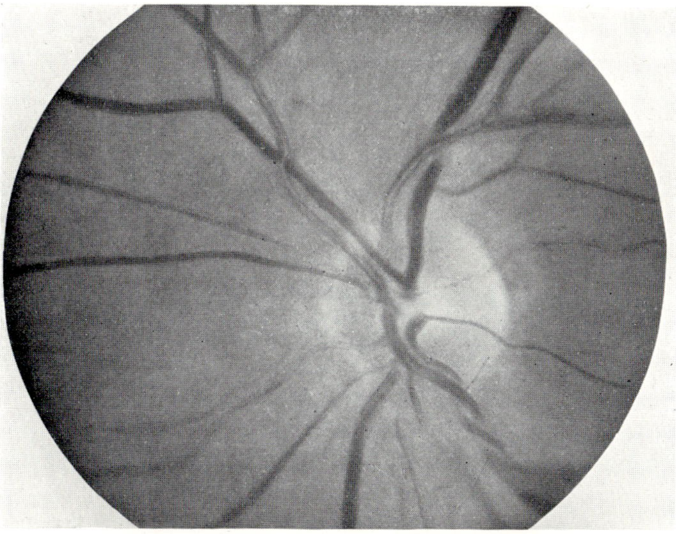

FIG. 1. Case 25 (1948). A man aged 46 years. Left eye showing vascular changes only (note venous compression). Blood-pressure 180–210/110–120

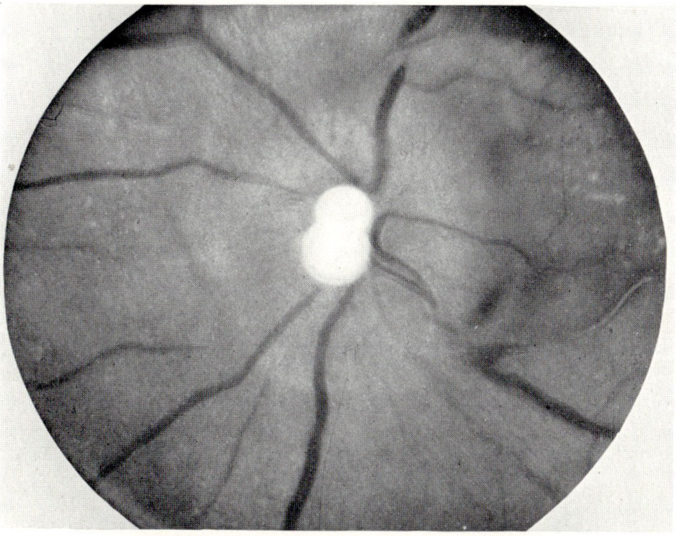

FIG. 2. The same, March 1951. Papilloedema with a few 'hard' exudates. Blood-pressure 220/145

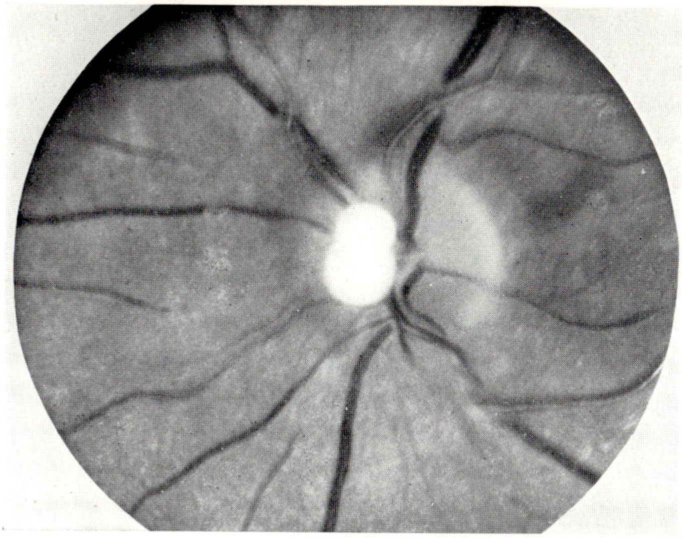

FIG. 3. The same, September 1951, after six months' treatment. Papilloedema has subsided

Note. The white double disk which shows in the centre of each photograph (except the Figs. 1 and 4) is a reflex from the lens of camera, unavoidable with this model. Figs. 1 and 4 were taken with a camera kindly lent to the Department by Messrs. Dixey.

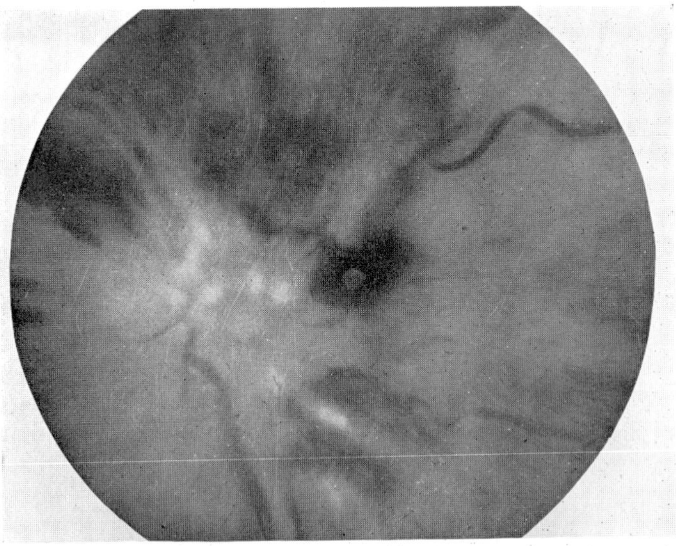

FIG. 4. M. C., aged 59 years. Thrombosis of central retinal vein

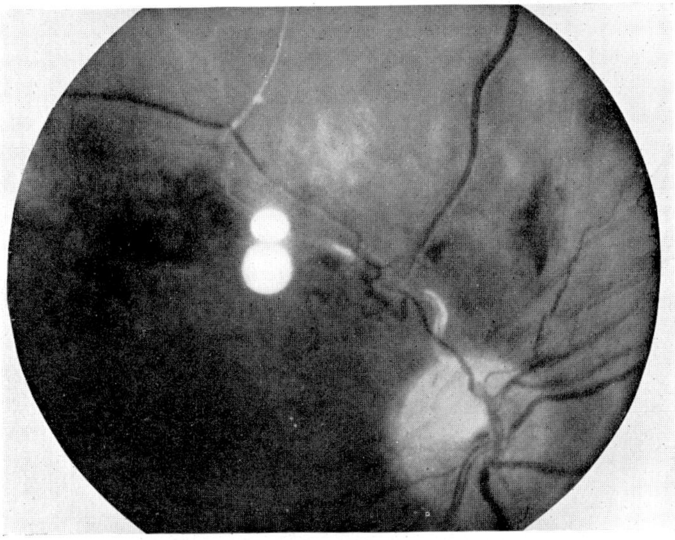

FIG. 5. G. B., a man aged 52 years. Right eye. Thrombosis of superior temporal branches of retinal artery and vein (for details see text)

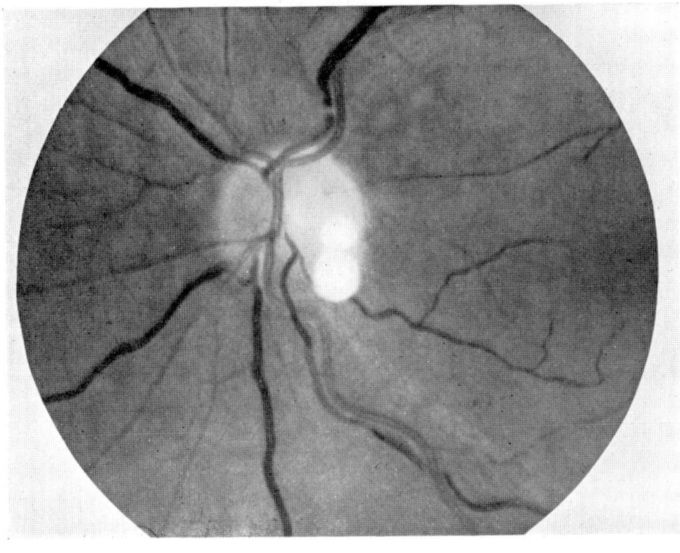

FIG. 6. Left eye of the same patient showing vascular sclerosis only

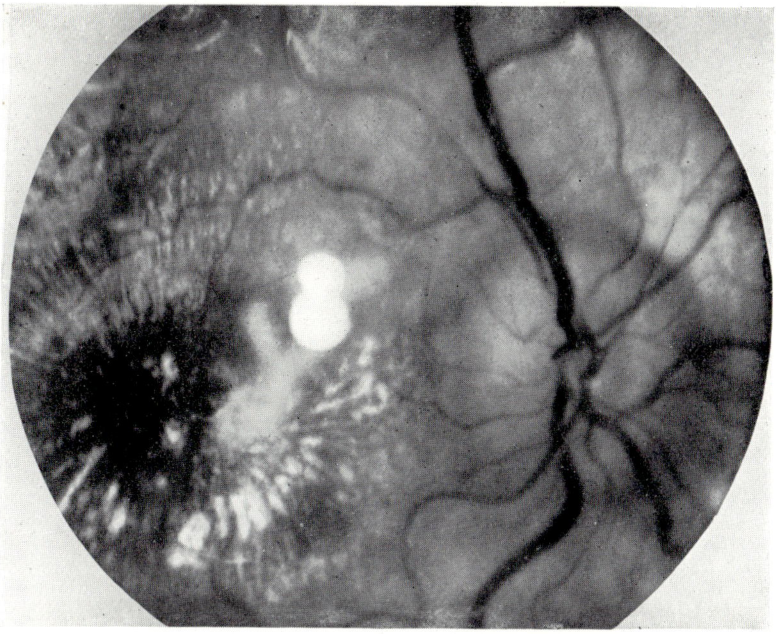

FIG. 7. Case 26. A boy aged 13 years. Right eye, May 1952. Gross papilloedema and macular star. Blood-pressure 220/170 (see text)

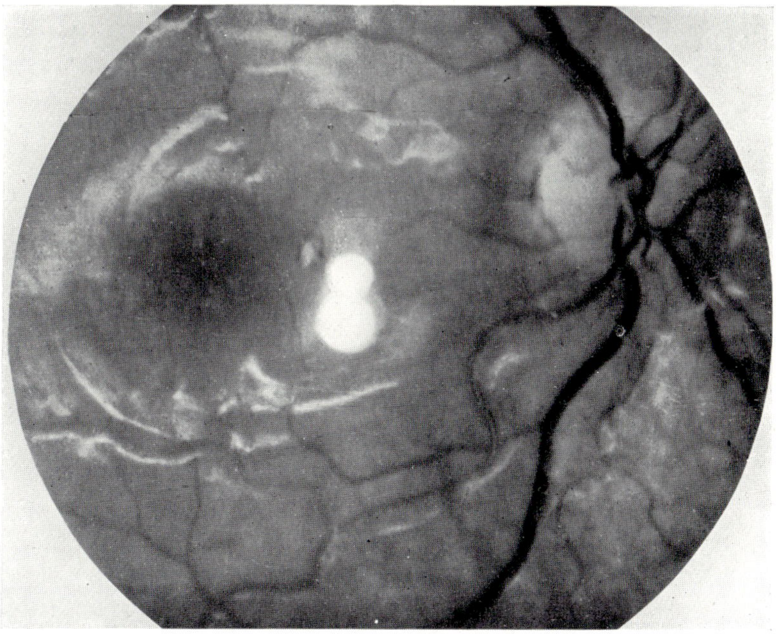

FIG. 8. The same. September 1953 (after treatment)

Note. Figs. 8 and 10 show a bright retinal reflection or 'shine' frequently seen in normal retinae especially of young people. In photographs it might almost be mistaken for exudate

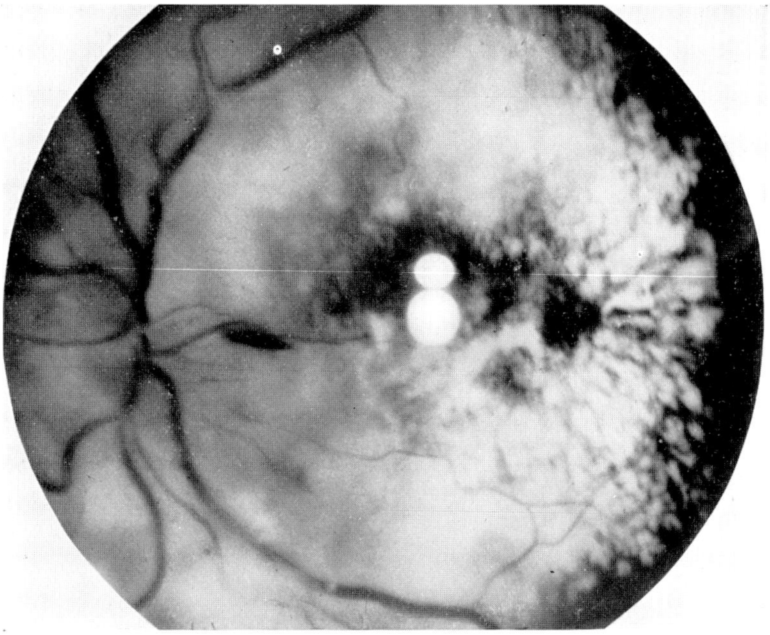

FIG. 9. The same patient (Case 26). Left eye, May 1952

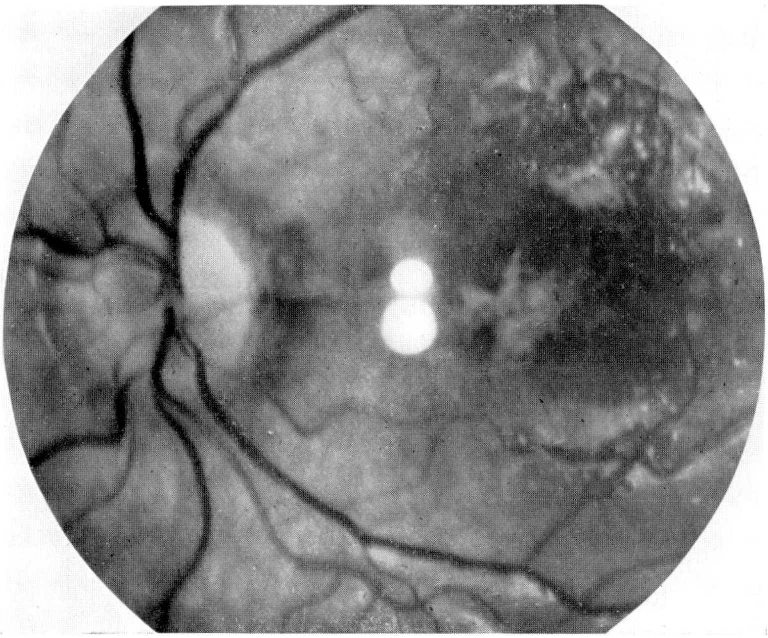

FIG. 10. The same, September 1953 (after treatment. A scar is present at the macula, but subjective vision is normal in both eyes.) See note to Fig. 8

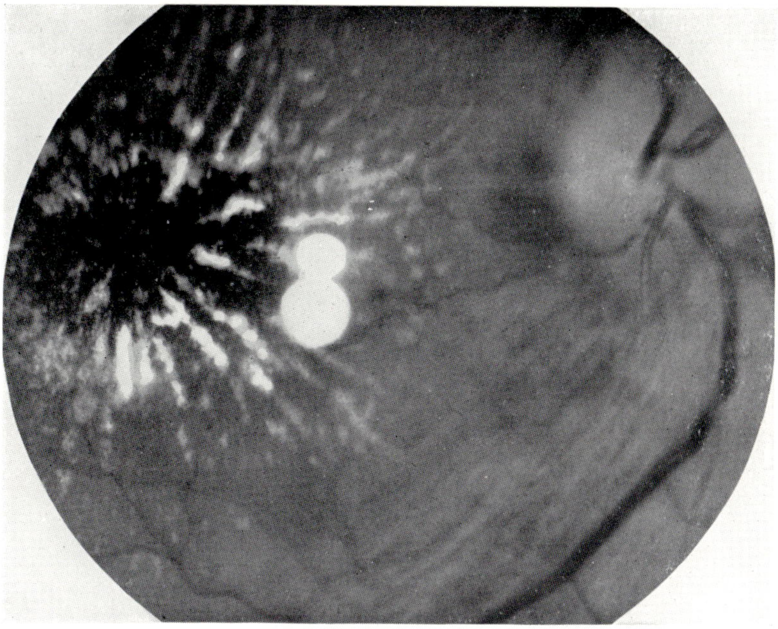

FIG. 11. Case 37. A man aged 58 years. Right eye shows papilloedema and macular star. Blood-pressure 220/140

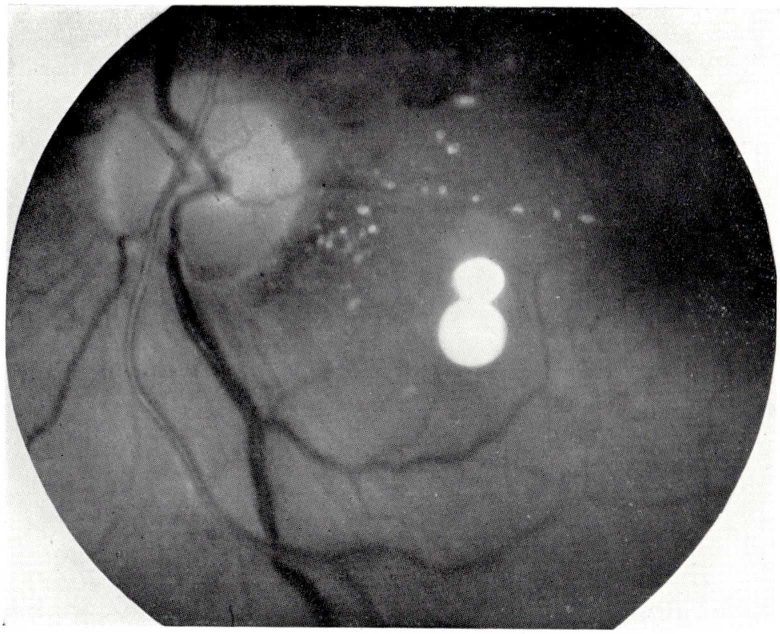

FIG. 12. The same patient. Left eye (same date) shows no papilloedema, but some small exudates (see text)

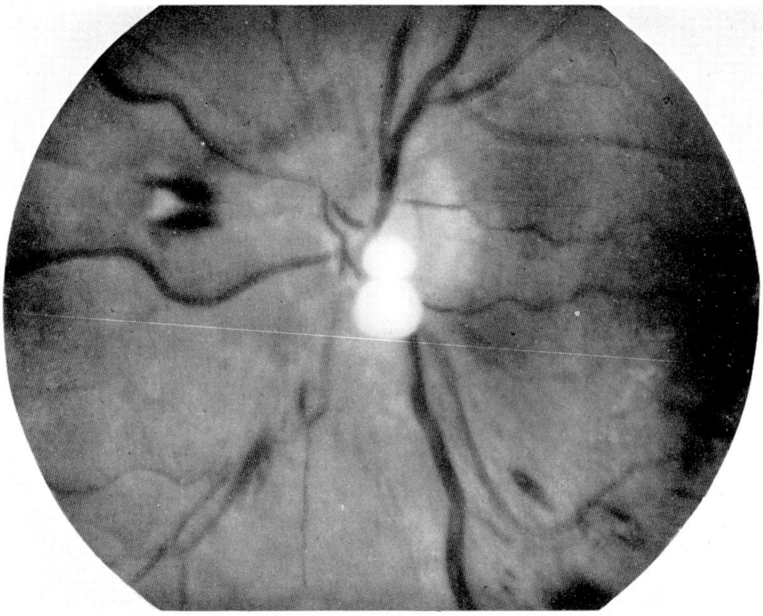

Fig. 13. Case 24. A man aged 42 years, April 1952. Left eye showing early papilloedema and haemorrhages. Blood-pressure 230/145

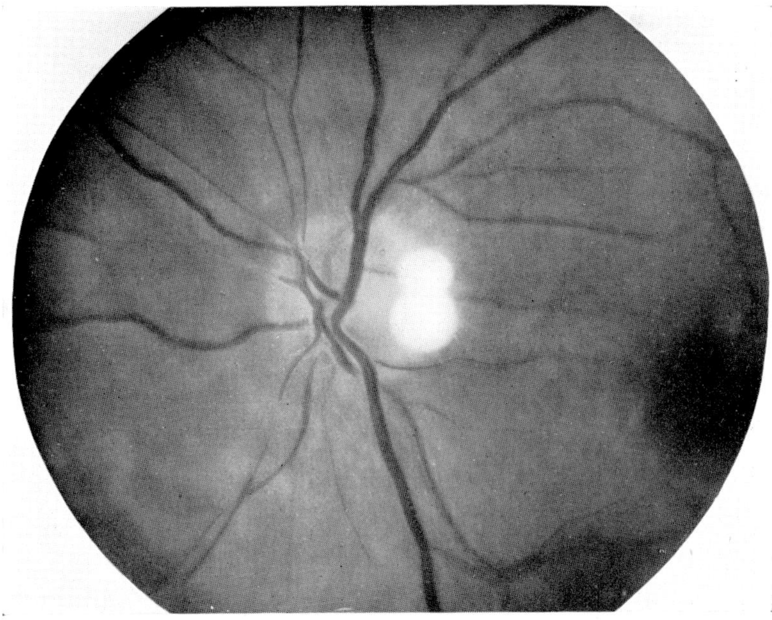

Fig. 14. The same, September 1953 (after treatment)

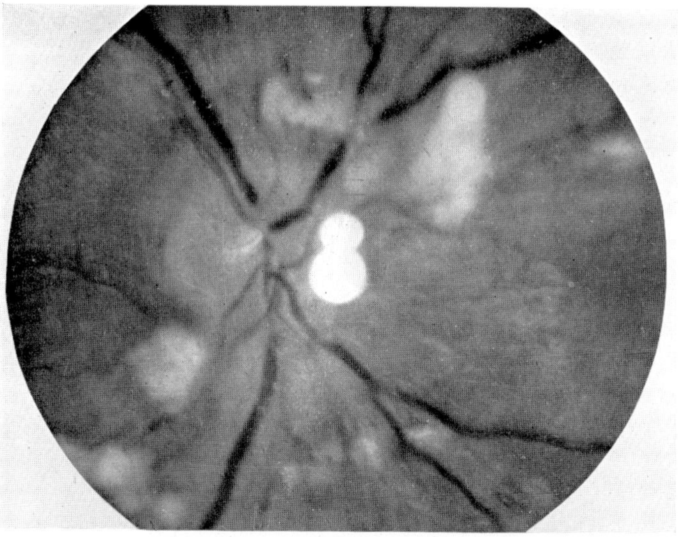

FIG. 15. Case 33. A man aged 38 years (see text). Right eye, December 1953. General retinal oedema; 'cotton-wool' exudates. Vision rapidly failing. Blood-pressure 270/160

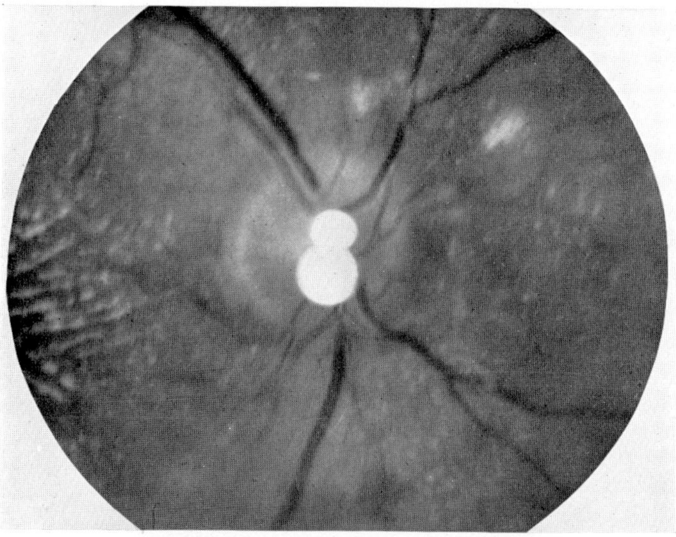

FIG. 16. The same. February 1954, after treatment. Vision nearly normal. The exudates have 'hardened', papilloedema has cleared, and a macular star has formed

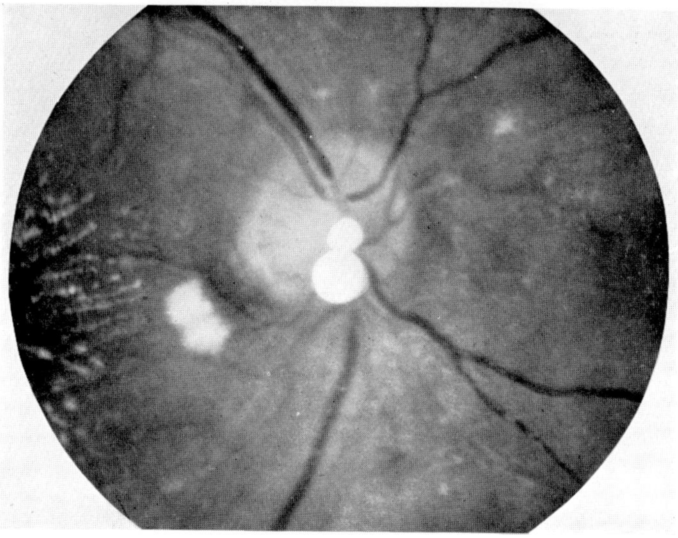

FIG. 17. The same, March 1954

FIGS. 18, 19, 20. The same as Figs. 15, 16, 17 respectively, but showing the macula. Note macular oedema, but no star, when vision was at its worst (Fig. 18)

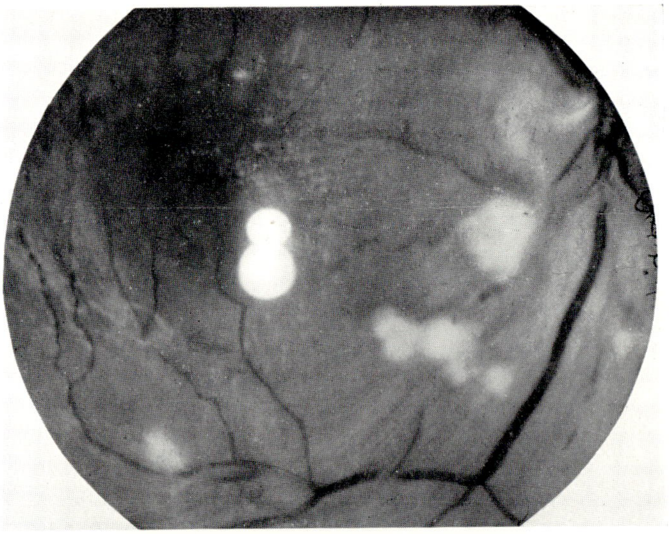

FIG. 18

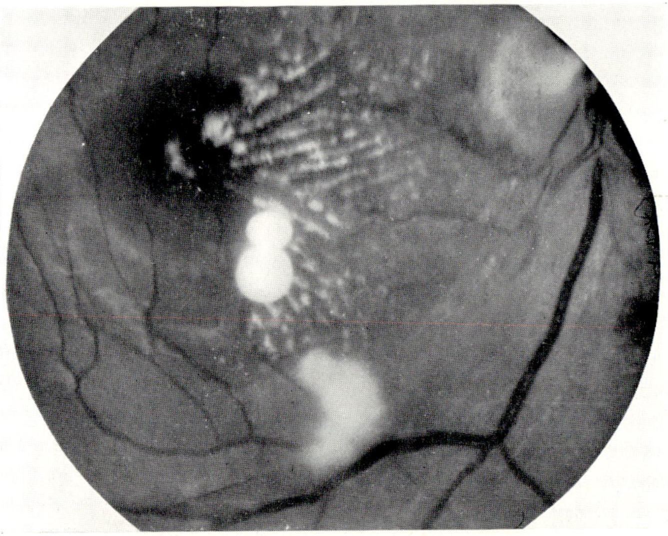

FIG. 19

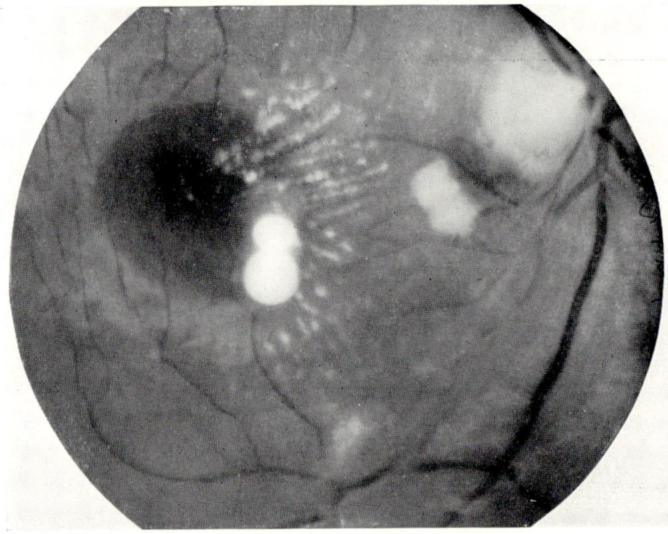

FIG. 20

THE ASSOCIATION OF PHYSICIANS OF GREAT BRITAIN AND IRELAND

1954

FORTY-EIGHTH ANNUAL GENERAL MEETING

The Forty-Eighth Annual General Meeting was held in Dublin on Friday and Saturday, June 4 and 5, 1954 in the Physics Theatre, University College. The attendance book was signed by 145 members and 12 visitors. The proceedings began at 9.30 a.m.

The President, Professor F. J. Nattrass, was in the Chair.

The Minutes of the last Annual General Meeting, having been published in the *Quarterly Journal of Medicine*, were taken as read, confirmed, and signed. The election of Officers, Executive Committee, Honorary Members, and Ordinary Members then followed.

Executive Committee

President.	Professor V. M. Synge.
President-Elect.	Professor J. Crighton Bramwell.
Treasurer.	Dr. C. Newman.
Secretary.	Dr. C. M. Fletcher.
Members for England.	Professor C. Bruce Perry. Dr. N. Lloyd Rusby. Dr. E. N. Chamberlain. Professor A. P. Thomson. Dr. E. R. Boland. Professor G. W. Pickering.
Members for Scotland.	Professor Stanley G. Graham. Professor I. G. W. Hill. Dr. J. G. M. Hamilton.
Members for Ireland.	Dr. O. Fitzgerald. Dr. R. W. M. Strain. Professor G. M. Bull.

Election of Honorary Members

(*Original Members*).	Lord Horder. Dr. T. P. C. Kirkpatrick. Dr. R. Barclay Ness. Professor W. H. Wynn. Sir Robert Young.
(*Ordinary Members*).	Professor J. Crighton Bramwell. Dr. S. B. Boyd Campbell. Dr. C. G. Imrie. Dr. F. G. Lescher. Dr. Robert Marshall. Professor F. J. Nattrass. Dr. P. T. J. O'Farrell.
Election of Editor.	Dr. D. H. Brinton.

Election of Ordinary Members

George Fowler Adams, M.D., M.R.C.P., Physician (Geriatrics), Belfast City Hospital.

Richard Ian Samuel Bayliss, M.D., M.R.C.P., Lecturer in Medicine, Postgraduate Medical School of London.

Hugh Conway, M.B., M.R.C.P., Physician, Royal Alexandra Infirmary, Paisley.

Raymond Daley, M.D., M.R.C.P., Physician, St. Thomas's Hospital.

Michael Ivo Drury, M.D., F.R.C.P.I., Assistant Physician, Mater Misericordiae Hospital.

John James Reid Duthie, M.B., F.R.C.P.E., Senior Lecturer in Rheumatism, Edinburgh University.

Paul Fourman, M.D., M.R.C.P., M.R.C. Department of Experimental Medicine, Cambridge.

Frances Gardner, M.D., F.R.C.P., Assistant Physician, Royal Free Hospital.

Kenneth David Keele, M.D., F.R.C.P., Physician, Ashford Hospital, Middlesex.

Malcolm Davenport Milne, M.D., M.R.C.P., Lecturer in Medicine, Postgraduate Medical School of London.

John Michael Naish, M.D., M.R.C.P., Lecturer in Medicine, Bristol University.

Howard Nicholson, M.D., F.R.C.P., Physician, University College Hospital.

Michael O'Donnell, M.D., F.R.C.P.I., Professor of Medicine, University of Galway.

Sydney William Stanbury, M.B., M.R.C.P., Lecturer in Medicine, Manchester University.

Graham Malcolm Wilson, M.D., F.R.C.P.E., Professor of Pharmacology, Sheffield University.

Alan Waller Woodruff, M.D., F.R.C.P., Professor of Tropical Medicine, London University.

The Treasurer, Dr. Charles Newman, presented his report for 1953, which showed an opening balance of £527 and a closing balance of £805. The accounts were adopted by the Association.

The Association agreed to amend the wording of *Rule 2* from '. . . on reaching the age of 65' to '. . . at the end of the Calendar year in which they reach the age of 65'. The Treasurer reported a suggestion of the Executive Committee that it would be advantageous to certain places of meeting, such as universities, to hold the Annual General Meeting on the week-end after Easter rather than at Whitsun, because this would make lecture theatres and halls of residence more easily available. It had been thought that it might also be a convenience to members to hold the Annual General Meeting in the Easter holiday, rather than disturb the work of the summer term. The Association agreed that *Rule 12* should be amended to read: 'A General Meeting shall be held once a year, at Whitsuntide or during the Easter Vacation, the actual date to be decided by the Executive Committee in consultation with the local Committee.' It was left to the Secretaries of the Association and to the local Committees to make the decision on each occasion. It was left with the secretaries of the specialist Societies to arrange for the convenient relation of the dates of their respective meetings.

Place of Meeting, 1955 and 1956. The Association confirmed that the 1955 meeting should be held in Manchester and the 1956 anniversary meeting should be held in London.

The Treasurer read an apology for absence from the Secretary, Dr. Charles Fletcher, and a reply from Dr. Parkes Weber to the Association's message of congratulations to him on his 90th birthday.

It was decided that the local Committee and the Executive Committee should consider before each Annual Meeting whether the proceedings should include a symposium, a demonstration, or some other activity, and they should be free to make what arrangements they thought best in view of local circumstances.

Professor V. M. Synge then took the Chair. He conveyed the thanks of the Association to Professor Nattrass for all the work and assistance which he had given to the Association during his year of presidency.

SCIENTIFIC BUSINESS

Friday Morning, June 4

1. Professor V. M. Synge gave a talk on the *Dublin Medical Schools*. He said that Dublin had a population of approximately half a million, and in it were three medical schools. 1. University College, Dublin was a constituent college of the National University, the other constituent colleges in Cork and Galway each having a medical school of their own. The National University had come into being in 1908, but the medical school in Dublin was a hundred years old, since it was the continuation of Newman's Catholic University medical school. 2. The Conjoint Board of the Royal College of Physicians and the Royal College of Surgeons was more than a hundred and fifty years old, and in the last century had absorbed several private medical schools. 3. Dublin University had only one college—Trinity College. The University had been opened in 1594, but it had had no medical school until 1711. The average annual number of students qualifying

during the period 1945–9 had been 121 at University College, Dublin; 60 at the Conjoint Board; 56 at Trinity College. There were 10 general teaching hospitals in Dublin, with 2,350 beds altogether. There were also 10 hospitals in which special subjects were taught. Lantern slides were shown of some of the Dublin hospitals, including the Rotunda, founded in 1745 by Mosse, one of the first obstetric hospitals in these islands; the Mater, the largest of the general teaching hospitals (500 beds); the Meath, made famous in the last century by Graves and Stokes; Steevens's, one of the oldest of the Dublin hospitals, founded in 1720; and St. Patrick's, for mental diseases, opened in 1757, built with the legacy which Jonathan Swift left 'to build a house for fools and mad'.

2. Dr. J. St. P. Cowell (introduced) discussed *B.C.G.—Selective versus Mass Vaccination.* He said that in Britain B.C.G. vaccine was being used selectively, while in Ireland a scheme for mass vaccination had been operated for the past five years. There were various reasons for these contrasting attitudes. By graphical comparison of mortality rates and the distribution of 'natural' tuberculous infection in similar age-groups and occupations in Britain and in Ireland, it appeared that two different epidemiological problems existed. In Ireland the predominantly rural population was largely non-infected. Fifty-five per cent. of young adults of between 18 and 30 years in the emigrant areas were still tuberculin-negative. For generations many of these highly susceptible young adults had tended to emigrate to areas of high tuberculous prevalence, and had thus acquired delayed primary infection which frequently advanced to progressive phthisis. In Britain tuberculous infection was more widespread, occurred earlier, and was frequent amongst young country children, the deduction being that bovine infection was responsible. There was no equivalent emigration problem. Differences in the prevalence of tuberculin sensitivity were demonstrated in: (*a*) Ordinary residents of Ireland and of Britain (higher sensitivity in Britain at all ages); (*b*) Irish workers employed at home and Irish workers employed in Britain (sensitivity in the latter invariably higher); (*c*) Irish rural and urban residents and British equivalents. Such evidence, and consideration of the Irish social and economic background, suggested that greater benefit was likely to accrue from mass B.C.G. vaccination in Ireland than from its selective use. One hundred and eighty thousand vaccinations had already been carried out.

Dr. W. F. Gaisford commented on the poor conversion rate after vaccination of new-born infants in Dr. Cowell's survey as compared with his experience in Manchester, where the conversion was 100 per cent. This was an important matter, because any increased resistance to infection afforded during the first two years of life was more vital than at any other time and was the chief justification for mass vaccination. The conversion rate at this age-period undoubtedly depended primarily upon the type of vaccine used. In Dr. Cowell's survey the strikingly increased incidence in the five-year-old group, attending school for the first time, suggested, in view of the non-infectivity of the primary infection in children, an infectious school-teacher, and once more drew attention to the urgent need for X-raying all school-teachers' chests at regular intervals.

Dr. Brendan O'Brien reminded the meeting of the rapidity with which tuberculous lesions could develop, so that a teacher with a clear X-ray who was infected might rapidly become dangerous. This risk could be reduced by universal early B.C.G. vaccination. At the Meath Hospital there had been no tuberculosis in the nurses since its introduction, although open tubercle was treated in that hospital.

Dr. R. W. Parnell thought that Dr. Cowell was right to stress the epidemiological situation, which he contrasted with quite a different situation. Under 10 per cent. of entrants to the University of Minnesota in recent years had been tuberculin-positive. This low proportion had been brought about gradually by mass radiography, tuberculin testing, and other preventive measures; B.C.G. had not been used. Now it seemed that if B.C.G. were used at Minnesota it would most probably be to protect students visiting the United Kingdom.

Dr. J. C. Gilson suggested that the differences between the tuberculin-sensitivity figures of the National B.C.G. Committee and those of the Prophit Survey could be accounted for by the elapse of 12 years between the surveys.

Dr. K. D. Keele asked whether milk was supplied in school meals in Ireland and, if so, whether this would not influence infection rates.

Dr. Cowell, replying to Dr. Gilson, said he did not think that the time interval would make much difference. While there were no big tuberculin surveys in Ireland with which to compare the present one, it was a well-known fact for many years among Irish physicians that a returned emigrant suffering from tuberculosis was all too likely to infect a houseful of tuberculin-negative siblings. Likewise English physicians would recollect that the Irish probationer nurse, inevitably tuberculin-negative before the advent of B.C.G., was a source of grave responsibility to any conscientious employer. To Dr. Keele he replied that pasteurized milk was supplied in the urban schools; in the schools of the Gaeltacht milk was also supplied. Because of local farming economy the only cow possessed by a family might be 'dry' for part of the year. Even if this milk was loose it would not provide an immunizing factor, because bovine tuberculosis was rare along the west coast of Ireland.

3. Dr. A. L. Cochrane (introduced), making an *Assessment of an Attempt to Control Tuberculosis in a Mining Community*, said that, as part of a long-term epidemiological investigation into the aetiology of progressive massive fibrosis (the more severe form of coal-workers' pneumoconiosis), the M.R.C. Pneumoconiosis Research Unit and the Welsh Regional Hospital Board had attempted to X-ray all the 25,000 inhabitants over the age of five years of a Welsh mining valley, the Rhondda Fach. In the winter of 1950–1, 90 per cent. of these people had been X-rayed. The films had been read in duplicate, sputum investigations had been carried out on a large scale, and persons considered to be suffering from infectious tuberculosis had immediately been taken into hospital. Special home-visiting arrangements were made after their discharge. In this way the valley could be said to have had radical therapy for tuberculosis. Last summer the population had again been X-rayed to reinforce and assess the effect of the first survey. Provisional results showed such a fall in the women's death-rate that no woman had died of tuberculosis during the past year. Similarly the prevalence of infectious tuberculosis had been markedly reduced. Some new cases of tuberculosis had appeared between the two surveys, but it was estimated that the attack rate of tuberculosis had been reduced to less than half of what it had been in the five-year period before the first survey. The importance of these findings was discussed.

Professor John Crofton asked about the type of new case that had appeared since the first survey, and whether the origin of the infection in such cases had been traced. Dr. Alice Stewart asked what factors were responsible for the unwillingness of those who refused to be X-rayed. Dr. Wade inquired whether legal compulsion could not be used.

In reply to Professor Crofton, Dr. Cochrane said that the analysis was not yet complete, but that the majority of cases had occurred among contacts some considerable time after the contact had been broken by removing the infectious patient to hospital. A few others had occurred among those working outside the valley, particularly in Cardiff. In reply to Dr. Stewart, he said that all the factors governing the refusal rate were not yet known, but it appeared that age, sex, and compensation for industrial disease were all important. There also appeared to be an 'economic factor', in that the professional classes were rather more difficult to persuade than others. Doctors and school-teachers were particularly difficult! In reply to Dr. Wade, he said that a compulsory X-ray scheme was apparently working well in Australia. His experience of Australians as prisoners of war suggested that they were very much more individualistic than people of the United Kingdom, so that if the Australians put up with it he did not doubt the British would do so.

4. Dr. R. W. D. Turner and Dr. H. Fraser (introduced) discussed *Auricular Fibrillation in Rheumatic Heart Disease*. Auricular fibrillation had been present in 42 per cent. of 200 cases of mitral valvular disease treated by operation, and in 84 per cent. of a parallel series of 105 cases considered too severe or too complex for surgical treatment. The incidence of fibrillation increased with age, but 33 per cent. of such patients were under 40 years old. No correlation could be established between the incidence of fibrillation and the size of the mitral orifice, the degree of mitral regurgitation, or the severity of pulmonary hypertension. Cardiac and left atrial size tended to be greater than in patients with sinus rhythm, but these increases in size were not primary factors in determining the incidence of fibrillation, nor did they directly result therefrom. Rheumatic carditis was probably the most important factor, but histological evidence was unsatisfactory. The onset of fibrillation might cause acute dyspnoea, syncope, palpitation, or anxiety. Dangers included pulmonary infarction, systemic embolism, and cardiac failure. Disadvantages included a decreased capacity for effort and more frequent cardiac failure during pregnancy. Fibrillation was a disadvantage, but not in itself a contra-indication to valvotomy. The incidence of intracardiac thrombosis was much higher than in patients with sinus rhythm, and so was that of systemic embolism at operation. Clot had been found in 40 per cent. of the 85 cases of fibrillation and in 1·7 per cent. of the 115 cases of sinus rhythm. Systemic

embolism had occurred in 12 cases. In 24 clot had been successfully evacuated before undertaking valvotomy. Fibrillation had developed a few days after operation in 33 per cent. of patients in sinus rhythm. Prophylactic quinidine, even in high dosage, was often ineffective. Quinidine begun soon after the 10th day after operation was the best régime, and had been successful in restoring normal rhythm in all but two of the 39 cases.

Dr. J. F. Goodwin said that in his experience patients who developed auricular fibrillation after mitral valvotomy might revert spontaneously to sinus rhythm after a longer interval—in one case six weeks after operation—so that attempts to convert fibrillation to sinus rhythm with drugs might be delayed longer than 10 days after operation. He added that it was his practice to give anticoagulants before attempting conversion, and that he had not seen any instance of embolism with this régime. At operation Mr. Cleland had noticed that patients with auricular fibrillation who had suffered previous embolisms usually had organized thrombus in the auricle but no free thrombus, whereas patients with fibrillation but without a history of emboli often had friable, easily detachable, recent thrombus in the auricle.

Dr. K. W. Donald said he and his colleagues had studied the cardiac output of a patient with idiopathic auricular fibrillation, and had found that the response to exercise was almost normal.

Dr. P. T. O'Farrell said that in 50 mitral valvotomies performed by Mr. T. O'Connell at St. Vincent's Hospital, Dublin, the incidence of auricular fibrillation after operation had been high, and he asked how long auricular fibrillation should be allowed to persist before attempts were made to restore normal rhythm. He was interested to hear that signs of active rheumatic infection in biopsy material from atrial appendices were difficult to identify microscopically. American observers apparently did not meet with this particular difficulty, and their reports seemed to indicate that Aschoff nodes were frequently found when active infection had not been thought to be present before operation. Did Dr. Turner think that, if these findings were correct, the operation of valvotomy might be better performed at an earlier age than was now the custom?

Drs. L. Abrahamson, E. G. L. Bywaters, J. C. Gilson, E. N. Chamberlain, M. I. A. Hunter, and J. F. Pantridge also asked questions.

Dr. Fraser, in reply, said that, with regard to Dr. Goodwin's point, he and Dr. Turner had always attempted reversal of rhythm early, and had not waited after fibrillation had persisted for 14 days. Out of 39 cases of fibrillation following operation, only one had returned spontaneously to normal rhythm in the first 14 days. Access to the mitral valve had on several occasions necessitated disturbance of fixed clot, and loose clot had often appeared to be engrafted on the fixed clot, so that both constituted hazards of embolus formation. Anticoagulants had not been used in any of the 36 cases in which clot had been found at operation. Embolism had occurred only once after operation, and this had been on the fifth day, much too soon after the operation for anticoagulant therapy to be used. In reply to Dr. O'Farrell he stated that 30 per cent. of the patients who developed auricular fibrillation after operation gave no history of having had paroxysmal fibrillation before operation. With regard to the age distribution of their cases, it was clear that the majority of operations for mitral stenosis were being carried out too late, and this was why valves whose structure precluded technically satisfactory valvotomy were encountered so often. He said that Aschoff bodies had been present in left atrial biopsy specimens in 33 cases, and in an additional 36 there were cellular aggregates of various degrees of development which were accepted by the pathologists as indicating active rheumatism, although the cellular architecture did not amount to a classical Aschoff body. Thus positive results from biopsy of the left atrial appendage had been found in 49 per cent. of cases when the several histological standards of positivity were accepted. No differences between younger and older age groups had been noticed in the histological appearances on biopsy of the left atrial appendage. In reply to Dr. Hunter it was stated that a few patients had shown evidence of recurrence of mitral stenosis after mitral valvotomy, but that biopsy findings in the left atrial appendix had not been positive in all of them. Surgical technique had improved substantially after the first 40 to 50 cases, and it was not surprising that a few patients treated by the earlier, less radical mitral valvotomy should show evidence of re-stenosis after two to three years. This should occur less commonly in patients treated by the method used in the last 150 cases. The effect of further rheumatic inflammation would be more likely to cause significant re-stenosis in the earlier cases than in those treated more recently by radical valvotomy. He could not explain Dr. Abrahamson's greater difficulty in restoring normal rhythm with quinidine. When quinidine was first given between the 10th and 14th days after operation, normal rhythm could usually be established with moderate doses, but in a few cases fairly large doses had been necessary, for example 50 gr. per day as opposed to the usual dose of 24 to 36 gr. per day.

5. Dr. K. W. Donald, Dr. O. L. Wade, and Dr. J. M. Bishop (introduced) described the *Effect of Mitral Valvulotomy on the Haemodynamic and Ventilatory Response to Exercise.* The response to exercise of the arteriovenous oxygen difference, the oxygen uptake, and the cardiac output had been studied minute by minute in 10 patients with chronic rheumatic heart disease before and after valvotomy, mixed venous samples being drawn from the pulmonary artery throughout five minutes of exercise and five minutes of recovery. Six patients had mitral stenosis, two had mitral and aortic stenosis, and two had mitral stenosis with predominating mitral regurgitation. In patients in whom the result of operation was classified as 'very good' there had been improvement in the arteriovenous oxygen difference, the cardiac output, the ventilation, and the percentage extraction of oxygen from inspired air. In patients in whom the clinical result had been less good, in particular in the two patients with mitral regurgitation, there was little or no change. Changes in pulmonary arterial pressure subsequent to the operation had been small, and seemed unrelated to clinical improvement. In one subject in whom the pulmonary arterial pressure on exercise had not fallen after the operation, but in whom a far higher cardiac output was achieved, the work of the right ventricle was greatly increased at a level of exertion which would be frequently encountered during his daily life.

6. Dr. G. Wade (introduced) reported clinical, radiological, electrocardiographic, and dynamic studies in seven cases with the *Clinical Syndrome of Primary Pulmonary Hypertension.* In all cases the diagnosis had been confirmed by cardiac catheterization, and in five there had been an autopsy. The disease affected young adults of either sex, and ran a rapidly progressive course to intractable right heart failure and death within two to three years. The clinical syndrome, in conjunction with the radiological and electrocardiographic findings, was sufficiently distinctive for diagnosis. The genesis of the symptoms and signs was briefly discussed. Evidence was brought forward suggesting that the site of the lesion was either the pulmonary arterioles or the pre-capillaries. In view of the short and progressive course it was suggested that the disease was acquired. The aetiology was uncertain, but the finding of a positive differential agglutination test (highly specific for rheumatoid arthritis) in three out of five cases suggested that in some cases the condition might be a connective-tissue disorder characterized by fibrinoid change.

In the ensuing discussion Professor Melville Arnott commented on the dynamics of the pulmonary circulation in this disease, and Professor J. H. Kellgren discussed the differential agglutination test in diseases other than rheumatoid arthritis.

Dr. J. F. Goodwin said that two other conditions which might cause difficulty in making a clinical diagnosis were patent ductus arteriosus with reversed shunt, and thrombosis of the main pulmonary arteries; the latter condition was frequently associated with right ventricular failure, fainting on exertion, and praecordial pain. He asked Dr. Wade whether he had tried the methonium group of drugs as a therapeutic measure, since it had been shown that hexamethonium was capable of reducing the pulmonary arterial pressure in other forms of pulmonary hypertension.

Professor J. McMichael pointed out the difficulties of confirming the diagnosis of primary pulmonary hypertension. At post-mortem terminal pulmonary embolism could obscure the whole picture. One case diagnosed in life was proved by angiocardiography to be a case of Eisenmenger's complex. Patent ductus arteriosus could also become complicated by pulmonary hypertension. There was no *a priori* reason for low arterial oxygen saturation in these cases. What was the explanation ?

Dr. E. G. L. Bywaters, Professor F. T. G. Prunty, Dr. Frances Gardner, and Dr. B. Schlesinger also contributed to the discussion. In reply Dr. Wade said that he had not tried the effect of methonium drugs. He thought the slight arterial unsaturation might be due to the opening up of pulmonary arteriovenous shunts of the type demonstrated by Tobin (1952). In most cases there was evidence of poor peripheral circulation, and a slight polycythaemia was a common finding. In three cases a search for the L. E. phenomenon was negative. The short duration, symptomatology, and radiological appearances serve to differentiate the disease from cases of tight mitral stenosis without murmurs. He did not know how long pulmonary hypertension had existed prior to the onset of symptoms.

7. DR. DONALD HUNTER described *Chronic Cadmium Poisoning in the Manufacture of Copper Alloys.* In the manufacture of the overhead wires for electric railways copper was alloyed with one per cent. of cadmium, for by this means the strength and resistance to wear are greatly improved without serious impairment of electrical conductivity. Four men, from 49 to 58 years of age, exposed in this process to cadmium oxide fume for 32, 17, 13, and 11 years respectively, had been under observation. One showed chronic enphysema but no proteinuria, one showed proteinuria but no emphysema, and the other two showed both. The amount of cadmium excreted in the urine in 24 hours varied from 40 to 870 micrograms. The protein was not obtained on boiling the urine, but was precipitated by trichloracetic acid. It showed an electrophoretic mobility lower than that of ordinary albumin, and examination by the ultracentrifuge indicated that its molecular weight might be about 30,000. In one of the cases it had been associated with a rising blood-urea and a fatal result. Neither rhinitis nor anosmia had occurred in any of the four cases. In the manufacture of copper alloys the installation of devices to remove cadmium fume by exhaust ventilation would suffice to prevent the disease. A detailed survey of the health hazards in the electrical copper industry in Great Britain had been carried out by Dr. J. A. Bonnell, the results of which would be published in the Proceedings of the Eleventh International Congress of Industrial Medicine, Naples, 1954.

The meeting adjourned to lunch at the Royal College of Surgeons, and reassembled for the Afternoon Session at 2.15. The session consisted of a symposium on *Vascular Hypertension.*

In introducing the discussion PROFESSOR G. W. PICKERING dealt with some *Basic Considerations which Affect the Management of Patients with Hypertension.* Broadly speaking, such patients fell into two classes: those in whom a specific cause for the hypertension could be recognized and removed, and those in whom this could not be done. The first group included coarctation of the aorta, phaeochromocytoma, unilateral renal disease, and probably Cushing's syndrome. Estimation of the urinary excretion of pressor amines was the one certain method of recognizing phaeochromocytoma. The removal of such tumours abolished paroxysmal hypertension, but in his experience left a substantial number of those who previously had sustained hypertension largely unchanged. Removal of a unilaterally diseased kidney was well recognized as an effective method of reducing high blood-pressure. So far as we knew this only worked if the other kidney was free from gross disease, usually pyelonephritis. In his experience of 10 cases of apparently unilateral pyelonephritis the arterial pressure had been substantially reduced in only five. It would seem, therefore, that in human hypertension, as in experimental hypertension, removal of the original cause of a prolonged hypertension might not reduce it substantially. When Cushing's syndrome was due to an adrenal tumour, the removal of this might cure the disease, but unfortunately a substantial number of these tumours were malignant. When no tumour existed, the removal of one adrenal and three-quarters of the other might abolish the hypertension in some cases.

The second group, in which the cause could not be removed, included nephritis, bilateral chronic pyelonephritis, polycystic kidney, and polyarteritis nodosa; but the great majority of cases were classified by exclusion as essential hypertension, which constituted the chief problem in management of hypertension. In saying a few words about its nature and aetiology, he would present his conclusions before the evidence. They were firstly, that so-called essential hypertension was not a well-defined condition but merely represented the higher ranges of arterial pressure for which no discrete cause could be found; secondly, that its cause was to be found in the genetic and environmental factors which affected the population as a whole. At the present time two factors, heredity and age, were partly understood; the effect of environment was understood not at all. The evidence for these statements was derived from measurements of the casual arterial pressure in a sample of the population and in first-degree relatives of subjects with so-called essential hypertension and subjects with normal pressures respectively. Distribution curves of systolic and diastolic pressures for both sexes in decades showed a continuous distribution, with no division into two populations. As age increased the curves spread out and shifted to the right, that is, arterial pressure rose with age more in some people than in others. Any division between so-called normal and high pressures was purely arbitrary. The frequency-distribution curves of arterial pressures in the relatives of normal subjects were approximately the same as those in the population sample. The pressures of relatives of hypertensive subjects were in general higher throughout the age-range from the second to the eighth decade. This suggested that the factor of inheritance in hypertension was no more than a tendency of relatives to resemble each other in blood-pressure, as in height and other features, and that arterial pressure, like height, was a graded characteristic. This resemblance had been estimated by a regression coefficient of 0·2, which meant that if one member of a family had an arterial pressure 10 mm. above the mean for that age, the other members would tend to have pressures averaging 2 mm. above the mean. The remaining factors determining arterial pressure were presumably environmental, but they had not been identified. Short of choosing our parents there was little or nothing that we could do at the present time to avoid hypertension.

Professor Pickering then turned to consider how far hypertension caused disability and death. Insurance companies' records showed that expectation of life was inversely proportional to pressure, and this relationship held down to quite low values. The great contribution of Volhard and Fahr had been to point out that the whole course of hypertension might be stable for many years, or might be rapidly progressive to renal failure within the year. The clinical distinction between these two courses was based on the fundus oculi, the malignant form presenting hypertensive neuroretinopathy, a bilateral condition characterized by papilloedema and exudates which were often, but not always, ill defined. In the benign form there was either no retinal lesion, apart from vascular change, or retinopathy which tended to be unilateral, without disk-swelling and with small and sharply defined exudates. The malignant course of hypertension was the result of arteriolar necroses found most frequently in the kidneys, and less extensively in gut, pancreas, adrenal, brain, heart, and eye, but not in skin or muscle. These necroses stopped the blood-flow and killed the tissues which the arterioles supplied. There was an increasing body of evidence suggesting that an important factor in the production of these lesions was the intensity of the hypertension, so that the malignant phase was essentially a consequence of the degree of hypertension rather than of its kind. It had been known to occur not only in essential hypertension but in all the other varieties, with the single exception of coarctation of the aorta. Death in the benign phase occurred chiefly from heart failure, and to a less extent from apoplexy, but about one-third of patients with essential hypertension died not of their disease but of something else. The exact cause of heart failure and of apoplexy was not fully explained, but atheroma and other forms of arterial degeneration were probably important. These forms of arterial disease occurred in the absence of hypertension, but were more frequent and severe in its presence. In the management of patients a distinction should be drawn between those in the malignant and those in the benign phase. In the malignant phase urgent and considerable reduction of arterial pressure was the first aim of management, since this often seemed to be able to arrest the course of the arteriolar lesions which would otherwise kill the patient. In the benign form indications were less clear, since the condition was comparatively stable and the influence of arterial pressure less obvious. All the treatments which were effective in reducing arterial pressure had a nuisance value, which might be far from negligible, and some treatments might convert the patient to a neurotic invalid. It was the essence of good management that a balance should be struck between the gains and the losses that the particular therapy was likely to confer. Here lay the rub. Even in the long-standing and much-used method, that of ablation of the sympathetic nerves, there had never been a proper clinical trial. Although treated and untreated cases had been compared, they had never been selected in precisely the same way and allocated at random before the treatment had been begun. It was therefore uncertain how far the difference in results between treated and untreated cases was the consequence of the initial selection or of the treatment employed.

Professor J. McMichael spoke on the *Place of Hypotensive Drugs*. At present parenterally administered methonium compounds were the most effective agents. Phasic reduction of blood-pressure produced improvement in retinitis, in cardiac failure, and in headache. Occlusive vascular changes were not affected. The following favourable results had been achieved in malignant hypertension: 15 out of 22 patients had survived beyond nine months, and six were now living after more than two years. Notable regression of retinitis had taken place in all, and in those surviving longest it had disappeared completely. Heart size was often reduced, but electrocardiographic improvement was less striking. An organizing fibrinous oedema of the lungs was the major untoward development. Measures for dealing with side-effects of methonium treatment included special glasses, β-methylcholine, belladonna, and interruption of dosage. Other hypotensive agents such as veratrum, hydralazine, and ergot alkaloids had been less satisfactory. Rauwolfia alkaloids might find a place in the treatment of less severe hypertensive illness. Statistically satisfactory evidence of drug efficacy in benign hypertension, however, was lacking. Methonium trials had proved that blood-pressure control was a worthwhile objective. It relieved certain manifestations of hypertensive vascular disease, and re-established a benign course in some cases of malignant hypertension.

Professor Robert Platt discussed the *Optic Fundus as a Guide to Management*. He suggested that the retinal changes of hypertension might be classified as follows: 1. Vascular changes (constriction, tortuosity, venous compression). 2. Vascular accidents (arterial and venous thrombosis, central or peripheral). These were as unpredictable as strokes and coronary thromboses in the course of hypertension. They had no important bearing on prognosis, but might leave permanent visual defects. 3. Hypertensive neuroretinopathy. This was the most important evidence of the malignant phase in hypertension, and demanded the use of measures to reduce blood-pressure, unless such treatment was otherwise contra-indicated. 4. Arteriosclerotic retinopathy (haemorrhages and hard exudates without papilloedema) which overlapped with (3) but, if typical, denoted a more gradual and not necessarily malignant course (Fishberg and Oppenheimer). 5. Papilloedema might occur without (or before) the development of diffuse neuroretinopathy in some cases.

Diffuse hypertensive neuroretinopathy almost never occurred unless the diastolic pressure was 140 or over (the reverse was not true). It should therefore recover, if not too far advanced, if the hypertension could be controlled at a lower level. A series of 39 unselected cases of hypertensive neuroretinopathy had been observed over the last three years. Some of them were of renal origin, and some showed advanced renal failure. For this or other reasons five patients had not been treated with hypotensive drugs. The remainder had been given hexamethonium or ansolysen by injection. The results might be summarized as follows:

Died without treatment	3
Died without significant retinal improvement	7
Died, but after significant retinal improvement	6
Not treated (living)	2
Treatment discontinued	5
Too recent to assess	2
Retina and vision significantly improved	4
Great improvement in severe retinopathy	10
	39

Illustrative fundus photographs were shown.

PROFESSOR M. L. ROSENHEIM, reviewing the *Dietary Management of Hypertension*, said that it had long been recognized that rigid restriction of sodium would lead to a lowering of the blood-pressure in many hypertensive patients. The Kempner rice diet owed its effect to its very low sodium content. Few patients, however, could tolerate extreme limitation of sodium intake for long, and less strict diets were ineffective, though they might benefit hypertensive cardiac failure. More recently cation exchange resins had been used to increase the hypotensive effect of diets moderately low in sodium. Extreme restriction of sodium was dangerous in the presence of renal failure, for, unless the tubular conservation of sodium was excellent, complications due to sodium deficiency arose. The diet could therefore not often be used in the malignant phase of hypertension. Although reduction in weight was probably without effect on the level of blood-pressure, it was of considerable benefit to the patient in early cardiac failure, and might provide symptomatic relief. There was as yet no satisfactory evidence that rigid restriction of lipoid intake affected the ultimate prognosis of the hypertensive patient.

MR. PATRICK FITZGERALD (introduced) discussed the *Surgical Treatment of Hypertension*. He had found that the first class of hypertensive patients referred to by Professor Pickering, in which the cause was directly amenable to surgery, was less than one per cent. of all cases. In essential hypertension, surgical therapy was based on supposed overactivity of the sympathetic nervous system. In considering the selection of cases the first group of surgical patients must be separated. In the remainder contra-indications to sympathectomy must be assessed, and then the type of sympathectomy most suitable for the patient's degree of vascular damage must be determined. To this end a careful family history and a history of cerebral, cardiac, and renal events was taken. Among miscellaneous symptoms special note was taken of paroxysmal attacks, sweating, epistaxis, and visual defects. Fatigue and associated states indicated psychiatric advice. Apart from general physical examination the following tests were of especial value: 1. Retinal grading. 2. Conway renal function test. 3. Postural effect on blood-pressure. 4. Rogitine test. In 300 tests only one significant drop had been obtained which was proved accurate at operation. The cases were classified on a system based on that of Smithwick, with special emphasis on eye changes. Operation was contra-indicated in patients with severe cerebral, cardiac, or renal damage. A Conway urea clearance below 40 was an absolute contra-indication. A Smithwick thoracolumbar sympathectomy was performed, removing the chain from T7 to L2 or L3 and the associated splanchnics, with an interval of 14 days between operations. Whenever there was a history of angina, a trans-thoracic operation was done and in addition the chain was removed up to T2, for cardiac denervation, by Dickson Wright's technique. The results of 13 years' experience of these methods, compared with medical treatment, were shown.

DR. T. B. COUNIHAN (introduced) described the *Effects of Resection of Coarctation of the Aorta on the Blood-pressure*. The development of the operation for relief of coarctation of the aorta had raised hopes that it might constitute an effective line of therapy for hypertension in the upper half of the body, which was associated with this condition. While there were some surgical claims of good results, adequate follow-up figures regarding the blood-pressure were lacking. In 20 cases of coarctation of the aorta blood-pressure readings over periods extending from three months to five years after operation were available. Adequate resection was indicated by a rise in femoral blood-pressure and the disappearance of collateral vessels and of delay in the femoral pulse-wave. Brachial blood-pressure on the average had been lower after operation, but restoration to normal had been rare. After operation the children in this series had shown a greater fall in blood-pressure than adults, but their pressures remained greater than the expected mean for their age. Collateral evidence of left ventricular hypertrophy from clinical, X-ray, and electrocardiographic signs had indicated in all cases but one that the strain on the left heart remained after operation. Failure of the blood-pressure to return to normal despite eradication of the primary cause was now recognized both clinically and experimentally.

DR. MAURICE SOKOLOW (introduced) discussed the *Psychological Aspects of Treatment of Hypertension*. Physicians for years had appreciated that hypertensive patients frequently showed maladjustment of their personality. Indeed, many attempts had been made to define this abnormality by psychiatric interviews, psychological testing, and studies involving experimental stress. Most investigators had found differences between hypertensive and normotensive subjects, but the role of psychological factors in hypertension had not been established either in terms of aetiology or as regards their effect on the course of the disease. Psychotherapy had rarely lowered the blood-pressure to normal, despite pertinent evidence of 'character neurosis' revealed by the analysis. As a result physicians rarely used psychiatric consultation in hypertensive patients, unless the indications for it were such as to require it regardless of the blood-pressure. It was accepted practice for physicians to advise hypertensive patients to adopt a calm, unhurried way of life and to see problems in their proper perspective. The fact that hypertensive patients have problems in special spheres of activity, about which they have little insight, was often unappreciated. The physician might be of considerable help in recognizing and dealing with these conflicts. Many studies, including his own, had demonstrated that hypertensive patients, with an outward façade of normality, had intense feelings of anger and had difficulty in expressing anger. They showed 'subnormal assertiveness'. In addition, resolution of dependence-independence conflicts was difficult for the hypertensive. Attempts to relate the onset of hypertensive crises (such as severe headache, encephalopathy, or the malignant phase) temporally to significant emotional events had often shown a close association. The physician could at times prevent recurrences by determining the causative emotional event and attempting to 'manipulate' the environment. A strong, confident, optimistic physician, who used explanation and reassurance about daily variations in pressure, and upon whom the patient could lean, might by his very presence relieve symptoms, decrease invalidism, and permit the patient to live a happier life.

In summing-up, PROFESSOR L. J. WITTS commented on the fact that the three last annual symposia had dealt with conditions (chronic bronchitis, fibrositis, and high blood-pressure) which were all probably multi-determined in aetiology, and which were more profitably studied as disturbances of homoeostasis than as simple disease entities. The assessment of therapy in such conditions was particularly difficult, and was best arrived at by isolating defined sub-groups for study. Treatment should also be assessed in terms of cost and practicability, and at the present time surgical treatment, as by sympathectomy or subtotal adrenalectomy, might be better for some patients than the difficult régime entailed by the use of hypotensive drugs. Hexamethonium bromide and ansolysen were a most promising advance in therapeutics, but they could be recommended for general use only in malignant hypertension and hypertensive encephalopathy. In other forms of hypertension their value still remained to be determined by research.

At 4.30 the meeting moved to St. Vincent's Hospital, where tea was provided and where the following demonstrations were exhibited:

DR. L. ABRAHAMSON and DR. M. L. ABRAHAMSON (introduced): 'Chronic anaemia associated with hypopituitarism'.

DR. S. J. BOLAND (introduced) and DR. O. FITZGERALD: 'Chronic relapsing pancreatitis'.

DR. J. ST. P. COWELL (introduced) and DR. E. T. FREEMAN: 'B.C.G. vaccination'.

DR. S. P. DUNDON and DR. F. J. GEOGHEGAN (introduced): 'Haemolytic disease of the newborn'.

MR. P. FITZGERALD: 'Surgical treatment of hypertension'.

DR. E. T. FREEMAN: 'Muscular dystrophy'.

PROFESSOR D. K. O'DONOVAN: 'Canities and hyperthyroidism'.

DR. J. P. R. REES (introduced) and PROFESSOR R. H. MICKS: 'Idiopathic hypoparathyroidism'.

DR. J. A. WALLACE (introduced) and PROFESSOR R. H. MICKS: 'A peculiar dysgraphia'.

Annual Dinner

The Annual Dinner was held at the Gresham Hotel. The local members kindly provided a sherry party beforehand. The President, PROFESSOR V. M. SYNGE, was in the Chair. The toast of the Association was proposed by the President, and that of the guests by PROFESSOR L. S. P. DAVIDSON. MR. W. DOOLIN replied, and the toast of the President was proposed by DR. ROBERT MARSHALL. The President responded.

Saturday, 9.30 a.m. Morning Session

8. DR. SHEILA SHERLOCK, and DR. W. H. J. SUMMERSKILL and DR. L. P. WHITE (introduced), described *Cerebral Disturbance with Altered Nitrogen Metabolism in Liver Disease.* It was suggested that toxic nitrogenous substances, passing from the portal vein to the systemic circulation through a damaged liver, portal venous collateral channels, or both, might effect a diffuse cerebral disturbance. Ammonia had been incriminated, and elevated blood-ammonia levels in hepatic and peripheral veins had been found in 15 patients with neurological complications of liver disease. The relative influence of liver damage and collateral short-circuiting vessels on these values could be shown by simultaneous sampling from peripheral and hepatic veins after an oral dose of ammonium chloride. The neurological syndrome consisted in a characteristic disorder of consciousness and of the motor system with electroencephalographic changes, and was uniform despite varied aetiology of the liver disease. In cases of liver disease with or without a collateral circulation, it might be precipitated by agents which increased the nitrogenous content of the intestine (including high-protein diet, ammonium chloride, and methionine) or by impaired liver function. Signs might be terminal, transient, or persistent. Patients with thrombosis of the portal vein or portocaval shunts might exhibit chronic nervous disorder, and a film was shown demonstrating the benefit of protein restriction in such patients.

DR. R. S. ALLISON inquired about the neurological sequelae of portocaval shunt operations, and whether hypoglycaemia occurred in any patient. He also drew attention to the fluctuation in electroencephalographic patterns.

DR. G. S. HALL stressed the importance of excluding Wilson's disease in patients with persistent signs, and said that he had found abnormal Lange curves in such patients.

PROFESSOR P. C. P. CLOAKE asked about the occurrence of mild variations of this syndrome in patients with chronic liver disease, who might show ataxia and coarse kinetic tremor over a period of years with recurrent short periods of drowsiness and mental confusion.

PROFESSOR F. J. NATTRASS suggested that high-protein diet in the treatment of liver disease should be reviewed.

SIR WALTER RUSSELL BRAIN commented on the characteristic variation in the neurological signs; he urged that the adjective 'flapping' should not be perpetuated as a description of the characteristic tremor exhibited by some patients with liver disease.

DR. A. M. COOKE wondered how closely a deranged ammonia metabolism was connected with the nervous disorder, and asked whether antibiotics had any beneficial effect.

DR. A. G. OGILVIE inquired about the incidence of cranial nerve lesions in this condition.

DR. OLIVER FITZGERALD asked what method had been used to determine blood-ammonia. He also asked about the possible significance of the methionine effect, which seemed in terms of the dose used to be very powerful. It was difficult to understand how methionine could give an effect, at least through formation of ammonia, for it required deamination in the liver before formation of ammonia. This function would presumably be grossly interfered with in liver disease.

Replying, Dr. Summerskill said that some observers estimated the incidence of neurological sequelae after portocaval shunt operations at 10 per cent., and that some deaths after operation might result from cerebral intoxication. None of the patients described had been hypoglycaemic, and Wilson's disease had been excluded in the chronic group by urinary copper estimations. No abnormality of the Lange curve had been found, and no cranial nerve lesions observed. It was considered that mild forms of the syndrome were common, especially following incidents likely to precipitate neurological disturbance. No apparent benefit from very high protein diet had been observed in liver disease, though, as had been shown, deterioration might occur in some patients. The effect of antibiotics was under consideration, but so far uncertain. The relationship between deranged ammonia metabolism and the cerebral disturbance was complex; peripheral venous ammonia levels depended on several factors, and were unlikely to reflect accurately changes within the brain-cells. The action of methionine could not be explained satisfactorily on the basis of deamination. Ammonia had been measured after 15 minutes' microdiffusion with Conway's technique.

9. Professor P. C. P. Cloake, Dr. W. T. Cooke, and Dr. G. S. Hall (introduced) discussed *Neurological Disorders associated with Steatorrhoea.* Cases had been collected from two sources. The first group had presented as neurological cases—neuropathy or atypical subacute combined degeneration—found on investigation to be associated with steatorrhoea. The second group had come from a large series of patients presenting general manifestations of steatorrhoea, among whom some had nervous degeneration. The neurological syndromes found were peripheral neuropathy, cerebellar ataxia, sensory ataxia, and pyramidal degeneration, alone or in various combinations. There were 18 patients, of whom one had optic atrophy and two had receptive deafness. These syndromes were compared with nutritional neuropathies in prisoners of war, similarities and differences being indicated. Two other patients had the 'burning feet' sydrome, with only slight evidence of organic nervous degeneration. Steatorrhoea in this association was regarded as an indication of the presence of defective intestinal absorption or defective utilization of essential nutritional elements, and the neurological disorder might have similar causes. Among associated disorders in these cases a history of diarrhoea was common but not invariable, macrocytic anaemia occurred in one-half, and gastric achlorhydria was present in six instances. No case had all the essential characteristics of true subacute combined degeneration of the spinal cord. Treatment had not been quite uniform, but all patients had been placed on a high-protein, low-fat diet, all but one had had crude liver or vitamin B_{12}, and some had had other elements of the vitamin-B complex. Results varied unaccountably. Three patients lost their symptoms, but five deteriorated steadily.

10. Dr. J. Badenoch and Dr. P. D. Bedford (introduced) reported two patients with *Massive Diverticulosis of the Upper Intestine presenting with Steatorrhoea and Megaloblastic Anaemia.* They gave reasons for believing that the diverticulosis was the cause of both the anaemia and the failure of fat-absorption. In both patients the course of the illness had been unlike that of idiopathic steatorrhoea, and the steatorrhoea had developed suddenly when the patients were 58 and 64 years old respectively. The first patient had had episodes of recurrent abdominal pain, severe melaena, and an attack of intestinal obstruction. The second patient had had diarrhoea and abdominal pain, which had proved unusually difficult to control. In both cases massive diverticulosis of the upper intestine, with retention of barium within the pouches, had been demonstrated radiologically. In one, post-mortem examination had confirmed these findings; the other patient was still alive. It was suggested that the numerous diverticula with their stagnant contents might exert an effect similar to that of a blind loop of small intestine. Bacteria would flourish within them, and infected or toxic material would spill over into the lumen of the bowel. This could impair its function and lead to a failure of absorption of many substances, including fat and those necessary for normal haemopoiesis. The association between diverticulosis of the jejunum and steatorrhoea or atypical megaloblastic anaemia did not appear to have been noted previously.

In discussing these two communications, Professor B. G. Maegraith asked whether any of the cases had been diagnosed as tropical sprue.

Dr. Hugh Conway asked whether any of the neurological complications had followed treatment with folic acid. He had had a patient with steatorrhoea who developed a syndrome indistinguishable from subacute combined degeneration after three years' treatment with folic acid. Free hydrochloric acid was present at first, but after the neurological condition had developed there was histamine-fast achlorhydria. When vitamin B_{12} was substituted for folic acid the nervous damage improved, but haematological relapse occurred.

Dr. J. N. Cruickshank referred to an example of defective fat-absorption with megaloblastic anaemia, achlorhydria, and neurological signs of pyramidal and posterior-column damage. There was a flat glucose-tolerance curve, and the vitamin-B_{12} assay at first showed gross deficiency (70), but after the administration of cytamen reached high normal levels (410 to 360). This patient had been treated with folic acid for over a year before he came under observation, and during that time his condition had steadily deteriorated. Improvement in nutrition and in the blood picture followed treatment with cytamen, but the neurological lesions did not respond. The absence of paraesthesia, the presence of increased protein in the cerebrospinal fluid (35 mg. per 100 ml.), and irregularity of the pupils, suggested that the condition was not an uncomplicated posterolateral sclerosis. It was possible that this malabsorption syndrome might not be identical with the classical subacute combined degeneration associated with pernicious anaemia.

Dr. J. Badenoch (introduced) said that two patients with steatorrhoea who had neurological symptoms had been studied in Professor Witts's Department at Oxford. One had had a peripheral neuropathy, and the other subacute combined degeneration. The symptoms of both patients had responded to vitamin B_{12} by injection. Gastric biopsy had shown that in neither case was there a severe atrophy of the mucosa of the body of the stomach, as seen in pernicious anaemia. In one patient studies using vitamin B_{12} labelled with ^{60}Co had shown that its absorption was within the normal range. In the other patient its absorption was reduced, but could not be increased by the addition of a potent source of intrinsic factor.

Dr. A. M. Cooke reminded the meeting that myopathy complicating sprue was described many years ago in a paper which was one of the few references he was able to remember—*Quarterly Journal of Medicine*, Volume I, page 1.

In his reply Dr. W. T. Cooke said that there had been no patients with tropical sprue in the group. Potassium deficiency, as assessed by the result of potassium-space estimates, muscle biopsy, and prolonged potassium administration, had not appeared to cause the neuropathy. The effect of prolonged mild potassium deficiency, such as tended to occur in these patients, in the production of organic nerve changes could not be evaluated at present. The group as a whole had been relatively well nourished. Folic acid was not given to any of the patients.

In the discussion, Dr. W. T. Cooke said that one of his patients with neuropathy had severe diverticulosis of the small intestine. Though she had been virtually bed-ridden 11 years ago, she had made a good recovery and was still ambulant. She had also had episodes of intestinal obstruction, but only in association with electrolyte depletion. It could not be emphasized too much that such episodes in the steatorrhoea syndrome were almost synonymous with potassium deficiency. Since they had studied cases with intestinal diverticula without abnormalities of fat-excretion, it might perhaps be doubted whether the diverticula were the cause of the symptoms in these two patients; they did, however, underline the unsatisfactory nature of the diagnosis of idiopathic steatorrhoea.

Dr. P. Fourman asked whether in some cases the steatorrhoea might be the result and not the cause of a neuromuscular disorder. Drs. Avery Jones, F. T. G. Prunty, R. Bodley Scott, and G. S. Hall also spoke.

11. Dr. J. R. Fountain (introduced) described *Clinical Observations in the Treatment of Leukaemia with 6-Mercaptopurine*. Twenty-four patients had been treated. Of 11 patients with acute leukaemia five had developed complete clinical and haematological remissions, and two had shown clinical and haematological improvement. The remissions had been temporary, and varied in duration, the longest being seven months. Remissions had been observed in both children and adults. Four patients had failed to respond to 6-mercaptopurine, two dying within the first week of treatment. Six out of seven patients with chronic myeloid leukaemia, including one in the acute terminal phase, had shown a fall in the leucocyte count, with a diminution in size of the spleen, liver, and lymph-nodes, and symptomatic improvement. Relapse had tended to occur a few weeks after treatment was discontinued, but by the use of maintenance therapy it seemed probable that this might be prevented. One patient had died of a cerebral thrombosis within a week of starting treatment. The same scheme of initial dosage had been used in the treatment of both

acute and chronic leukaemia, viz. 2·5 mg. per kg. A delay of one to four weeks generally occurred before the drug became effective. Serious toxic manifestations had not been encountered, although excessive dosage might lead to severe depression of haematopoiesis. Two patients with chronic lymphatic leukaemia, two with multiple myeloma, and one with a reticulosis of the skin had failed to show any satisfactory improvement. One patient with mycosis fungoides had appeared to be temporarily benefited on two occasions by a course of 6-mercaptopurine.

Dr. R. Bodley Scott said that he had used 6-mercaptopurine in 12 cases of leukaemia; 10 of these were acute, and two were of the chronic myeloid variety in the terminal myeloblastic phase. In both of the latter a precipitous fall in white blood-cells occurred without significant clinical improvement. In only two of the acute cases had even partial remission been noted, and in neither was its duration more than three weeks. His experience did not encourage him to share the optimism of the speaker.

Dr. J. F. Wilkinson also reported unsatisfactory experiences with 6-mercaptopurine.

Professor Robert Platt said that the most interesting fact which seemed to emerge from the treatment of leukaemia was that, although the disease might respond to a first course of treatment, it usually failed to respond to subsequent courses. This had been found to be true of treatment with several different drugs; it was reminiscent of bacterial resistance, and might be due to similar causes, for instance genetic differences in cell nuclei. He asked whether the haematologists tried giving several drugs together, in the way that streptomycin and PAS or INH were combined.

Dr. Fountain, in replying, was unable to account for Dr. Bodley Scott's and Dr. Wilkinson's unsatisfactory results with 6-mercaptopurine. He referred to the findings, recently reported in America, that the remission rate in acute leukaemia with 6-mercaptopurine was equal to that which followed aminopterin or amethopterin therapy. In addition the fact that 6-mercaptopurine did not result in serious toxic manifestations was of considerable importance. With regard to the question of ultimate resistance to 6-mercaptopurine, and to chemotherapeutic agents as a whole, Dr. Fountain agreed with Professor Platt that this was a very important subject, and stressed the fact that much research was being undertaken in this field.

12. Dr. D. G. James and Dr. A. D. Thomson (introduced) described the *Kveim Test in the Diagnosis of Sarcoidosis.* The antigen they had used consisted of a saline emulsion of sarcoid tissue obtained from affected lymph-nodes or spleen. The response consisted of the torpid development of a bluish-red nodule at the site of intradermal injection during the ensuing weeks. Biopsy of the nodule revealed the characteristic histological features of sarcoidosis. In the dermis there were numerous epithelioid cells, occasional giant cells of the Langhans type, and a sparse peripheral rim of lymphocytes, but no collagen necrosis or caseation. The test had been positive clinically and histologically in 12 out of 16 cases of sarcoidosis, but negative in 47 control subjects including 28 patients with tuberculosis. In all 12 positive cases intrathoracic sarcoidosis had been associated with other widely disseminated lesions. The test had been negative in four cases of healed sarcoidosis. When there were no conveniently available lymph-glands or skin lesions to provide histological confirmation of sarcoidosis, this test was a safe, simple, and specific out-patient alternative to liver or intrathoracic biopsy. It was an index of progress, and serial biopsy provided a means of evaluating therapy. In two patients treated with cortisone, streptomycin, and INH, histological evidence of sarcoidosis had still been present at the Kveim site three months after starting treatment.

13. Dr. S. W. Stanbury spoke on *Renal Osteodystrophy.* Long-term clinical observations, with radiological study and histological examination of biopsy or necrosy specimens of bone, had demonstrated that several types of skeletal disease might arise in the course of azotaemic renal failure. Osteomalacia (or rickets), osteitis fibrosa, and osteosclerosis had been seen in both children and adults with chronic nitrogen retention. One patient, followed from the age of 13 to 20 years, had shown radiological evidence at first of rickets, which healed with osteitis fibrosa; osteosclerosis succeeded, with skeletal deformity from the earlier conditions. Other patients had shown evidence of subperiosteal new bone formation. It did not seem impossible to anticipate the nature of the skeletal changes from the clinical history and blood examination alone. The distinction of 'essentially tubular' or 'essentially glomerular' renal insufficiency as causes of particular forms of skeletal disease appeared to be an over-simplification.

14. Dr. W. E. Miall (introduced) discussed the *Relationship between Chest X-ray Abnormalities and Rheumatoid Arthritis in a Welsh Mining Population.* In a previous publication a correlation had been established between the characteristic type of nodular fibrosis of the lung in coal-miners, described by Caplan, and rheumatoid arthritis. There was at present no epidemiological, clinical, or pathological evidence to suggest that these lesions differed aetiologically from the ordinary progressive massive fibrosis of coal-workers' pneumoconiosis. The relationship between chest X-ray abnormalities and rheumatoid arthritis had been investigated in a complete mining community in the Rhondda Fach, and the prevalence of this type of arthritis among miners and ex-miners had not been found to differ significantly from that in men who were not miners; as progressive massive fibrosis was very common among the miners (over 20 per cent. in the older age-group) it seemed unlikely that massive fibrosis predisposed to rheumatoid arthritis. In 26 out of 52 miners with rheumatoid arthritis chest X-rays had shown massive fibrosis, compared with 10 out of 52 miners in an age-standardized control group without arthritis. Preliminary results also indicated more prevalent radiological evidence of pulmonary tuberculosis in the rheumatoid arthritis group, and similar findings had been made in women with rheumatoid arthritis, compared with an age-balanced group without arthritis; the fact was stressed that few of these tuberculous lesions were of clinical significance. There was already considerable evidence of a 'rheumatoid diathesis', and that the genetic factor might be of importance in Caplan's syndrome was shown by illustrative cases. The simplest explanation of the findings was that the rheumatoid diathesis was associated with an altered type of tissue-resistance to pulmonary tuberculosis, or among miners to progressive massive fibrosis, and that this altered type of reaction might be responsible for the characteristic type of pulmonary fibrosis which developed in some coal-miners with rheumatoid arthritis.

15. Dr. E. A. Spriggs (introduced) presented Mr. O. A. Marxer's radiographs and drawings to show *Twisting, Kinking, and Rotation of the Stomach.* The deformities, which were also demonstrated on a flexible model, included 'cascade' stomach, 'jack-knife' stomach, chronic and recurrent gastric volvulus round different axes, and 'torsion' of the stomach. Records of 44 patients with florid abnormalities of this sort had been compared with records of a similar number of patients without them; most of the patients had had opaque meals with follow-through, and only a small proportion had had gastric disease. The following conclusions had been reached from the comparison: 1. Patients in whom kinking, rotation, or twisting were found in a routine opaque meal were unlikely to become surgical emergencies, and many of them described no relevant symptoms. 2. Such patients not infrequently suffered from severe attacks of epigastric distension, and they might burst abdominal wounds after laparotomy. 3. Occasionally retrosternal pain was described, with radiation similar to that of cardiac ischaemia. 4. There was a significant relation between the presence of these deformities and the X-ray appearance of pneumatosis of the stomach and of the left colic flexure.

16. Professor A. A. Moncrieff described three instances of *Sucrosuria with Mental Defect and Hiatus Hernia.* They had occurred in early childhood, and thus there were three types of congenital abnormality in the same subject—inborn metabolic error, mental defect, and an anatomical abnormality. Autopsy in one case had revealed a congenital defect in the brain, thus ruling out the hypothesis that the mental retardation might be due to the sucrosaemia. It was concluded that the sucrosuria resulted essentially from rapid absorption of the unsplit disaccharide, but technical difficulties had made it impossible to investigate further the failure of splitting or its degree. The previous scanty reports dealt mostly with similar instances of exogenous origin, as far as the sucrosuria was concerned. Careful study of the sugars ingested and subsequently passed in the urine had revealed a more complicated story than that of excessive alimentary absorption of sucrose and urinary excretion. Provisional 'normal' values for urinary sugars obtained by chromatography were suggested. The close association of lactose and sucrose in the diet, in relation to the occurrence of sucrose in the urine, seemed definitely established in these cases. Glucose metabolism had been unaffected.

Time did not allow discussion of the last five communications.

On Saturday afternoon a party of visitors was taken in cars, by the local members, to Glendalough, and another party attended the Leopardstown Races.

INDEX

Addison's disease, non-tuberculous, and its relationship to 'giant-cell granuloma' and multiple glandular disease, 403; incidence of non-tuberculous Addison's disease, 408; aetiology of non-tuberculous Addison's disease, 408.

Adenoma sebaceum in cases of pulmonary tuberous sclerosis, 114.

Anaemia, macrocytic, ascorbic acid requirements and urinary excretion of *p*-hydroxyphenylacetic acid in, 307.

Antirabic treatment, 'neuroparalytic accidents' of, 16.

Ascorbic acid requirements and urinary excretion of *p*-hydroxyphenylacetic acid in steatorrhoea and macrocytic anaemia, 307.

Biological actions and therapeutic applications of nitrogen mustard, 231; chemical reactions, 232; biological actions, 232; therapeutic applications, 235.

Blood-pressure of obese hypertensive women, the effect of weight reduction upon, 331.

Clinical diagnosis of pulmonary hypertension in patients with mitral stenosis, 105.

Diabetes insipidus: water-losing nephritis, a syndrome simulating, 147.

Diphtheria immunization, 15.

Effect of weight reduction upon the blood-pressure of obese hypertensive women, 331.

Effects of peripheral arterial embolism, 73.

Electrolyte depletion in pyloric stenosis, 367; plan of study and technical methods, 367; serum-electrolytes, 369; sodium balance, 370; potassium balance, 371; chloride balance, 371; interrelations, 372.

Embolism, peripheral arterial, effects of, 73.

Familial factor V deficiency: the pattern of heredity, 323.

Five-year assessment of patients in a controlled trial of streptomycin in pulmonary tuberculosis, 347; plan and conduct of the trial, 347; comparability of the two treatment series, 348; results during the five-year period, 350; prognostic factors in acute bilateral pulmonary tuberculosis in young adults, 356.

Ganglion-blocking agents in the treatment of pink disease, 223.

Gastro-intestinal disorders, studies of uropepsinogen excretion in, 291.

'Giant-cell granuloma' and multiple glandular disease: non-tuberculous Addison's disease and its relationship to, 403; and the other pituitary granulomata, 425.

Heart failure, congestive, complicating chronic lung disease: pulmonary hypertension in, 57.

Heredity, the pattern of: familial factor V deficiency, 323.

Hydroxyphenylic acids, paper-chromatographic technique for identification of, 307.

Hypertension, pulmonary, in congestive heart failure complicating chronic lung disease, 57.

—, —, in patients with mitral stenosis: clinical diagnosis of, 105.

Hypertensive retinopathy and its medical treatment, 441.

Hypoparathyroidism, idiopathic, 383; pseudohypoparathyroidism, 393; biochemical findings, 394.

Idiopathic hypoparathyroidism, 383; pseudohypoparathyroidism, 393; biochemical findings, 394.

Inoculation, pertussis, 12.

—, prophylactic, neurological sequelae of, 1; neurological complications of serum administration, 2; typhoid-paratyphoid vaccine (T.A.B.), 9; tetanus toxoid, 12; pertussis inoculation, 12; diphtheria immunization, 15; 'neuroparalytic accidents' of antirabic treatment, 16; miscellaneous immunizing agents, 18; neurological sequelae of skin-testing, 19.

Kidney, polyuria in certain other conditions affecting the, 159.

Lung disease, chronic, pulmonary hypertension in congestive heart failure complicating, 57.

Macrocytic anaemia, ascorbic acid requirements and urinary excretion of *p*-hydroxyphenylacetic acid in, 307.
Meningitis, tuberculous, spinal complications of, 275; definition and incidence, 275; clinical picture of transverse myelitis, 277; relationship of transverse myelitis to the presence of spinal block, 285; relationship of spinal block to mortality, 286.
Mental deficiency in cases of pulmonary tuberous sclerosis, 114.
Mitral stenosis, clinical diagnosis of pulmonary hypertension in patients with, 105.
Myelitis, transverse, clinical picture of, 277; relationship of, to the presence of spinal block, 285.
Myelomatosis, renal changes in, 158.

Nephritis, water-losing, 147; renal changes in myelomatosis, 158; polyuria in certain other conditions affecting the kidney, 159; pathogenesis, 161.
Neurological sequelae of prophylactic inoculation, 1; neurological complications of serum administration, 2; typhoid-paratyphoid vaccine (T.A.B.), 9; tetanus toxoid, 12; pertussis inoculation, 12; diphtheria immunization, 15; 'neuroparalytic accidents' of antirabic treatment, 16; miscellaneous immunizing agents, 18; neurological sequelae of skin-testing, 19.
Nitrogen mustard, biological actions and therapeutic applications of, 231; chemical reactions, 232; biological actions, 232; therapeutic applications, 235.
Non-tuberculous Addison's disease and its relationship to 'giant-cell granuloma' and multiple glandular disease, 403; incidence of non-tuberculous Addison's disease, 408; aetiology of non-tuberculous Addison's disease, 408.

Osteomalacia in steatorrhoea, 165.

Paper-chromatographic technique for identification of hydroxyphenylic acids, 307.
Peripheral arterial embolism, effects of, 73.
Pertussis inoculation, 12.
p-hydroxyphenylacetic acid in steatorrhoea and macrocytic anaemia, ascorbic acid requirements and urinary excretion of, 307.
Pink disease, the autonomic disorder and its treatment with ganglion-blocking agents, 215; the normal response in relation to age, 217; the response in cases of pink disease, 219; ganglion-blocking agents in pink disease, 223.
Pituitary gland, granulomata of, 428.
Polycythaemia vera, treatment of, with radiophosphorus, 91; haematological results, 94; clinical results, 101.
Polyuria, in water-losing nephritis, 147; in certain other conditions affecting the kidney, 159.
Proceedings of the Association of Physicians of Great Britain and Ireland, 1954: Forty-eighth Annual General Meeting, 451.
Prophylactic inoculation, *see* inoculation.
Pulmonary hypertension in congestive heart failure complicating chronic lung disease, 57.
— — in patients with mitral stenosis, clinical diagnosis of, 105.
— tuberculosis, five-year assessment of patients in a controlled trial of streptomycin in, 347; plan and conduct of the trial, 347; comparability of the two treatment series, 348; results during the five-year period, 350; prognostic factors in acute bilateral pulmonary tuberculosis in young adults, 356.
— tuberous sclerosis, 113.
Pyloric stenosis, electrolyte depletion in, 367; plan of study and technical methods, 367; serum-electrolytes, 369; sodium balance, 370; potassium balance, 371; chloride balance, 371; interrelations, 372.

Radiophosphorus, treatment of polycythaemia vera with, 91; haematological results, 94; clinical results, 101.
Retinopathy, hypertensive, and its medical treatment, 441.

Rheumatic fever, salicylates in, an attempt to assess their value, 177.

Salicylates in rheumatic fever, an attempt to assess their value, 177.
Sarcoidosis, 29; presenting symptoms and signs, 31; organs involved, 32; histology, 35; tuberculin test, 39; treatment, 49.
Sclerosis, tuberous, historical review of, 113; forms of, 124; nature of, 136.
—, —, pulmonary, 113.
Sequential tests in prophylactic and therapeutic trials, 255.
Serum administration, neurological complications of, 2.
Skin-testing, neurological sequelae of, 19.
Spinal block, relationship of transverse myelitis to the presence of, 285; relationship of, to mortality, 286.
— cord complications of tuberculous meningitis, 275; definition and incidence, 275; clinical picture of transverse myelitis, 277; relationship of transverse myelitis to the presence of spinal block, 285; relationship of spinal block to mortality, 286.
Steatorrhoea, ascorbic acid requirements and urinary excretion of *p*-hydroxyphenylacetic acid in, 307.
— osteomalacia in, 165.
Stenosis, mitral, clinical diagnosis of pulmonary hypertension in patients with, 105.
—, pyloric, electrolyte depletion in, 367; plan of study and technical methods, 367; serum-electrolytes, 369; sodium balance, 370; potassium balance, 371; chloride balance, 371; interrelations, 372.
Streptomycin in pulmonary tuberculosis, five-year assessment of patients in a controlled trial of, 347; plan and conduct of the trial, 347; comparability of the two treatment series, 348; results during the five-year period, 350; prognostic factors in acute bilateral pulmonary tuberculosis in young adults, 356.
Studies of uropepsinogen excretion in gastro-intestinal disorders, 291.

T.A.B., 9.
Tetanus toxoid, 12.
Treatment of polycythaemia vera with radiophosphorus, 91; haematological results, 94; clinical results, 101.
Tuberculin test for sarcoidosis, 39.
Tuberculosis Chemotherapy Trials Committee of the Medical Research Council, Report to the, 347.
Tuberculosis, pulmonary, five-year assessment of patients in a controlled trial of streptomycin in, 347; plan and conduct of the trial, 347; comparability of the two treatment series, 348; results during the five-year period, 350; prognostic factors in acute bilateral pulmonary tuberculosis in young adults, 356.
Tuberculous meningitis, spinal cord complications of, 275; definition and incidence, 275; clinical picture of transverse myelitis, 277; relationship of transverse myelitis to the presence of spinal block, 285; relationship of spinal block to mortality, 286.
Tuberous sclerosis, historical review of, 113; forms of, 124; nature of, 136.
— —, pulmonary, 113.
Typhoid-paratyphoid vaccine (T.A.B.), 9.

Urinary excretion of *p*-hydroxyphenylacetic acid in steatorrhoea and macrocytic anaemia, ascorbic acid requirements and, 307.
Uropepsinogen excretion in gastro-intestinal disorders, studies of, 291.

Water-losing nephritis, 147; renal changes in myelomatosis, 158; polyuria in certain other conditions affecting the kidney, 159; pathogenesis, 161.
Weight reduction, effect of, upon the blood-pressure of obese hypertensive women, 331.
Women, obese hypertensive, the effect of weight reduction upon the blood-pressure of, 331.